Clinical Diagnosis and Treatment of Pulmonary Diseases

Clinical Diagnosis and Treatment of Pulmonary Diseases

Editor: Beatrice Gunther

AMERICAN
MEDICAL PUBLISHERS
www.americanmedicalpublishers.com

AMERICAN
MEDICAL PUBLISHERS
www.americanmedicalpublishers.com

Cataloging-in-Publication Data

Clinical diagnosis and treatment of pulmonary diseases / edited by Beatrice Gunther.
p. cm.
Includes bibliographical references and index.
ISBN 979-8-88740-566-7
1. Lungs--Diseases. 2. Lungs--Diseases--Diagnosis. 3. Lungs--Diseases--Treatment. I. Gunther, Beatrice.
RC756 .P85 2023
616.24--dc23

American Medical Publishers,
41 Flatbush Avenue,
1st Floor, New York,
NY 11217, USA

ISBN 979-8-88740-566-7 (Hardback)

Contents

Preface

The main aim of this book is to educate learners and enhance their research focus by presenting diverse topics covering this vast field. This is an advanced book which compiles significant studies by distinguished experts in the area of analysis. This book addresses successive solutions to the challenges arising in the area of application, along with it; the book provides scope for future developments.

Pulmonary diseases are a group of disorders that affect the lungs and other parts of the respiratory system. Some of the major causes of pulmonary diseases include infection, tobacco smoke and other forms of air pollution. They can be classified into several types, such as asthma, lung cancer, chronic obstructive pulmonary disease (COPD), pneumonia and pulmonary fibrosis. Several diagnostic tests can be used to diagnose pulmonary diseases, including biopsy of the lung or pleura, blood test, bronchoscopy, chest X-ray, CT scan, pulmonary function test, etc. The treatment of pulmonary disorders depends on the type of disease. Pulmonary rehabilitation, lung transplant and oxygen therapy are some common treatment options available for the clinical management of pulmonary fibrosis. This book outlines the diagnosis and treatment of pulmonary diseases in detail. A number of latest researches have been included to keep the readers up-to-date with the major concepts in this area of study. With state-of-the-art inputs by acclaimed pulmonologists, this book targets medical students and professionals.

It was a great honour to edit this book, though there were challenges, as it involved a lot of communication and networking between me and the editorial team. However, the end result was this all-inclusive book covering diverse themes in the field.

Finally, it is important to acknowledge the efforts of the contributors for their excellent chapters, through which a wide variety of issues have been addressed. I would also like to thank my colleagues for their valuable feedback during the making of this book.

Editor

1

An Illustrated Guide to the Imaging Evolution of COVID in Non-Epidemic Areas of Southeast China

*Lihua Wang[1], Yeerfan Jiaerken[1], Qian Li[1], Peiyu Huang[1], Zhujing Shen[1], Tongtong Zhao[2], Hanpeng Zheng[3], Wenbin Ji[4], Yuantong Gao[5], Junli Xia[6], Jianmin Cheng[7], Jianbing Ma[8], Jun Liu[9], Yongqiang Liu[10], Miaoguang Su[11], Guixiang Ruan[12], Jiner Shu[13], Dawei Ren[14], Zhenhua Zhao[15], Weigen Yao[16], Yunjun Yang[17] and Minming Zhang[1]**

[1]Department of Radiology, Second Affiliated Hospital, School of Medicine, Zhejiang University, Hangzhou, China, [2]Fuyang Second People's Hospital, Fuyang, China, [3]Yueqing People's Hospital, Yueqing, China, [4]Zhejiang Taizhou Hospital, Taizhou, China, [5]Radiology Department, Third Affiliated Hospital of Wenzhou Medical University, Wenzhou, China, [6]Bozhou Bone Trauma Hospital Image Center, Bozhou, China, [7]Department of Radiology, Second Affiliated Hospital and Yuying Children's Hospital of Wenzhou Medical University, Wenzhou, China, [8]First Hospital of Jiaxing, Jiaxing, China, [9]Second Xiangya Hospital, Central South University, Changsha, China, [10]Quzhou Kecheng People's Hospital, Quzhou, China, [11]Pingyang County People's Hospital, Wenzhou, China, [12]Yuhang First People's Hospital, Hangzhou, China, [13]Jinhua Central Hospital, Jinhua, China, [14]Ningbo First Hospital, Ningbo, China, [15]Shaoxing People's Hospital, Shaoxing, China, [16]Yuyao People's Hospital, Yuyao, China, [17]Radiology Department, First Affiliated Hospital of Wenzhou Medical University, Wenzhou, China

***Correspondence:**
Minming Zhang
zhangminming@zju.edu.cn

Purpose: By analyzing the CT manifestations and evolution of COVID in non-epidemic areas of southeast China, analyzing the developmental abnormalities and accompanying signs in the early and late stages of the disease, providing imaging evidence for clinical diagnosis and identification, and assisting in judging disease progression and monitoring prognosis.

Methods: This retrospective and multicenter study included 1,648 chest CT examinations from 693 patients with laboratory-confirmed COVID-19 infection from 16 hospitals of southeast China between January 19 and March 27, 2020. Six trained radiologists analyzed and recorded the distribution and location of the lesions in the CT images of these patients. The accompanying signs include crazy-paving sign, bronchial wall thickening, microvascular thickening, bronchogram sign, fibrous lesions, halo and reverse-halo signs, nodules, atelectasis, and pleural effusion, and at the same time, they analyze the evolution of the abovementioned manifestations over time.

Result: There were 1,500 positive findings in 1,648 CT examinations of 693 patients; the average age of the patients was 46 years, including 13 children; the proportion of women was 49%. Early CT manifestations are single or multiple nodular, patchy, or flaky ground-glass–like density shadows. The frequency of occurrence of ground-glass shadows (47.27%), fibrous lesions (42.60%), and microvascular thickening (40.60%) was significantly higher than that of other signs. Ground-glass shadows increase and expand 3–7 days after the onset of symptoms. The distribution and location of lesions were not significantly related to the appearance time. Ground-glass shadow is the most common lesion, with an average absorption time of 6.2 days, followed by consolidation, with an absorption time of about 6.3 days. It takes about 8 days for pure ground-glass lesions to absorb. Consolidation change into ground glass or pure ground glass takes

10–14 days. For ground-glass opacity to evolve into pure ground-glass lesions, it takes an average of 17 days. For ground-glass lesions to evolve into consolidation, it takes 7 days, pure ground-glass lesions need 8 days to evolve into ground-glass lesions. The average time for CT signs to improve is 10–15 days, and the first to improve is the crazy-paving sign and nodules; while the progression of the disease is 6–12 days, the earliest signs of progression are air bronchogram signs, bronchial wall thickening, and bronchiectasis. There is no severe patient in this study.

Conclusion: This study depicts the CT manifestation and evolution of COVID in non-epidemic origin areas, and provides valuable first-hand information for clinical diagnosis and judgment of patient's disease evolution and prediction.

Keywords: COVID, image, CT, evolution, multicenter

INTRODUCTION

Coronavirus disease 2019 (COVID-19), an acute respiratory infectious disease in 2019–2020, is becoming more and more serious. Although the epidemic situation in China has been well controlled, the number of cases in the world is increasing, and it is still in a pandemic state. With the continuous accumulation and comprehensive understanding of disease prevention, control, diagnosis, and treatment experience, research on the disease evolution, including the risk factors for patients progressed from mild-to-severe even critical illness, risk factors for death and related early warning models, is actively processing. Imaging plays an important role in disease diagnosis, clinical decision-making, treatment, and clinical outcome evaluation. The occurrence and development of imaging is of great significance for us to understand the characteristics of the disease and to guide clinical practice. The combination of imaging findings and the nucleic acid test as a means of diagnosis program aimed to make up for missed diagnosis of early nucleic acid–negative cases, and can also be used to evaluate curative effect, and it has now become a consensus in the treatment of COVID-19. This study collects imaging and clinical data of patients with confirmed COVID-19 in 16 hospitals in southeast China outside of the epidemic area; uses big data analysis to find the early and late development; explores the correlation among imaging performance, developmental trend, and patient basic diseases; describes the characteristics and evolution of the imaging manifestations with the time of onset; displays the imaging map of new coronary pneumonia; provides imaging clues for clinical diagnosis and identification; and provides assistance in disease progression and prognostic monitoring.

METHODS

Patients Information

The study was conducted in accordance with the Declaration of Helsinki (as revised in 2013). This retrospective multicenter study was approved by the Institutional Review Board of each participating hospital. Written informed consent was waived. A total of 693 patients came from the southeastern region of China outside of the epidemic-intensive areas, with an average age of 46 years, including 13 children; the proportion of women was 49%. They were all imported second-generation confirmed cases. This study included 1,648 chest CT examinations at 16 hospitals between January 19 and March 27, 2020. The median CT follow-up period was 10 days from symptom onset (IQR, 6–16; range, 0–58 days). All patients were recovered after treatment, and there are no clinically critically ill patients in this study.

CT Protocol

CT examinations were performed using 16-slice to 128-slice CT scanners of different manufacturers, including SIEMENS, GE, TOSHIBA, and PHILIPS. Chest CT examinations were performed with a varying slice thickness from 1 to 5 mm. Standard lung algorithm settings were used as follows: tube voltage, 100–130 kV; tube current, 100–440 mAs; section thickness, 1–5 mm; and reconstruction matrix, 512 × 512.

CT Image Recording Method

All CT images were read by six attending doctors with qualifications. The density of lesions was divided into pure ground-glass shadow (completely ground-glass density), ground-glass lesions (referring to ground-glass lesions containing consolidation lesions not exceeding one-half of the total volume), and consolidation lesions (completely solidified lesions or contained ground-glass opacity not exceeding one-half of the total volume). At the same time, the lobe location and distribution characteristics of the lesions were recorded: subpleural distribution pattern defined as lesions distributed within 2 cm of the subpleural area on both sides; diffuse distribution refers to the involvement of multiple lobes in both lungs; distribution along the bronchial vascular bundle pattern refers to the lesions distributed along the bronchial vascular bundle. Signs within the lesion were recorded, such as bronchogram sign, paving stone sign (shown as mosaic ground-glass shadow with thickened interlobular septum), thickened microvessels, halo and reversal halo signs, nodules, fibrous foci, and other manifestations such as pleural effusion and pericardium effusion, and old lesions. In the follow-up CT, the outcome of the above-observed lesion was recorded once more, in

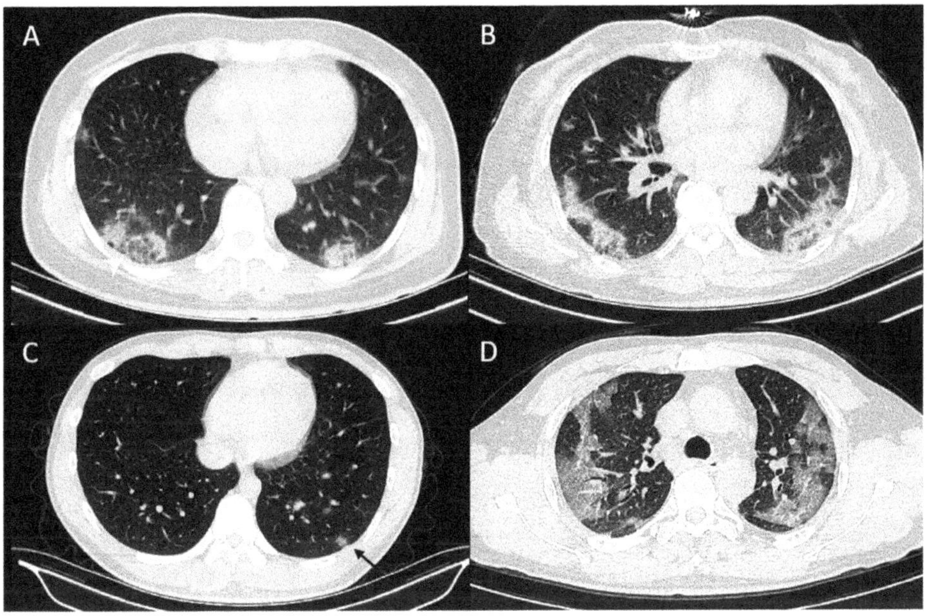

FIGURE 1 | CT signs of reversed hollow sign **(A)**, bilateral distribution of lesion **(B)**, and nodule with hollow sign **(C)**, and crazy-paving sign **(D)**.

addition to the improvement and progress of the lesion. The form of lesion improvement is explained as the reduction of lesion area and density, including ground-glass and consolidation shadow absorption, and any kinds of density decreased and area reduced. The form of lesion progression is explained as the increase in the range and/or density of the original lesion, including pure ground-glass lesions that progress to ground-glass lesions, and ground-glass lesions that progress to consolidation lesions; disappearance of signs means improvement, and reappearance of signs means progress. The first examination was negative, and the reexamination showed that the lesion appeared and was recorded as a new lesion. The days of improvement, absorption, and progression of different density lesions and signs were recorded.

Statistical Analysis

The differences in the frequency of the CT signs were tested with the chi-square test. The differences between the days of the onset between different CT signs were tested with the ANOVA test. The differences in the demographic data between groups were also tested with the ANOVA test. Data normality was tested with the K-W test. All statistical analyses were performed with MATLAB 2019b on windows platform. A corrected p value of < 0.05 was considered as statistically significant.

RESULT

Examination Information

The average time for the first CT examination was 6.5 days after the onset of the disease, and the longest CT examination was 58 days after the onset of the disease; the median number of follow-ups was two, and the maximum number of follow-ups was 10; the average follow-up interval was 5.3 days; and there were positive findings in 1,500 CT examinations.

Basic CT Manifestations

All 1,500 CT examinations with positive signs were included, and the distribution, density, accompanying signs, and extrapulmonary manifestations were analyzed. The basic CT manifestations are as follows: 1. The distribution is mainly under the pleura, more often on the dorsal side or the lower lobes of the lungs. The lesions are mostly localized, mainly subsegmental or segmental. 2. Single or multiple nodular, patchy, or ground-glass density shadows, with or without intralobular reticular shadows, thickening of the lobular septa, and thickened microvessels and paving stone sign inside (**Figures 1A–D**). Consolidation was accompanied by bronchogram, internal bronchiectasis, and with or without subsegmental or lobular atelectasis, which was manifested as a fusiform, flat, or strip-shaped shadow connected to the bronchovascular bundle under the pleura (**Figure 2**). 3. As the course of the disease progresses and treatment measures follow-up, the ground-glass shadow or consolidation completely or partially absorbed, and was transformed into lobular atelectasis or fibrosis. Extrapulmonary manifestations including pleural effusion, pericardial effusion, and lymphadenopathy are rare.

Frequency Analysis of Lesions

CT lesion distribution and imaging manifestation frequency analysis are shown in **Table 1**. The results of the chi-square test showed that the distribution of lesions was mainly subpleural (82.33%), which was significantly more than the distribution of bronchial vascular bundles or diffuse distribution, and diffuse

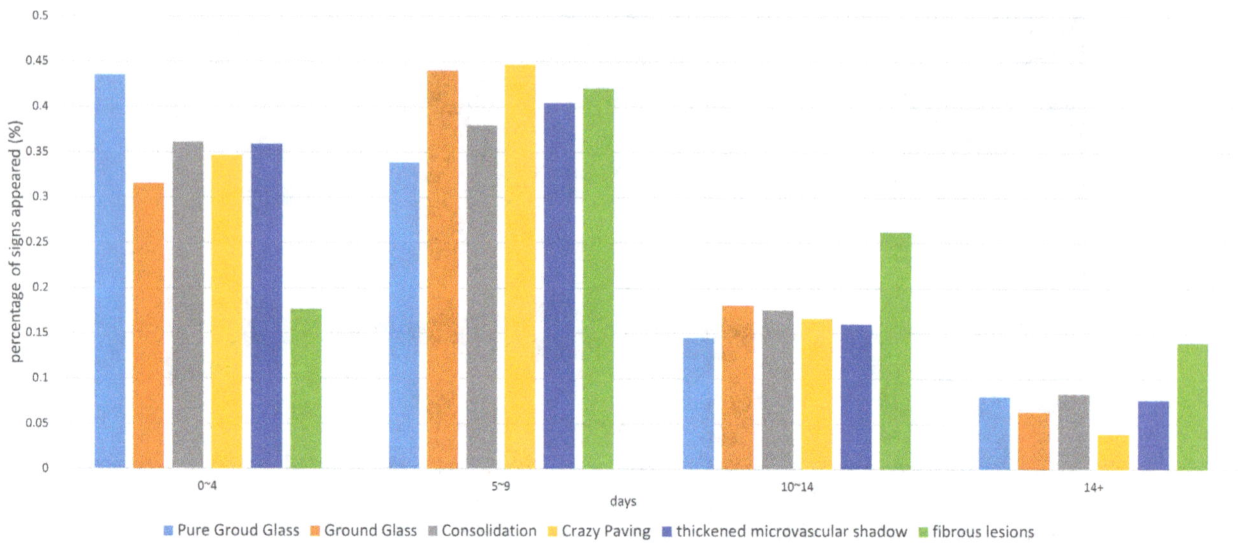

FIGURE 2 | The percentage of time at each CT sign. The horizontal axis is the date of onset, and the vertical axis represents the percentage of the number of positive cases with the corresponding sign to all cases with the sign on that date.

TABLE 1 | The frequency of CT lesion distribution, location, intensity, and signs.

CT lesion description	Number (%)
CT lesion distribution	
Under the pleura	1,235 (82.33)[a]
Along bronchovascular bundle	573 (38.20)[b]
Diffused distribution	102 (6.80)[c]
CT lesion location	
Right upper lobe	920 (61.33)[a]
Left upper lobe	993 (66.20)[a]
Right middle lobe	773 (51.53)[b]
Right lower lobe	1,279 (85.27)[c]
Left lower lobe	1,251 (83.40)[c]
CT lesion intensity	
Ground-glass opacity	709 (47.27)[a]
Consolidation	507 (33.80)[b]
Pure ground-glass opacity	378 (25.20)[c]
CT signs of changes in the lung	
Fibrous lesions	639 (42.60)[a]
Thickened small vessel	609 (40.60)[a]
Air bronchogram	478 (31.87)[b]
Bronchial dilating and wall thickening	383 (25.53)[c]
Halo sign	309 (20.60)[c]
Crazy-paving sign	264 (17.60)[d]
Nodule	231 (15.40)[d]
Inversed halo	60 (4.00)[e]
Lobular atelectasis	29 (1.93)[f]
Pulmonary fibrosis	23 (1.53)[f]
Pulmonary emphysema	33 (2.20)[e,f]
CT signs of changes outside the lung	
Pleural effusion	21 (1.40)[a]
Pericardial effusion	3 (0.20)[b]
Enlargement of lymph nodes	32 (2.13)[b]

Frequency (%) of CT lesion distribution, location, intensity, and signs of changes in and outside the lung were shown. Within a same sub-table, the pair with the same superscript letter (a,b,c...) showed no statistically significant differences, while the pair with different superscript letter had significant differences (chi-square test, Bonferroni corrected $p < 0.05$).

distribution was rare. The lesions are mainly seen in the two lower lungs, and there is no obvious difference between the left and right lungs. The frequency of lesions in the middle lobe of the right lung is relatively low (51.53%); the most common manifestation is ground-glass density shadow (47.27%). The first three signs with higher frequency were fibrous lesions (42.60%), microvascular thickening (40.60%), and air bronchogram (31.87%). There was no significant difference among the three. In other accompanying signs, the paving stone sign is about 17%, and the antihalo sign is less, which is about 4%.

Analysis of Follow-Up Outcome

The first CT examination showed significant differences in the appearance time of lesions and signs with different densities ($p = 0.014$). The average time of appearance of pure ground-glass, ground-glass lesions, and consolidation and accompanying signs including paving stone, bronchogram, thickened microvessels, nodules, halo and reversed halo signs was about 6–7 days (**Table 2**); among them, pure ground-glass lesions appear earliest, with the highest peak at 0–4 days (43.54% of pure ground-glass lesions appear in this period), and it took about 8 days for pure ground-glass lesions to absorb, while progress into consolidation needs 11 days (**Figure 3**). It takes 8 days for pure ground-glass disease to progress to ground-glass lesions. The first examination was negative, and among them, 18 patients showed original pure ground-glass lesions after 16 days of reexamination (**Figure 4**), 16 cases showed ground-glass lesions, and 24 cases showed consolidation lesions in about 13 days. The number of ground-glass lesions was the largest (216 cases), and the peak appeared on the sixth day. The average absorption time was 6.2 days, or

TABLE 2 | Comparison of time and clinical data between different outcome groups.

Trend	Lesion development	Mean days between visit	Number of cases
Recovery	Consolidation turned negative	6.37	181
	Consolidation to ground-glass opacity	10.66	71
	Consolidation to pure ground-glass opacity	13.78	23
	Ground-glass opacity turned negative	6.21	216
	Ground-glass opacity to pure ground-glass opacity	17.14	29
	Pure ground-glass opacity turned negative	7.99	78
Progressed	New pure ground-glass opacity	15.78	18
	Pure ground-glass opacity to ground glass opacity	8.73	13
	Pure ground-glass opacity to consolidation	11.07	15
	New ground-glass opacity	11.75	16
	Ground-glass opacity to consolidation	7.35	54
	New consolidation lesion	12.92	24

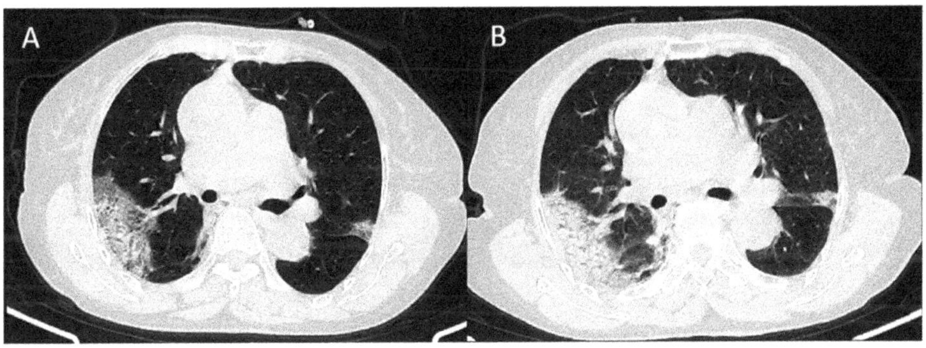

FIGURE 3 | CT signs of a 74-year-old female showed subpleural distributed ground-glass opacity in 13 days **(A)** and 16 days **(B)** from onset.

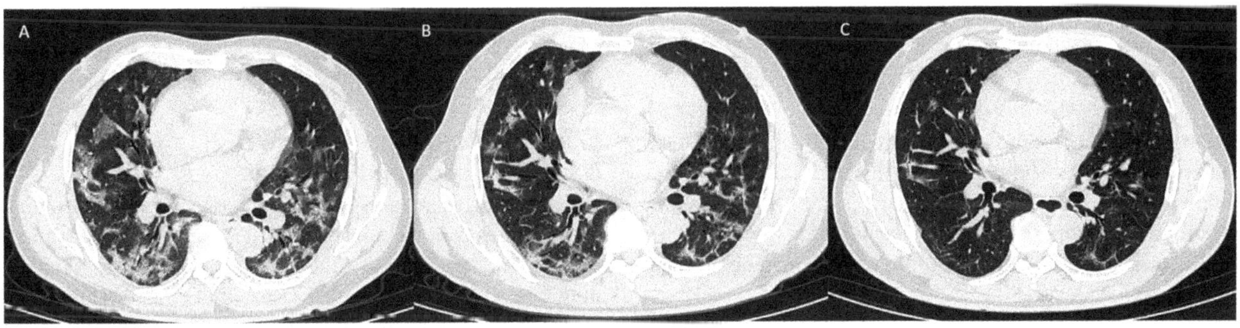

FIGURE 4 | CT signs of a 47-year-old male on day 1 **(A)**, day 5 **(B),** and day 17 **(C)** showed bilateral ground-glass opacity absorbed and fibrosis formation.

it progressed to consolidation in 7 days. There were 29 cases of ground-glass lesions that evolved into pure ground-glass lesions, and the lesions took the longest time to be absorbed, which is about 17 days. Among the 29 cases, 11 patients had underlying diseases (37.93%), which was significantly higher than the other groups, including two cases of diabetes, two cases of hypertension with diabetes, two cases of hypertension, two cases of tuberculosis, two cases of spinal surgery, and one case of chronic nettle. As for age, gender, body temperature, and the proportion of neutrophils and lymphocytes, there was no significant difference between these 29 patients compared with the ground-glass absorption group.

The absorption time of consolidation lesions is about 6.3 days. It takes 10–14 days for consolidation to transform into ground-glass or pure ground-glass lesions. Most of the peaks of accompanying signs are on the 5th to 9th days, such as paving stone sign, microvascular thickening, and fibrous lesions (**Table 3**). The average time for improvement is 10–15 days. The first improvement is the paving stone sign and nodules; the time for signs to progress is 6–12 days. The earliest signs of progress are bronchogram, bronchial wall thickening, and

TABLE 3 | Development of CT signs.

CT signs	From positive to negative		From negative to positive	
	Mean days between visit	**Number of cases (%)**	**Mean days between visit**	**Number of cases (%)**
Crazy-paving	10.14 a	62 (19.50)	10.15 b	17 (6.67)
Air bronchogram	11.32 a	79 (24.84)	6.20 b	23 (9.02)
Fibrous lesions	15.08 a	13 (4.09)	10.12 b	133 (52.15)
Bronchial dilating and wall thickening	12.88 a	56 (17.61)	9.12 b	34 (13.33)
Thickened small vessel	13.26 a	74 (23.27)	8.56 b	25 (9.80)
Nodule	10.82 a	34 (10.69)	11.48 a,b	23 (9.02)
Halo sign	11.44	54 (14.52)	9.78	16 (6.40)

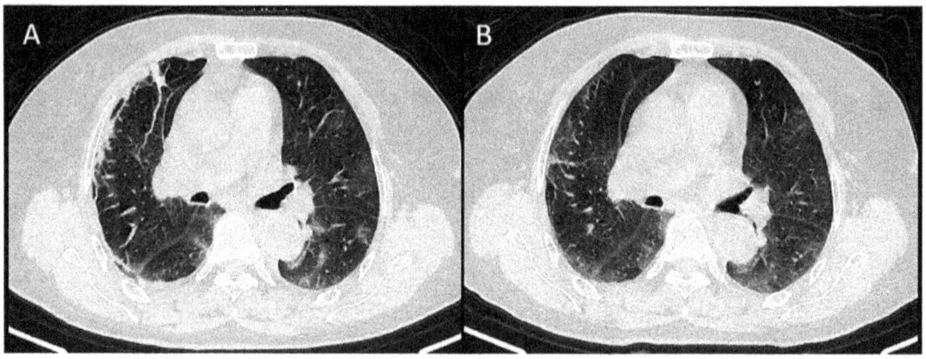

FIGURE 5 | A 68-year-old female showed lobular atelectasis in the subpleural area of the right upper lobe on day 3 from onset **(A)** and disappeared on day 6 **(B)**.

bronchiectasis. Fibrous lesions appear less frequently in 0–4 days (17.68%), but the duration is long, and there is still 26.12% in 10–14 days, which is higher than other signs (**Figure 5**).

DISCUSSION

This article summarizes and analyzes the imaging manifestation in non-epidemic areas, summarizes the image characteristics and evolution time of sporadic cases, describes the accompanying signs of the images, provides clinical diagnosis for sporadic cases and mild patients, and provides comprehensive imaging data for efficacy clinical evaluation.

Selection of Imaging Methods

Chest CT is the first choice for screening and evaluating new coronary pneumonia (Wong et al., 2019). It is recommended to use a volumetric CT scan, the scan thickness is 5 mm (16-slice CT and above are acceptable), and the reconstruction is a thin layer of 1.0–1.5 mm. Multi-planar reconstruction (cross-sectional, sagittal, and coronal) was based on thin-slice CT. At present, the latest guidelines have not yet reached a consensus on the timing of the use of low-dose CT (LDCT) examination and the time interval for reexamination of CT. Early CT findings of some patients with new coronary pneumonia are negative, and positive findings gradually appear in the lungs as the disease progresses (Minming and Bin, 2020). We agree with opinions as follows: reports of the various CT features of COVID-19 pneumonia are an important first step in helping radiologists identify patients who may have COVID-19 pneumonia in the appropriate clinical environment. CT should be reserved for evaluation of complications of COVID-19 pneumonia or for assessment if alternative diagnoses are suspected (Raptis et al., 2020).

CT Manifestations

Density Change and Evolution

Density changes include ground-glass opacity and consolidation; ground-glass opacity indicated slight increase in density as a hazy cloud-like change that does not cover the accompanying pulmonary vascular shadows in the lungs. Consolidation means a significant increase in the density of lung parenchyma, and the pulmonary blood vessels and airway walls are unclear due to the lack of alveolar gas contrast (Adam et al., 2020). The imaging manifestations depend on the pathology. The pathology of COVID-19 shows that the lungs exhibited different degrees of consolidation, mainly showing diffuse alveolar injury and exudative alveolitis. Pulmonary lesions in different areas are complex and diverse, with the new and the old lesions alternating. The formation of serous/fibrinous exudate and transparent membrane in the alveolar cavity can show consolidation of different densities in imaging. Infiltrating cells are mainly monocytes and macrophages. Type-II alveolar epithelial cell hyperplasia, alveolar septal hyperemia and edema, and some alveolar hyperinflation, forming airspace-containing cavity, can form lobular septal thickening and paving stone signs. Bronchioles and small bronchi are easy to see mucus thrombosis, pulmonary vasculitis and thrombosis, and embolism, which can explain the signs of microvascular thickening. With the developement of the disease, it can be seen that the alveolar cavity exudate is organized (meat change) and the pulmonary interstitial fibrosis, so the later stage could find the formation of fibrous bands (Minming and Bin, 2020).

The results showed that the lesions were mainly distributed under the two lower lobes, followed by the two upper lobes, and the right middle lobe was the least involved (Fan et al., 2020; Minming and Bin, 2020; Salehi et al., 2020). The frequency of ground-glass opacity is the highest, and the peak time is 0–4 days, which is consistent with many literature reports outside Hubei Province and can have no clinical symptoms (Ai et al., 2020; Xiong et al., 2020; Zhao et al., 2020). Meng et al. (2020) reported asymptomatic cases with normal laboratory findings confirmed by nucleic acid testing show CT findings as ground-glass opacity (GGO) (94.8%) with peripheral (75.9%) distribution, unilateral location (58.6%), and mostly involving one or two lobes (65.5%).

The most rapid absorption of lesion density evolution was ground glass–based lesions, with an average transformation time of 6.2 days, followed by consolidation, with an absorption time of about 6.3 days, which was also the shortest absorption time, which did not match the 3.5-day average prognosis time reported by Li et al. (2020). Shi et al. (2020) reported a case of Wuhan with pure ground-glass shadow absorption for 13 days, which the author believes is related to clinical treatment and individual differences in patients and virus virulence. It may be due to different areas of the patient. Xiong et al. (2020) reported that in Wuhan, 83% of patients, which is more than that in our observation, progressed to opacifications, consolidation, interstitial thickening, fibrous strips, and air bronchogram signs during a mean follow-up period of 4.5 and 11.6 days.

According to our result, it takes about 7–11 days for ground-glass or pure ground-glass lesions to switch to consolidation. Wang et al. (2020) reported that the ground-glass lesions progressed to a mixed type for about 12–17 days. The progression of the lesion is based on pure ground-glass opacity and develops into ground glass in turn, followed by consolidation. It is speculated that density increase is related to the increase in exudate and cells in the lung, the thickening of the interlobular septum, and the formation of fibrosis. It takes about 10–14 days for consolidation absorption to turn into ground-glass or pure ground-glass opacity; ground-glass lesions evolve into pure ground-glass and also indicate that the lesions improve absorption, but it takes as long as 17 days. The reason is that this group of patients has underlying diseases, such as hypertension, diabetes, or a history of surgery. It is speculated that the immune function of the patients may delay the absorption of the lesion. Relevant literature on clinical indicators predicting lesion progression predicted that patients with imaging progression had significantly higher frequency of chronic inflammatory manifestation than those without imaging progression (Yang et al., 2020). This may be related to the pathological basis of pulmonary edema, protein exudation, and thickening of pulmonary interstitium, which may play a role, resulting in the formation of ground-glass opacity. Among them, edema and protein exudation are absorbed faster, while the lung interstitium thickness process is relatively slow, which can explain the different results of ground-glass shadow absorption in some patients. Similarly, consolidation may be caused by multiple pathological factors. After pulmonary edema and exudation are absorbed, the density of the lesion decreases, and the interstitial thickening maintains the ground-glass density and enters a slow absorption period, which can evolve into fibrotic lesions in the later stage.

Accompanying Signs and Evolution

Accompanying signs include paving stone sign, microvascular thickening, bronchogram sign, halo sign, reversed halo sign, tree-in-bud sign, nodules, and traction bronchiectasis. Most signs merged in 5–9 days and accompanied with the absorption and evolution of the lesions; only fibrotic lesions appear on the 9th day. The average time for improvement is 10–15 days, and the first to get better is the paving stone sign. The progression time of signs is 6–12 days, and the relatively earlier signs are bronchogram, bronchial wall thickening, and traction bronchiectasis.

What needs to be emphasized is the paving stone sign. Some researchers believe that this sign indicates the progress of the disease; we have different opinions. The crazy-paving pattern demonstrates as thickened interlobular septa and intralobular lines with superimposition on a GGO background, resembling irregular paving stones (Cheng et al., 2020; Fan et al., 2020; Qi et al., 2020; Raptis et al., 2020; Wang et al., 2020; Ye et al., 2020). The early pathological changes of COVID-19 include pulmonary edema, protein exudation, thickening of the lung interstitium, and infiltration of multinucleated giant cells and macrophages in the alveolar cavity. Pan et al. (2020) mentioned that in 22 cases of observation, the paving stone sign appeared in 5–8 days from the symptom and continued to be absorbed after 13 days, and the lesion progression was accompanied by more paving stone signs. Salehi et al. (2020) indicated follow-up CT in the intermediate stage of disease shows an increase in the number and size of GGOs and progressive transformation of GGO into multifocal consolidative opacities, septal thickening, and development of a crazy-paving pattern, with the greatest severity of CT findings visible around day 10 after the symptom onset. There were no severe cases in this study, the paving stone sign improved in about 10 days in 20% of the patients, only 6% cases progressed, and the average progression time was also about 10 days. Relatively speaking, bronchial wall thickening appeared more frequently. In many progressive cases, thickening of the bronchial wall and microvessel signs had larger frequency and may be predictive signs of critically ill patients. The paving stone sign has been used to distinguish it from viral pneumonia. While a cluster-like pattern and bronchial wall thickening were more frequently seen in influenza pneumonia(Wang et al., 2020), we considered that the imaging manifestations of COVID and avian influenza, influenza B, and influenza A have a large overlap, and the performance is similar, and the differential diagnosis depends on clinical microbiological tests. YU reported (Yu et al., 2020) interlobular septal thickening (75%), air bronchogram (70%), and pleural effusion (40%) were more likely to manifest in patients with severe form. Wang et al. (2020) also reported heavy/critical-type COVID-19 was associated with multiple lobe involvement and the presence of consolidation, the crazy-paving sign, interlobular septal thickening, pleural thickening, and pleural effusion.

Halo sign, reversed-halo sign, tree-in-bud sign, and nodules are rare manifestations. Halo sign refers to a circle of ground-glass density shadow around the nodules or patchy opacity on CT. It was first used to describe the exudation around the focal invasive *Aspergillus* nodule. The pathological mechanism is bleeding around the lesion and so was a nonspecific sign. To COVID-19, it shows ill-defined cloud-like inflammatory exudation around the lesion, which is similar to other opacity. As for reversed-halo sign, there is a certain difference between the traditional appearance and COVID-19. The center of the reversed-halo sign showed a ground-glass density shadow, the surrounding appearance is ring or crescent, and the density of the ring in COVID-19 is lower than that of the ring in others, such as organized pneumonia. The pathological mechanism of GGO-like banding needs further explanation (Guan et al., 2020). It is reported that reversed halo sign was observed in approx. 5% of patients (Hamer et al., 2020). In the early CT images, nodules with a diameter of ≤3 cm can be solid nodules, partial solid nodules, and pure ground-glass nodules, with clear or fuzzy boundaries. As for the tree-in-bud sign, the initial lesion was a solitary sub-centimeter ground-glass nodule distributed in the boundary between the outer one-third and inner two-thirds of pulmonary lobes, along with adjacent bronchovascular bundles, and the lesion progressed over a period of 2–3 days, presenting as an enlarged nodule with a blurred margin on CT (Xia et al., 2020). Current pathological studies believe that COVID-19 mainly causes inflammatory reactions characterized by deep airway and alveolar damage. However, individual COVID-19 cases showed tree-in-bud signs, suggesting that the disease involves bronchioles (Güneyli et al., 2020).

Fibrous lesions appeared with a low frequency (17.68%) in 0–4 days, and 26.12% in 10–14 days, which is higher than that in other signs. The frequency of fibrotic lesions in the disease outcome of this study was higher, which may be due to different interpretations: some fiber streaks disappeared in the later period, and two cases of streaks were reported to be absorbed in 19 days (Jiang et al., 2020). Guan et al. (2020) reported a delay in the changes on CT and evidence of lesion absorption. During the absorption period, the patchy lung consolidations gradually absorbed and shrank, but the subpleural line was still present 22 days after admission. It is suggested that the stripe shadow displayed in the previous stage is atelectasis or segmental atelectasis. Lobular atelectasis refers to complete atelectasis or results in swelling of the lung caused by bronchial obstruction or contraction of scar tissue in the lung, which is caused by bronchiolitis. The resulting inflammation is absorbed, the lumen of the bronchioles reopens, and the lung is recruited to expand. The unabsorbable fiber strips are the real scars. Pleural effusion and enlargement of lymph nodes appear less generally. Traction bronchiectasis may appear in the consolidation area on CT or in the fibrous cord shadow.

RESEARCH LIMITATIONS

This study mainly describes the imaging manifestations and evolution of COVID-19, and does not include the treatment and the clinical evolution of the patient. The reason is that the current treatment is basically the same, and the difference is the patient's individual response and immune status. Therefore, the image analysis of big data shows that the overall development of new coronary pneumonia has a certain degree of representativeness.

SUMMARY

This study describes the CT manifestation and evolution of COVID-19 in non-epidemic areas of southeast China, and provides valuable first-hand information for clinical diagnosis and judgment of disease evolution and prediction.

AUTHOR CONTRIBUTIONS

All authors listed have made a substantial, direct, and intellectual contribution to the work and approved it for publication.

REFERENCES

Adam, B., Mei, X., Huang, M., Yang, Y., Fayad, Z. A., Zhang, N., et al. (2020). Chest CT Findings in Coronavirus Disease-19 (COVID-19): Relationship to Duration of Infection. *Radiol.* 295, 200463. doi:10.1148/radiol.2020200463

Ai, T., Yang, Z., Hou, H., Zhan, C., Chen, C., Lv, W., et al. (2020). Correlation of Chest CT and RT-PCR Testing for Coronavirus Disease 2019 (COVID-19) in China: A Report of 1014 Cases. *Radiol.* 296, E32, 2020 . Online ahead of print. doi:10.1148/radiol.2020200642

Cheng, Z., Qin, L., Cao, Q., Dai, J., Pan, A., Yang, W., et al. (2020). Quantitative Computed Tomography of the Coronavirus Disease 2019 (COVID-19) Pneumonia. *Radiol. Infect. Dis.* 7 (2), 55–61. Epub 2020 Apr 28. doi:10.1016/j.jrid.2020.04.004

Fan, N., Fan, W., Li, Z., Shi, M., and Liang, Y. (2020). Imaging Characteristics of Initial Chest Computed Tomography and Clinical Manifestations of Patients with COVID-19 Pneumonia. *Jpn. J. Radiol.* 38 (6), 533–538. doi:10.1007/s11604-020-00973-x

Guan, C. S., Lv, Z. B., Yan, S., Du, Y. N., Chen, H., Wei, L. G., et al. (2020b). Imaging Features of Coronavirus Disease 2019 (COVID-19): Evaluation on Thin-Section CT. *Acad. Radiol.* 27, 609–613. doi:10.1016/j.acra.2020.03.002

Guan, W., Liu, J., and Yu, C. (2020a). CT Findings of Coronavirus Disease (COVID-19) Severe Pneumonia. *Am. J. Roentgenol.* 214, W85–W86. doi:10.2214/ajr.20.23035 0361–803X/20/2145–W85.

Güneyli, S., Atçeken, Z., Atceken, Z., Dogan, H., Altinmakas, E., and Atasoy, K. C. (2020). Radiological Approach to COVID-19 Pneumonia with an Emphasis on Chest CT. *Diagn. Interv. Radiol.* 26 (4), 323–332. doi:10.5152/dir.2020.20260

Hamer, O. W., Salzberger, B., Gebauer, J., Stroszczynski, C., and Pfeifer, M. (2020). CT Morphology of COVID-19: Case Report and Review of Literature. *Fortschr Röntgenstr* 192, 386–392. Published online: 26.3.2020. doi:10.1055/a-1142-4094

Jiang, X., Yin, Z., Wang, T., Zhai, N., Lu, F., Zhan, C., et al. (2020). COVID-19 Dynamic Computed Tomography (CT) Performance and Observation of Some Laboratory Indicators. *Med. Sci. Monit.* 26, e924403. doi:10.12659/MSM.924403

Li, X., Zeng, W., Li, X., Chen, H., Shi, L., Li, X., et al. (2020). CT Imaging Changes of Corona Virus Disease 2019(COVID-19): A Multi-Center Study in Southwest China. *J. Transl Med.* 18 (1), 154. doi:10.1186/s12967-020-02324-w

Meng, H., Xiong, R., He, R., Lin, W., Hao, B., Zhang, L., et al. (2020). CT Imaging and Clinical Course of Asymptomatic Cases with COVID-19 Pneumonia at Admission in Wuhan, China. *J. Infect.* 81 (1), e33–e39. Epub 2020 Apr 12. doi:10.1016/j.jinf.2020.04.004

Minming, Z., and Bin, L. (2020). *Diagnostic Imaging of Novel Coronavirus Pneumonia | SpringerLink*. Singapore: Springer.

Pan, F., Ye, T., Sun, P., Gui, S., Liang, B., Li, L., et al. (2020). Time Course of Lung Changes at Chest CT during Recovery from Coronavirus Disease 2019 (COVID-19). *Radiol.* 295, 715–721. Online ahead of print. doi:10.1148/radiol.2020200370

Qi, X., Lei, J., Yu, Q., Xi, Y., Wang, Y., and Ju, S. (2020). CT Imaging of Coronavirus Disease 2019 (COVID-19): from the Qualitative to Quantitative. *Ann. Transl Med.* 8 (5), 256. doi:10.21037/atm.2020.02.91

Raptis, C. A., Hammer, M. M., Short, R. G., Shah, A., Bhalla, S., Bierhals, A. J., et al. (2020). Chest CT and Coronavirus Disease (COVID-19): A Critical Review of the Literature to Date. *AJR* 215, 1–4. doi:10.2214/AJR.20.23202 0361–803X/20/2154–1.

Salehi, S., Abedi, A., Balakrishnan, U., and Ali, G. (2020). Coronavirus Disease 2019 (COVID-19): A Systematic Review of Imaging Findings in 919 Patients. *AJR* 215, 1–7. doi:10.2214/AJR.20.23034

Shi, H., Han, X., and Zheng, C. (2020). Evolution of CT Manifestations in a Patient Recovered from 2019 Novel Coronavirus (2019-nCoV) Pneumonia in Wuhan, China. *Radiol.* 295, 20. doi:10.1148/radiol.2020200269

Wang, H., Wei, R., Rao, G., Zhu, J., and Song, B. (2020a). Characteristic CT Findings Distinguishing 2019 Novel Coronavirus Disease (COVID-19) from Influenza Pneumonia. *Eur. Radiol.* 30, 4910–4917. doi:10.1007/s00330-020-06880-z

Wang, J., Xu, Z., Wang, J., Feng, R., An, Y., Ao, W., et al. (2020b). CT Characteristics of Patients Infected with 2019 Novel Coronavirus: Association with Clinical Type. *Clin. Radiol.* 75 (6), 408–414. Epub 2020 Apr 7. doi:10.1016/j.crad.2020.04.001

Wang, Y., Dong, C., Hu, Y., Li, C., Ren, Q., Zhang, X., et al. (2020c). Temporal Changes of CT Findings in 90 Patients with COVID-19 Pneumonia: A Longitudinal Study. *Radiol.* 296, E55–E64. Online ahead of print. doi:10.1148/radiol.2020200843

Wong, H. Y. F., Lam, H. Y. S., Fong, A. H., Leung, S. T., Chin, T. W., Lo, C. S. Y., et al. (2019). Frequency and Distribution of Chest Radiographic Findings in COVID-19 Positive Patients. *Radiol.* 296, 201160. doi:10.1148/radiol.2020201160

Xia, T., Li, J., Gao, J., and Xu, X. (2020). Small Solitary Ground-Glass Nodule on CT as an Initial Manifestation of Coronavirus Disease 2019 (COVID-19) Pneumonia. *Korean J. Radiol.* 21 (5), 545–549. doi:10.3348/kjr.2020.0240

Xiong, Y., Sun, D., Liu, Y., Fan, Y., Zhao, L., Li, X., et al. (2020). Clinical and High-Resolution CT Features of the COVID-19 Infection. *Invest. Radiol.* 55 (6), 332–339. doi:10.1097/RLI.0000000000000674

Yang, Z., Shi, J., He, Z., Lü, Y., Xu, Q., Ye, C., et al. (2020). Predictors for Imaging Progression on Chest CT from Coronavirus Disease 2019 (COVID-19) Patients. *Aging* 12 (7), 6037–6048. Epub 2020 Apr 10. doi:10.18632/aging.102999

Ye, Z., Zhang, Y., Wang, Y., Huang, Z., and Song, B. (2020). Chest CT Manifestations of New Coronavirus Disease 2019 (COVID-19): a Pictorial Review. *Eur. Radiol.* 30 (8), 4381–4389. doi:10.1007/s00330-020-06801-0

Yu, M., Xu, D., Lan, L., Tu, M., Liao, R., Cai, S., et al. (2020). Thin-section Chest CT Imaging of Coronavirus Disease 2019 Pneumonia: Comparison between Patients with Mild and Severe Disease. *Radiol.* 2 (2), e200126. doi:10.1148/ryct.2020200126

Zhao, W., Zhong, Z., Xie, X., Yu, Q., and Liu, J. (2020). Relation between Chest CT Findings and Clinical Conditions of Coronavirus Disease (COVID-19) Pneumonia: A Multicenter Study. *Am. J. Roentgenol.* 214, 1072–1077. doi:10.2214/ajr.20.22976

2

Gremlin2 Activates Fibroblasts to Promote Pulmonary Fibrosis through the Bone Morphogenic Protein Pathway

Caijuan Huan[1†], Wangting Xu[1†], Yaru Liu[2], Kexin Ruan[1], Yueli Shi[3], Hongqiang Cheng[2], Xue Zhang[2], Yuehai Ke[2] and Jianying Zhou[1]*

[1]Department of Respiratory Medicine, The First Affiliated Hospital, Zhejiang University School of Medicine, Hangzhou, China, [2]Department of Pathology and Pathophysiology, Zhejiang University School of Medicine, Hangzhou, China, [3]The Fourth Affiliated Hospital, Zhejiang University School of Medicine, Yiwu, China

***Correspondence:**
Jianying Zhou
zjyhz@zju.edu.cn

[†]These authors have contributed equally to this work and share first authorship

Idiopathic pulmonary fibrosis (IPF) is a progressive lung disease causing unremitting extracellular matrix deposition. Transforming growth factor-β (TGF-β) superfamily involves bone morphogenetic proteins (BMPs) and TGF-β, and the balance between the activation of TGF-β-dependent SMADs (Smad2/3) and BMP-dependent SMADs (Smad1/5/8) is essential for fibrosis process. *GREM2*, initially identified as a TGF-β-inducible gene, encodes a small secreted glycoprotein belonging to a group of matricellular proteins, its role in lung fibrosis is not clear. Here, we identified Gremlin2 as a key regulator of fibroblast activation. Gremlin2 was highly expressed in the serum and lung tissues in IPF patients. Bleomycin-induced lung fibrosis model exhibited high expression of Gremlin2 in the bronchoalveolar lavage fluid (BALF) and lung tissue. Isolation of primary cells from bleomycin-induced fibrosis lung showed a good correlation of Gremlin2 and Acta2 (α-SMA) expressions. Overexpression of Gremlin2 in human fetal lung fibroblast 1 (HFL-1) cells increased its invasion and migration. Furthermore, Gremlin2 regulates fibrosis functions through mediating TGF-β/BMP signaling, in which Gremlin2 may activate TGF-β signaling and inhibit BMP signaling. Therefore, we provided *in vivo* and *in vitro* evidence to demonstrate that Gremlin2 may be a potential therapeutic target for the treatment of IPF.

Keywords: IPF (idiopathic pulmonary fibrosis), gremlin2, BMP antagonists, P-smad1, fibroblast

INTRODUCTION

Idiopathic pulmonary fibrosis (IPF), is the most common form of interstitial pneumonia (ATS/ERS, 2000), which deteriorates rapidly in a short period of time (Martinez et al., 2005) and the median survival is only 2–3 years (Raghu et al., 2011).Tissue fibrosis is an increasing cause of severe morbidity and mortality with limited therapeutic options, and IPF is characterized by patchy subpleural parenchymal fibrosis with pathological features including the accumulation of myofibroblasts, the formation of fibroblast foci, distortion of pulmonary architecture, and increased collagen deposition (Noble et al., 2012). Mechanisms leading to severe and progressive fibrosis are not entirely understood. Previous studies demonstrated that fibroblasts from patients with IPF acquire an invasive phenotype that is essential for severe fibrogenesis (Li et al., 2011; Lovgren et al., 2011; Ahluwalia et al., 2016; Chen et al., 2016).

Fibroblasts are the main effector cells in fibrosis. They migrate from different sources to damaged sites, such as resident stromal fibroblasts, circulating fibroblasts, as well as epithelial cells and pericytes, and they are eventually activated as myofibroblasts (Andersson-Sjöland et al., 2008; Fernandez and Eickelberg, 2012; Wolters et al., 2014; Bagnato and Harari, 2015), which secrete excessive extracellular matrix (ECM), resulting in increased tissue hardness and loss of alveolar tissue function.

The progression of fibrosis is regulated by the transforming growth factor-β (TGF-β)/bone morphogenic protein (BMP) family.

After an injury to the airway epithelium, important profibrotic mediators, such as TGF-β, are released from many types of lung cells, involving myofibroblasts and epithelial cells (Li et al., 2017). Their regulation on progenitor cells also affects fibrosis progression. TGF-β is very important for the progression of pulmonary fibrosis in mice, as it regulates fibroblast proliferation, collagen synthesis and myofibroblast differentiation (Bonniaud et al., 2004; Bonniaud et al., 2005; Kang et al., 2007).The other important fibrosis regulator is BMP family, especially BMP4/7, which is considered to be an important regulatory molecule for anti-fibrosis (Hinck and Huang, 2013; Huan et al., 2015; Chanda et al., 2019). In recent years, antagonists of the BMP family gradually become the center of research for fibrosis treatment. For example, Gremlin1 and Follistatin-like 1 were proved to participate in and affect pulmonary fibrosis (Dong et al., 2015; Church et al., 2017; Myllärniemi, et al., 2008a; Mezzano et al., 2018).

Overall, the balance between the activation of BMP-dependent SMADs (SMAD1/5/8) and TGF-β-dependent (SMAD2/3) plays a great role in fibrosis process.

Gremlin2 (*GREM2*), also known as PRDC, located on human chromosome 1Q43 (CKTSF1B2) (Katoh and Katoh, 2004), is a highly conserved secretory glycoprotein in the DAN region. Gremlin2 was first discovered as a protein associated with embryonic development (Hsu et al., 1998; Stanley et al., 1998). In recent years, its highly stable dimer structure formed via non-disulfide bonds has led scientists to further explore its structure (Kattamuri et al., 2012; Hinck and Huang, 2013; Nolan et al., 2016). Heparin-competitive antagonistic combination of Gremlin2 and BMP provides a new idea for Gremlin2 targeted therapy and the exploration of its structure (Nolan et al., 2013; Kattamuri et al., 2017). As a development-related protein, Gremlin2 is highly expressed during embryonic development but its high levels in adults may imply a severe disease state. It is known that Gremlin2 plays a crucial role in kidney development and kidney injury (Wen et al., 2019). Furthermore, as a strong antagonist of the BMP family, Gremlin2 has a strong effect on gastric cancer and myocardial fibrosis, but its effect on pulmonary fibrosis has not been reported (Sanders et al., 2016; Ran et al., 2019). However, the ability of Gremlin2 to regulate fibroblast activity in pathological settings has not been investigated.

Our previous study showed that Gremlin2 is highly expressed in myofibroblasts in single-cell sequencing (Xie et al., 2018). Data showed Gremlin2 expression is significantly high in myofibroblasts, which is consistent with specific myofibroblast markers Acta2 and Myh11 (Hsia et al., 2016; Hinz et al., 2007). Meanwhile, in other mesenchymal cells, Gremlin2 expression is low, indicating that Gremlin2 has a functional role in myofibroblasts.

Therefore, here, we aimed to show the effect of Gremlin2 in IPF via *in vivo* and *in vitro* studies, as well as through database investigations and understand the potential of it as a therapeutic target.

MATERIALS AND METHODS

Mice

C57/BL6 male mice (6–8 weeks old) were purchased from GemPharmatech Co., Ltd., Jiangsu, China. All mice were housed and cared for in a pathogen-free facility at Zhejiang University. All animal protocols were approved by the animal care and use committee of the Zhejiang University School of Medicine.

Lungs were removed from mice at the age of 8-12 weeks after appropriate treatment. The tissues were minced, digested, and cultured in DMEM supplemented with 10% fetal bovine serum (FBS) and antibiotics-antimycotics (Thermo Fisher Scientific).

Idiopathic Pulmonary Fibrosis Samples From Patients

Lung tissue samples were obtained from surgical lung biopsies or lung transplant explants from patients with IPF or other types of pulmonary fibrosis. IPF diagnosis was performed according to standard accepted American Thoracic Society recommendations (ATS/ERS, 2000). Human blood samples were obtained from the Clinical Laboratory. All samples were collected from the First Affiliated Hospital of Zhejiang University.

Bleomycin Administration and Bronchoalveolar Lavage Fluid

Bleomycin was injected intratracheally at 2.5 U/kg body weight. Mice exposed to the same volume of PBS were used as controls and sacrificed via pentobarbital injection after 7, 14, and 21 days. Lungs were harvested for RNA preparation, protein isolation or fibroblast isolation. For bronchoalveolar lavage, the trachea was lavaged three times with 0.8 ml sterile saline at room temperature. Samples were centrifuged at 1,500 rpm for 5 min, and the supernatant was collected and stored at −80°C until further use.

Enzyme-Linked Immunosorbent Assay of Serum and Bronchoalveolar Lavage Fluid

The mice were anesthetized with 1% pentobarbital at a dose of 50 mg/kg, and the apical blood was obtained in a sterile environment and kept at 4°C overnight. The next day, the blood was centrifuged at 4°C for 15 min at 3,000 × g. The supernatant was removed and stored separately below −70°C

TABLE 1 | Reagent and antibody.

Product name	Company	Catalog	Lot
Rabbit polyclonal to PRDC-C-terminal	Abcam, cambridge, MA	Cat#ab228736	Lot# GR3209267-6
GREM2 antibody	CUSABIO	Catalog#CSB-PA107590	Lot#10902Y
Rabbit polyclonal to fibronectin	Abcam, cambridge, MA	Cat# ab2413, RRID:AB_2262874	Lot#GR3323518-2
Anti-alpha smooth muscle actin antibody	Abcam, cambridge, MA	Cat# ab7817, RRID:AB_262054	Lot# GR3257713-10
Mouse PRDC/GREM2 antibody	R And D systems	Cat# AF 2069, RRID:AB_2263614	Lot#USW0114091
Mouse PRDC/GREM2 biotinylated antibody	R And D systems	Cat# BAF 2069, RRID:AB_2279268	Lot#UUB0112051
Phospho-Smad1(Ser463/465) /Smad5(Ser463/465) /Smad9(Ser465/467) (D5B10)Rabbit mAb	Cell signaling TECHNOLOGY	Cat# 13820T	Lot#3
Smad1(D59D7)Rabbit mAb	Cell signaling TECHNOLOGY	Cat# 6944T	Lot#5
Phospho-SMAD2(Ser465/467) (E8F3R)	Cell signaling TECHNOLOGY	Cat# 188338T	Lot#3
Smad2 (D43B4) XP® rabbit mAb	Cell signaling TECHNOLOGY	Cat#5339T	Lot#6
Rabbit anti-P-Smad3(S423/425)		Cat# ET1609	Lot#HM0708
Human Gremlin-2 ELISA kit	Biolebo, beijing, China	ZN2207	Lot#TF0611
Recombinant human PRDC/GREM2 protein, CF	R&D systems	Catalog #8436-PR-050	Lot#DEUB0220071
HRP labeled goat anti-rabbit IgG(H + L)	BIOKER BIOTECHNOLOGY	Catalog #BK-R050	Lot#2313

before detection. BALF from each mouse was collected as mentioned in 2.3. Before measurement, the BALF supernatant of each mouse was stored at −70°C. Gremlin2 levels in the serum and BALF supernatant were measured using Mouse Gremlin-2 ELISA Kit (Biolebo, Beijing, China), according to the manufacturer's instructions.

Lung Histology and Immunohistochemistry

Mice were sacrificed at different time points after bleomycin treatment under anesthesia. The left lung of each mouse was fixed with 10% neutral buffer formalin overnight, then embedded in paraffin using standard procedures. Tissues were sectioned to 5 μm slices for hematoxylin and eosin, Masson's Trichrome, and Gremlin2 staining (**Table 1**).

The alveolar wall thickness and alveolar space were photographed and measured using DP2-BSW software (Olympus, Tokyo, Japan). Slides were screened in a blinded manner and six lungs were observed in areas that did not contain bronchi or major pulmonary vessels. A total of 20 random measurements of alveolar wall thickness were recorded in each field.

Immunohistochemistry Score

We selected five sections randomly from each slide at 200× magnification for IHC score statistics as follows: negative, 1 point (less than 5% of cells); weak positive 2 points (5–25% of cells); positive, 3 points (25–50% of cells); strong positive, 4 points (50–75% of cells). IHC score staining degree and multiple cell ratio score of each section were added, the average of the five visual fields was accepted as the IHC score of the slide, and the average score of each slide was taken after two investigators agreed.

Immunofluorescence

For cell immunofluorescence, after 48 h of TGF-β1 stimulation, fibroblasts were washed in PBS preheated at 37°C, fixed in 4% paraformaldehyde for 20 min, and permeated with 0.1% Triton X-100 for 20 min. Cells were blocked in 10% FBS at room temperature for 1 h, and fibroblasts were incubated overnight with antibodies against Gremlin2 or α-SMA (**Table 1**). On the second day, fibroblasts were washed with PBS, and 488 goat anti-rabbit/rat IgG (Invitrogen, Fisher Scientific, California, United States) was added for 1 h at room temperature. Cells were then washed with PBS, then immersed in DAPI to stain the nuclei. The staining was performed using a positive two-photon confocal microscope (Olympus BX61).

For tissue immunofluorescence, paraffin sections were baked, dewaxed, and hydrated after microwave antigen repair. They were then incubated in 0.5% Triton-TBS for 20 min and 5% goat serum for 30 min. Anti-Gremlin2 and α-SMA antibodies were added at 4°C overnight. The next day, slides were washed with PBS and incubated for 2 h at room temperature with 488/576 goat anti-rabbit/rat IgG (Invitrogen, Fisher Scientific, California, United States), then washed with PBS, and immersed in DAPI to observe the nuclei. Imaging was performed using a positive two-photon confocal microscope (Olympus BX61).

Quantitative Real-Time Polymerase Chain Reaction

Total RNA was extracted from tissues or cells using TRIzol (Invitrogen, Carlsbad, CA, United States) according to the manufacturer's protocol. RNA concentration was measured using a spectrophotometer (Eppendorf, Hamburg, Germany). Reverse transcription of total RNA (2 g) 20 μL was performed using PrimeScript II 1st Strand cDNA Synthesis Kit (Takara, Otsu, Japan). Quantitative real-time PCR was performed using FastStart universal SYBR Green Master Kit (Mannheim Roche, Germany). Sequences of specific primers used are shown in **Table 2**.

Western Blotting

The cells were washed with cold PBS and lysed with NP−40, then 6X loading buffer was added. Equivalent proteins were separated

TABLE 2 | Sequences of specific primers.

	Sense strand (5′ to 3′)	Anti-sense strand (5′ to 3′)
Gremlin2(mouse)	GGTAGCTGAAACACGGAAGAA	TCTTGCACCAGTCACTCTTGA
GAPDH(mouse)	AATGCATTTGGACGCATTGGT	TTTGCACTGGTACGTGTTGAT
Col1a1(mouse)	CCAAGAAGACATCCCTGAAGTCA	TGCACGTCATCGCACACA
Col1a2(mouse)	CGGAGAAGCTGGATCTGC	CAGGAGGACCCATTACACCA
Gremlin2(human)	ATCCCCTCGCCTTACAAGGA	TCTTGCACCAGTCACTCTTGA
GAPDH(human)	TGTGGGCATCAATGGATTTGG	ACACCATGTATTCCGGGTCAAT
Col1(human)	GTTGCTGCTTGCAGTAACCTT	AGGGCCAAGTCCAACTCCTT
ACTA2(human)	GACAATGGCTCTGGGCTCTGTAA	CTGTGCTTCGTCACCCACGTA
Fibronectin(human)	CAGGATCACTTACGGAGAAACAG	GCCAGTGACAGCATACACAGTG

via SDS-PAGE, then transferred to a cellulose nitrate membrane (Pall, Port Washington, NY) and incubated with the relevant primary antibodies (anti-Gremlin2, anti-α-Tubulin, anti-fibronectin, anti-collagen1, anti-α-SMA). This protocol was performed in three replicates. Shorter exposures were selected for optical density analysis to ensure that the band strength was within the linear range, and the integral density of the specified band was calculated using the ImageJ software.

Transwell Assay

For cell migration, 5×10^4 cells were resuspended in 200 µl starvation medium and seeded into the upper chamber. In the lower chamber, 600 µl of complete medium containing 10% FBS was added. After 24 h, the medium was removed, the upper chamber was washed twice with PBS, and cells were fixed with 4% PFA at room temperature for 30 min. The cells were stained with crystal violet. Three fields were randomly selected under 100× magnification and cells were counted in each field for statistical analysis.

For cell invasion, the matrigel was diluted in Ham's F-12K (Kaighn's) Medium (1:32) (Gibco, Thermo Fisher, United States), added to the upper chamber one day in advance, and blow-dried overnight under ultraviolet light. 2×10^5 cells were resuspended in 100 µl starvation medium and added to the superior lumen. Exactly 600 µl of medium containing 10% FBS was added to the lower chamber. After 48 h, the cells were collected, and the same steps were performed as the migration experiment.

GEO Database Analysis

The original data in the GEO database were homogenized. We used R language (R i386 3.6.1.Ink) and GEO2R analysis software provided by the GEO website for group analysis. Then, the data for different groups were plotted using GraphPad Prism (version 5) and paired t-test was performed for statistical analysis.

Lentiviral Infection

To knock out *GREM2* in fibroblasts, shRNA-Gremlin2-plko.1 and a control lentiviral vector [(RRID:Addgene_23,260), Sigma-Aldrich] were obtained. 293T (RRID:CVCL_LF41) cells were transfected with pMD2. G and psPAX2 were prepared using Lipofectamine 3,000 reagent (Invitrogen, Addgene, Cambridge, MA). After 48 and 72 h, the virus superfluids were collected and filtered through a 0.22 µm filter, and added to fibroblasts. After 12 h, the culture medium was changed to allow the cells to grow until treatment and analysis.

Statistical Analysis

All the results were expressed as the mean ± SD, calculated using the statistical program of GraphPad Prism version 5. Student's t-test (two-tailed) was used and $p < 0.05$ was considered statistically significant.

RESULTS

High Expression of Gremlin2 has a Strong Correlation With Idiopathic Pulmonary Fibrosis in the Fibrotic Area

To discern the importance of Gremlin2 in pulmonary fibrosis, we evaluated the expression of Gremlin2 using the GEO database and selected two fibrosis-related databases, GSE99621 (https://www.ncbi.nlm.nih.gov/geo/query/acc.cgi?acc=GSE99621) and GSE10667 (https://www.ncbi.nlm.nih.gov/geo/query/acc.cgi). GSE10667 exhibited that the transcription level of Gremlin2 in the lung tissues of patients with IPF was significantly higher than that of healthy people (**Figure 1A**, $p < 0.001$). In GSE99621, we divided the data into Group1 (**Figure 1B**), patients with fibrosis, and healthy controls, and Group2 (**Figure 1B**), fibrosis foci and non-fibrosis foci of patients. Gremlin1 ($p = 0.0011$) (Myllärniemi et al., 2008a; Myllärniemi et al., 2008b) and Gremlin2 ($p < 0.001$) expressions in Group 1 (**Figure 1B**) were significantly high in the lung tissues of patients with fibrosis, while there was no difference in the expression of another BMP strong antagonist CHRD ($p = 0.1819$) between healthy people and patients with fibrosis. In Group2 (**Figure 1C**), only Gremlin2 ($p = 0.032$) expression was significantly higher in the fibrotic scar area than that in the non-fibrotic scar area of patients with IPF. Meanwhile, Gremlin1 ($p = 0.2622$) and CHRD ($p = 0.7755$) expressions showed no statistical significance. These two databases suggested that there was a strong relationship between Gremlin2 and IPF.

Gremlin2 Expression is Increased in Patients With Idiopathic Pulmonary Fibrosis

To verify the data obtained from databases, we collected blood samples from four patients with non-IPF fibrosis and three

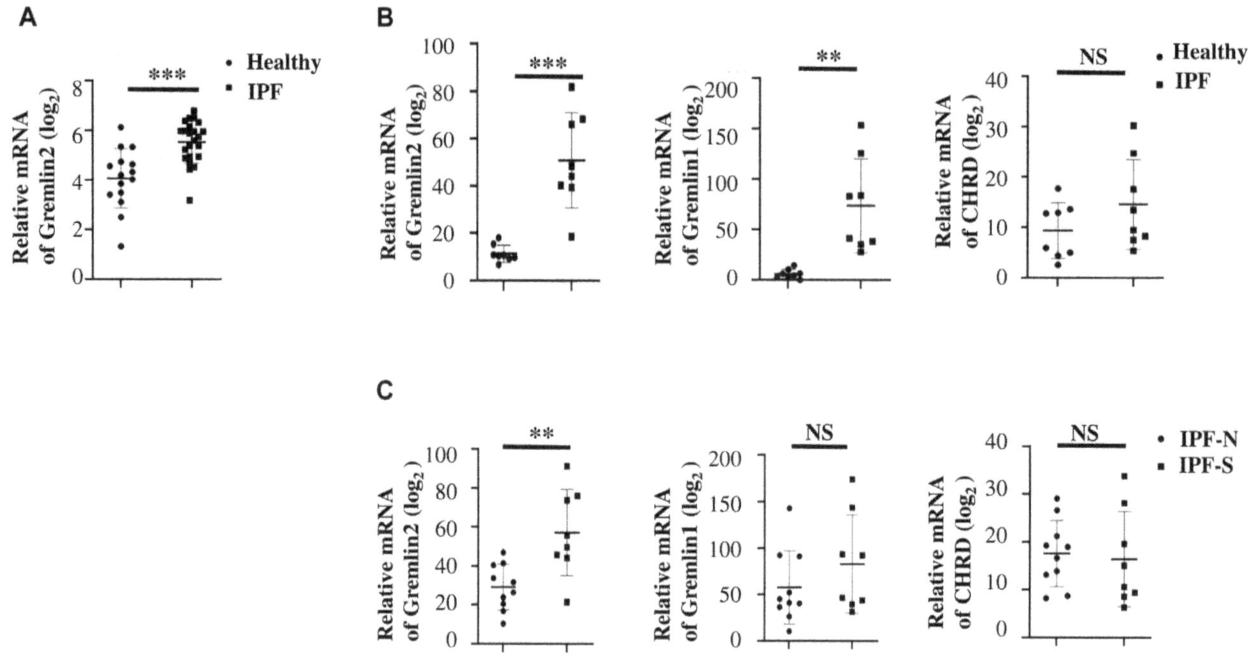

FIGURE 1 | High expression of Gremlin2 in the fibrotic area obtained from IPF databases **(A)** The mRNA expression of Gremlin2 in patients with IPF and healthy people in database GSE10667. The data has been log_2 processed. **(B)** The mRNA expression levels of Gremlin2, Gremlin1, and CHORD in the lung tissues of eight IPF patients and eight healthy people using the GSE99621 database. The data has been log_2 processed. **(C)** mRNA expression levels of Gremlin2, Gremlin1, and CHORD in the GSE99621 database in the scar regions of eight IPF patients and ten non-scar regions of patients with IPF. The data has been log2 processed.NS stands for $p > 0.05$, $^{*}p < 0.05$, $^{**}p < 0.01$, $^{***}p < 0.001$. Student's t-test was used for statistics. IPF-N, non-fibrosis lung area of IPF patients; IPF-S, fibrosis lung area of patients with IPF.

patients with IPF, and measured the concentration of Gremlin2 in the blood serum. These IPF patients were first diagnosed with IPF and had not received anti-fibrosis therapy. The concentration of Gremlin2 in the peripheral blood serum was detected using ELISA (**Figure 2A**), which showed that Gremlin2 expression was high in patients with IPF and low in non-IPF patients.

To further detect the expression of Gremlin2 in the lung tissue, IHC was performed using the lung tissue samples from 20 patients with fibrosis, and the expression of Gremlin2 was compared with that of 16 healthy lung tissues. The patient information is shown in **Table 3**. Gremlin2 expression was hardly detected in healthy lung tissues but was high in the fibrotic foci (**Figure 2B**). IHC score (**Figure 2C**) showed that Gremlin2 expression was statistically high in fibrotic lung tissues ($p < 0.001$). To verify whether myofibroblasts are the main effector cells of Gremlin2, we detected the morphology of cells with high Gremlin2 expression (**Figure 2D**) and co-stained cells with a myofibroblasts marker. We observed the strong positive cells, which showed the long spindle shape characteristic of myofibroblast cells and were concentrated in the fibroblast lesions (**Figure 2D**). At the same time, Gremlin2 and α-SMA expressions were observed in the adjacent regions (**Figure 2E**). The precise localization of Gremlin2 is somewhat difficult, as it is a secreted protein, just like another secreted protein IL-11 (Ng et al., 2019).

These clinical data were consistent with the databases analysis results, suggesting the possibility of clinical transformation of Gremlin2.

Gremlin2 Expression is High in Bleomycin-Induced Mice Lung Tissues

We treated C57BL/6 mice with bleomycin (Tashiro et al., 2017) and detected the expression levels of Gremlin2 at mRNA and protein levels in the lung tissue. Since Gremlin2 is a secretory glycoprotein, we collected mouse alveolar lavage fluid for the detection of Gremlin2 concentration using ELISA.

Bleomycin airway infusion (2.5 U/kg) was used to induce pulmonary fibrosis in mice, we detected fibrosis induction using Masson trichromatic staining (**Figure 3A**). The blue area represented collagen accumulation, suggesting a fibrotic condition. The expression of Gremlin2 in the lung tissue was detected using western blotting (**Figure 3B**). Compared with the commonly used fibrosis indexes involving collagenl (Coll) and fibronectin (FN), we found that the Gremlin2 expression level in the fibrosis model mice group increased more significantly, and was even more sensitive and indicative than the international indexes.

By detecting the mRNA level of Gremlin2 in the lung tissues at different time points, we found that the transcription level of Gremlin2 increased significantly on day 14, while there was no statistical difference between the pulmonary tissues of fibrotic

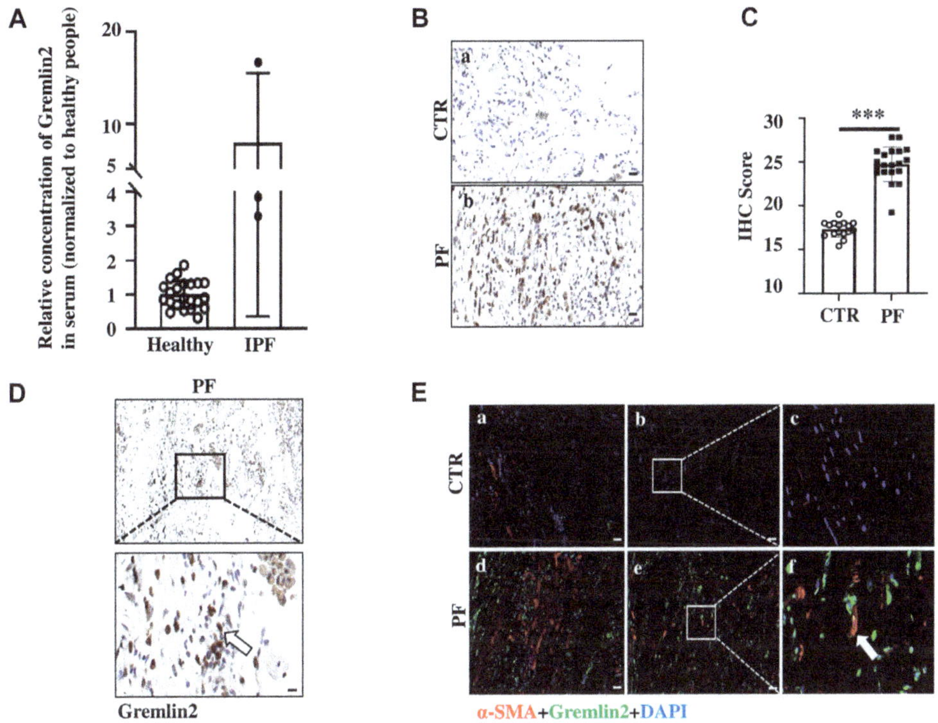

FIGURE 2 | Gremlin2 expression is increased in patients with IPF **(A)** Expression of Gremlin2 in the blood serum detected using ELISA, CTR (healthy control) $n = 22$, IPF $n = 3$. **(B)** Representative pictures of IHC showing Gremlin2 expression in the lung tissue. Scale Bar = 50 μm. **(C)** IHC score of patients via immunohistochemical staining grading, CTR (normal) $n = 16$, PF $n = 20$, $^{***}p < 0.001$, paired t-test. **(D)** Representative photos of Gremlin2 immunohistochemical staining in the fibrotic lung tissue samples of the patient. Lower graph shows the strong positive area of Gremlin2 magnified from upper graph, white arrow shows the strong positive cells of Gremlin2. Scale Bar = 20 μm. **(E)** Gremlin2 was co-localized with α-SMA in fibrotic foci. Representative images of immunofluorescence detection for α-SMA (red) and gremlin2 (green), and merged (yellow) images of normal subjects and patients with IPF. Graph **(2Ea–c)** showed the pulmonary tissue in the fibrotic area of normal lung tissues near the fibrotic area of patients with IPF; graph **(2Ed,e)**, f showed the fibrotic lung tissue of patients with IPF; graph **(2Ec,f)** showed the locally enlarged view in the white box in graph **(2Eb,e)**; white arrow points to the cells with high co-expression of α-SMA and Gremlin2. CTR is the normal tissue around the pulmonary tissue of patients with fibrosis, and PF is the lung tissue section of patients with lung fibrosis. Scale Bar = 50 μm. NS stands for $p > 0.05$, $^{*}p < 0.05$, $^{**}p < 0.01$, $^{***}p < 0.001$. Student's t-test was used for statistics.

mice and the control group on day 21 (**Figure 3C**, $p = 0.0534$). This suggested that the transcription level of Gremlin2 increased during the acute progression of fibrosis, thus affecting the process. Gremlin2 content of mouse alveolar lavage fluid was traced using ELISA. As shown in **Figure 3D**, the concentration of Gremlin2 in the alveolar lavage fluid was significantly increased ($p = 0.0102$). Using IHC, we observed that the expression of Gremlin2 in the fibrotic lung tissue was significantly increased (**Figure 3E**). The time course (day 0, day 7, day 14, day 21) data of Gremlin2 mRNA, protein, and BALF were shown in **Supplementary Figure S2**. Overall, Gremlin2 expression was high in the bleomycin-induced pulmonary fibrosis mouse model.

Myofibroblasts Express High Levels of Gremlin2 in Bleomycin-Induced Lung Fibrosis Mouse Model

To investigate whether the cells with high Gremlin2 expression were activated fibroblasts or not, immunofluorescence staining was used. It was difficult to identify the precise location of Gremlin2, as it is secreted. Co-localization of α-SMA and Gremlin2 in bleomycin-induced fibrosis lung of mice was observed (**Figure 4A**).

Then we isolated lung fibroblasts on day 14 after treatment with PBS or bleomycin to detect Gremlin2 expression. After culturing for 5 days, we examined the expression of α-SMA and Gremlin2 in lung fibroblasts through western blotting (**Figure 4B**) and immunofluorescence detection (**Figure 4C**). **Figures 4B,C** both show the high relevance between the expressions of α-SMA and Gremlin2, indicating myofibroblasts were the effector cells of Gremlin2 expression.

Gremlin2 is an Activated Regulator to Fibroblasts

We used TGF-β1 (Li et al., 2014; Meng et al., 2016) to stimulate fibroblasts and mimic the activation of fibroblasts *in vivo* (Xie et al., 2018). Protein and mRNA levels of Gremlin2 were measured after TGF-β1 treatment in fibroblasts (**Figures 5A,B**). Gremlin2 expression increased significantly upon activation of fibroblasts, and the mRNA levels increased in line with the ECM production ($p < 0.05$). The well-known

TABLE 3 | Patients' information of IPF and other types of pulmonary fibrosis.

IHC of patients' slices

Pathology number	Gender	Age (years old)	Pathological diagnosis	Sample site
2019106687–5	Male	51	Pulmonary fibrosis nodules with charcoal deposition	Middle lobe of right lung
2019106687–6				Adjacent area of fibrosis
2019112471–3	Male	40	Fibrotic nodules	Inferior lobe of right lung
2019112471–5				Adjacent area of fibrosis
2019112971–3	Female	56	Chronic inflammatory fibrosis	Upper lobe of left lung
2019112971–4				Adjacent area of fibrosis
2019116608–9	Female	72	Fibrotic nodules	Inferior lobe of right lung
2019116608–8				Adjacent area of fibrosis
2019117672–9	Male	67	Chronic mucosal inflammation with pulmonary fibrosis nodules	Upper lobe of right lung
2019117672–13				Adjacent area of fibrosis
2020000937–3	Female	65	Fibrotic nodules	Middle lobe of right lung
2020000937–4				Adjacent area of fibrosis
2020001297–2	Female	49	Fibrotic nodules	Upper lobe of left lung
2020001297–5				Adjacent area of fibrosis
2020003176–2	Female	69	Fibrotic collagenous nodules	The proper segment of the upper lobe of the left lung
2020003176–3				Adjacent area of fibrosis
2020006458–10	Male	55	Chronic inflammation of lung tissue with collagen fibrotic nodules	Inferior lobe of left lung
2020006458–11				Adjacent area of fibrosis
2020009101–2	Male	44	Chronic inflammation of lung tissue with fibrotic nodules	Inferior lobe of right lung
2020009101–3				Adjacent area of fibrosis
2020009493–3	Male	51	Fibrotic nodules	Upper lobe of right lung
2020009493–8				Adjacent area of fibrosis
2020009765–3	Female	74	Chronic inflammatory fibrosis	Upper lobe of right lung
2020009765–7				Adjacent area of fibrosis
2020012831–1	Male	55	Fibrosis and degenerative necrotic nodules	Inferior lobe of right lung
2020012831–2				Adjacent area of fibrosis
2020020563–3	Male	70	Fibrotic nodules with charcoal deposition	Upper lobe of left lung
2020020563–4				Adjacent area of fibrosis
2020037421–1	Male	68	Interstitial pulmonary fibrosis	Inferior lobe of right lung
2020037421–2				Adjacent area of fibrosis
201651141	Male	64	Chronic interstitial pneumonia with fibrosis	Right lung
201709433	Female	69	Chronic interstitial pneumonia with fibrosis	Right lung
201713228	Male	67	Chronic interstitial pneumonia with fibrosis	Right lung
201722515	Male	58	Interstitial pulmonary fibrosis	Right lung

Blood serum of IPF patients

Medical record number	Gender	Age (years old)	Clinical diagnosis	Illness stage
5057536	Female	62	IPF	Recurring fever with fatigue for a year, acute exacerbation
3165154	Female	66	IPF	Repeated cough for three years, chest tightness for two years, aggravation for half a year, with respiratory failure
4141982	Male	83	IPF	Repeated shortness of breath for three years, acute exacerbation with respiratory failure for one week

markers of fibroblast activation, including FN, Col1, and α-SMA (ACTA2) were chosen to verify the activation. Similarly, α-SMA and Gremlin2 staining was used to detect expression levels with or without TGF-β1 treatment (**Figure 5C**). We obtained similar results using immunofluorescence and western blotting, where TGF-β1 activated fibroblasts showed upregulated Gremlin2 expression.

Next, we wanted to explore whether Gremlin2 expression affected the activation of fibroblasts. First, α-SMA expression was detected in fibroblast via cellular immunofluorescence (**Figure 5D**). We found that after Gremlin2 overexpression, fibroblasts were spontaneously activated into myofibroblasts. The expression of α-SMA in human fetal lung fibroblast 1 (HFL-1) (ATCC Cat# CCL-153, RRID:CVCL_0298) cells or MRC-5 (ATCC Cat# CCL-171, RRID:CVCL_0440) showed high fluorescence intensity after Gremlin2 overexpression. However, fluorescence intensity did not increase further in Gremlin2-overexpressing HFL-1 cells after TGF-β1 stimulation, which might indicate that Gremlin2 and TGF-β1 counteract each other in fibroblast activation, as shown in **Supplementary Figure S3**.

To explore the effect of Gremlin2 deficiency, we used an adenovirus containing shGremlin2 and detected changes in fibroblasts stimulated by TGF-β1 after Gremlin2 knockdown (**Figure 5E**). After knockdown of Gremlin2, α-SMA expression decreased simultaneously, and fibroblasts were significantly less activated by TGF-β1 than control fibroblasts. Overall, these might indicate that the presence of Gremlin2 was crucial for fibroblast activation.

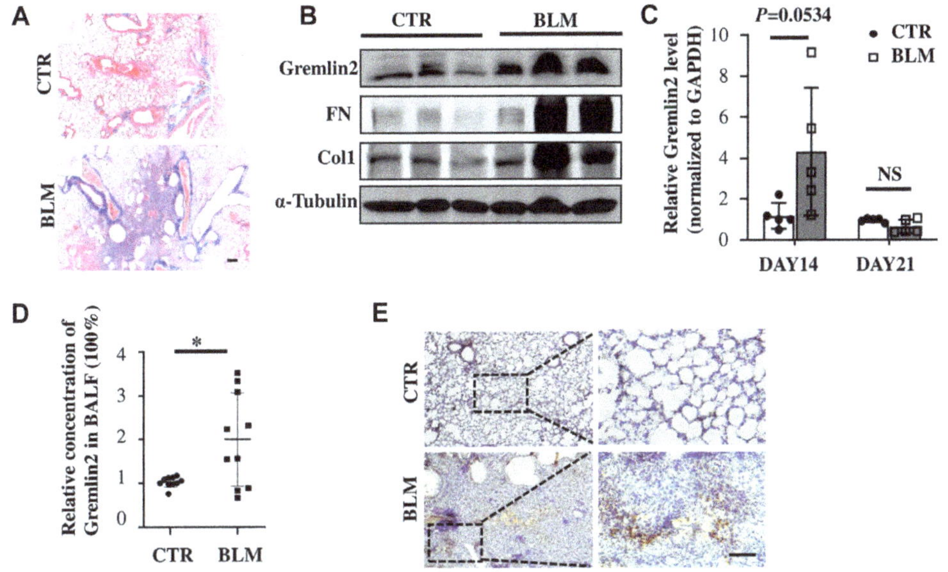

FIGURE 3 | Increased expression of Gremlin2 in the lung tissue of bleomycin-induced pulmonary fibrosis mice **(A)** Masson's trichrome staining of the lung tissue in the bleomycin-treated mice and PBS-treated control mice. **(B)** 21 days after bleomycin (BLM) or PBS (CTR) treatment mice were sacrificed. Western blotting was performed using the lung tissue homogenates. α-tubulin was used as a reference collagen1 (Col1) and fibronectin (FN) were detected as indicators of fibrosis, and Gremlin2 (Grem2) was used as the target protein. **(C)** Following the same operation method as **(B)**, the corresponding mRNA was extracted from the lung tissue of mice treated for 14 and 21 days, and real-time-quantitative PCR was used to detect the mRNA expression levels of Gremlin2. Day 14 CTR $n = 5$, BLM $n = 5$, $p = 0.0534$, student's paired t-test; day 21 CTR $n = 5$, BLM $n = 5$, NS $p > 0.05$, student's paired t-test. **(D)** Expression level of Gremlin2 in alveolar lavage fluid. CTR $n = 10$, BLM $n = 10$, $^*p = 0.0102$, student t paired test. **(E)** Representative images of control lung tissue sections (CTR) and fibrotic lung tissue (BLM) assessed using immunohistochemical staining with anti-Gremlin2 antibody. The right two pictures are 10 x magnified versions of the left two corresponding pictures. The relative content of Gremlin2 was obtained after standardized numerical treatment. Use the Student's bilateral t-test. Scale bar = 50 μm. CTR, control with PBS-treated group; and BLM, bleomycin-treated group.

We obtained the same results from primary lung fibroblasts of bleomycin-induced lung fibrosis mouse model and activated HFL-1 cells. We observed the same upward trend in α-SMA and Gremlin2 expressions. Compared to classic lung biopsy for IPF diagnosis, it was more convenient to detect Gremlin2 expression from BALF, which could be used as a detection method to indicate the occurrence and development of fibrosis.

Gremlin2 Regulates Migration and Invasion of Fibroblasts

Next, we identified the functional role of Gremlin2 in lung fibroblasts by investigating whether Gremlin2 expression regulates the invasion and migration of fibroblasts. Gremlin2 overexpression in lung fibroblasts showed a significant increase in fibroblast migration (**Figures 6A,B**; $p = 0.0024$) and invasion (**Figures 6C,D**; $p = 0.0054$). We also examined Col1 mRNA expression levels and found that there was a strong correlation between Gremlin2 and Col1 expression (**Figure 6E**). This suggested that Gremlin2 might control migration and invasion by increasing ECM production. To identify the function of Gremlin2, we used the recombinant human Gremlin2/rPRDC to stimulate HFL-1 cells. Gremlin2/rPRDC activated fibroblasts, inducing high expression of FN and Col1 (**Figure 6F**). α-SMA expression also increased, which was similar to TGF-β1 stimulation (**Figure 6G**). These results revealed that high expression of Gremlin2 in the activated fibroblasts affected their migration and invasion, and Gremlin2 acted on the inactive fibroblasts after secretion, exerting a positive feedback effect.

Gremlin2 Activates Fibroblasts Through the Bone Morphogenic Protein Signaling Pathway

We used Gremlin2 overexpression plasmid in fibroblasts and verified it at mRNA and protein levels (**Figures 7A,B**; $p < 0.001$). When Gremlin2 was overexpressed in fibroblasts, phosphorylation of Smad1 was decreased, while phosphorylation of Smad2 was not significantly changed (**Figure 7C**). To visualize the changes in Smad1 and Smad2 phosphorylation, we detected *p*-Smad1 and *p*-Smad2 through immunofluorescence. The fluorescence intensity in the nucleus represented the level of phosphorylation. The results showed that Gremlin2 overexpression affected the Smad1 phosphorylation, leading to low expression of *p*-Smad1. However, Gremlin2 overexpression had an insignificant effect on Smad2 phosphorylation (**Figure 7D**).

To explore the effect of Gremlin2 deficiency, we infected fibroblasts with Gremlin2-specific adenovirus and validated the knockdown efficiency at transcription and translation levels (**Figures 7E,F**). When Gremlin2 was knocked down, Smad1 phosphorylation increased, while Smad2 phosphorylation did not significantly change. To visualize the change in Smad1 and

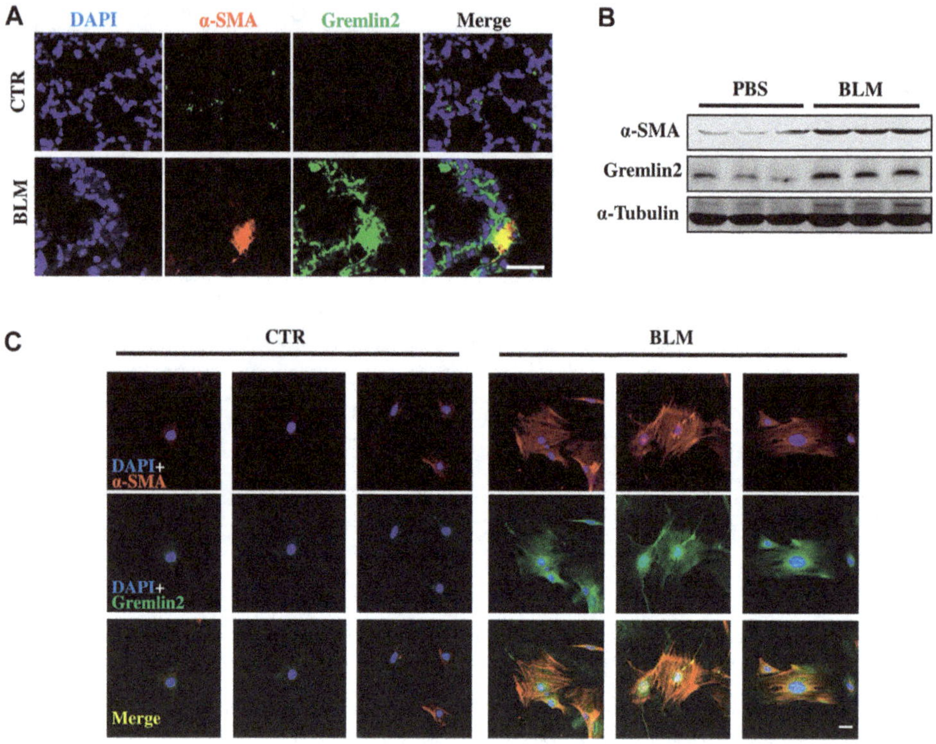

FIGURE 4 | Myofibroblast expresses high level of Gremlin2 in bleomycin induced lung fibrosis model through co-localization **(A)** Immunofluorescence shows co-localization of fibroblast activation marker (α-SMA) and Gremlin2 in lungs of bleomycin-induced fibrosis mice, Gremlin2 (Green), and α-SMA (Red), DAPI (Blue), Yellow (Merge), scale bar = 10 μm. **(B)** Fibroblasts were isolated from mice after PBS or bleomycin treatment on day 14, then western blotting was performed to detect the expression of Gremlin2, and α-SMA. Every group contained three mice. CTR n = 3, BLM n = 4. **(C)** Following the same operation method as **(B)**, then immunofluorescence was performed to detect the expression of Gremlin2 (Green), and α-SMA (Red). DAPI (Blue) indicated the nucleus. Scale bar = 20 μm. CTR n = 3, BLM n = 4. CTR, control with PBS-treated group; and BLM, bleomycin-treated group.

Smad2 phosphorylation, we located *p*-Smad1 and *p*-Smad2 through immunofluorescence. The results showed that Gremlin2 knockdown upregulated the phosphorylation of Smad1, but had little effect on the phosphorylation level of Smad2 (**Figure 7H**). As shown in **Figures 7E–H**, the HFL-1 fibroblast cell line was selected for Gremlin2 knockdown, and fibroblast activation was not performed during this process. Even in the inactive state, Gremlin2 knockdown also affected the Smad1 phosphorylation level, indicating that baseline Gremlin2 expression might regulate the BMP signaling. To prove that Gremlin2 affects Smad1 phosphorylation, we knocked down Gremlin2 in TGF-β1-activated HFL-1 cells, and the same trend was observed (**Figure 7G**). Smad1 phosphorylation was upregulated in activated fibroblasts (**Supplementary Figure S4**).

Overall, overexpression of Gremlin2 in HFL-1 cells affected the phosphorylation of Smad1 to mediate the BMP signaling pathway.

DISCUSSION

Here, we achieved overexpression of Gremlin2 (gain of function) and downregulation of Gremlin2 using specific shRNA (loss of function), which showed that Gremlin2 knockdown upregulated the phosphorylation of Smad1 and Gremlin2 overexpression downregulated the phosphorylation of Smad1. In the mice model, the phosphorylation of Smad1 in primary lung fibroblast was upregulated in the bleomycin treatment group shown in **Supplementary Figures S6E–G**. These results suggest that Gremlin2 might regulate fibrosis via controlling the phosphorylation of Smad1 to mediate the BMP signaling pathway.

IPF is a progressive, fatal disorder that presents a major challenge for clinicians, and the mechanisms that control IPF are not fully understood (King et al., 2011). The main pathological manifestations of IPF are characteristic fibroblast foci composed of major effector fibroblasts (ATS/ERS, 2000). There have been many studies on fibroblasts, including the senescence phenotype of fibroblasts (Waters et al., 2018), tumor-related fibroblasts (Woodcock et al., 2019), and activation of fibroblasts. Myofibroblasts are key effector cells involved in ECM deposition in various fibrotic conditions, including IPF. Our studies demonstrated the profibrotic role of Gremlin2 in pulmonary fibrosis. We provided data at the cellular, molecular, and animal levels to support a role of Gremlin2 as a therapeutic target candidate for lung fibrosis.

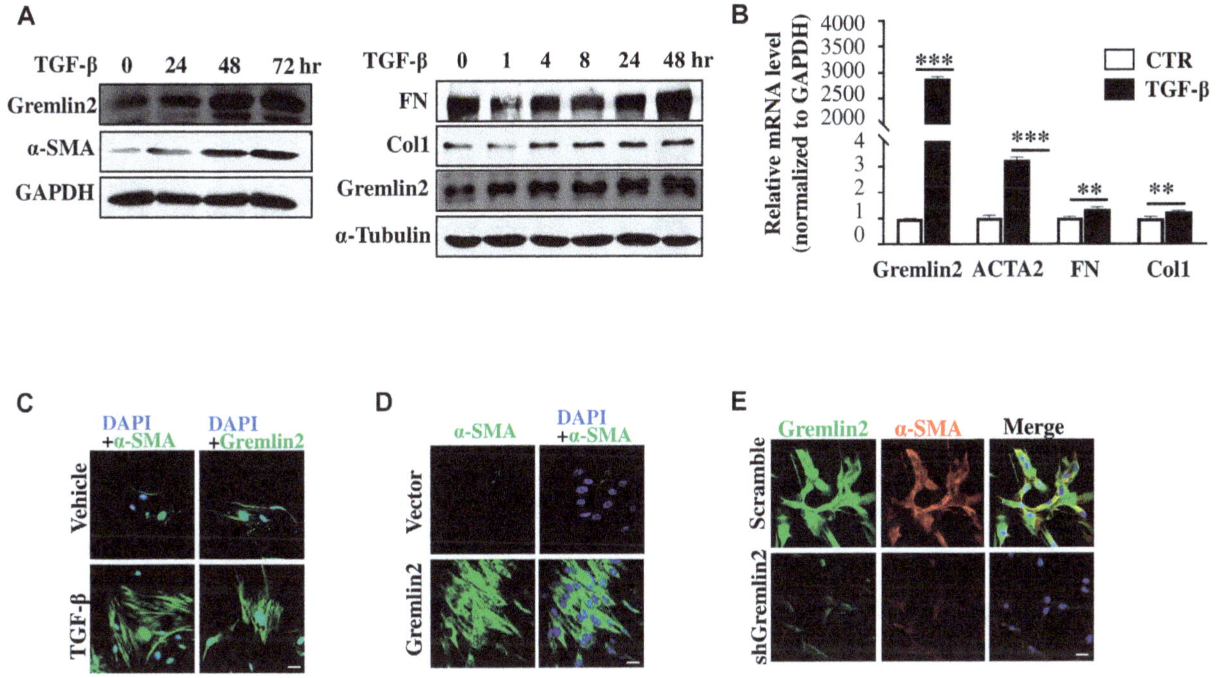

FIGURE 5 | Gremlin2 is an activated regulator to fibroblast **(A)** HFL-1 were collected after treatment with TGF-β1 at 5 ng/mL for 0, 24, 48, and 72 h. Protein expression was detected using western blotting, with GAPDH as a quantitative indicator protein, α-SMA as an indicator of fibroblast activation, and Gremlin2 as a target protein (this experiment was repeated three times). The same treatment applied to HFL-1 cells with TGF-β1 at 5 ng/mL for 0, 1, 4, 8, 24, and 48 h. Western blotting was used to detect fibronectin and collagen1 expression. α-Tubulin was used as the quantitative indicator protein. **(B)** The mRNA was extracted after treatment of HFL-1 cells with TGF-β1 (5 ng/mL) for 24 h, and then real-time quantitative PCR was performed to detect the corresponding mRNA expression levels. α-SMA (ACTA2), fibronectin (FN), and collagen1 (Col1) were used as indicators of fibroblast activation (this experiment was repeated three times). Gremlin2 ****p* < 0.0001, Acta2 ****p* = 0.0002, FN ***p* = 0.0037, Col1 ***p* = 0.0069. **(C)** Immunofluorescence staining was performed on HFL-1 cells were treated with 5 ng/mL TGF-β1 for 24 h to reveal the content of target antigens in the cells. Blue (DAPI) represents the nucleus, green represents the target antigen (α-SMA/Gremlin2). The control group (CTR) received the same treatment without TGF-β1 (the same experiment was performed using HFL-1). Scale bar = 20 μm. **(D)** Gremlin2 was overexpressed in HFL-1, the control group was transfected with empty-load pcDNA3.1, and TGF-β1 stimulation was performed. Immunofluorescence staining was used to detect the content of target antigens in the cells, with DAPI representing the nucleus and α-SMA representing the target antigen in green as an indicator of fibroblast activation. Scale bar = 20 μm. **(E)** Gremlin2 knockdown in MRC-5 cells using shGremlin2, the control group transfected with plko.1. Immunofluorescence staining showed DAPI in blue indicating the nucleus, Gremlin2 in green, and α-SMA in red. Scale bar = 20 μm. All the experiments have been repeated three times.

First, through the known databases GSE10667 and GSE99621, we found that the expression of Gremlin2 in the fibrotic lung tissue was significantly higher than that in the healthy tissue. Second, Gremlin2 mRNA and protein levels were high in IPF lung tissues and blood serum compared to healthy people. The data collected from the GEO database, including GSE10667 and GSE99621, are shown in **Figure 1**, while all the samples collected from patients primarily diagnosed with IPF or those who had a lung transplant due to interstitial pulmonary disease with fibrosis are shown in **Figure 2**. The GSE10667, the dataset contained data of samples collected after a biopsy or lung transplant from patients with IPF at the University of Pittsburgh Health Sciences Tissue Bank. The GSE99621 dataset contained the samples of healthy lung tissues from healthy controls and affected or unaffected lung tissues from patients with IPF. Because of the low incidence of IPF (2–60 cases per 100,000 persons per year) (Martinez et al., 2017), it was difficult to collect enough samples of lung tissue samples to meet the IPF diagnosis standard. As the focus of our research was Gremlin2 expression in myofibroblasts and fibroblasts around fibrotic lesions, which are pathological features of the fibrotic region, we collected the fibrotic lesion transplant samples not only from patients with IPF but also from those with other types of lung fibrosis. Therefore, we defined the collective tissue samples as pulmonary fibrosis (PF) samples. Third, when fibroblasts were treated with TGF-β1, Gremlin2 expression increased, which correlated with ECM production. When the expression of Gremlin2 was inhibited through shRNA knockdown, ECM production decreased. We verified the function of upregulating Gremlin2 in mice lung fibroblast in **Supplementary Figure S6**. The primary lung fibroblasts in bleomycin treatment mice lung showed the high capacity of migration and invasion shown in **Supplementary Figures S6A–D**. One hypothesis has emerged that links IPF and cancer due to their similar hallmark pathological alterations, such as aberrant myofibroblast proliferation and apoptosis and ECM invasion (Vancheri et al., 2010). Studies showed that cell invasion increases in IPF fibroblasts (Li et al., 2011). Moreover, IPF lung fibroblasts have an increased migratory capacity compared to healthy lung fibroblasts (Cai et al., 2010). We showed here that Gremlin2

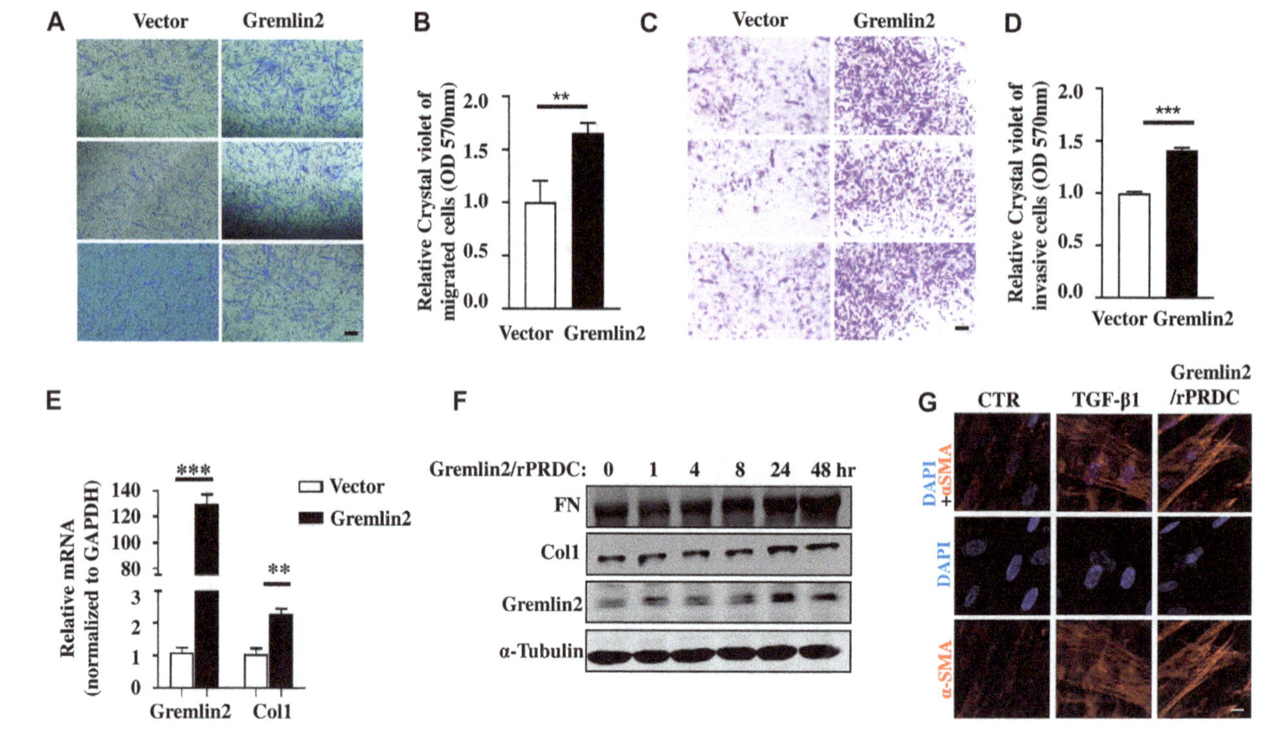

FIGURE 6 | Overexpression of Gremlin2 increases the migration and invasion of fibroblasts. **(A)** Transwell cell migration experiment after Gremlin2 overexpression in fibroblasts. The lower chamber was stained with crystal violet 24 h later, and three fields were randomly selected for imaging under 100× magnification. Scale bar = 100 μm. The experiment was repeated three times. **(B)** The value of OD570 after elution of crystal violet, normalized to that of the control group, $^{**}p = 0.072$. Unpaired student t test. **(C)** Transwell cell invasion experiment after 1:32 matrix glue was laid. After 48 h, crystal violet staining was carried out on the lower layer of the chamber. Scale bar = 100 μm. The experiment was repeated three times. **(D)** The value of OD570 after elution of crystal violet, normalized to that of the control group. $^{***}p < 0.001$. Unpaired student t test. **(E)** HFL-1 cells transfected with Gremlin2 expression plasmid for 24 h, and mRNA was extracted. Then, real-time quantitative PCR was performed to detect the corresponding mRNA expression levels. Using student's t-test, $^{***}p < 0.001$, $^{**}p < 0.01$. Scale bar = 100 μm. **(F)** Recombinant human PRDC (rPRDC)/GREM2 was added to HFL-1 cells for 0, 1, 4, 8, 24, and 48 h, then western blotting was performed to detect the expression of fibronectin, collagen1, and Gremlin2. **(G)** TGF-β1 or recombinant human PRDC (rPRDC)/GREM2 was added to HFL-1 cells for 48 h, then immunofluorescence was performed to detect the expression of α-SMA (Red). DAPI (Blue) shows the nucleus. Scale bar = 20μm. All the experiments have been repeated three times.

overexpression in lung fibroblasts increased the migration and invasion of them. Although we showed that Gremlin2 was upregulated in IPF lung tissues and myofibroblasts, but the role of Gremlin2 in alveolar type II cells was not investigated.

Co-labeling via immunofluorescence showed that Gremlin2 was expressed not only in myofibroblasts but also in the injured epithelial cells. Based on the results of **Figure 4A**, these α-SMA-negative cells expressing gremlin2 might have involved epithelial cells, shown in **Supplementary Figure S1**. We used E-Cadherin as an indicator of epithelial cells and co-localized it with Gremlin2 immunofluorescence staining in mice fibrosis lung tissue. **Supplementary Figure S1** showed epithelial cells could express Gremlin2. We selected different visual fields for analysis. **Supplementary Figure S1A** showed some epithelial cells expressed Gremlin2 with the white arrow pointing to the merge part. **Supplementary Figure S1B** was hardly any cell co-expressed Gremlin2 and E-Cadherin, indicating that there were other types of cells expressing Gremlin2 in the fibrotic area and not all epithelial can express Gremlin2. Overall, the epithelial cells, possibly the injured epithelial expressed Gremlin2, indicating that injured epithelial cells might play role in the process of fibrosis. This suggested that Gremlin2 might cause the process of pulmonary fibrosis through the migration and invasion of fibroblasts and epithelial injury repair. In this article, we focused on the function of Gremlin2 in fibroblasts; meanwhile, the role of Gremlin2 in epithelial injury repair should also be investigated.

Type II alveolar epithelial (AT-II) cells play a key role in the regulation of alveolar physiology (Zhang et al., 2012). Dysfunctional AEC2 should regenerate damaged cells, leading to insufficient repair ability. Persistent epithelial injury is a key mechanism of severe fibrosis in patients with IPF (Liang et al., 2016). Therefore, exploring the function of Gremlin2 in alveolar epithelial cells might reveal if Gremlin2 is involved in other aspects of fibrosis as well.

Here, we provided another hypothesis that injured epithelial cells expressing Gremlin2 might be another possible mechanism of IPF.

The TGF-β superfamily, which includes the BMP family, is an important regulator of fibrosis (Henderson et al., 2020). In bleomycin-induced lung fibrosis, TGF-β and BMP signaling follow an inverse course, with dynamic activation of TGF-β

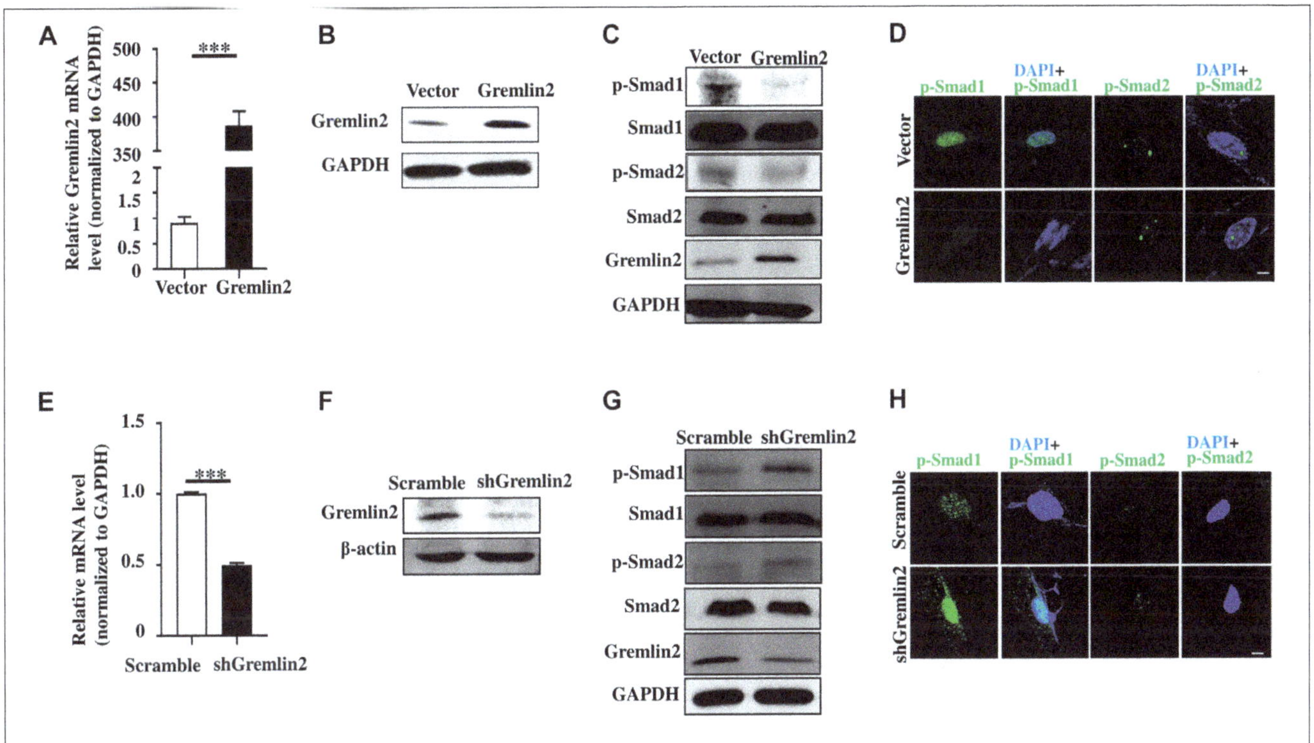

FIGURE 7 | Gremlin2 regulates fibroblast activation through the TGF-β/BMP signaling pathway. **(A)** The mRNA level of Gremlin2 after HFL-1 cells were transfected with Gremlin2 or empty-load plasmid for 24 h. **(B)** The expression level of Gremlin2 after HFL-1 were transfected with Gremlin2 or empty-load plasmid for 72 h detected using western blotting. **(C)** Detection of the p-Smad1 and p-Smad2 in the control group and fibroblasts overexpressing Gremlin2, Smad1 and Smad2 were used as the overall control group. **(D)** Expression level of p-Smad1 and p-Smad2 in the control group and fibroblasts overexpressing Gremlin2 using immunofluorescence. Green represents p-Smad1 and p-Smad2, and blue represents DAPI (nucleus). Scale bar = 5μm. **(E)** The mRNA expression of Gremlin2 after HFL-1 cells were treated with shRNA of Gremlin2 for 24 h, and the control group was infected with plko.1 no-load virus without the target gene, and the corresponding mRNA expression level was standardized to that of GAPDH. **(F)** Protein concentration in the cells was detected using western blotting with actin as the quantitative indicator protein and Gremlin2 as the target protein. **(G)** Expression level of p-Smad1 and p-Smad2 in the control group and the Gremlin2 knockdown HFL-1 cells with Smad1 and Smad2 as the overall control. **(H)** The expression of p-Smad1 and p-Smad2 in the control group and Gremlin2 knockdown fibroblasts, and the expression level of target antigen. Green represents p-Smad1 and p-Smad2 and blue represents DAPI (nucleus). Scale bar = 5 m. ***$p < 0.001$, Student's t test bilateral was used to analyze. Experiments were repeated three times.

signaling and repression of BMP signaling. Modulating the balance between BMP and TGF-β may be a therapeutic target in fibrotic lung disease (De Langhe et al., 2015). BMP-7 expression decreases in patients with IPF (Gu et al., 2014) and BMP-7 supplementation significantly reduces the hydroxyproline content in mice treated with aseptic materials (Myllärniemi et al., 2008a). Strong antagonists of the BMP family also include Gremlin1 and CHORD. Previous studies have shown that Pirfenidone can reduce the activity of fibroblasts induced by TGF-β, and the upregulation of BMP4/Gremlin1 can be detected (Jin et al., 2019), while Gremlin-1 regulates the recruitment of inflammatory cells and the production of anti-fibrosis chemokines in the lung (Koli et al., 2016).

However, we also recognized there are a few limitations to the current investigation. Studies showed that Fstl1 promoted TGF-β signaling and inhibits BMP signaling in epithelial cells, whereas in fibroblasts Fstl1 promotes TGF-β signaling without altering BMP signaling (Geng et al., 2011; Zheng et al., 2017). Therefore, further investigation into the mechanisms under which Gremlin2 regulates lung fibrosis could provide a novel target for the development of therapeutics for patients with pulmonary fibrosis. Gremlin2 is a secreted glycoprotein, meaning that it is not only expressed in a specific area but also can be detected in the bloodstream. As a development-related protein, it is highly expressed during embryonic development but its expression is low in adulthood. The high expression of it in adults might imply a severe disease state. We detected the concentration of Gremlin2 in the blood serum of healthy control samples, and the low expression verified that Gremlin2 low-expression was stable in the healthy control group. The increase in the expression of Gremlin2 can be easily detected via its increased secretion into the bloodstream. Moreover, compared to the golden criteria of a lung biopsy for IPF diagnosis, the detection of biomarkers in the blood serum is more convenient for patients. Less invasive techniques are more appliable in IPF screening at the early stage, therefore, biomarkers, such as Gremlin2, should be further investigated for their potential clinical application.

Besides, in mice model, we found that Gremlin2 showed an upregulated tendency after 2.5 units of bleomycin treatment with time going on. More interestingly, the concentration of Gremlin2 in BALF after 5 units of bleomycin treatment showed an exaggerated increase on day 7 shown in **Supplementary Figure S5A**. We tried to explore the origin by immunohistochemistry and cell immunofluorescence. By immunofluorescence co-staining CD11b and Gremlin2, we found a significant co-staining relationship between them showed in **Supplementary Figure S5B** in the 5 units bleomycin-treated 7 days group. But the control group treated with PBS showed no this phenomenon shown in **Supplementary Figure S5C**. Furthermore, we got the cells in BALF from the bleomycin-treated mouse group, the Giemsa staining showed a great amount of macrophage shown in **Supplementary Figure S5D**. Cell immunofluorescence co-staining CD11b and Gremlin2 also showed the great consistency shown in **Supplementary Figure S5E**. Besides, we constructed the one-day model treated by LPS for the acute inflammation model to explore the neutrophils would express Gremlin2 or not. The result showed in **Supplementary Figure S5F** may indicate the low expression of Gremlin2 in neutrophils. In all, we found the macrophage may contribute to the high expression of Gremlin2 in BALF of the 5-units bleomycin-treated group. Mice treated with 5 units of bleomycin began to die after 7 days showed high expression of Gremlin in BALF. Gremlin2 was first found as a development-related protein, the high expression of Gremlin2 in adulthood might indicate a severe disease condition. Our experiments have confirmed that fibroblasts can be activated by Gremlin2 to form myofibroblasts shown in **Figures 6F,G**, and a large amount of Gremlin2 production in early macrophages may contribute to the activation of fibroblasts and the progression of fibrosis.

We have constructed Gremlin2 knockout mice and will continue to explore the role of Gremlin2 in pulmonary fibrosis in future studies. Further, we have confirmed that Gremlin2 caused the increased invasive fibroblasts phenotypes, but more *in vivo* evidence is needed to verify that it affects mouse lung fibrosis through myofibroblasts. α-SMA-positive myofibroblasts or Col1a1-positive fibroblasts both originate from cells expressing Tbx4, can be applied as a general marker of fibroblasts (Xie et al., 2016). TBX4-creER, Gremlin2$^{flox/flox}$ mouse model would further verify the role of Gremlin2 in promoting fibrosis through mesenchymal cells.

ETHICS STATEMENT

The studies involving human participants were reviewed and approved by Clinical Trial Ethics Committee of the First Hospital of Zhejiang University. The patients/participants provided their written informed consent to participate in this study. The animal study was reviewed and approved by animal care and use committee of the Zhejiang University School of Medicine. Written informed consent was obtained from the owners for the participation of their animals in this study. Written informed consent was obtained from the individual(s) for the publication of any potentially identifiable images or data included in this article.

AUTHOR CONTRIBUTIONS

CH and WX co-wrote the manuscript. YL contributed to statistical work and rechecked the text composition. KR collected patient information and samples. YS, XZ, HC, and YK were occupied for logical comments of the article. WX accomplished all experimental design and operation. CH and JZ designed and directed the article.

SUPPLEMENTARY MATERIAL

Supplementary Figure S1 | Epithelial cells express Gremlin2. Immunofluorescence shows the co-localization of the epithelial cell marker E-Cadherin and Gremlin2 in the lungs of bleomycin-induced fibrosis mice. Gremlin2 (Green), and E-Cadherin (Red), DAPI (Blue), Yellow (Merge), scale bar = 20 μm. **(A)** The white arrow pointed to the co-labeled cells. **(B)** The high expression of Gremlin2 or E-Cadherin.

Supplementary Figure S2 | Gremlin2 expression at mRNA and protein levels and its levels in BALF of mice on day 0, 7, 14, 21 after bleomycin treatment. The relative concentration of Gremlin2 in the BALF, and its expression at mRNA and protein levels in the lung tissues of mice on **(A)** day 0 (CTR, $n = 5$; BLM, $n = 5$), **(B)** day 7 (CTR, $n = 5$; BLM, $n = 4$), **(C)** day 14 (CTR, $n = 5$; BLM, $n = 5$), **(D)** day 21 (BALF CTR, $n = 10$; BLM, $n = 10$, mRNA and protein levels CTR $n = 5$, BLM $n = 5$) after bleomycin (BLM) or PBS (CTR) treatment. Student's unpaired t-test.

Supplementary Figure S3 | Gremlin2 is overexpressed in HFL-1 cells. The control group was transfected with empty-load pcDNA3.1 with or without TGF-β1 treatment. Immunofluorescence staining was used to detect the content of target antigens in the cells, with DAPI representing the nucleus and α-SMA representing the target antigen in green as an indicator of fibroblast activation. Scale bar = 20 μm.

Supplementary Figure S4 | Gremlin2 activates fibroblasts through the BMP signaling pathway. Expression level of p-Smad1 and p-Smad2 in the control group and the Gremlin2-knockdown HFL-1 cells after 48 h of TGF-β1 treatment with Smad1 and Smad2, as the overall control.

Supplementary Figure S5 | Macrophages contribute to the high expression of Gremlin2 in BALF. **(A)** The relative concentration of Gremlin2 in BALF at day7 days after 5 units bleomycin (BLM) or PBS (CTR) treatment mice were sacrificed. CTR $n = 5$, BLM $n = 4$, student's unpaired t-test. $p = 0.0073$. **(B)** Gremlin2 (Green) and CD11b (Red) were co-stained by immunofluorescence of bleomycin **(a)** or PBS **(b)** treated mouse lungs. The right pictures are the enlargement of the white frame area in the left picture. White scale bar = 100 μm, yellow scale bar = 20 μm. **(C)** The Giemsa staining of cells from mice BALF. Black scale bar= 20μm. **(D)** Gremlin2 (Green) and CD11b (Red) were co-stained by immunofluorescence of cells in BALF from bleomycin treated mice. The right pictures are the enlargement of the white frame area in the left picture. White scale bar = 40 μm, yellow scale bar = 10 μm. **(E)** Gremlin2 (Green) and CD11b (Red) were co-stained by immunofluorescence of cells in BALF from one-day LPS treated mice. The right pictures are the enlargement of the white frame area in the left picture. White scale bar = 40 μm, yellow scale bar = 10 μm.

Supplementary Figure S6 | *p*-Smad1 is upregulated in activated mice lung fibroblasts after bleomycin treatment. **(A)** Transwell cell migration experiment of mice lung fibroblasts after PBS or bleomycin treatment. The lower chamber was stained with crystal violet 24 h later, and three fields were randomly selected for imaging under 100x magnification. Scale bar =100 μm. CTR $n = 2$, BLM $n = 2$. **(B)** The value of OD570 after elution of crystal violet, normalized to that of the control group, $^{**}p = 0.001$. Unpaired student t test. **(C)** Transwell cell invasion experiment of mice lung fibroblasts after PBS or bleomycin treatment. The lower chamber was stained with crystal violet 24 h later, and three fields were randomly selected for imaging under 100x magnification. Scale bar = 100 μm. CTR $n = 2$, BLM $n = 2$. **(D)** The value of OD570 after elution of crystal violet, normalized to that of the control group, $^{***}p < 0.001$. Unpaired student t test. **(E)** Detection of the p-Smad1 and p-Smad2 in the fibroblasts from PBS or bleomycin treatment group, Smad1 and Smad2 were used as the overall control group. CTR $n = 3$, BLM $n = 3$. Paired student t test was used, $p = 0.0011$. **(F)** Expression level of p-Smad1 in the fibroblasts from PBS or bleomycin treatment group using immunofluorescence. Green represents p-Smad1 and p-Smad2, and blue represents DAPI (nucleus). Scale bar = 10 μm. CTR $n = 3$, BLM $n = 5$. Scale bar = 10 μm. **(G)** Expression level of p-Smad2 in the fibroblasts from PBS or bleomycin treatment group using immunofluorescence. Green represents p-Smad1 and p-Smad2, and blue represents DAPI (nucleus). Scale bar = 10 μm. CTR $n = 3$, BLM $n = 5$. Scale bar = 10 μm. CTR presented as PBS treatment group, BLM presented as the bleomycin treatment group.

REFERENCES

Ahluwalia, N., Grasberger, P. E., Mugo, B. M., Feghali-Bostwick, C., Pardo, A., Selman, M., et al. (2016). Fibrogenic Lung Injury Induces Non-cell-autonomous Fibroblast Invasion. *Am. J. Respir. Cel Mol Biol.* 54, 831–842. doi:10.1165/rcmb.2015-0040OC

Andersson-Sjöland, A., de Alba, C. G., Nihlberg, K., Becerril, C., Ramírez, R., Pardo, A., et al. (2008). Fibrocytes Are a Potential Source of Lung Fibroblasts in Idiopathic Pulmonary Fibrosis. *Int. J. Biochem. Cel Biol.* 40, 2129–2140. doi:10.1016/j.biocel.2008.02.012

ATS/ERS (2000). American Thoracic Society. Idiopathic Pulmonary Fibrosis: Diagnosis and Treatment. International Consensus Statement. American Thoracic Society (ATS), and the European Respiratory Society (ERS). *Am. J. Respir. Crit. Care Med.* 161, 646–664. doi:10.1164/ajrccm.161.2.ats3-00

Bagnato, G., and Harari, S. (2015). Cellular Interactions in the Pathogenesis of Interstitial Lung Diseases. *Eur. Respir. Rev.* 24, 102–114. doi:10.1183/09059180.00003214

Bonniaud, P., Kolb, M., Galt, T., Robertson, J., Robbins, C., Stampfli, M., et al. (2004). Smad3 Null Mice Develop Airspace Enlargement and Are Resistant to TGF-β-Mediated Pulmonary Fibrosis. *J. Immunol.* 173, 2099–2108. doi:10.4049/jimmunol.173.3.2099

Bonniaud, P., Margetts, P. J., Kolb, M., Schroeder, J. A., Kapoun, A. M., Damm, D., et al. (2005). Progressive Transforming Growth Factor β1-induced Lung Fibrosis Is Blocked by an Orally Active ALK5 Kinase Inhibitor. *Am. J. Respir. Crit. Care Med.* 171, 889–898. doi:10.1164/rccm.200405-612OC

Cai, G.-q., Zheng, A., Tang, Q., White, E. S., Chou, C.-F., Gladson, C. L., et al. (2010). Downregulation of FAK-Related Non-kinase Mediates the Migratory Phenotype of Human Fibrotic Lung Fibroblasts. *Exp. Cel Res.* 316, 1600–1609. doi:10.1016/j.yexcr.2010.01.021

Chanda, D., Otoupalova, E., Smith, S. R., Volckaert, T., De Langhe, S. P., and Thannickal, V. J. (2019). Developmental Pathways in the Pathogenesis of Lung Fibrosis. *Mol. Aspects Med.* 65, 56–69. doi:10.1016/j.mam.2018.08.004

Chen, H., Qu, J., Huang, X., Kurundkar, A., Zhu, L., Yang, N., et al. (2016). Mechanosensing by the α6-integrin Confers an Invasive Fibroblast Phenotype and Mediates Lung Fibrosis. *Nat. Commun.* 7, 12564. doi:10.1038/ncomms12564

Church, R. H., Ali, I., Tate, M., Lavin, D., Krishnakumar, A., Kok, H. M., et al. (2017). Gremlin1 Plays a Key Role in Kidney Development and Renal Fibrosis. *Am. J. Physiology-Renal Physiol.* 312, F1141–f1157. doi:10.1152/ajprenal.00344.2016

De Langhe, E., Cailotto, F., De Vooght, V., Aznar-Lopez, C., Vanoirbeek, J. A., Luyten, F. P., et al. (2015). Enhanced Endogenous Bone Morphogenetic Protein Signaling Protects against Bleomycin Induced Pulmonary Fibrosis. *Respir. Res.* 16, 38. doi:10.1186/s12931-015-0202-x

Dong, Y., Geng, Y., Li, L., Li, X., Yan, X., Fang, Y., et al. (2015). Blocking Follistatin-like 1 Attenuates Bleomycin-Induced Pulmonary Fibrosis in Mice. *J. Exp. Med.* 212, 235–252. doi:10.1084/jem.20121878

Fernandez, I. E., and Eickelberg, O. (2012). New Cellular and Molecular Mechanisms of Lung Injury and Fibrosis in Idiopathic Pulmonary Fibrosis. *The Lancet* 380, 680–688. doi:10.1016/s0140-6736(12)61144-1

Geng, Y., Dong, Y., Yu, M., Zhang, L., Yan, X., Sun, J., et al. (2011). Follistatin-like 1 (Fstl1) Is a Bone Morphogenetic Protein (BMP) 4 Signaling Antagonist in Controlling Mouse Lung Development. *Proc. Natl. Acad. Sci.* 108, 7058–7063. doi:10.1073/pnas.1007293108

Gu, P., Luo, B., Yi, X., Zhu, H., Li, S., Yu, X., et al. (2014). The Expressions and Meanings of BMP-7 and TGF-β in Idiopathic Pulmonary Fibrosis and Idiopathic Nonspecific Interstitial Pneumonia. *Zhonghua Jie He He Hu Xi Za Zhi* 37, 664–670.

Henderson, N. C., Rieder, F., and Wynn, T. A. (2020). Fibrosis: from Mechanisms to Medicines. *Nature* 587, 555–566. doi:10.1038/s41586-020-2938-9

Hinck, A. P., and Huang, T. (2013). TGF-β Antagonists: Same Knot, but Different Hold. *Structure* 21, 1269–1270. doi:10.1016/j.str.2013.07.015

Hinz, B., Phan, S. H., Thannickal, V. J., Galli, A., Bochaton-Piallat, M.-L., and Gabbiani, G. (2007). The Myofibroblast. *Am. J. Pathol.* 170, 1807–1816. doi:10.2353/ajpath.2007.070112

Hsia, L.-t., Ashley, N., Ouaret, D., Wang, L. M., Wilding, J., and Bodmer, W. F. (2016). Myofibroblasts Are Distinguished from Activated Skin Fibroblasts by the Expression of AOC3 and Other Associated Markers. *Proc. Natl. Acad. Sci. USA.* 113, E2162–E2171. doi:10.1073/pnas.1603534113

Hsu, D. R., Economides, A. N., Wang, X., Eimon, P. M., and Harland, R. M. (1998). The Xenopus Dorsalizing Factor Gremlin Identifies a Novel Family of Secreted Proteins that Antagonize BMP Activities. *Mol. Cel.* 1, 673–683. doi:10.1016/s1097-2765(00)80067-2

Huan, C., Yang, T., Liang, J., Xie, T., Cheng, L., Liu, N., et al. (2015). Methylation-mediated BMPER Expression in Fibroblast Activation *In Vitro* and Lung Fibrosis in Mice *In Vivo*. *Sci. Rep.* 5, 14910. doi:10.1038/srep14910

Jin, J., Togo, S., Kadoya, K., Tulafu, M., Namba, Y., Iwai, M., et al. (2019). Pirfenidone Attenuates Lung Fibrotic Fibroblast Responses to Transforming Growth Factor-B1. *Respir. Res.* 20, 119. doi:10.1186/s12931-019-1093-z

Kang, H.-R., Cho, S. J., Lee, C. G., Homer, R. J., and Elias, J. A. (2007). Transforming Growth Factor (TGF)-β1 Stimulates Pulmonary Fibrosis and Inflammation via a Bax-dependent, Bid-Activated Pathway that Involves Matrix Metalloproteinase-12. *J. Biol. Chem.* 282, 7723–7732. doi:10.1074/jbc.M610764200

Katoh, M., and Katoh, M. (2004). Identification and Characterization of Human CKTSF1B2 and CKTSF1B3 Genes In Silico. *Oncol. Rep.* 12, 423–427.

Kattamuri, C., Luedeke, D. M., Nolan, K., Rankin, S. A., Greis, K. D., Zorn, A. M., et al. (2012). Members of the DAN Family Are BMP Antagonists that Form Highly Stable Noncovalent Dimers. *J. Mol. Biol.* 424, 313–327. doi:10.1016/j.jmb.2012.10.003

Kattamuri, C., Nolan, K., and Thompson, T. B. (2017). Correction: Analysis and Identification of the Grem2 Heparin/heparan Sulfate-Binding Motif. *Biochem. J.* 474, 1529. doi:10.1042/bcj-2016-1050_cor

King, T. E., Jr., Pardo, A., and Selman, M. (2011). Idiopathic Pulmonary Fibrosis. *The Lancet* 378, 1949–1961. doi:10.1016/s0140-6736(11)60052-4

Koli, K., Sutinen, E., Rönty, M., Rantakari, P., Fortino, V., Pulkkinen, V., et al. (2016). Gremlin-1 Overexpression in Mouse Lung Reduces Silica-Induced Lymphocyte Recruitment - A Link to Idiopathic Pulmonary Fibrosis through Negative Correlation with CXCL10 Chemokine. *PLoS One* 11, e0159010. doi:10.1371/journal.pone.0159010

Li, S., Wang, L., Zhao, Q., Liu, Y., He, L., Xu, Q., et al. (2014). SHP2 Positively Regulates TGFβ1-Induced Epithelial-Mesenchymal Transition Modulated by its Novel Interacting Protein Hook1*. *J. Biol. Chem.* 289, 34152–34160. doi:10.1074/jbc.M113.546077

Li, X., Yang, L., Sun, X., Wu, J., Li, Y., Zhang, Q., et al. (2017). The Role of TGFβ-HGF-Smad4 axis in Regulating the Proliferation of Mouse Airway Progenitor Cells. *Mol. Med. Rep.* 16, 8155–8163. doi:10.3892/mmr.2017.7636

Li, Y., Jiang, D., Liang, J., Meltzer, E. B., Gray, A., Miura, R., et al. (2011). Severe Lung Fibrosis Requires an Invasive Fibroblast Phenotype Regulated by Hyaluronan and CD44. *J. Exp. Med.* 208, 1459–1471. doi:10.1084/jem.20102510

Liang, J., Zhang, Y., Xie, T., Liu, N., Chen, H., Geng, Y., et al. (2016). Hyaluronan and TLR4 Promote Surfactant-Protein-C-Positive Alveolar Progenitor Cell Renewal and Prevent Severe Pulmonary Fibrosis in Mice. *Nat. Med.* 22, 1285–1293. doi:10.1038/nm.4192

Lovgren, A. K., Kovacs, J. J., Xie, T., Potts, E. N., Li, Y., Foster, W. M., et al. (2011). -Arrestin Deficiency Protects against Pulmonary Fibrosis in Mice and Prevents Fibroblast Invasion of Extracellular Matrix. *Sci. Translational Med.* 3, 74ra23. doi:10.1126/scitranslmed.3001564

Martinez, F. J., Collard, H. R., Pardo, A., Raghu, G., Richeldi, L., Selman, M., et al. (2017). Idiopathic Pulmonary Fibrosis. *Nat. Rev. Dis. Primers* 3, 17074. doi:10.1038/nrdp.2017.74

Martinez, F. J., Safrin, S., Weycker, D., Starko, K. M., Bradford, W. Z., King, T. E., Jr., et al. (2005). The Clinical Course of Patients with Idiopathic Pulmonary Fibrosis. *Ann. Intern. Med.* 142, 963–967. doi:10.7326/0003-4819-142-12_part_1-200506210-00005

Meng, X.-m., Nikolic-Paterson, D. J., and Lan, H. Y. (2016). TGF-β: the Master Regulator of Fibrosis. *Nat. Rev. Nephrol.* 12, 325–338. doi:10.1038/nrneph.2016.48

Mezzano, S., Droguett, A., Lavoz, C., Krall, P., Egido, J., and Ruiz-Ortega, M. (2018). Gremlin and Renal Diseases: Ready to Jump the Fence to Clinical Utility? *Nephrol. Dial. Transpl.* 33, 735–741. doi:10.1093/ndt/gfx194

Myllärniemi, M., Lindholm, P., Ryynänen, M. J., Kliment, C. R., Salmenkivi, K., Keski-Oja, J., et al. (2008a). Gremlin-mediated Decrease in Bone Morphogenetic Protein Signaling Promotes Pulmonary Fibrosis. *Am. J. Respir. Crit. Care Med.* 177, 321 329. doi:10.1164/rccm.200706-945OC

Myllärniemi, M., Vuorinen, K., Pulkkinen, V., Kankaanranta, H., Aine, T., Salmenkivi, K., et al. (2008b). Gremlin Localization and Expression Levels Partially Differentiate Idiopathic Interstitial Pneumonia Severity and Subtype. *J. Pathol.* 214, 456–463. doi:10.1002/path.2300

Ng, B., Dong, J., D'Agostino, G., Viswanathan, S., Widjaja, A. A., Lim, W.-W., et al. (2019). Interleukin-11 Is a Therapeutic Target in Idiopathic Pulmonary Fibrosis. *Sci. Transl. Med.* 11, eaaw1237. doi:10.1126/scitranslmed.aaw1237

Noble, P. W., Barkauskas, C. E., and Jiang, D. (2012). Pulmonary Fibrosis: Patterns and Perpetrators. *J. Clin. Invest.* 122, 2756–2762. doi:10.1172/jci60323

Nolan, K., Kattamuri, C., Luedeke, D. M., Deng, X., Jagpal, A., Zhang, F., et al. (2013). Structure of Protein Related to Dan and Cerberus: Insights into the Mechanism of Bone Morphogenetic Protein Antagonism. *Structure* 21, 1417–1429. doi:10.1016/j.str.2013.06.005

Nolan, K., Kattamuri, C., Rankin, S. A., Read, R. J., Zorn, A. M., and Thompson, T. B. (2016). Structure of Gremlin-2 in Complex with GDF5 Gives Insight into DAN-Family-Mediated BMP Antagonism. *Cel Rep.* 16, 2077–2086. doi:10.1016/j.celrep.2016.07.046

Raghu, G., Collard, H. R., Egan, J. J., Martinez, F. J., Behr, J., Brown, K. K., et al. (2011). An Official ATS/ERS/JRS/ALAT Statement: Idiopathic Pulmonary Fibrosis: Evidence-Based Guidelines for Diagnosis and Management. *Am. J. Respir. Crit. Care Med.* 183, 788–824. doi:10.1164/rccm.2009-040GL

Ran, A., Guan, L., Wang, J., and Wang, Y. (2019). GREM2 Maintains Stem Cell-like Phenotypes in Gastric Cancer Cells by Regulating the JNK Signaling Pathway. *Cell Cycle* 18, 2414–2431. doi:10.1080/15384101.2019.1646561

Sanders, L. N., Schoenhard, J. A., Saleh, M. A., Mukherjee, A., Ryzhov, S., McMaster, W. G., Jr., et al. (2016). BMP Antagonist Gremlin 2 Limits Inflammation after Myocardial Infarction. *Circ. Res.* 119, 434–449. doi:10.1161/circresaha.116.308700

Stanley, E., Biben, C., Kotecha, S., Fabri, L., Tajbakhsh, S., Wang, C.-C., et al. (1998). DAN Is a Secreted Glycoprotein Related to Xenopus Cerberus. *Mech. Develop.* 77, 173–184. doi:10.1016/s0925-4773(98)00139-7

Tashiro, J., Rubio, G. A., Limper, A. H., Williams, K., Elliot, S. J., Ninou, I., et al. (2017). Exploring Animal Models that Resemble Idiopathic Pulmonary Fibrosis. *Front. Med.* 4, 118. doi:10.3389/fmed.2017.00118

Vancheri, C., Failla, M., Crimi, N., and Raghu, G. (2010). Idiopathic Pulmonary Fibrosis: a Disease with Similarities and Links to Cancer Biology. *Eur. Respir. J.* 35, 496–504. doi:10.1183/09031936.00077309

Waters, D. W., Blokland, K. E. C., Pathinayake, P. S., Burgess, J. K., Mutsaers, S. E., Prele, C. M., et al. (2018). Fibroblast Senescence in the Pathology of Idiopathic Pulmonary Fibrosis. *Am. J. Physiology-Lung Cell Mol. Physiol.* 315, L162–l172. doi:10.1152/ajplung.00037.2018

Wen, H., Kumar, V., Mishra, A., Song, S., Aslam, R., Hussain, A., et al. (2019). Grem2 Mediates Podocyte Apoptosis in High Glucose Milieu. *Biochimie* 160, 113–121. doi:10.1016/j.biochi.2019.02.015

Wolters, P. J., Collard, H. R., and Jones, K. D. (2014). Pathogenesis of Idiopathic Pulmonary Fibrosis. *Annu. Rev. Pathol. Mech. Dis.* 9, 157–179. doi:10.1146/annurev-pathol-012513-104706

Woodcock, H. V., Eley, J. D., Guillotin, D., Platé, M., Nanthakumar, C. B., Martufi, M., et al. (2019). The mTORC1/4E-BP1 axis Represents a Critical Signaling Node during Fibrogenesis. *Nat. Commun.* 10, 6. doi:10.1038/s41467-018-07858-8

Xie, T., Liang, J., Liu, N., Huan, C., Zhang, Y., Liu, W., et al. (2016). Transcription Factor TBX4 Regulates Myofibroblast Accumulation and Lung Fibrosis. *J. Clin. Invest.* 126, 3063–3079. doi:10.1172/jci85328

Xie, T., Wang, Y., Deng, N., Huang, G., Taghavifar, F., Geng, Y., et al. (2018). Single-Cell Deconvolution of Fibroblast Heterogeneity in Mouse Pulmonary Fibrosis. *Cel Rep.* 22, 3625–3640. doi:10.1016/j.celrep.2018.03.010

Zhang, X., Zhang, Y., Tao, B., Teng, L., Li, Y., Cao, R., et al. (2012). Loss of Shp2 in Alveoli Epithelia Induces Deregulated Surfactant Homeostasis, Resulting in Spontaneous Pulmonary Fibrosis. *FASEB j.* 26, 2338–2350. doi:10.1096/fj.11-200139

Zheng, X., Qi, C., Zhang, S., Fang, Y., and Ning, W. (2017). TGF-β1 Induces Fstl1 via the Smad3-C-Jun Pathway in Lung Fibroblasts. *Am. J. Physiology-Lung Cell Mol. Physiol.* 313, L240–l251. doi:10.1152/ajplung.00523.2016

3

The Potential Role of Extracellular Vesicles in COVID-19 Treatment: Opportunity and Challenge

Yan-yan Yan[1†], Wen-min Zhou[2†], Yu-qing Wang[2†], Qiao-ru Guo[2,3], Fu-xi Zhao[1], Zhuang-yan Zhu[1], Yan-xia Xing[1], Hai-yan Zhang[1], Mohamad Aljofan[4], Alireza Mosavi Jarrahi[5], Bolat Makabel[3] and Jian-ye Zhang[2]**

[1]School of Medicine, Shanxi Datong University, Datong, China, [2]Key Laboratory of Molecular Target and Clinical Pharmacology and the State Key Laboratory of Respiratory Disease, School of Pharmaceutical Sciences and the Fifth Affiliated Hospital, Guangzhou Medical University, Guangzhou, China, [3]Xinjiang Institute of Materia Medica, Urumqi, China, [4]Department of Biomedical Sciences, School of Medicine, Nazarbayev University, Nur-Sultan, Kazakhstan, [5]School of Medicine, Shahid Beheshti University of Medical Sciences, Tehran, Iran

***Correspondence:**
Bolat Makabel
kzkt@163.com
Jian-ye Zhang
jianyez@163.com

†These authors have contributed equally to this work and share first authorship.

SARS-CoV-2 infection has become an urgent public health concern worldwide, severely affecting our society and economy due to the long incubation time and high prevalence. People spare no effort on the rapid development of vaccine and treatment all over the world. Amongst the numerous ways of tackling this pandemic, some approaches using extracellular vesicles (EVs) are emerging. In this review, we summarize current prevalence and pathogenesis of COVID-19, involving the combination of SARS-CoV-2 and virus receptor ACE2, endothelial dysfunction and micro thrombosis, together with cytokine storm. We also discuss the ongoing EVs-based strategies for the treatment of COVID-19, including mesenchymal stem cell (MSC)-EVs, drug-EVs, vaccine-EVs, platelet-EVs, and others. This manuscript provides the foundation for the development of targeted drugs and vaccines for SARS-CoV-2 infections.

Keywords: COVID-19, SARS-CoV-2, extracellular vesicles (EVs), mesenchymal stem cell (MSC), immunomodulation, ACE2

OVERVIEW OF COVID-19

Current Prevalence of COVID-19

COVID-19, named Coronavirus Infectious Disease 2019 by the World Health Organization (Zhou, et al., 2020a; Zhu, et al., 2020), is an infectious disease caused by the severe acute respiratory syndrome coronavirus type 2 (SARS-CoV-2), which was first reported in Wuhan, China, in December 2019. COVID-19 infection is now a pressing global public health problem. As of today, 23 March 2021, more than 124 million people have been infected with SARS-CoV-2 and more than 2.7 million have died. In addition to having an unprecedented impact on global health care systems, COVID-19 has profound socioeconomic consequences (Nicola, et al., 2020).

Clinically, COVID-19 mainly affects the lungs. Although the majority of COVID-19 victims may show asymptomatic or mild symptoms, interstitial pneumonia (IP) and acute respiratory distress syndrome (ARDS) requiring mechanical ventilation in the intensive care units can occur in approximately 15% of cases (Cascella, et al., 2021), especially in the elderly and individuals with underlying diseases. COVID-19 also has systemic manifestations, affecting multiple organ systems containing cardiovascular, gastrointestinal, hematopoietic, renal, and immune systems (Yi, et al., 2020). In severe cases, COVID-19 can lead to severe cytokine storm or cytokine release syndrome (CRS) (Cascella, Rajnik, 2021), sepsis, multiple organ failure and even death.

SARS-CoV-2 is by far the seventh human coronavirus discovered to date. Four viruses (HCoV-NL63, HCoV-229E, HCoV-OC43, and HKU1) persist in human population and cause mild common cold symptoms (Fung,and Liu, 2019). The other two are similar to SARS-CoV-2, named SARS-CoV and Middle East Respiratory Syndrome (MERS)-CoV, and both of them lead to acute respiratory disease (Cui, et al., 2019). SARS-CoV-2 is a spherical or pleomorphic enveloped virus particle with a typical diameter range of 80–120 nm. This virus contains a 30 kB positive single-stranded RNA which surrounded by a membrane embedded with a variety of viral proteins, especially the Spike (S) protein (Mousavizadeh, and Ghasemi, 2020). Studies shown that the Spike protein in SARS-CoV-2 shared a high degree of structural homology with that in SARS-CoV (Li, et al., 2005; Xu, et al., 2020b). SARS-CoV-2 virus infect into human cells by recognizing the angiotensin converting enzyme 2 (ACE2) receptor of host cells. A recent study by Wan et al. reported that SARS-CoV-2 had a stronger binding ability with ACE2 than with SARS-CoV, promoting the infection and transmission capacity of the virus (Wan, et al., 2020).

Pathogenesis of COVID-19

ACE2 Plays a Key Role in SARS-CoV-2 Invasion

In 2020, using cryopreserved electron microscopy, Zhou Qiang Laboratory of Westlake University successfully analyzed the full-length structure of ACE2 (Yan, et al., 2020), the receptor protein of SARS-CoV-2. This is the first time of the world that the full-length structure of ACE2 has been resolved. As SARS-CoV-2 invades the body, ACE2 acts like a "doorknob," the virus grabs it and opens the door to the recipient cells. In addition, interestingly, it has recently been demonstrated that transmembrane protease serine 2 (TMPRSS2) incises the Spike protein during the internalization of SARS-CoV-2 which fuses with host cell membrane (Scheller, et al., 2019). This process is necessary for SARS-CoV-2 to enter into recipient cells (Devaux, et al., 2020). After fusing with the human cell membrane, the virus genome enters into the recipient/host cell. The virus then begins to replicate, mature and leave the host cells to infect new healthy cells. SARS-CoV-2 enters the respiratory system from the upper respiratory tract and eventually infects alveolar cells, causing angiectasis of alveolar cells, increased capillary permeability, decreased pulmonary surface active substances with infiltration of lymphocytes and monocytes. As ACE2 and TMPRSS2 are abundant in type II alveolar and endothelial cells (Hamming, et al., 2004), pulmonary vessels are susceptible to SARS-CoV-2-induced inflammation and injury (Zhao, et al., 2020). Other than the respiratory tract, SARS-CoV-2 infection can cause parts of the body damage, such as the cardiovascular system. Therefore, COVID-19 patients may present with severe forms of myocarditis and endocarditis besides respiratory dysfunction (Guzik, et al., 2020).

ACE2 is located in various types of epithelial cells (lung, kidney, heart, intestinal) and endothelial cells. In recent years, studies have shown that ACE2 played roles in the cardiovascular, renal and respiratory system, and was associated with hypertension and diabetes. ACE2 has a protective effect on a variety of lung diseases, such as acute lung injury, asthma, ARDS, pulmonary hypertension and chronic obstructive pulmonary disease (Jia, 2016). More importantly, ACE2 was identified as a SARS-CoV and SARS-CoV-2 receptor, which played a protective role in the pathogenesis of SARS and COVID-19. As the first homolog of ACE, ACE2 regulates the renin angiotensin system (RAS) by balancing the ACE activity. The binding complex of Spike protein with ACE2 can induce the cell membrane ACE2 down-regulation (Glowacka, et al., 2010), contributing to the imbalance of ACE and ACE2 activity, and therefore leading to acute lung injury (Zhang, et al., 2020a).

COVID-19 Is Associated With Endothelial Dysfunction and Micro-thrombosis

Patients with COVID-19 have a high incidence of thrombotic events (Berger, et al., 2020). About the mechanism of thrombosis in COVID-19, there are a lot of speculations, such as coagulation and platelet activation, endothelial cell activation, inflammation and complement system activation, etc (Mackman, et al., 2020). Varga and colleagues demonstrated that SARS-CoV-2 presented in the endothelial cells of various human organs (Varga, et al., 2020). In addition, evidence of alveolar capillary micro-thrombosis and endothelial injury associated with intracellular viruses has been noted in autopsy analyses of infected lungs (Ackermann, et al., 2020). Due to ACE2 show high-expression in vascular endothelial cells, viral infection of the circulatory system directly leads to excessive coagulation in COVID-19 patients (Varga, Flammer, 2020). In addition, the number of peripheral blood mononuclear cells decreased significantly in patients with respiratory failure 7–14 days after the onset of SARS-CoV-2 infection (Yi, Lagniton, 2020). High level of D-dimer was found to presence for the moment, which was associated with severe hypercoagulation and indicated a poor prognosis (Yi, Lagniton, 2020). As a major activator of the coagulation cascade (Grover, and Mackman, 2018), several studies have speculated that the induction of tissue factor (TF) might play an important role in the COVID-19-related thrombosis (Bautista-Vargas, et al., 2020; Grover and Mackman, 2018; Mackman, Antoniak, 2020). Axel Rosell et al. developed a method to determine the activity of TF in plasma EVs in 100 patients with moderate to severe COVID-19. The results showed that the level of EVs-TF activity was significantly higher in COVID-19 patients than in the normal individuals. In addition, the level of EVs-TF activity was associated with disease severity, mortality, and several plasma markers, including D-dimer. These findings suggest that SARS-CoV-2 infection induces the release of TF-positive EVs into the circulation, and possibly cause thrombosis in patients infected with COVID-19 (Rosell, et al., 2020).

Cytokine Storm: Immune Response to SARS-CoV-2 Is a Major Driving Force of Disease Severity

Because SARS-CoV-2 entry into cells depend on binding to its receptor, ACE2, the RAS and various inflammatory cascades are connected with the pathobiology of COVID-19 (Bourgonje, et al., 2020). The SARS-CoV-2 can also activate the innate and adaptive immune response in patients with COVID-19 (Yang, et al., 2020a). The immune effector cells release a large amount of proinflammatory cytokines and chemokines (Tukmechi, et al., 2014), such as tumor necrosis factor (TNF), interleukin 1 (IL-1), interleukin 6 (IL-6), interleukin 7 (IL-7) and granulocyte colony stimulating factor (Pedersen and Ho, 2020), inducing an uncontrolled CRS, and leading to various clinical manifestations, such as high fever, hepatosplenomegaly, cytopenia, central nervous system abnormalities, hypoalbuminaemia and capillary leakage (England, et al., 2021; Gao, et al., 2021). A previously published study showed that identifying circulating protein biomarkers in COVID-19 patients used an ultra-high-throughput serum and plasma proteomics technology (Messner, et al., 2020). Recently, Balaji Krishnamachary et al. indicated that EVs from patients affected by the SARS-CoV-2 might alter the pro-inflammatory response, blood coagulation disorders, and endothelium damage. They found that EVs of serious cases of COVID-19 carried higher levels of cytokines, including the IL-6 family, TNF superfamily, chemokines (MCP-1 and CXCL16), and proteases and peptidases (Cathepsin L1), compared with that of patients with moderate COVID-19 or asymptomatic individuals (Krishnamachary, et al., 2020). Therefore, the use of appropriate immunosuppressive and immunomodulatory agents to address the potential inflammatory complications of COVID-19 is currently being explored, which might improve clinical outcomes and ultimately reduce COVID-19 mortality (Stebbing, et al., 2020). Because ACE2 receptors are widely distributed in human alveolar type II cells and capillary endothelial cells (Hamming, Timens, 2004), the lungs are exceptionally sensitive to SARS-CoV-2 infection. In fact, recently published researches have shown that a substantial portion of the lungs were impacted by this disease, leading to an extensive damage that could subsequently result in permanent change of lung function. A recent MRI study in a 59-year-old man who diagnosed with COVID-19, suggested that this disease was not restricted to any specific area in the lung, but spread to the entire lung. In fact, this symptom is not composed directly arouse the SARS-CoV-2 virus, but a host immune response that causes a resistless cytokine storm in lungs. Overexpression of cytokines such as the interleukin family (IL-2, IL-6, IL-7), GSCF, IP10, MCP1, MIP1A, and TNF-α leads to edema and impairs oxygen exchange, which may lead to ARDS with potential acute cardiac injury, secondary infection and death (Huang, et al., 2020a).

EVS ARE THE PROMISING NEW THERAPEUTIC MEANS OF COVID-19

There is currently no specific therapeutic for COVID-19. Conventional treatment includes infection prevention, supportive care that invloving supplement of oxygen and mechanical ventilation support (Grasselli, et al., 2020; Marini, and Gattinoni., 2020). Currently, drugs against COVID-19 are evaluated worldwide, including antiviral drugs, anti-malarial drugs and anti-inflammatory drugs, such as radecivir (Beigel, et al., 2020), chloroquine (Zhou, et al., 2020b) and hydroxychloroquine (HCQ) (Soy, et al., 2020), anthropoized anti-IL-6 receptor antibody tocilizumab (Perrone, et al., 2020; Toniati, et al., 2020; Xu, et al., 2020c), recombinant human IL-1 receptor antagonist Anakinra (Cavalli, et al., 2020; Huet, et al., 2020), etc. Although these treatment strategies improved patient recovery and survival, they do not definitively restore lung damage caused by the virus. In addition, a range of anti-inflammatory drugs have been tested to inhibit the cytokine storm and multiple organ failure caused by the worsening immune response in severe patients, but the effect has not been significant. In recent years, increasing researches reported that the role of EVs in the treatment of inflammation (Lasser, et al., 2016; Martinez-Bravo, et al., 2017), injury (Lanyu, and Feilong, 2019), and lung and respiratory viral infection (Scheller, Herold, 2019; van Dongen, et al., 2016; Yoshikawa, et al., 2019). It was reported that EVs promoted the pathogenesis of diseases such as in infectious diseases and cancers (Fleming, et al., 2014; Han, et al., 2019). The interesting interaction between EVs and the virus provides a new perspective on the treatment of COVID-19 (Dogrammatzis, et al., 2020). Viral infection may affect the exosomal-loading mechanisms of the host cells, resulting in changes in protein and nucleic acid content of EVs. It means the infected cells release modified EVs, not rely on virus contents. Therefore, compared with EVs without infected cells, these modified EVs may modulate the host immune response. Besides, EVs may act as a negatively regulatory element in the transmission of viral infection, and induce the immune system to respond to the virus. There are three types of EVs, including exosomes (20–150 nm), microvesicles (MVs) (100–1,000 nm in diameter), and apoptotic vesicles (1,000–5,000 nm) (Maione, et al., 2020; Raposo and Stoorvogel, 2013). EVs, as a carrier for cell-to-cell transfer of biomolecules, is an important mode of cell-to-cell communication (Huang, et al., 2020b). EVs are present in a variety of biological fluids, such as blood, tissue fluid, pleural fluid, bronchoalveolar lavage fluid (BAL), peritoneal fluid, saliva, urine, breast milk, cerebrospinal fluid, amniotic fluid and so on (Kowal, et al., 2014; Rezaie, et al., 2019). EVs can be transported or accumulated not only in biological liquids but also in solid tissues. In solid tissue, EVs deliver their contents, such as proteins, miRNAs, mRNAs, and lncRNAs, to adjacent or distant cells and reprogram the target cells in fate, function, and morphology, resulting in physiological or pathological effects (Kowal, Tkach, 2014; Maas, et al., 2017; Statello, et al., 2018).

Exosomes, also referred to as intraluminal vesicles (ILVs), are a subtype of EV formed by an endosomal route, which are surrounded by a phospholipid bilayer, and have been found in biological liquids (Raposo and Stoorvogel, 2013). Exosomal vesicles form through inward budding of the limiting membrane of early endosomes, which mature into multivesicular bodies (MVBs) (Huang, Yan, 2020b). MVBs play a significant role in the endocytic and trafficking functions of the cell material, such as protein sorting, recycling, storage, transport, and release (Babaei, and Rezaie, 2021). Release of exosomes into the extracellular space is facilitated by the fusion of the MVB limiting membrane with the plasma membrane. Researches showed that exosomes participated in cell communication, cell maintenance, and tumor progression (Rezaie, et al., 2021). Balaji Krishnamachary et al. explored EVs isolated from plasma of patients with COVID-19 to identify some potential biomarkers which influence the disease severity and to analyze its role in the pathogenesis of this disease (Krishnamachary, Cook, 2020). Plasma-derived EVs were separated from 53 COVID-19 patients in hospital and compared depending on the severity of their disease. Analysis of inflammation and cardiovascular protein loading in large EVs suggested significant differences in protein expression across disease subgroups. Prominently, the TNF superfamily and IL-6 family members were upregulated in severe and moderate disease patients who need oxygen supplement. EVs in severe patients also shown enhancement of prothrombotic or endothelial injury factors (TF, t-PA, and VWF) and cardiovascular pathology-related proteins (MB, PRSS8, REN, and HGF). There were significantly higher levels of TF, CD163, and EN-RAGE has been observed in EVs from patients with severe disease compared to moderate disease. EVs also play a key role in transmitting viral infection (Owczarek, et al., 2018). It was found that EVs and viruses shared similar physicochemical properties. They are small in size and have common biogenesis and cell entry mechanisms (van Dongen, Masoumi, 2016). The virus enters the uninfected cell *via* the endocytosis pathway and then exits the host cell by budding directly through the cell membrane. A new study found that EVs acted as the tool of virus export to cell, and the EVs depend virus entry mechanisms for cargo transport. EVs are the delivery vectors of viral contents. EVs released from virus-infected cells can infect healthy cells by transferring viral components, for example, virus-derived miRNAs and viral proteins, etc. (Ali, et al., 2010; Arenaccio, et al., 2015; Nolte-'t Hoen, et al., 2016). EVs separated from infected cells may also activate humoral and cellular immune responses by transferring viruses and autoantigens in the host (Fleming, Sampey, 2014; Gunasekaran, et al., 2017). In addition, EVs release from virus-infected cells can also transfer viral receptors and pro-inflammatory factors to the recipient cells, leading to the transmitting of viral infection and worsening of tissue damage (Mack, et al., 2000). Studies have shown that the number of EVs secreted from the SARS-CoV-2 infected cells increased significantly during the virus infection, and EVs still played an important role in the pathogenesis of diseases (Yoshikawa, Teixeira, 2019). Lanyu et al. emphasized the role of EVs play which secreted by lung cells and alveolar epithelial cells in lung injury and inflammation (Lanyu and Feilong, 2019). According to report, EVs secreted from broncho alveolar lavage fluid are involved in the pathogenesis of idiopathic pulmonary fibrosis through the signaling regulation mediators such as Wnt5a (Martin-Medina, et al., 2018). The latest research showed EVs derived from epithelial cells which transduced by lentiviral overexpressing SARS-CoV-2 gene could transfer viral genes to recipient cardiomyocytes, leading to increased expression of inflammatory genes (Kwon, et al., 2020).

EVs may contribute to the infection, internalization and transmission of SARS-CoV-2 virus. Some components such as miRNAs, viral proteins and viral receptor ACE2 could be packed into EVs (Wang, et al., 2020), that render the recipient cells sensitive to viral invasion (**Figure 1**). In this review, we discuss the current EVs based COVID-19 treatment strategies, including MSC and its EVs, EVs based drug delivery systems, EVs based vaccine, platelet EVs and inhibition of EVs intake, etc.

EVS-BASED COVID-19 THERAPY

MSC and MSC-EVs

MSCs are heterogeneous cells, including stromal cells, progenitor cells, fibroblasts, and stem cells (Dominici, et al., 2006; Galderisi and Giordano, 2014). The MSCs can be isolated from many tissues, such as bone marrow, placenta, adipose tissue, and umbilical cord blood. They are currently used as therapeutics at the present time, and meanwhile being tested in multiple clinical trials across the world (Meng, et al., 2020). MSCs are safe and possess immunomodulatory and tissue regeneration capabilities (Gao, et al., 2016; Thompson, et al., 2020). Studies suggested that the prospective therapeutic products based on MSCs were success, despite the apparent heterogeneity origin and lacking in specific biomarkers to predict, once implanted, MSCs could show strong regulate ability in immunomodulatory, antioxidant, and angiogenesis. MSCs and MSC-EVs have emerged as promising novel therapies that can not only reduce inflammation, but also regenerate and repair lung damage, and may therefore be used alone or in combination with other therapeutic agents to benefit patients with COVID-19.

Due to MSCs lack the expression of membrane bound molecules involved in immune rejection which enable their allogenic transplantation, the clinical applications of MSC-based therapy have witnessed an outstanding achievement (Ahmadi and Rezaie, 2021). Nevertheless, in the long-term follow up, safety issues regarding MSCs-based therapy are still a matter of debate. It is worth noting that MSCs have the capacity to differentiate into endothelial cells and to create a capillary network, and the inhibitory effect of MSCs in anti-tumor immune response results an increased tumor growth, which promotes tumor growth and metastasis (Kolios and Moodley, 2013). In addition, it was reported that local microenvironment in which MSCs engraft contained factors that induced unwanted differentiation of transplanted MSCs *in vivo*. Therefore, several factors and signaling pathways regarding MSCs therapy after their *in vivo* administration should be focused. Medical staff should abide by moral and ethical norms, so that the public and government administrators can clearly comprehend the nature and functions of MSCs, and understand the potential risks of treatment, and avoid deviating by non-standard clinical trials (Volarevic, et al., 2018).

The membrane of MSC-EVs is rich in cholesterol, sphingomyelin, ceramide and lipid raft proteins, which enables membrane fusion with target cells. After fusion, MSC-EVs may trigger signaling pathways through the receptor ligand interaction, or be internalized by endocytosis to deliver contents, such as mRNAs, miRNAs, enzymes, cytokines, etc. (Harrell, et al., 2019). Compared with homocellular transport, MSC-EVs overcome safety concerns regarding the long-term survival of engrafted MSCs due to its composition (Rezaie, et al., 2018). Thus, MSC-EVs therapy is a new remedy in cell-free treatment of autoimmune and inflammatory diseases.

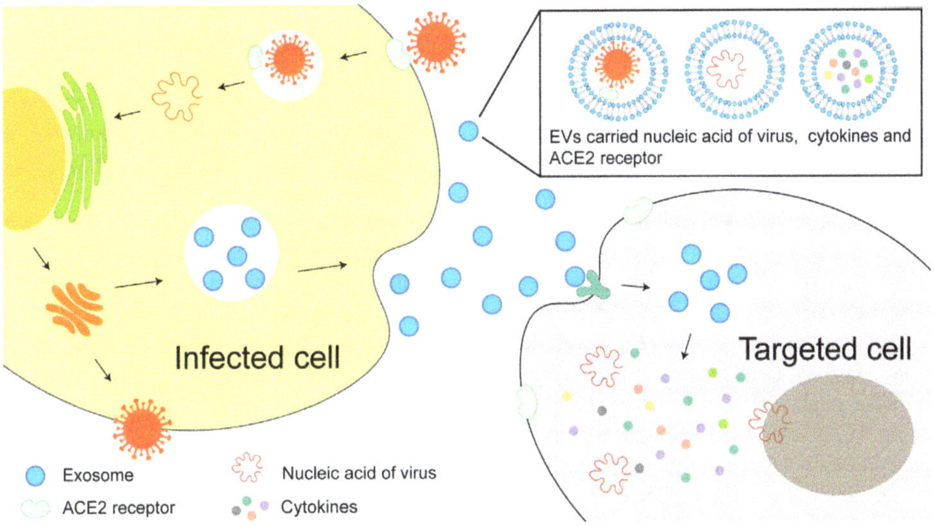

FIGURE 1 | The role of EVs in SARS-CoV-2 virus internalization and infection. EVs may contribute to the transmission of SARS-CoV-2 virus. The virus may enter the recipient cells through internalization. Virus components, such as miRNAs, viral proteins and viral receptor ACE2, are packaged into the EVs and make the healthy cells sensitive to viral invasion.

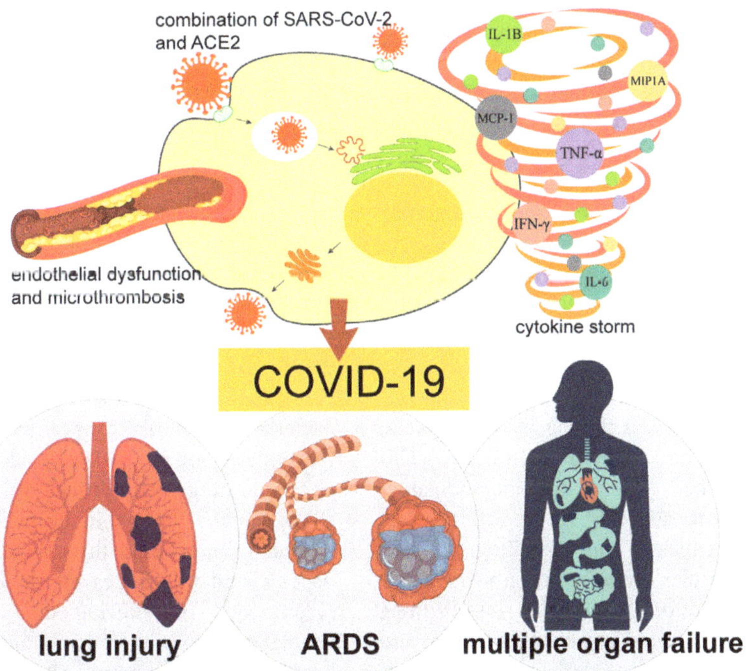

FIGURE 2 | Pathogenesis of COVID-19. The combination of SARS-CoV-2 and virus receptor ACE2, endothelial dysfunction and micro thrombosis, together with cytokine storm leads to COVID-19, causing a series of clinical manifestations such as lung injury, ARDS, and even systemic multiple organ failure.

Application of MSCs in Pulmonary Diseases

Inflammatory cytokines play a leading role in the development of COVID-19-caused lung injury (**Figure 2**). Immunotherapy that reduce the cytokine storm could be the key treatment option. However, traditional immunotherapy usually targeted one or two factors and may not produce enough response. MSCs have been shown to have powerful and extensive immunomodulatory and anti-inflammatory capabilities (Abdi, et al., 2008; Wada, et al., 2000).

Bone marrow MSCs therapy has evolved from preclinical trials to clinical trials for different diseases states in recent years. In animal models, MSCs significantly improve lung pathological change (Cruz and Rocco, 2020) and inhibit immune cell-mediated inflammation induced by influenza virus (Khatri, et al., 2018). Bhattacharya et al. demonstrated that bone marrow MSCs could stabilize endothelial cells and maintain alveolar-capillary barrier function, which is essential for maintaining or reducing inflammation-induced lung permeability, thereby mitigating the development of interstitial pulmonary edema (Bhattacharya and Matthay, 2013). Li et al. reported that MSCs could alleviate acute lung injury caused by H9N2 and H5N1 viruses in mice by reducing the secretion of pro-inflammatory chemokines and cytokines, and inhibiting migration of inflammatory cells to the lungs (Li, et al., 2016). Currently, there are several ongoing clinical trials using MSCs for a variety of pulmonary diseases, such as obstructive bronchiolitis idiopathic pulmonary fibrosis (NCT02013700), chronic obstructive pulmonary disease (NCT01849159), and bronchial dysplasia (NCT01175655) (Wecht and Rojas, 2016), as well as for ARDS (NCT02097641) (Matthay, et al., 2019) and septic shock (NCT02421484) (McIntyre, et al., 2018). Specifically, Leng et al. found that there were no ACE2 and TMPRSS2 receptors express in MSCs, which indicated that the virus should not infect this cell population (Leng, et al., 2020). In a rat model of hyperoxia-induced lung injury, MSCs reduced overexpression of hyperoxia-induced angiotensin and angiotensin type 1 receptor (AT1R), and reduced ACE to normal level (Chen and Chou, 2018). Recently, Simonson et al. reported a long-term follow-up study on two severe ARDS patients, who required ECMO support and combined mechanical ventilation during the acute phase (Simonson, et al., 2020). After receiving a single systemic infusion of allogeneic MSCs, both patients fully recovered their physical and mental abilities. Remarkably, a dual-energy CT scan showed no signs of pulmonary fibrosis after 5 yr of MSCs treatment.

Application of MSCs in the Treatment of COVID-19

MSCs therapy is considered a promising strategy for the treatment of COVID-19. The potential of MSCs for the treatment of COVID-19 is based on two benefits: *1*) induction of the regenerative program of lung epithelial and endothelial cells, and *2*) synchronous modulation of the inflammatory response. MSCs secrete multiple kinds of cytokines and paracrine factors which interact with immune cells directly, including T cells, B cells, dendritic cells, macrophages, and natural killer cells. This combined effect enables MSCs have immunomodulatory capability, which contributes to suppressing overactivation of the immune system. By producing and recruiting different growth factors such as vascular endothelial growth factor (VEGF), epidermal growth factor (EGF) and transforming growth factor (TGF), MSCs promote tissue regeneration and thus improve the microenvironment (Atluri, et al., 2020). It prevents uncontrolled inflammatory cascades while reducing pulmonary fibrosis and pulmonary dysfunction following COVID-19 infection (Mo, et al., 2020; Sun, et al., 2020; Thille, et al., 2013). Particularly, the lacking of ACE2 ensures the injected MSCs achieve immunomodulatory effects free from being destroyed by virus. MSCs from human umbilical cord origin were reported in a recent clinical trial, compared to the placebo group, they were associated with the increase of peripheral lymphocyte count and the decrease of systemic inflammatory biomarkers (ChiCTR2000029990) (Leng, et al., 2020). MSC infusion alleviated cytokine storm syndrome and significantly improved outcomes in patients with severe COVID-19.

Application of MSC-EVs in Lung Diseases

Most of the therapeutic progress of MSCs are achieved through paracrine mechanisms, including EVs secretion that contain cell protective factors such as keratinocyte growth factor (KGF), anti-inflammatory mediators (PGE2 or lipid A4), anti-osmotic factors (Angl) and others (Doorn, et al., 2012; Gnecchi, et al., 2008; Li, et al., 2014; Silini, et al., 2017). There have been reports of some limitations of using MSCs. For instance, intravenous administration of MSCs may induce particle aggregation leading to embolism; and some MSCs, especially those from embryonic tissues, may carry a risk of mutagenicity and tumorigenicity. Therefore, MSC derivatives such as SECRETOME (Bari, et al., 2019) and EVs (Tsiapalis and O'Driscoll, 2020) have been suggested as alternatives to MSC therapy. In addition, account of the low immunogenicity and tumorigenicity, simplicity of operation, and low cost, MSC-EVs therapy has significant advantages over MSC therapy. According to the report recently published, MSC-EVs could be administered by inhalation or injection (Bari, Ferrarotti, 2019). Preliminary studies have shown that MSC-EVs might also be effective against COVID-19 (Bari, et al., 2020). MSC-derived EVs have been demonstrated to induce similar influence to parent cells. In animal models, they can be store for a longer time safely without losing their biological function, on the other hand, they have been indicated similar or better indications than MSCs (Tsiapalis and O'Driscoll, 2020).

Some researchers have demonstrated the immunomodulatory effects of MSC-derived EVs *in vitro* (Budoni, et al., 2013; Del Fattore, et al., 2015; Di Trapani, et al., 2016; Henao Agudelo, et al., 2017; Liu, et al., 2012), and have shown significant anti-inflammatory and regenerative abilities in several diseased animal models (Fierabracci, et al., 2015; Phinney and Pittenger, 2017). Specifically, researchers showed demonstration that in animal models of lung injury, the efficacy of MSC-EVs was effective like in hyperoxia (Braun, et al., 2018; Porzionato, et al., 2019; Willis, et al., 2018), severe bacterial pneumonia (Monsel, et al., 2015), and viral pneumonia (Khatri, Richardson, 2018). In addition, MSC-EVs has beneficial effects on lung perfusion *ex vivo* with severe *E. coli* pneumonia (Park, et al., 2011). Finally, MSC-EVs can effectively repair marginal donor lungs through several methods, the first one is dose-dependently increasing the clearance of alveolar fluid; the second one is reducing lung weight after perfusion and ventilation; and the third one is improving airway and hemodynamic parameters (Ragni, et al., 2017). On the basic of these useful and promising results, the role of MSC-EVs in alleviating and repairing ARDS lung injury is gaining increasing attention (Lee, et al., 2019; Li, Huang, 2014; Monsel, Zhu, 2015; Shah, et al., 2019). Notably, fibrosis sequelae with reduced pulmonary function have been reported in patients recovering from COVID-19 pneumonia. Indeed, there is an increased risk of idiopathic pulmonary fibrosis following viral infection (Sheng, et al., 2020), as a long-term complication, it has been reported in parts of SARS infected patients (Zhang, et al., 2020b). MSC-EVs prevent fibrosis following experimental lung injury, which is similar to the cells of their origin (Cargnoni, et al., 2009; Mansouri, et al., 2019). In fact, there is a growing interest in the new potential application of EV as a disease treatment strategy. EVs are considered safe, easy and cheap to produce, isolate, store and manage (Muraca, et al., 2017), which could reduce costs and improve product availability. It is worth mentioning that EVs seem to be a very generic product that it has application diversity and can be modified by various technologies, for example, manipulating their parent cells use genetic engineering, and then integrated into the secreted EVs by introducing exogenous substances (Armstrong, et al., 2017; Vader, et al., 2016; Wiklander, et al., 2019). A similar method has been demonstrated to deliver exogenous miRNA-Let-7c to alleviate renal fibrosis *via* MSC-EVs in the mice model of unilateral ureteral obstruction (Wang, et al., 2016). On the other hand, studies also suggested that EVs could be loaded with therapeutic molecules form a polymer complex to improve its targeting activity (Cappariello, et al., 2018; Pascucci, et al., 2014; Vader, Mol, 2016; van der Meel, et al., 2014).

The pulmonary pathology of COVID-19 critically ill patients includes the exudation and proliferation phase of diffuse alveolar injury, and microvascular thrombosis that suggest early ARDS (Wichmann, et al., 2020; Xu, et al., 2020d). The pathogenesis includes change of alveolar permeability and neutrophils infiltration (Zemans and Matthay, 2017). Several studies showed that MSC-EVs could reduce alveolar permeability and increase alveolar fluid clearance, in an vitro model of human perfusion lung injury with severe *E. coli* pneumonia (Gennai, et al., 2015; Lee, et al., 2009; Park, et al., 2019). Interestingly, there were antibacterial substances in the culture medium of the bacteria-stimulated MSCs (Krasnodembskaya, et al., 2010). In a mouse sepsis model, treatment with MSCs could increase bacterial clearance, part of the reason is it increased phagocytic activity of host immune cells (Mei, et al., 2010). In addition, MSC-EVs demonstrated antiviral activity *in vitro* by inhibiting replication of influenza virus in lung epithelial cells, meanwhile by reducing viral load in an influenza-induced lung injury model of pigs (Khatri, Richardson, 2018).

Application of MSC-EVs in the Treatment of COVID-19

Recently, Sengupta, et al. published the safety and efficacy of allogeneic bone marrow MSC-derived EVs in 24 patients with COVID-19 severe pneumonia that they have been treated with hydroxychloroquine and azithromycin (Sengupta, et al., 2020). It was interesting to note that inflammatory biomarkers and absolute neutrophilic counts were decreased prominently, while the counts of total lymphocyte and $CD8^+$ were increased prominently within 5 days after EVs injection. In addition, D-dimer was significantly reduced. Although this EVs treatment resulted about 71% of patients recovery to health, it is not clear whether the recovery was attributable to EVs treatment, because of the lack of a matched control group and the lack of reported protein or microRNA composition of EVs used in the study. In summary, we would like to underline that there has been currently no approved MSC-based approach in preventing and treating the COVID-19, either with MSCs or MSCs-derived EVs. Clinical trials using EVs should be carried out with great caution, as their cargo determines the functional impact. Consequently, before MSC-derived EVs used in clinic, standardized protocols need to be developed, including mass production, isolation, functional evaluation, and batch-to-batch consistency. Some clinical trials using MSC-EVs in COVID-19 is currently underway and are summarized in **Table 1**.

Preliminary studies demonstrated that intravenous injection of MSCs and MSC-EVs possessed an enormous potential in treatment for COVID-19 patients. So far, no adverse events were found during MSCs and MSC-EVs treatment and follow-up period, suggesting that this therapy is safe and effective for COVID-19 patients (Akbari and Rezaie, 2020). However, MSCs express tissue factors and accumulate mainly in pulmonary capillaries, which may increase the risk of pulmonary embolism and other thromboembolic events. The effects of administration time, dose, frequency and route of MSCs and MSC-EVs need further study. Though clinical outcomes are promising, the limited literature still warrants more studies to establish safety and efficacy of MSCs and MSC-EVs to treat and manage symptoms associated with COVID-19 infection (Hamdan, et al., 2021).

Drug-EVs

One interesting approach of using EVs as therapeutic agents is its drug delivery potential (Gnecchi, et al., 2006; Lamichhane, et al., 2016; Lv, et al., 2012). EVs have a cellular origin, such as MSCs, and therefore offer greater safety and stability than other delivery systems such as liposomes (Malhotra, et al., 2016). Selectable compounds or genetically engineered molecules may loading with EVs in the nanocarriers to enhance the targeting ability for tissue/cell infection, suggesting that EVs-based nanocarriers can be used to treat infectious diseases. Some studies have used EV as an effective carrier of tumor-targeted anticancer drugs curcumin, doxorubicin, and paclitaxel (Kim, et al., 2016). Therefore, an EV-based drug delivery system has great potential to increase drug loading in targeting cells and inhibit off-target effects. EVs may be used to deliver therapeutic drugs or biomodulators to inhibiting the spread and replication of virus in the recipient cells (Romagnoli, et al., 2014). The development of safe and efficient nanocarriers is the main goal of nanomedicine. Therefore, the development of EVs-based nanocarriers offers a promising opportunity for therapeutic drug delivery. However, most of the studies have been conducted *in vitro* and *in vivo* experimental models, but it remains a mystery of the safety, specificity, and efficiency of the method in clinical trials.

Another attractive treatment option is to use the blood products of convalescent patients, such as the whole blood, plasma or serum. The EVs containing neutralizing antibodies in convalescent blood products were transferred into patients, and we benefit tremendously with this treatment by promoting immune regulation and lung tissue wound healing. Kesimer et al. proved that EVs derived from culture medium of human tracheobronchial epithelial cells showed a neutralizing effect on human influenza virus (Kesimer, et al., 2009). Studies have proved that plasma-derived EVs also carry an amount of cell growth factors, and these factors could induce the activation of cellular signaling pathways, change vascular reactivity, induce angiogenesis and promote tissue repair (Guo, et al., 2017; Tao, et al., 2017; Torreggiani, et al., 2014).

TABLE 1 | Ongoing clinical trials of MSC-EVs in COVID-19.

Registration number	Study title	Number enrolled	Interventions	Purposes
NCT04276987	A pilot clinical study on inhalation of mesenchymal stem cells exosomes treating severe novel coronavirus pneumonia	24	MSCs-derived exosomes	To explore the safety and efficiency of aerosol inhalation of the exosomes derived from allogenic adipose mesenchymal stem cells (MSCs-Exo)
NCT04798716	The use of exosomes for the treatment of acute respiratory distress syndrome or novel coronavirus pneumonia caused by COVID-19	55	MSC-exosomes delivered intravenously	To explore the safety and efficacy of an intravenous injection of MSC derived exosomes
NCT04491240	Evaluation of safety and efficiency of method of exosome inhalation in SARS-CoV-2 associated pneumonia. (COVID-19EXO)	30	EXO inhalation	To explore the safety and efficiency of aerosol inhalation of the exosomes
ChiCTR2000030261	A study for the key technology of mesenchymal stem cells exosomes atomization in the treatment of novel coronavirus pneumonia (COVID-19)	26	Aerosol inhalation of exosomes	To inhibit inflammatory factors and enhance the immunity of the body, promoting the early recovery of patients and reducing complications
ChiCTR2000030484	HUMSCs and exosomes treating patients with lung injury following novel coronavirus pneumonia (COVID-19)	90	Intravenous infusion of HUMSCs and exosomes	To evaluate the safety and efficacy of the treatment of human umbilical cord mesenchymal stem cells (MSCs)

Detailed information can be searched at https://clinicaltrials.gov and http://www.chictr.org.cn.

EVs Vaccines

The use of EVs as immunogenicity factors in the treatment of SARS coronavirus infection has been studied. EV might be used as a vaccine with its advantages of high stability, low toxicity and immunogenicity in circulation (Zhou, et al., 2020c). Kuate et al. analyzed exosome-based vaccines which containing the S protein of SARS-CoV-2. The S proteins-containing exosomes were procured by replacing the transmembrane and cytoplasmic domains of the S protein with those of VSV-G, and its immunogenicity and efficacy were tested in mice. After comparing it to an adenoviral vector vaccine expressing the S protein, it has been proved that both of the exosomes and the vaccine could induce neutralizing antibody titers. After priming with the SARS-S protein exosomal vaccine and boosting with the adenoviral vector the neutralizing antibody titers of using SARS-S protein exosomal vaccine exceeded those observed in the convalescent serum of SARS patients (Kuate, et al., 2007). In addition, the treatment of EVs has been shown to be more effective than that of soluble protein subunit vaccines, which might be due to the fact that the expression of multiple copies of the same viral protein exposed on the EVs surface promotes the cross-linking between EVs and the B cell receptor (Gyorgy, et al., 2015).

Platelet-derived EVs

Platelets are small (2–4 μm), and they are the anuclear cellular fragments of megakaryocytes from bone marrow and lung (Lefrancais, et al., 2017; Machlus, and Italiano, 2013). There are almost one trillion platelets patrol in the blood to hold the vascular system integrity. Once blood vessels are damaged, platelets will form a thrombus to prevent subsequent hemorrhage (Davi and Patrono, 2007). Platelet mediated thrombosis may also involve EVs (micro particles or micro vesicles), that provide anionic phospholipids such as phosphatidylserine to support the blood coagulation cascade (Ridger, et al., 2017). In addition to playing a role in hemostasis and thrombosis, platelets contribute to inducing the immune and inflammatory response (Kapur, et al., 2015; Li, et al., 2012; Morrell, et al., 2014; Semple, et al., 2011). The exosmosis and invasion to inflammatory tissues of neutrophils require interaction with activated platelets (Imhof, et al., 2016; Sreeramkumar, et al., 2014). The release of extracellular DNA (NETosis) by neutrophils was observed in patients with COVID-19 (Barnes, et al., 2020; Middleton, et al., 2020; Zuo, et al., 2020). NETosis requires platelets and may result in thrombosis (Constantinescu-Bercu, et al., 2020; Martinod, and Wagner, 2014). Some immune and inflammatory molecules have been found to express in platelets, such as IL-1; besides some immune receptors have been detected, such as CD40L, Toll-like receptors (TLR), and Fc receptors (Karas, et al., 1982; Lindemann, et al., 2001; Semple, Italiano, 2011).

Serological findings in patients with symptomatic COVID-19 include severe leukopenia and lymphocytopenia (Arentz, et al., 2020; Connors and Levy, 2020; Tang, et al., 2020). Low platelet count is closely associated with an increased risk of death for the in-hospital COVID-19 patients, although platelet levels are not generally considered clinically relevant. This finding suggests that SARS-CoV-2 infection may decrease platelet production and/or increase the damage of platelet. Patients with COVID-19 are more likely increase platelet consumption because of the platelet activation and thrombosis (Al-Samkari, et al., 2020; Liao, et al., 2020; Lippi and Favalora, 2020a; Lippi, et al., 2020b; Liu, et al., 2020; Xu, et al., 2020a; Yang, et al., 2020b).

Since thrombus and clotting are mainly controlled by platelets (Roberts, et al., 2006), it is critical to determine the status of platelets in COVID-19. Platelet-EVs delivers molecules from the mother platelet. They transport platelet-derived cytokines and other pro-inflammatory molecules, such as damage-associated molecular patterns (DAMPs) (Boudreau, et al., 2014; Maugeri, et al., 2018; Melki, et al., 2017). SARS-CoV-2 enters the ACE2-expressed endothelial cells. The loss of endothelial integrity may facilitate the recruitment of circulating platelets to the infected site, causing platelet activation and degranulation. Through analysis of platelet degranulation and cytokine release, Zaid et al. observed an evident increase in platelet-EVs firstly in platelet-EVs in patients with COVID-19 (Zaid, et al., 2020). This increase may be due to increased production of megakaryocytes or platelets, reduced clearance, or a combination of the two. Surprisingly, the level of platelet-EVs was significantly lower in severely ill patients than in non-critically ill patients. In severe COVID-19 cases, the number of platelets decreases. They reported that platelets were at the forefront of COVID-19 because they release various molecules at different stages of the disease. Thus, it is possible that platelets, which are associated with SARS-CoV-2 RNA and are highly activated in COVID-19, may be involved in the overwhelming thrombosis of COVID-19. Platelet overactivation may be involved in the systemic inflammatory response and thrombosis events observed in this disease. Therefore, inhibition of pathways associated with platelet activation may improve prognosis during COVID-19.

Giuseppe Cappellano et al. (Cappellano, et al., 2021) showed that platelet-EVs counts were higher in SARS-CoV-2 positive patients compared with SARS-CoV-2-negative patients, while platelet counts were not changed. What is particularly interesting is that the level of PLT-EVs was strongly associated with SARS-CoV-2 infection by a multivariate analysis, which independent from any confounding factors (age, sex, comorbidity, etc.). There was a very good diagnostic performance in ROC curve analysis, with sensitivity of 75% and specificity of 74%.

Platelet-derived EVs can be used to develop novel treatment strategies for COVID-19 patients. A study showed that engineered platelet-derived EVs loaded with TPCA-1 were effective in treating pneumonia (Ma, et al., 2020). In mouse models that selectively target inflammatory sites, platelet-derived EVs suppressed inflammation and reduced local cytokine storms.

Reduces EVs Secreted by Virus-infected Cells Into Receptor Cells

EVs secreted from virus-infected cells contribute to promoting viral infection and inhibiting immune cell response. Therefore, it may be a new useful method to overcome viral transmission by inhibiting the uptake of EVs (Li, et al., 2019; Schneider, et al., 2017).

OPPORTUNITIES AND CHALLENGES

Understanding the roles of EVs in COVID-19 infection could increase our knowledge of the dynamics of the virus and help developing effective prevention and treatment modalities. The above-mentioned findings provide a basis for future research on the dynamics of SARS-CoV-2 virus infection and its inhibition. However, it is worth noting that no EVs-based treatment has been approved to date. Significant barriers remain for the development of MSC-EVs as a therapeutic tool (Tsiapalis and O'Driscoll, 2020). Currently, we do not have any information on the possible side effects of EVs treatment against COVID-19. First, there are the similarities between EVs and viruses, both of them interact with the endosomal system which is responsible for synthesis of EVs. Some viruses may use this mechanism to pack viral proteins and RNA into vesicles in infected cells, subsequently released into the extracellular space, then facilitate the spread of the virus to uninfected cells (Gould, et al., 2003). This process has been demonstrated in HIV infection, but has not been elucidated in coronavirus infection (Arenaccio, Anticoli, 2015; Giannessi, et al., 2020). Second, the heterogeneity of EVs is a big challenge (Tkach, et al., 2018). Up to now, all published studies using heterogeneous EVs in some cases using the part size (<200 nm "small" EVs). Because the origin, size, composition and functional characteristics of the EVs are different, the source selection should be carefully described when using them for treatment. It is important to note that different sizes EVs of dendritic cells can induce the activation of T cells with different polarization mode (Kowal, et al., 2016). Third, due to the lack of standardization for accurate counting EV, as well as the current equipment does not differentiate between vesicles and non-vesicular granules, the quantitation of EV preparation is also an unsolved problems (Tkach, Kowal, 2018). For example, Campanella et al. reported that autologous exosomes were safer than allogeneic plasma exosomes in regenerative medicine (Campanella, et al., 2019). Soni et al. demonstrated that alveolar macrophages produce EVs might have a proinflammatory or anti-inflammatory effects, depending on the separation time of EVs in the process of acute lung injury (Soni, et al., 2016). Fourth, variability of tissue of origin and culture conditions (Patel, et al., 2018; Pittenger, et al., 2019). Although the MSCs from different sources have different immunosuppression and differentiation ability, but the optimal source of immunomodulation has not yet been determined (Gao, Chiu, 2016). Chance et al. reported that MSC-EVs had higher thrombotic activity than BMMMSC-EVs (Chance, et al., 2019). Recently, Inal reported a specific EVs subgroup, especially the EVs-TF positive might be associated with venous thromboembolism in COVID-19 patients with hypertension and diabetes (Inal, 2020). Taken together, it is critical to emphasize that care should be taken in using EVs for disease treatment (Borger, et al., 2020). To ensure the curative effect and safety of using EVs for COVID-19, enormous efforts are required to improve the technology for the separation and identification of EVs.

AUTHOR CONTRIBUTIONS

Y-yY, W-mZ, and Y-qW wrote the first draft of manuscript, Q-rG, F-xZ, and Z-yZ designed the figures, Y-xX and H-yZ finished the table, MA and AMJ amended the text and figures, BM and J-yZ designed and revised the manuscript. All authors read and approved the final manuscript.

FUNDING

This work was supported by the National Natural Science Foundation of China (81902152, U1903126, 81773888 and 81903467), Open Founding of Key Laboratory Ethnomedicine Ministry of Education (KLEM-KF2019Y03), the Key Medical Science and Technology Project of Shanxi Province (2020 XM33-"Four Batches" of Science and Technology Medical Innovation Project of Shanxi Province), and the Fund of Shanxi Province Higher Education Technology Innovation Project (2019L0753).

REFERENCES

Abdi, R., Fiorina, P., Adra, C. N., Atkinson, M., and Sayegh, M. H. (2008). Immunomodulation by Mesenchymal Stem Cells: A Potential Therapeutic Strategy for Type 1 Diabetes. *Diabetes* 57, 1759–1767. doi:10.2337/db08-0180

Ackermann, M., Verleden, S. E., Kuehnel, M., Haverich, A., Welte, T., Laenger, F., et al. (2020). Pulmonary Vascular Endothelialitis, Thrombosis, and Angiogenesis in Covid-19. *N. Engl. J. Med.* 383, 120–128. doi:10.1056/NEJMoa2015432

Ahmadi, M., and Rezaie, J. (2021). Ageing and Mesenchymal Stem Cells Derived Exosomes: Molecular Insight and Challenges. *Cell Biochem Funct* 39, 60–66. doi:10.1002/cbf.3602

Akbari, A., and Rezaie, J. (2020). Potential Therapeutic Application of Mesenchymal Stem Cell-Derived Exosomes in SARS-CoV-2 Pneumonia. *Stem Cell Res. Ther.* 11, 356. doi:10.1186/s13287-020-01866-6

Al-Samkari, H., Karp Leaf, R. S., Dzik, W. H., Carlson, J. C. T., Fogerty, A. E., Waheed, A., et al. (2020). COVID-19 and Coagulation: Bleeding and Thrombotic Manifestations of SARS-CoV-2 Infection. *Blood* 136, 489–500. doi:10.1182/blood.2020006520

Ali, S. A., Huang, M.-B., Campbell, P. E., Roth, W. W., Campbell, T., Khan, M., et al. (2010). Genetic Characterization of HIV Type 1 Nef-Induced Vesicle Secretion. *AIDS Res. Hum. Retroviruses* 26, 173–192. doi:10.1089/aid.2009.0068

Arenaccio, C., Anticoli, S., Manfredi, F., Chiozzini, C., Olivetta, E., and Federico, M. (2015). Latent HIV-1 Is Activated by Exosomes from Cells Infected with Either Replication-Competent or Defective HIV-1. *Retrovirology* 12, 87. doi:10.1186/s12977-015-0216-y

Arentz, M., Yim, E., Klaff, L., Lokhandwala, S., Riedo, F. X., Chong, M., et al. (2020). Characteristics and Outcomes of 21 Critically Ill Patients with COVID-19 in Washington State. *JAMA* 323, 1612–1614. doi:10.1001/jama.2020.4326

Armstrong, J. P. K., Holme, M. N., and Stevens, M. M. (2017). Re-Engineering Extracellular Vesicles as Smart Nanoscale Therapeutics. *ACS Nano* 11, 69–83. doi:10.1021/acsnano.6b07607

Atluri, S., Manchikanti, L., and Hirsch, J. A. (2020). Expanded Umbilical Cord Mesenchymal Stem Cells (UC-MSCs) as a Therapeutic Strategy in Managing Critically Ill COVID-19 Patients: The Case for Compassionate Use. *Pain Physician* 23, E71–E83. doi:10.36076/ppj.2020/23/e71

Babaei, M., and Rezaie, J. (2021). Application of Stem Cell-Derived Exosomes in Ischemic Diseases: Opportunity and Limitations. *J. Transl Med.* 19, 196. doi:10.1186/s12967-021-02863-w

Bari, E., Ferrarotti, I., Saracino, L., Perteghella, S., Torre, M. L., and Corsico, A. G. (2020). Mesenchymal Stromal Cell Secretome for Severe COVID-19 Infections: Premises for the Therapeutic Use. *Cells* 9, 924. doi:10.3390/cells9040924

Bari, E., Ferrarotti, I., Torre, M. L., Corsico, A. G., and Perteghella, S. (2019). Mesenchymal Stem/stromal Cell Secretome for Lung Regeneration: The Long Way through "pharmaceuticalization" for the Best Formulation. *J. Control. Release* 309, 11–24. doi:10.1016/j.jconrel.2019.07.022

Barnes, B. J., Adrover, J. M., Baxter-Stoltzfus, A., Borczuk, A., Cools-Lartigue, J., Crawford, J. M., et al. (2020). Targeting Potential Drivers of COVID-19: Neutrophil Extracellular Traps. *J. Exp. Med.* 217, e20200652. doi:10.1084/jem.20200652

Bautista-Vargas, M., Bonilla-Abadía, F., and Cañas, C. A. (2020). Potential Role for Tissue Factor in the Pathogenesis of Hypercoagulability Associated with in COVID-19. *J. Thromb. Thrombolysis* 50, 479–483. doi:10.1007/s11239-020-02172-x

Beigel, J. H., Tomashek, K. M., Dodd, L. E., Mehta, A. K., Zingman, B. S., Kalil, A. C., et al. (2020). Remdesivir for the Treatment of Covid-19 - Final Report. *N. Engl. J. Med.* 383, 1813–1826. doi:10.1056/NEJMoa2007764

Berger, J. S., Kunichoff, D., Adhikari, S., Ahuja, T., Amoroso, N., Aphinyanaphongs, Y., et al. (2020). Prevalence and Outcomes of D-Dimer Elevation in Hospitalized Patients with COVID-19. *Arterioscler. Thromb. Vasc. Biol.* 40, 2539–2547. doi:10.1161/ATVBAHA.120.314872

Bhattacharya, J., and Matthay, M. A. (2013). Regulation and Repair of the Alveolar-Capillary Barrier in Acute Lung Injury. *Annu. Rev. Physiol.* 75, 593–615. doi:10.1146/annurev-physiol-030212-183756

Börger, V., Weiss, D. J., Anderson, J. D., Borràs, F. E., Bussolati, B., Carter, D. R. F., et al. (2020). International Society for Extracellular Vesicles and International Society for Cell and Gene Therapy Statement on Extracellular Vesicles from Mesenchymal Stromal Cells and Other Cells: Considerations for Potential Therapeutic Agents to Suppress Coronavirus Disease-19. *Cytotherapy* 22, 482–485. doi:10.1016/j.jcyt.2020.05.002

Boudreau, L. H., Duchez, A.-C., Cloutier, N., Soulet, D., Martin, N., Bollinger, J., et al. (2014). Platelets Release Mitochondria Serving as Substrate for Bactericidal Group IIA-Secreted Phospholipase A2 to Promote Inflammation. *Blood* 124, 2173–2183. doi:10.1182/blood-2014-05-573543

Bourgonje, A. R., Abdulle, A. E., Timens, W., Hillebrands, J. L., Navis, G. J., Gordijn, S. J., et al. (2020). Angiotensin-converting Enzyme 2 (ACE2), SARS-CoV -2 and the Pathophysiology of Coronavirus Disease 2019 (COVID -19). *J. Pathol.* 251, 228–248. doi:10.1002/path.5471

Braun, R. K., Chetty, C., Balasubramaniam, V., Centanni, R., Haraldsdottir, K., Hematti, P., et al. (2018). Intraperitoneal Injection of MSC-Derived Exosomes Prevent Experimental Bronchopulmonary Dysplasia. *Biochem. Biophys. Res. Commun.* 503, 2653–2658. doi:10.1016/j.bbrc.2018.08.019

Budoni, M., Fierabracci, A., Luciano, R., Petrini, S., Di Ciommo, V., and Muraca, M. (2013). The Immunosuppressive Effect of Mesenchymal Stromal Cells on B Lymphocytes Is Mediated by Membrane Vesicles. *Cell Transplant.* 22, 369–379. doi:10.3727/096368911X58276910.3727/096368911x582769b

Campanella, C., Caruso Bavisotto, C., Logozzi, M., Marino Gammazza, A., Mizzoni, D., Cappello, F., et al. (2019). On the Choice of the Extracellular Vesicles for Therapeutic Purposes. *Int. J. Mol. Sci.* 20, 236. doi:10.3390/ijms20020236

Cappariello, A., Loftus, A., Muraca, M., Maurizi, A., Rucci, N., and Teti, A. (2018). Osteoblast-Derived Extracellular Vesicles Are Biological Tools for the Delivery of Active Molecules to Bone. *J. Bone Miner Res.* 33, 517–533. doi:10.1002/jbmr.3332

Cappellano, G., Raineri, D., Rolla, R., Giordano, M., Puricelli, C., Vilardo, B., et al. (2021). Circulating Platelet-Derived Extracellular Vesicles Are a Hallmark of Sars-Cov-2 Infection. *Cells* 10, 85. doi:10.3390/cells10010085

Cargnoni, A., Gibelli, L., Tosini, A., Signoroni, P. B., Nassuato, C., Arienti, D., et al. (2009). Transplantation of Allogeneic and Xenogeneic Placenta-Derived Cells Reduces Bleomycin-Induced Lung Fibrosis. *Cell Transplant.* 18, 405–422. doi:10.3727/096368909788809857

Cascella, M., Rajnik, M., Cuomo, A., Dulebohn, S. C., and Di Napoli, R. (2021). *Features, Evaluation, and Treatment of Coronavirus (COVID-19).* Treasure Island, FL: StatPearls.

Cavalli, G., De Luca, G., Campochiaro, C., Della-Torre, E., Ripa, M., Canetti, D., et al. (2020). Interleukin-1 Blockade with High-Dose Anakinra in Patients with COVID-19, Acute Respiratory Distress Syndrome, and Hyperinflammation: A Retrospective Cohort Study. *Lancet Rheumatol.* 2, e325–e331. doi:10.1016/S2665-9913(20)30127-2

Chance, T. C., Rathbone, C. R., Kamucheka, R. M., Peltier, G. C., Cap, A. P., and Bynum, J. A. (2019). The Effects of Cell Type and Culture Condition on the Procoagulant Activity of Human Mesenchymal Stromal Cell-Derived Extracellular Vesicles. *J. Trauma Acute Care Surg.* 87, S74–S82. doi:10.1097/TA.0000000000002225

Chen, C. M., and Chou, H. C. (2018). Human Mesenchymal Stem Cells Attenuate Hyperoxia-Induced Lung Injury through Inhibition of the Renin-Angiotensin System in Newborn Rats. *Am. J. Transl Res.* 10, 2628–2635.

Connors, J. M., and Levy, J. H. (2020). COVID-19 and its Implications for Thrombosis and Anticoagulation. *Blood* 135, 2033–2040. doi:10.1182/blood.2020006000

Constantinescu-Bercu, A., Grassi, L., Frontini, M., Salles-Crawley, I. I., Woollard, K., and Crawley, J. T. (2020). Activated αIIbβ3 on Platelets Mediates Flow-dependent NETosis via SLC44A2. *Elife* 9, e53353. doi:10.7554/eLife.53353

Cruz, F. F., and Rocco, P. R. M. (2020). The Potential of Mesenchymal Stem Cell Therapy for Chronic Lung Disease. *Expert Rev. Respir. Med.* 14, 31–39. doi:10.1080/17476348.2020.1679628

Cui, J., Li, F., and Shi, Z.-L. (2019). Origin and Evolution of Pathogenic Coronaviruses. *Nat. Rev. Microbiol.* 17, 181–192. doi:10.1038/s41579-018-0118-9

Davì, G., and Patrono, C. (2007). Platelet Activation and Atherothrombosis. *N. Engl. J. Med.* 357, 2482–2494. doi:10.1056/NEJMra071014

Del Fattore, A., Luciano, R., Pascucci, L., Goffredo, B. M., Giorda, E., Scapaticci, M., et al. (2015). Immunoregulatory Effects of Mesenchymal Stem Cell-Derived Extracellular Vesicles on T Lymphocytes. *Cell Transplant.* 24, 2615–2627. doi:10.3727/096368915X687543

Devaux, C. A., Rolain, J.-M., and Raoult, D. (2020). ACE2 Receptor Polymorphism: Susceptibility to SARS-CoV-2, Hypertension, Multi-Organ Failure, and COVID-19 Disease Outcome. *J. Microbiol. Immunol. Infect.* 53, 425–435. doi:10.1016/j.jmii.2020.04.015

Di Trapani, M., Bassi, G., Midolo, M., Gatti, A., Takam Kamga, P., Cassaro, A., et al. (2016). Differential and Transferable Modulatory Effects of Mesenchymal Stromal Cell-Derived Extracellular Vesicles on T, B and NK Cell Functions. *Sci. Rep.* 6, 24120. doi:10.1038/srep24120

Dogrammatzis, C., Waisner, H., and Kalamvoki, M. (2020). Cloaked Viruses and Viral Factors in Cutting Edge Exosome-Based Therapies. *Front. Cell Dev. Biol.* 8, 376. doi:10.3389/fcell.2020.00376

Dominici, M., Le Blanc, K., Mueller, I., Slaper-Cortenbach, I., Marini, F. C., Krause, D. S., et al. (2006). Minimal Criteria for Defining Multipotent Mesenchymal Stromal Cells. The International Society for Cellular Therapy Position Statement. *Cytotherapy* 8, 315–317. doi:10.1080/14653240600855905

Doorn, J., Moll, G., Le Blanc, K., van Blitterswijk, C., and de Boer, J. (2012). Therapeutic Applications of Mesenchymal Stromal Cells: Paracrine Effects and Potential Improvements. *Tissue Eng. Part B Rev.* 18, 101–115. doi:10.1089/ten.TEB.2011.0488

England, J. T., Abdulla, A., Biggs, C. M., Lee, A. Y. Y., Hay, K. A., Hoiland, R. L., et al. (2021). Weathering the COVID-19 Storm: Lessons from Hematologic Cytokine Syndromes. *Blood Rev.* 45, 100707. doi:10.1016/j.blre.2020.100707

Fierabracci, A., Del Fattore, A., Luciano, R., Muraca, M., Teti, A., and Muraca, M. (2015). Recent Advances in Mesenchymal Stem Cell Immunomodulation: the Role of Microvesicles. *Cell Transplant.* 24, 133–149. doi:10.3727/096368913X675728

Fleming, A., Sampey, G., Chung, M.-C., Bailey, C., van Hoek, M. L., Kashanchi, F., et al. (2014). The Carrying Pigeons of the Cell: Exosomes and Their Role in Infectious Diseases Caused by Human Pathogens. *Pathog. Dis.* 71, 109–120. doi:10.1111/2049-632X.12135

Fung, T. S., and Liu, D. X. (2019). Human Coronavirus: Host-Pathogen Interaction. *Annu. Rev. Microbiol.* 73, 529–557. doi:10.1146/annurev-micro-020518-115759

Galderisi, U., and Giordano, A. (2014). The Gap Between the Physiological and Therapeutic Roles of Mesenchymal Stem Cells. *Med. Res. Rev.* 34, 1100–1126. doi:10.1002/med.21322

Gao, F., Chiu, S. M., Motan, D. A. L., Zhang, Z., Chen, L., Ji, H.-L., et al. (2016). Mesenchymal Stem Cells and Immunomodulation: Current Status and Future Prospects. *Cell Death Dis* 7, e2062. doi:10.1038/cddis.2015.327

Gao, Y. M., Xu, G., Wang, B., and Liu, B. C. (2021). Cytokine Storm Syndrome in Coronavirus Disease 2019: A Narrative Review. *J. Intern. Med.* 289, 147–161. doi:10.1111/joim.13144

Gennai, S., Monsel, A., Hao, Q., Park, J., Matthay, M. A., and Lee, J. W. (2015). Microvesicles Derived from Human Mesenchymal Stem Cells Restore Alveolar Fluid Clearance in Human Lungs Rejected for Transplantation. *Am. J. Transplant.* 15, 2404–2412. doi:10.1111/ajt.13271

Giannessi, F., Aiello, A., Franchi, F., Percario, Z. A., and Affabris, E. (2020). The Role of Extracellular Vesicles as Allies of HIV, HCV and SARS Viruses. *Viruses* 12, 571. doi:10.3390/v12050571

Glowacka, I., Bertram, S., Herzog, P., Pfefferle, S., Steffen, I., Muench, M. O., et al. (2010). Differential Downregulation of ACE2 by the Spike Proteins of Severe Acute Respiratory Syndrome Coronavirus and Human Coronavirus NL63. *J. Virol.* 84, 1198–1205. doi:10.1128/JVI.01248-09

Gnecchi, M., He, H., Noiseux, N., Liang, O. D., Zhang, L., Morello, F., et al. (2006). Evidence Supporting Paracrine Hypothesis for Akt-modified Mesenchymal Stem Cell-mediated Cardiac protection and Functional Improvement. *FASEB J.* 20, 661–669. doi:10.1096/fj.05-5211com

Gnecchi, M., Zhang, Z., Ni, A., and Dzau, V. J. (2008). Paracrine Mechanisms in Adult Stem Cell Signaling and Therapy. *Circ. Res.* 103, 1204–1219. doi:10.1161/CIRCRESAHA.108.176826

Gould, S. J., Booth, A. M., and Hildreth, J. E. K. (2003). The Trojan Exosome Hypothesis. *Proc. Natl. Acad. Sci. USA* 100, 10592–10597. doi:10.1073/pnas.1831413100

Grasselli, G., Zangrillo, A., Zanella, A., Antonelli, M., Cabrini, L., Castelli, A., et al. (2020). Baseline Characteristics and Outcomes of 1591 Patients Infected with SARS-CoV-2 Admitted to ICUs of the Lombardy Region. *Italy. JAMA.* 323, 1574–1581. doi:10.1001/jama.2020.539410.1001/jama.2020.4031

Grover, S. P., and Mackman, N. (2018). Tissue Factor: An Essential Mediator of Hemostasis and Trigger of Thrombosis. *Arterioscler. Thromb. Vasc. Biol.* 38, 709–725. doi:10.1161/ATVBAHA.117.309846

Gunasekaran, M., Xu, Z., Nayak, D. K., Sharma, M., Hachem, R., Walia, R., et al. (2017). Donor-Derived Exosomes with Lung Self-Antigens in Human Lung Allograft Rejection. *Am. J. Transplant.* 17, 474–484. doi:10.1111/ajt.13915

Guo, S.-C., Tao, S.-C., Yin, W.-J., Qi, X., Yuan, T., and Zhang, C.-Q. (2017). Exosomes Derived from Platelet-Rich Plasma Promote the Re-epithelization of Chronic Cutaneous Wounds via Activation of YAP in a Diabetic Rat Model. *Theranostics* 7, 81–96. doi:10.7150/thno.16803

Guzik, T. J., Mohiddin, S. A., Dimarco, A., Patel, V., Savvatis, K., Marelli-Berg, F. M., et al. (2020). COVID-19 and the Cardiovascular System: Implications for Risk Assessment, Diagnosis, and Treatment Options. *Cardiovasc. Res.* 116, 1666–1687. doi:10.1093/cvr/cvaa106

György, B., Hung, M. E., Breakefield, X. O., and Leonard, J. N. (2015). Therapeutic Applications of Extracellular Vesicles: Clinical Promise and Open Questions. *Annu. Rev. Pharmacol. Toxicol.* 55, 439–464. doi:10.1146/annurev-pharmtox-010814-124630

Hamdan, H., Hashmi, S. K., Lazarus, H., Gale, R. P., Qu, W., and El Fakih, R. (2021). Promising Role for Mesenchymal Stromal Cells in Coronavirus Infectious Disease-19 (COVID-19)-Related Severe Acute Respiratory Syndrome? *Blood Rev.* 46, 100742. doi:10.1016/j.blre.2020.100742

Hamming, I., Timens, W., Bulthuis, M., Lely, A., Navis, G., and van Goor, H. (2004). Tissue Distribution of ACE2 Protein, the Functional Receptor for SARS Coronavirus. A First Step in Understanding SARS Pathogenesis. *J. Pathol.* 203, 631–637. doi:10.1002/path.1570

Han, L., Lam, E. W.-F., and Sun, Y. (2019). Extracellular Vesicles in the Tumor Microenvironment: Old Stories, but New Tales. *Mol. Cancer* 18, 59. doi:10.1186/s12943-019-0980-8

Harrell, C. R., Jovicic, N., Djonov, V., Arsenijevic, N., and Volarevic, V. (2019). Mesenchymal Stem Cell-Derived Exosomes and Other Extracellular Vesicles as New Remedies in the Therapy of Inflammatory Diseases. *Cells* 8, 1605. doi:10.3390/cells8121605

Henao Agudelo, J. S., Braga, T. T., Amano, M. T., Cenedeze, M. A., Cavinato, R. A., Peixoto-Santos, A. R., et al. (2017). Mesenchymal Stromal Cell-Derived Microvesicles Regulate an Internal Pro-inflammatory Program in Activated Macrophages. *Front. Immunol.* 8, 881. doi:10.3389/fimmu.2017.00881

Huang, C., Wang, Y., Li, X., Ren, L., Zhao, J., Hu, Y., et al. (2020a). Clinical Features of Patients Infected with 2019 Novel Coronavirus in Wuhan, China. *Lancet* 395, 497–506. doi:10.1016/S0140-6736(20)30183-5

Huang, W., Yan, Y., Liu, Y., Lin, M., Ma, J., Zhang, W., et al. (2020b). Exosomes with Low miR-34c-3p Expression Promote Invasion and Migration of Non-small Cell Lung Cancer by Upregulating Integrin α2β1. *Signal Transduct. Target. Ther.* 5, 39. doi:10.1038/s41392-020-0133-y

Huet, T., Beaussier, H., Voisin, O., Jouveshomme, S., Dauriat, G., Lazareth, I., et al. (2020). Anakinra for Severe Forms of COVID-19: A Cohort Study. *Lancet Rheumatol.* 2, e393–e400. doi:10.1016/S2665-9913(20)30164-8

Imhof, B. A., Jemelin, S., Ballet, R., Vesin, C., Schapira, M., Karaca, M., et al. (2016). CCN1/CYR61-mediated Meticulous Patrolling by Ly6Clow Monocytes Fuels Vascular Inflammation. *Proc. Natl. Acad. Sci. USA* 113, E4847–E4856. doi:10.1073/pnas.1607710113

Inal, J. (2020). COVID-19 Comorbidities, Associated Procoagulant Extracellular Vesicles and Venous Thromboembolisms: A Possible Link with Ethnicity? *Br. J. Haematol.* 190, e218–e220. doi:10.1111/bjh.17011

Jia, H. (2016). Pulmonary Angiotensin-Converting Enzyme 2 (ACE2) and Inflammatory Lung Disease. *Shock* 46, 239–248. doi:10.1097/SHK.0000000000000633

Kapur, R., Zufferey, A., Boilard, E., and Semple, J. W. (2015). Nouvelle Cuisine: Platelets Served with Inflammation. *J. Immunol.* 194, 5579–5587. doi:10.4049/jimmunol.1500259

Karas, S., Rosse, W., and Kurlander, R. (1982). Characterization of the IgG-Fc Receptor on Human Platelets. *Blood* 60, 1277–1282. doi:10.1182/blood.v60.6.1277.bloodjournal6061277

Kesimer, M., Scull, M., Brighton, B., DeMaria, G., Burns, K., O'Neal, W., et al. (2009). Characterization of Exosome-like Vesicles Released from Human Tracheobronchial Ciliated Epithelium: A Possible Role in Innate Defense. *FASEB J.* 23, 1858–1868. doi:10.1096/fj.08-119131

Khatri, M., Richardson, L. A., and Meulia, T. (2018). Mesenchymal Stem Cell-Derived Extracellular Vesicles Attenuate Influenza Virus-Induced Acute Lung

Injury in a Pig Model. *Stem Cell Res. Ther.* 9, 17. doi:10.1186/s13287-018-0774-8

Kim, M. S., Haney, M. J., Zhao, Y., Mahajan, V., Deygen, I., Klyachko, N. L., et al. (2016). Development of Exosome-Encapsulated Paclitaxel to Overcome MDR in Cancer Cells. *Nanomedicine* 12, 655–664. doi:10.1016/j.nano.2015.10.012

Kolios, G., and Moodley, Y. (2013). Introduction to Stem Cells and Regenerative Medicine. *Respiration* 85, 3–10. doi:10.1159/000345615

Kowal, J., Arras, G., Colombo, M., Jouve, M., Morath, J. P., Primdal-Bengtson, B., et al. (2016). Proteomic Comparison Defines Novel Markers to Characterize Heterogeneous Populations of Extracellular Vesicle Subtypes. *Proc. Natl. Acad. Sci. USA* 113, E968–E977. doi:10.1073/pnas.1521230113

Kowal, J., Tkach, M., and Théry, C. (2014). Biogenesis and Secretion of Exosomes. *Curr. Opin. Cell Biol.* 29, 116–125. doi:10.1016/j.ceb.2014.05.004

Krasnodembskaya, A., Song, Y., Fang, X., Gupta, N., Serikov, V., Lee, J.-W., et al. (2010). Antibacterial Effect of Human Mesenchymal Stem Cells Is Mediated in Part from Secretion of the Antimicrobial Peptide LL-37. *Stem Cells* 28, 2229–2238. doi:10.1002/stem.544

Krishnamachary, B., Cook, C., Spikes, L., Chalise, P., and Dhillon, N. K. (2020). The Potential Role of Extracellular Vesicles in COVID-19 Associated Endothelial Injury and Pro-inflammation. medRxiv [Preprint]. Available at: https://www.ncbi.nlm.nih.gov/pmc/articles/PMC7480053/ (Accessed September 1, 2020). doi:10.1101/2020.08.27.20182808

Kuate, S., Cinatl, J., Doerr, H. W., and Überla, K. (2007). Exosomal Vaccines Containing the S Protein of the SARS Coronavirus Induce High Levels of Neutralizing Antibodies. *Virology* 362, 26–37. doi:10.1016/j.virol.2006.12.011

Kwon, Y., Nukala, S. B., Srivastava, S., Miyamoto, H., Ismail, N. I., Rehman, J., et al. (2020). Detection of Viral RNA Fragments in Human iPSC-Cardiomyocytes Following Treatment with Extracellular Vesicles from SARS-CoV-2 Coding-Sequence-Overexpressing Lung Epithelial Cells. bioRxiv [Preprint]. Available at: https://pubmed.ncbi.nlm.nih.gov/32637965/ (Accessed July 1, 2020). doi:10.1101/2020.05.14.093583

Lamichhane, T. N., Jeyaram, A., Patel, D. B., Parajuli, B., Livingston, N. K., Arumugasaamy, N., et al. (2016). Oncogene Knockdown via Active Loading of Small RNAs into Extracellular Vesicles by Sonication. *Cell. Mol. Bioeng.* 9, 315–324. doi:10.1007/s12195-016-0457-4

Lanyu, Z., and Feilong, H. (2019). Emerging Role of Extracellular Vesicles in Lung Injury and Inflammation. *Biomed. Pharmacother.* 113, 108748. doi:10.1016/j.biopha.2019.108748

Lässer, C., O'Neil, S. E., Shelke, G. V., Sihlbom, C., Hansson, S. F., Gho, Y. S., et al. (2016). Exosomes in the Nose Induce Immune Cell Trafficking and Harbour an Altered Protein Cargo in Chronic Airway Inflammation. *J. Transl Med.* 14, 181. doi:10.1186/s12967-016-0927-4

Lee, J. H., Park, J., and Lee, J.-W. (2019). Therapeutic Use of Mesenchymal Stem Cell-Derived Extracellular Vesicles in Acute Lung Injury. *Transfusion* 59, 876–883. doi:10.1111/trf.14838

Lee, R. H., Pulin, A. A., Seo, M. J., Kota, D. J., Ylostalo, J., Larson, B. L., et al. (2009). Intravenous hMSCs Improve Myocardial Infarction in Mice Because Cells Embolized in Lung Are Activated to Secrete the Anti-inflammatory Protein TSG-6. *Cell Stem Cell* 5, 54–63. doi:10.1016/j.stem.2009.05.003

Lefrançais, E., Ortiz-Muñoz, G., Caudrillier, A., Mallavia, B., Liu, F., Sayah, D. M., et al. (2017). The Lung Is a Site of Platelet Biogenesis and a Reservoir for Haematopoietic Progenitors. *Nature* 544, 105–109. doi:10.1038/nature21706

Leng, Z., Zhu, R., Hou, W., Feng, Y., Yang, Y., Han, Q., et al. (2020). Transplantation of ACE2- Mesenchymal Stem Cells Improves the Outcome of Patients with COVID-19 Pneumonia. *Aging Dis.* 11, 216–228. doi:10.14336/AD.2020.0228

Li, C., Li, J., Li, Y., Lang, S., Yougbare, I., Zhu, G., et al. (2012). Crosstalk Between Platelets and the Immune System: Old Systems with New Discoveries. *Adv. Hematol.* 2012, 1–14. doi:10.1155/2012/384685

Li, F., Li, W., Farzan, M., and Harrison, S. C. (2005). Structure of SARS Coronavirus Spike Receptor-Binding Domain Complexed with Receptor. *Science* 309, 1864–1868. doi:10.1126/science.1116480

Li, J., Huang, S., Wu, Y., Gu, C., Gao, D., Feng, C., et al. (2014). Paracrine Factors from Mesenchymal Stem Cells: A Proposed Therapeutic Tool for Acute Lung Injury and Acute Respiratory Distress Syndrome. *Int. Wound J.* 11, 114–121. doi:10.1111/iwj.12202

Li, S., Li, S., Wu, S., and Chen, L. (2019). Exosomes Modulate the Viral Replication and Host Immune Responses in HBV Infection. *Biomed. Res. Int.* 2019, 1–9. doi:10.1155/2019/2103943

Li, Y., Xu, J., Shi, W., Chen, C., Shao, Y., Zhu, L., et al. (2016). Mesenchymal Stromal Cell Treatment Prevents H9N2 Avian Influenza Virus-Induced Acute Lung Injury in Mice. *Stem Cell Res. Ther.* 7, 159. doi:10.1186/s13287-016-0395-z

Liao, D., Zhou, F., Luo, L., Xu, M., Wang, H., Xia, J., et al. (2020). Haematological Characteristics and Risk Factors in the Classification and Prognosis Evaluation of COVID-19: A Retrospective Cohort Study. *Lancet Haematol.* 7, e671–e678. doi:10.1016/S2352-3026(20)30217-9

Lindemann, S., Tolley, N. D., Dixon, D. A., McIntyre, T. M., Prescott, S. M., Zimmerman, G. A., et al. (2001). Activated Platelets Mediate Inflammatory Signaling by Regulated Interleukin 1β Synthesis. *J. Cell Biol.* 154, 485–490. doi:10.1083/jcb.200105058

Lippi, G., and Favaloro, E. J. (2020a). D-dimer Is Associated with Severity of Coronavirus Disease 2019: A Pooled Analysis. *Thromb. Haemost.* 120, 876–878. doi:10.1055/s-0040-1709650

Lippi, G., Plebani, M., and Henry, B. M. (2020b). Thrombocytopenia Is Associated with Severe Coronavirus Disease 2019 (COVID-19) Infections: A Meta-Analysis. *Clin. Chim. Acta* 506, 145–148. doi:10.1016/j.cca.2020.03.022

Liu, F. P., Dong, J. J., Sun, S. J., Gao, W. Y., Zhang, Z. W., Zhou, X. J., et al. (2012). Autologous Bone Marrow Stem Cell Transplantation in Critical Limb Ischemia: A Meta-Analysis of Randomized Controlled Trials. *Chin. Med. J. (Engl)* 125, 4296–4300. doi:10.3760/cma.j.issn.0366-6999.2012.23.024

Liu, Y., Sun, W., Guo, Y., Chen, L., Zhang, L., Zhao, S., et al. (2020). Association between Platelet Parameters and Mortality in Coronavirus Disease 2019: Retrospective Cohort Study. *Platelets* 31, 490–496. doi:10.1080/09537104.2020.1754383

Lv, L.-H., Wan, Y.-L., Lin, Y., Zhang, W., Yang, M., Li, G.-L., et al. (2012). Anticancer Drugs Cause Release of Exosomes with Heat Shock Proteins from Human Hepatocellular Carcinoma Cells that Elicit Effective Natural Killer Cell Antitumor Responses In Vitro. *J. Biol. Chem.* 287, 15874–15885. doi:10.1074/jbc.M112.340588

Ma, Q., Fan, Q., Xu, J., Bai, J., Han, X., Dong, Z., et al. (2020). Calming Cytokine Storm in Pneumonia by Targeted Delivery of TPCA-1 Using Platelet-Derived Extracellular Vesicles. *Matter* 3, 287–301. doi:10.1016/j.matt.2020.05.017

Maas, S. L. N., Breakefield, X. O., and Weaver, A. M. (2017). Extracellular Vesicles: Unique Intercellular Delivery Vehicles. *Trends Cell Biol.* 27, 172–188. doi:10.1016/j.tcb.2016.11.003

Machlus, K. R., and Italiano, J. E., Jr. (2013). The Incredible Journey: From Megakaryocyte Development to Platelet Formation. *J. Cell Biol.* 201, 785–796. doi:10.1083/jcb.201304054

Mack, M., Kleinschmidt, A., Brühl, H., Klier, C., Nelson, P. J., Cihak, J., et al. (2000). Transfer of the Chemokine Receptor CCR5 between Cells by Membrane-Derived Microparticles: A Mechanism for Cellular Human Immunodeficiency Virus 1 Infection. *Nat. Med.* 6, 769–775. doi:10.1038/77498

Mackman, N., Antoniak, S., Wolberg, A. S., Kasthuri, R., and Key, N. S. (2020). Coagulation Abnormalities and Thrombosis in Patients Infected with SARS-CoV-2 and Other Pandemic Viruses. *Arterioscler. Thromb. Vasc. Biol.* 40, 2033–2044. doi:10.1161/ATVBAHA.120.314514

Maione, F., Cappellano, G., Bellan, M., Raineri, D., and Chiocchetti, A. (2020). Chicken-or-egg Question: Which Came First, Extracellular Vesicles or Autoimmune Diseases? *J. Leukoc. Biol.* 108, 601–616. doi:10.1002/JLB.3MR0120-232R

Malhotra, H., Sheokand, N., Kumar, S., Chauhan, A. S., Kumar, M., Jakhar, P., et al. (2016). Exosomes: Tunable Nano Vehicles for Macromolecular Delivery of Transferrin and Lactoferrin to Specific Intracellular Compartment. *J. Biomed. Nanotechnol* 12, 1101–1114. doi:10.1166/jbn.2016.2229

Mansouri, N., Willis, G. R., Fernandez-Gonzalez, A., Reis, M., Nassiri, S., Mitsialis, S. A., et al. (2019). Mesenchymal Stromal Cell Exosomes Prevent and Revert Experimental Pulmonary Fibrosis through Modulation of Monocyte Phenotypes. *JCI Insight* 4, e128060. doi:10.1172/jci.insight.128060

Marini, J. J., and Gattinoni, L. (2020). Management of COVID-19 Respiratory Distress. *JAMA* 323, 2329–2330. doi:10.1001/jama.2020.6825

Martin-Medina, A., Lehmann, M., Burgy, O., Hermann, S., Baarsma, H. A., Wagner, D. E., et al. (2018). Increased Extracellular Vesicles Mediate WNT5A Signaling in Idiopathic Pulmonary Fibrosis. *Am. J. Respir. Crit. Care Med.* 198, 1527–1538. doi:10.1164/rccm.201708-1580OC

Martinez-Bravo, M.-J., Wahlund, C. J. E., Qazi, K. R., Moulder, R., Lukic, A., Rådmark, O., et al. (2017). Pulmonary Sarcoidosis Is Associated with Exosomal

Vitamin D-Binding Protein and Inflammatory Molecules. *J. Allergy Clin. Immunol.* 139, 1186–1194. doi:10.1016/j.jaci.2016.05.051

Martinod, K., and Wagner, D. D. (2014). Thrombosis: Tangled up in NETs. *Blood* 123, 2768–2776. doi:10.1182/blood-2013-10-463646

Matthay, M. A., Calfee, C. S., Zhuo, H., Thompson, B. T., Wilson, J. G., Levitt, J. E., et al. (2019). Treatment with Allogeneic Mesenchymal Stromal Cells for Moderate to Severe Acute Respiratory Distress Syndrome (START Study): A Randomised Phase 2a Safety Trial. *Lancet Respir. Med.* 7, 154–162. doi:10.1016/S2213-2600(18)30418-1

Maugeri, N., Capobianco, A., Rovere-Querini, P., Ramirez, G. A., Tombetti, E., Valle, P. D., et al. (2018). Platelet Microparticles Sustain Autophagy-Associated Activation of Neutrophils in Systemic Sclerosis. *Sci. Transl. Med.* 10, eaao3089. doi:10.1126/scitranslmed.aao3089

McIntyre, L. A., Stewart, D. J., Mei, S. H. J., Courtman, D., Watpool, I., Granton, J., et al. (2018). Cellular Immunotherapy for Septic Shock. A Phase I Clinical Trial. *Am. J. Respir. Crit. Care Med.* 197, 337–347. doi:10.1164/rccm.201705-1006OC

Mei, S. H. J., Haitsma, J. J., Dos Santos, C. C., Deng, Y., Lai, P. F. H., Slutsky, A. S., et al. (2010). Mesenchymal Stem Cells Reduce Inflammation while Enhancing Bacterial Clearance and Improving Survival in Sepsis. *Am. J. Respir. Crit. Care Med.* 182, 1047–1057. doi:10.1164/rccm.201001-0010OC

Melki, I., Tessandier, N., Zufferey, A., and Boilard, E. (2017). Platelet Microvesicles in Health and Disease. *Platelets* 28, 214–221. doi:10.1080/09537104.2016.1265924

Meng, F., Xu, R., Wang, S., Xu, Z., Zhang, C., Li, Y., et al. (2020). Human Umbilical Cord-Derived Mesenchymal Stem Cell Therapy in Patients with COVID-19: A Phase 1 Clinical Trial. *Signal Transduct. Target. Ther.* 5, 172. doi:10.1038/s41392-020-00286-5

Messner, C. B., Demichev, V., Wendisch, D., Michalick, L., White, M., Freiwald, A., et al. (2020). Ultra-High-Throughput Clinical Proteomics Reveals Classifiers of COVID-19 Infection. *Cell Syst.* 11, 11–24. doi:10.1016/j.cels.2020.05.012

Middleton, E. A., He, X.-Y., Denorme, F., Campbell, R. A., Ng, D., Salvatore, S. P., et al. (2020). Neutrophil Extracellular Traps Contribute to Immunothrombosis in COVID-19 Acute Respiratory Distress Syndrome. *Blood* 136, 1169–1179. doi:10.1182/blood.2020007008

Mo, X., Jian, W., Su, Z., Chen, M., Peng, H., Peng, P., et al. (2020). Abnormal Pulmonary Function in COVID-19 Patients at Time of Hospital Discharge. *Eur. Respir. J.* 55, 2001217. doi:10.1183/13993003.01217-2020

Monsel, A., Zhu, Y.-g., Gennai, S., Hao, Q., Hu, S., Rouby, J.-J., et al. (2015). Therapeutic Effects of Human Mesenchymal Stem Cell-Derived Microvesicles in Severe Pneumonia in Mice. *Am. J. Respir. Crit. Care Med.* 192, 324–336. doi:10.1164/rccm.201410-1765OC

Morrell, C. N., Aggrey, A. A., Chapman, L. M., and Modjeski, K. L. (2014). Emerging Roles for Platelets as Immune and Inflammatory Cells. *Blood* 123, 2759–2767. doi:10.1182/blood-2013-11-462432

Mousavizadeh, L., and Ghasemi, S. (2021). Genotype and Phenotype of COVID-19: Their Roles in Pathogenesis. *J. Microbiol. Immunol. Infect.* 54, 159–163. doi:10.1016/j.jmii.2020.03.022

Muraca, M., Piccoli, M., Franzin, C., Tolomeo, A., Jurga, M., Pozzobon, M., et al. (2017). Diverging Concepts and Novel Perspectives in Regenerative Medicine. *Int. J. Mol. Sci.* 18, 1021. doi:10.3390/ijms18051021

Nicola, M., Alsafi, Z., Sohrabi, C., Kerwan, A., Al-Jabir, A., Iosifidis, C., et al. (2020). The Socio-Economic Implications of the Coronavirus Pandemic (COVID-19): A Review. *Int. J. Surg.* 78, 185–193. doi:10.1016/j.ijsu.2020.04.018

Nolte-'t Hoen, E., Cremer, T., Gallo, R. C., and Margolis, L. B. (2016). Extracellular Vesicles and Viruses: Are They Close Relatives? *Proc. Natl. Acad. Sci. U S A.* 113, 9155–9161. doi:10.1073/pnas.1605146113

Owczarek, K., Szczepanski, A., Milewska, A., Baster, Z., Rajfur, Z., Sarna, M., et al. (2018). Early Events During Human Coronavirus OC43 Entry to the Cell. *Sci. Rep.* 8, 7124. doi:10.1038/s41598-018-25640-0

Park, J., Kim, S., Lim, H., Liu, A., Hu, S., Lee, J., et al. (2019). Therapeutic Effects of Human Mesenchymal Stem Cell Microvesicles in an Ex Vivo Perfused Human Lung Injured with Severe *E. coli* Pneumonia. *Thorax* 74, 43–50. doi:10.1136/thoraxjnl-2018-211576

Park, J. S., Shim, M.-S., Shim, S. H., Yang, H. N., Jeon, S. Y., Woo, D. G., et al. (2011). Chondrogenic Potential of Stem Cells Derived from Amniotic Fluid, Adipose Tissue, or Bone Marrow Encapsulated in Fibrin Gels Containing TGF-B3. *Biomaterials* 32, 8139–8149. doi:10.1016/j.biomaterials.2011.07.043

Pascucci, L., Coccè, V., Bonomi, A., Ami, D., Ceccarelli, P., Ciusani, E., et al. (2014). Paclitaxel Is Incorporated by Mesenchymal Stromal Cells and Released in Exosomes that Inhibit In Vitro Tumor Growth: A New Approach for Drug Delivery. *J. Control. Release* 192, 262–270. doi:10.1016/j.jconrel.2014.07.042

Patel, D. B., Santoro, M., Born, L. J., Fisher, J. P., and Jay, S. M. (2018). Towards Rationally Designed Biomanufacturing of Therapeutic Extracellular Vesicles: Impact of the Bioproduction Microenvironment. *Biotechnol. Adv.* 36, 2051–2059. doi:10.1016/j.biotechadv.2018.09.001

Pedersen, S. F., and Ho, Y.-C. (2020). SARS-CoV-2: A Storm Is Raging. *J. Clin. Invest.* 130, 2202–2205. doi:10.1172/JCI137647

Perrone, F., Piccirillo, M. C., Piccirillo, M. C., Ascierto, P. A., Salvarani, C., Parrella, R., et al. (2020). Tocilizumab for Patients with COVID-19 Pneumonia. The Single-Arm TOCIVID-19 Prospective Trial. *J. Transl Med.* 18, 405. doi:10.1186/s12967-020-02573-9

Phinney, D. G., and Pittenger, M. F. (2017). Concise Review: MSC-Derived Exosomes for Cell-free Therapy. *Stem Cells* 35, 851–858. doi:10.1002/stem.2575

Pittenger, M. F., Discher, D. E., Péault, B. M., Phinney, D. G., Hare, J. M., and Caplan, A. I. (2019). Mesenchymal Stem Cell Perspective: Cell Biology to Clinical Progress. *NPJ Regen. Med.* 4, 22. doi:10.1038/s41536-019-0083-6

Porzionato, A., Zaramella, P., Dedja, A., Guidolin, D., Van Wemmel, K., Macchi, V., et al. (2019). Intratracheal Administration of Clinical-Grade Mesenchymal Stem Cell-Derived Extracellular Vesicles Reduces Lung Injury in a Rat Model of Bronchopulmonary Dysplasia. *Am. J. Physiol. Lung Cell Mol. Physiol.* 316, L6–L19. doi:10.1152/ajplung.00109.2018

Ragni, E., Banfi, F., Barilani, M., Cherubini, A., Parazzi, V., Larghi, P., et al. (2017). Extracellular Vesicle-Shuttled mRNA in Mesenchymal Stem Cell Communication. *Stem Cells* 35, 1093–1105. doi:10.1002/stem.2557

Raposo, G., and Stoorvogel, W. (2013). Extracellular Vesicles: Exosomes, Microvesicles, and Friends. *J. Cell Biol.* 200, 373–383. doi:10.1083/jcb.201211138

Rezaie, J., Aslan, C., Ahmadi, M., Zolbanin, N. M., Kashanchi, F., and Jafari, R. (2021). The Versatile Role of Exosomes in Human Retroviral Infections: From Immunopathogenesis to Clinical Application. *Cell Biosci* 11, 19. doi:10.1186/s13578-021-00537-0

Rezaie, J., Mehranjani, M. S., Rahbarghazi, R., and Shariatzadeh, M. A. (2018). Angiogenic and Restorative Abilities of Human Mesenchymal Stem Cells Were Reduced Following Treatment with Serum from Diabetes Mellitus Type 2 Patients. *J. Cell. Biochem.* 119, 524–535. doi:10.1002/jcb.26211

Rezaie, J., Rahbarghazi, R., Pezeshki, M., Mazhar, M., Yekani, F., Khaksar, M., et al. (2019). Cardioprotective Role of Extracellular Vesicles: A Highlight on Exosome Beneficial Effects in Cardiovascular Diseases. *J. Cell. Physiol* 234, 21732–21745. doi:10.1002/jcp.28894

Ridger, V. C., Boulanger, C. M., Angelillo-Scherrer, A., Badimon, L., Blanc-Brude, O., Bochaton-Piallat, M.-L., et al. (2017). Microvesicles in Vascular Homeostasis and Diseases. *Thromb. Haemost.* 117, 1296–1316. doi:10.1160/TH16-12-0943

Roberts, H., Hoffman, M., and Monroe, D. (2006). A Cell-Based Model of Thrombin Generation. *Semin. Thromb. Hemost.* 32 (Suppl. 1), 32–38. doi:10.1055/s-2006-939552

Romagnoli, G. G., Zelante, B. B., Toniolo, P. c. A., Migliori, I. K., and Barbuto, J. A. M. (2014). Dendritic Cell-Derived Exosomes May Be a Tool for Cancer Immunotherapy by Converting Tumor Cells into Immunogenic Targets. *Front. Immunol.* 5, 692. doi:10.3389/fimmu.2014.00692

Rosell, A., Havervall, S., von Meijenfeldt, F., Hisada, Y., Aguilera, K., Grover, S. P., et al. (2021). Patients with COVID-19 Have Elevated Levels of Circulating Extracellular Vesicle Tissue Factor Activity that Is Associated with Severity and Mortality-Brief Report. *Arterioscler. Thromb. Vasc. Biol.* 41, 878–882. doi:10.1161/ATVBAHA.120.315547

Scheller, N., Herold, S., Kellner, R., Bertrams, W., Jung, A. L., Janga, H., et al. (2019). Proviral MicroRNAs Detected in Extracellular Vesicles from Bronchoalveolar Lavage Fluid of Patients with Influenza Virus-Induced Acute Respiratory Distress Syndrome. *J. Infect. Dis.* 219, 540–543. doi:10.1093/infdis/jiy554

Schneider, D. J., Speth, J. M., Penke, L. R., Wettlaufer, S. H., Swanson, J. A., and Peters-Golden, M. (2017). Mechanisms and Modulation of Microvesicle Uptake in a Model of Alveolar Cell Communication. *J. Biol. Chem.* 292, 20897–20910. doi:10.1074/jbc.M117.792416

Semple, J. W., Italiano, J. E., Jr, and Freedman, J. (2011). Platelets and the Immune Continuum. *Nat. Rev. Immunol.* 11, 264–274. doi:10.1038/nri2956

Sengupta, V., Sengupta, S., Lazo, A., Woods, P., Nolan, A., and Bremer, N. (2020). Exosomes Derived from Bone Marrow Mesenchymal Stem Cells as Treatment for Severe COVID-19. *Stem Cells Dev.* 29, 747–754. doi:10.1089/scd.2020.0080

Shah, T. G., Predescu, D., and Predescu, S. (2019). Mesenchymal Stem Cells-derived Extracellular Vesicles in Acute Respiratory Distress Syndrome: A Review of Current Literature and Potential Future Treatment Options. *Clin. Transl. Med.* 8, 25. doi:10.1186/s40169-019-0242-9

Sheng, G., Chen, P., Wei, Y., Yue, H., Chu, J., Zhao, J., et al. (2020). Viral Infection Increases the Risk of Idiopathic Pulmonary Fibrosis. *Chest* 157, 1175–1187. doi:10.1016/j.chest.2019.10.032

Silini, A. R., Magatti, M., Cargnoni, A., and Parolini, O. (2017). Is Immune Modulation the Mechanism Underlying the Beneficial Effects of Amniotic Cells and Their Derivatives in Regenerative Medicine? *Cell Transplant.* 26, 531–539. doi:10.3727/096368916X693699

Simonson, O. E., Ståhle, E., Hansen, T., Wedin, J. O., Larsson, A., Mattsson, M., et al. (2020). Five-Year Follow-Up After Mesenchymal Stromal Cell-Based Treatment of Severe Acute Respiratory Distress Syndrome. *Am. J. Respir. Crit. Care Med.* 202, 1051–1055. doi:10.1164/rccm.202003-0544LE

Soni, S., Wilson, M. R., O'Dea, K. P., Yoshida, M., Katbeh, U., Woods, S. J., et al. (2016). Alveolar Macrophage-Derived Microvesicles Mediate Acute Lung Injury. *Thorax* 71, 1020–1029. doi:10.1136/thoraxjnl-2015-208032

Soy, M., Keser, G., Atagündüz, P., Tabak, F., Atagündüz, I., and Kayhan, S. (2020). Cytokine Storm in COVID-19: Pathogenesis and Overview of Anti-inflammatory Agents Used in Treatment. *Clin. Rheumatol.* 39, 2085–2094. doi:10.1007/s10067-020-05190-5

Sreeramkumar, V., Adrover, J. M., Ballesteros, I., Cuartero, M. I., Rossaint, J., Bilbao, I., et al. (2014). Neutrophils Scan for Activated Platelets to Initiate Inflammation. *Science* 346, 1234–1238. doi:10.1126/science.1256478

Statello, L., Maugeri, M., Garre, E., Nawaz, M., Wahlgren, J., Papadimitriou, A., et al. (2018). Identification of RNA-Binding Proteins in Exosomes Capable of Interacting with Different Types of RNA: RBP-Facilitated Transport of RNAs into Exosomes. *PLoS One* 13, e0195969. doi:10.1371/journal.pone.0195969

Stebbing, J., Phelan, A., Griffin, I., Tucker, C., Oechsle, O., Smith, D., et al. (2020). COVID-19: Combining Antiviral and Anti-inflammatory Treatments. *Lancet Infect. Dis.* 20, 400–402. doi:10.1016/S1473-3099(20)30132-8

Sun, P., Qie, S., Liu, Z., Ren, J., Li, K., and Xi, J. (2020). Clinical Characteristics of Hospitalized Patients with SARS-CoV-2 Infection: A Single Arm Meta-analysis. *J. Med. Virol.* 92, 612–617. doi:10.1002/jmv.25735

Tang, N., Li, D., Wang, X., and Sun, Z. (2020). Abnormal Coagulation Parameters Are Associated with Poor Prognosis in Patients with Novel Coronavirus Pneumonia. *J. Thromb. Haemost.* 18, 844–847. doi:10.1111/jth.14768

Tao, S.-C., Guo, S.-C., and Zhang, C.-Q. (2017). Platelet-derived Extracellular Vesicles: An Emerging Therapeutic Approach. *Int. J. Biol. Sci.* 13, 828–834. doi:10.7150/ijbs.19776

Thille, A. W., Esteban, A., Fernández-Segoviano, P., Rodriguez, J.-M., Aramburu, J.-A., Vargas-Errázuriz, P., et al. (2013). Chronology of Histological Lesions in Acute Respiratory Distress Syndrome with Diffuse Alveolar Damage: A Prospective Cohort Study of Clinical Autopsies. *Lancet Respir. Med.* 1, 395–401. doi:10.1016/S2213-2600(13)70053-5

Thompson, M., Mei, S. H. J., Wolfe, D., Champagne, J., Fergusson, D., Stewart, D. J., et al. (2020). Cell Therapy with Intravascular Administration of Mesenchymal Stromal Cells Continues to Appear Safe: An Updated Systematic Review and Meta-Analysis. *EClinicalMedicine* 19, 100249. doi:10.1016/j.eclinm.2019.100249

Tkach, M., Kowal, J., and Théry, C. (2018). Why the Need and How to Approach the Functional Diversity of Extracellular Vesicles. *Philos. Trans. R. Soc. Lond. B Biol. Sci.* 373, 20160479. doi:10.1098/rstb.2016.0479

Toniati, P., Piva, S., Cattalini, M., Garrafa, E., Regola, F., Castelli, F., et al. (2020). Tocilizumab for the Treatment of Severe COVID-19 Pneumonia with Hyperinflammatory Syndrome and Acute Respiratory Failure: A Single center Study of 100 Patients in Brescia, Italy. *Autoimmun. Rev.* 19, 102568. doi:10.1016/j.autrev.2020.102568

Torreggiani, E., Perut, F., Perut, F., Roncuzzi, L., Zini, N., Baglìo, S., et al. (2014). Exosomes: Novel Effectors of Human Platelet Lysate Activity. *Eur. Cell Mater.* 28, 137–151. doi:10.22203/ecm.v028a11

Tsiapalis, D., and O'Driscoll, L. (2020). Mesenchymal Stem Cell Derived Extracellular Vesicles for Tissue Engineering and Regenerative Medicine Applications. *Cells* 9, 991. doi:10.3390/cells9040991

Tukmechi, A., Rezaee, J., Nejati, V., and Sheikhzadeh, N. (2013). Effect of Acute and Chronic Toxicity of Paraquat on Immune System and Growth Performance in Rainbow trout, *Oncorhynchus mykiss*. *Aquac. Res.* 45, 1737–1743. doi:10.1111/are.12118

Vader, P., Mol, E. A., Pasterkamp, G., and Schiffelers, R. M. (2016). Extracellular Vesicles for Drug Delivery. *Adv. Drug Deliv. Rev.* 106, 148–156. doi:10.1016/j.addr.2016.02.006

van der Meel, R., Fens, M. H. A. M., Vader, P., van Solinge, W. W., Eniola-Adefeso, O., and Schiffelers, R. M. (2014). Extracellular Vesicles as Drug Delivery Systems: Lessons from the Liposome Field. *J. Control. Release* 195, 72–85. doi:10.1016/j.jconrel.2014.07.049

van Dongen, H. M., Masoumi, N., Witwer, K. W., and Pegtel, D. M. (2016). Extracellular Vesicles Exploit Viral Entry Routes for Cargo Delivery. *Microbiol. Mol. Biol. Rev.* 80, 369–386. doi:10.1128/MMBR.00063-15

Varga, Z., Flammer, A. J., Steiger, P., Haberecker, M., Andermatt, R., Zinkernagel, A. S., et al. (2020). Endothelial Cell Infection and Endotheliitis in COVID-19. *Lancet* 395, 1417–1418. doi:10.1016/S0140-6736(20)30937-5

Volarevic, V., Markovic, B. S., Gazdic, M., Volarevic, A., Jovicic, N., Arsenijevic, N., et al. (2018). Ethical and Safety Issues of Stem Cell-Based Therapy. *Int. J. Med. Sci.* 15, 36–45. doi:10.7150/ijms.21666

Wada, N., Gronthos, S., and Bartold, P. M. (2013). Immunomodulatory Effects of Stem Cells. *Periodontol. 2000* 63, 198–216. doi:10.1111/prd.120242013

Wan, Y., Shang, J., Graham, R., Baric, R. S., and Li, F. (2020). Receptor Recognition by the Novel Coronavirus from Wuhan: An Analysis Based on Decade-Long Structural Studies of SARS Coronavirus. *J. Virol.* 94, e00127-20. doi:10.1128/JVI.00127-20

Wang, B., Yao, K., Huuskes, B. M., Shen, H.-H., Zhuang, J., Godson, C., et al. (2016). Mesenchymal Stem Cells Deliver Exogenous MicroRNA-Let7c via Exosomes to Attenuate Renal Fibrosis. *Mol. Ther.* 24, 1290–1301. doi:10.1038/mt.2016.90

Wang, J., Chen, S., and Bihl, J. (2020). Exosome-Mediated Transfer of ACE2 (Angiotensin-Converting Enzyme 2) from Endothelial Progenitor Cells Promotes Survival and Function of Endothelial Cell. *Oxid. Med. Cell Longev.* 2020, 1–11. doi:10.1155/2020/4213541

Wecht, S., and Rojas, M. (2016). Mesenchymal Stem Cells in the Treatment of Chronic Lung Disease. *Respirology* 21, 1366–1375. doi:10.1111/resp.12911

Wichmann, D., Sperhake, J.-P., Lütgehetmann, M., Steurer, S., Edler, C., Heinemann, A., et al. (2020). Autopsy Findings and Venous Thromboembolism in Patients with COVID-19. *Ann. Intern. Med.* 173, 268–277. doi:10.7326/M20-2003

Wiklander, O. P. B., Brennan, M. Á., Lötvall, J., Breakefield, X. O., and El Andaloussi, S. (2019). Advances in Therapeutic Applications of Extracellular Vesicles. *Sci. Transl. Med.* 11, eaav8521. doi:10.1126/scitranslmed.aav8521

Willis, G. R., Fernandez-Gonzalez, A., Anastas, J., Vitali, S. H., Liu, X., Ericsson, M., et al. (2018). Mesenchymal Stromal Cell Exosomes Ameliorate Experimental Bronchopulmonary Dysplasia and Restore Lung Function through Macrophage Immunomodulation. *Am. J. Respir. Crit. Care Med.* 197, 104–116. doi:10.1164/rccm.201705-0925OC

Xu, P., Zhou, Q., and Xu, J. (2020a). Mechanism of Thrombocytopenia in COVID-19 Patients. *Ann. Hematol.* 99, 1205–1208. doi:10.1007/s00277-020-04019-0

Xu, X., Chen, P., Wang, J., Feng, J., Zhou, H., Li, X., et al. (2020b). Evolution of the Novel Coronavirus from the Ongoing Wuhan Outbreak and Modeling of its Spike Protein for Risk of Human Transmission. *Sci. China Life Sci.* 63, 457–460. doi:10.1007/s11427-020-1637-5

Xu, X., Han, M., Li, T., Sun, W., Wang, D., Fu, B., et al. (2020c). Effective Treatment of Severe COVID-19 Patients with Tocilizumab. *Proc. Natl. Acad. Sci. USA* 117, 10970–10975. doi:10.1073/pnas.2005615117

Xu, Z., Shi, L., Wang, Y., Zhang, J., Huang, L., Zhang, C., et al. (2020d). Pathological Findings of COVID-19 Associated with Acute Respiratory Distress Syndrome. *Lancet Respir. Med.* 8, 420–422. doi:10.1016/S2213-2600(20)30076-X

Yan, R., Zhang, Y., Li, Y., Xia, L., Guo, Y., and Zhou, Q. (2020). Structural Basis for the Recognition of SARS-CoV-2 by Full-Length Human ACE2. *Science* 367, 1444–1448. doi:10.1126/science.abb2762

Yang, L., Liu, S., Liu, J., Zhang, Z., Wan, X., Huang, B., et al. (2020a). COVID-19: Immunopathogenesis and Immunotherapeutics. *Signal Transduct. Target. Ther.* 5, 128. doi:10.1038/s41392-020-00243-2

Yang, X., Yang, Q., Wang, Y., Wu, Y., Xu, J., Yu, Y., et al. (2020b). Thrombocytopenia and its Association with Mortality in Patients with COVID-19. *J. Thromb. Haemost.* 18, 1469–1472. doi:10.1111/jth.14848

Yi, Y., Lagniton, P. N. P., Ye, S., Li, E., and Xu, R.-H. (2020). COVID-19: What Has Been Learned and to Be Learned about the Novel Coronavirus Disease. *Int. J. Biol. Sci.* 16, 1753–1766. doi:10.7150/ijbs.45134

Yoshikawa, F. S. Y., Teixeira, F. M. E., Sato, M. N., and Oliveira, L. M. d. S. (2019). Delivery of MicroRNAs by Extracellular Vesicles in Viral Infections: Could the News Be Packaged? *Cells* 8, 611. doi:10.3390/cells8060611

Zaid, Y., Puhm, F., Allaeys, I., Naya, A., Oudghiri, M., Khalki, L., et al. (2020). Platelets Can Associate with SARS-Cov-2 RNA and Are Hyperactivated in COVID-19. *Circ. Res.* 127, 1404–1418. doi:10.1161/CIRCRESAHA.120.317703

Zemans, R. L., and Matthay, M. A. (2017). What Drives Neutrophils to the Alveoli in ARDS? *Thorax* 72, 1–3. doi:10.1136/thoraxjnl-2016-209170

Zhang, H., Penninger, J. M., Li, Y., Zhong, N., and Slutsky, A. S. (2020a). Angiotensin-converting Enzyme 2 (ACE2) as a SARS-CoV-2 Receptor: Molecular Mechanisms and Potential Therapeutic Target. *Intensive Care Med.* 46, 586–590. doi:10.1007/s00134-020-05985-9

Zhang, P., Li, J., Liu, H., Han, N., Ju, J., Kou, Y., et al. (2020b). Long-term Bone and Lung Consequences Associated with Hospital-Acquired Severe Acute Respiratory Syndrome: A 15-year Follow-Up from a Prospective Cohort Study. *Bone Res.* 8, 8. doi:10.1038/s41413-020-0084-5

Zhao, Y., Zhao, Z., Wang, Y., Zhou, Y., Ma, Y., and Zuo, W. (2020). Single-Cell RNA Expression Profiling of ACE2, the Receptor of SARS-CoV-2. *Am. J. Respir. Crit. Care Med.* 202, 756–759. doi:10.1164/rccm.202001-0179LE

Zhou, P., Yang, X.-L., Wang, X.-G., Hu, B., Zhang, L., Zhang, W., et al. (2020a). A Pneumonia Outbreak Associated with a New Coronavirus of Probable Bat Origin. *Nature* 579, 270–273. doi:10.1038/s41586-020-2012-7

Zhou, W., Wang, H., Yang, Y., Chen, Z.-S., Zou, C., and Zhang, J. (2020b). Chloroquine Against Malaria, Cancers and Viral Diseases. *Drug Discov. Today* 25, 2012–2022. doi:10.1016/j.drudis.2020.09.010

Zhou, X., Xie, F., Wang, L., Zhang, L., Zhang, S., Fang, M., et al. (2020c). The Function and Clinical Application of Extracellular Vesicles in Innate Immune Regulation. *Cell Mol Immunol* 17, 323–334. doi:10.1038/s41423-020-0391-1

Zhu, F.-C., Guan, X.-H., Li, Y.-H., Huang, J.-Y., Jiang, T., Hou, L.-H., et al. (2020). Immunogenicity and Safety of a Recombinant Adenovirus Type-5-Vectored COVID-19 Vaccine in Healthy Adults Aged 18 Years or Older: A Randomised, Double-Blind, Placebo-Controlled, Phase 2 Trial. *Lancet* 396, 479–488. doi:10.1016/S0140-6736(20)31605-6

Zuo, Y., Yalavarthi, S., Shi, H., Gockman, K., Zuo, M., Madison, J. A., et al. (2020). Neutrophil Extracellular Traps in COVID-19. *JCI Insight* 5, e138999. doi:10.1172/jci.insight.138999

4

Targeting M2 Macrophages Alleviates Airway Inflammation and Remodeling in Asthmatic Mice *via* miR-378a-3p/GRB2 Pathway

Qiujie Wang[1,2,3†], Luna Hong[1,2,3†], Ming Chen[1,2,3], Jiangting Shi[1,2,3], Xiaoling Lin[1,2,3], Linjie Huang[1,2,3], Tiantian Tang[1,2,3], Yimin Guo[1,2,3], Xiaoqing Yuan[2,4] and Shanping Jiang[1,2,3]**

[1]Division of Pulmonary and Critical Care Medicine, Sun Yat-sen Memorial Hospital, Sun Yat-sen University, Guangzhou, China, [2]Guangdong Provincial Key Laboratory of Malignant Tumor Epigenetics and Gene Regulation, Medical Research Center, Sun Yat-Sen Memorial Hospital, Sun Yat-sen University, Guangzhou, China, [3]Institute of Pulmonary Diseases, Sun Yat-sen University, Guangzhou, China, [4]Breast Tumor Center, Sun Yat-Sen Memorial Hospital, Sun Yat-Sen University, Guangzhou, China

***Correspondence:**
Xiaoqing Yuan
yuanxq_1986@163.com
Shanping Jiang
jiangshp@mail.sysu.edu.cn

†These authors have contributed equally to this work and share first authorship

Background: Asthma is a complex respiratory disease characterized by airway inflammation and remodeling. MicroRNAs (miRNAs) mediate various cellular processes including macrophage polarization and play an important role in the pathogenesis of asthma. In present study, we aimed to screen miRNA profiling involved in macrophage polarization and investigate its possible functions and mechanisms.

Methods: An OVA-sensitized mouse model was established and 2-chloroadenosine (2-CA) was used to interfere with macrophages. The airway inflammation and remodeling were assessed. The identification and function of M2 alveolar macrophages were assessed by flow cytometry, RT-qPCR, arginase activity and co-culture experiment. Microarray screening was used to select miRNAs which were related to macrophage polarization and RNA interference (RNAi) technique was performed to confirm the function of the selected miRNA and its target gene.

Results: Alveolar macrophages of asthmatic mice showed significant M2 polarization. 2-CA alleviated airway inflammation and remodeling as well as M2 polarization. *In vitro*, IL-4-induced M2 macrophages promoted the proliferation of α-SMA-positive cells. And miRNA profiling showed a remarkable increased expression of miR-378a-3p in IL-4 induced M2 macrophages. Dual luciferase reporter assay confirmed growth factor receptor binding protein 2 (GRB2) was a target gene of miR-378a-3p. A miR-378a-3p inhibitor and knockdown of GRB2 repolarized alveolar macrophages from M1 to M2 phenotype.

Conclusion: Our findings suggest that miR-378a-3p/GRB2 pathway regulates the polarization of alveolar macrophages which acts as a potential therapeutic target for airway inflammation and remodeling in asthma.

Keywords: asthma, airway inflammation, airway remodeling, M2 macrophages, miR-378a-3p, GRB2

Abbreviations: AMs, alveolar macrophages; BALF, bronchoalveolar lavage fluid; GRB2, growth factor receptor binding protein 2; miRNAs, microRNAs; MH-S, murine alveolar macrophages; M1, classically activated macrophages; M2, alternatively activated macrophages; OVA, ovalbumin; 2-CA, 2-chloroadenosine.

INTRODUCTION

Asthma is a chronic inflammatory airway disorder in which eosinophils, neutrophils, macrophages and $CD4^+$ T cells migrate into the airways and release powerful mediators which lead to airway inflammation and remodeling (Anderson 2008; Holgate 2012; Fehrenbach et al., 2017). One of the most notable features of remodeling is airway smooth muscle cells hyperplasia, which strongly predicts airflow limitation and contributes to narrow airways (Brightling et al., 2012; James et al., 2012; Collaborators 2017).

Alveolar macrophages (AMs) have been recognized to play an important role in maintaining immunological homeostasis and host defense in the lungs. It has been reported that the depletion of AMs in mice with asthma attenuated airway inflammation and remodeling (Lee et al., 2015). 2-CA, a purine analog, might cause a competitive reduction in intracellular adenosine content once phagocytized by macrophages, thus reducing the viability of macrophages (Ohtani et al., 1982; Saito and Yamaguchi 1985). Kubota et al. reported that 2-CA would deplete the number of AMs in the bronchoalveolar lavage fluid of mice without any effect on neutrophil or lymphocyte counts (Kubota et al., 1999). Additionally, Hadjigol et al. found that the depletion of pulmonary macrophages by administration of 2-CA into the lungs suppressed airway hyperresponsiveness and reduced the expression of IL-13, TNF-α and IFN-γ (Hadjigol et al., 2020). Macrophages can be polarized into different phenotypes. M1 or 'classically activated' macrophages have high microbicidal and tumoricidal activity, as exemplified by the production of nitric oxide and pro-inflammatory cytokines such as IL-12 and TNF-α, while M2 or 'alternatively activated' macrophages have antiparasitic and tissue remodeling activity, characterized by the production of Arg-1, CD206, FIZZ1, Ym1, CCL17, and CCL24 (Liu and Yang 2013). It has been recognized that M2 macrophages were mainly activated by Th2 cytokines such as IL-4 and IL-13 (Gordon and Martinez 2010; Van Dyken and Locksley 2013). M2 macrophages have been known to facilitate the Th2 immune response and the secretion of chemokines and cytokines which regulate airway inflammation, tissue repair and airway remodeling in the lung (Murray and Wynn 2011; Yang et al., 2012; Byrne et al., 2015). Holtzman reported that the differentiation and accumulation of M2 macrophages might be a hallmark of allergic airway disease (Holtzman 2012).

miRNAs are noncoding small RNAs of 19–25 nucleotide in length which regulate characters of target sites, thus being responsible for diverse biological processes (Shenoy and Blelloch 2014). In our previous study, we have identified that miR-142-5p and miR-130a-3p regulated M2 macrophage polarization and promoted the expression of profibrogenic genes in chronic inflammation (Su et al., 2015). The expression of miRNAs in M2 alveolar macrophages and the mechanisms regarding its polarization require further investigation. In the present study, we aimed to screen miRNA profiling involved in macrophage polarization and investigate its possible functions and mechanisms. Through microarray screening, we identified the candidate miRNA responsible for macrophage polarization and confirmed its target gene.

MATERIALS AND METHODS

Materials

OVA and 2-CA were purchased from Sigma (Missouri, United States). Recombinant murine IL-4 was sourced from Peprotech (New-Jersey, United States). Anti-CD80-PE, anti-CD206-BV650 and anti-CCR3-BV421 were purchased from Biolegend (California, United States). Antibodies for α-SMA and GRB2 were purchased from Abcam (Cambridge, England), F4/80 from Servicebio (Hangzhou, China), ECP-1 from Bioss (Beijing, China). The FISH kit, miRNA mimics, miRNA inhibitor and siRNAs were all purchased from GenePharma (Shanghai, China). The primers for PCR were synthesized by BGI (Beijing, China). The lipofectamine RNAiMax was purchased from Invitrogen (California, United States) while the X-tremeGENE HP DNA Transfection Reagent was purchased from Roche (Basel, Switzerland). The arginase assay kit was obtained from BioAssay (California, United States) and the Cell-Light Edu Apollo567 *In Vitro* Kit was purchased from Ribobio (Guangzhou, China). ELISA kits of IL-4 were from BD Biosciences (New-Jersey, United States) and the dual-Glo®Luciferase assay system was from Promega (Wisconsin, United States).

Animals

Male BALB/c mice aged 6–8 weeks were obtained from the Beijing Vital River Laboratory Animal Technology Company and maintained in the Laboratory Animal Center of Sun Yat-sen University. All the experiments were performed in accordance with the protocol approved by the Institutional Animal Care and Use Committee at the Medical College of Sun Yat-sen University (Approval Number: 2017189).

Establishment of Murine Model With Chronic Asthma

To produce further insights into the macrophage phenotype of asthma, an asthmatic model was established, and 2-CA was used to interfere with macrophages. Male BALB/c mice were randomly divided into three groups with eight mice in each group and treated as follows. 1) The control group were sham sensitized and boosted with normal saline. 2) In OVA group, mice were sensitized and challenged with OVA as previously described (Chen et al., 2011). They were sensitized by intraperitoneal injection (*i.p.*) of 10 μg of OVA emulsified in 1 mg of aluminium hydroxide in a total volume of 200 μl on Day-1 and Day-14. 7 days after the last sensitization (Day-21), mice were in atomization to 2.5% OVA aerosol for up to 30 min every 3 days for 8 weeks. 3) The 2-CA group was comprised of mice that were sensitized and challenged as in the OVA group described above and were additionally treated with 2 μM of 2-CA *via* intratracheal aerosolization using a compressor nebulizer (Dalian, China) before every subsequent three challenges of OVA. The mice were sacrificed 24 h after the final OVA challenge.

BALF Analysis

Bronchoalveolar lavage fluid (BALF) was collected by lavage of lungs with 5 ml of precooled PBS *via* a tracheal cannula and centrifuged (3,000 rpm, 10 min, 4°C). The cells were used to detect the expression of CD80, CD206, and CCR3 by flow cytometry and the supernatants were analyzed for IL-4 by ELISA.

Histology and Blood Analysis

The left lung lobes were harvested for histological analysis and the right lobes were snap-frozen in liquid nitrogen and stored at −80°C for RNA analysis. The blood was collected within heparinized tubes for flow cytometry analysis, while the plasma was kept at −80°C.

Cell Culture and Differentiation

The murine alveolar macrophages (MH-S) purchased from ATCC (Cat. No.: CRL-2019) were maintained in RPMI 1640 containing 10% FBS supplemented with 1% penicillin/streptomycin and incubated at 37°C in a humidified incubator containing 5% CO_2. To obtain M2 alveolar macrophages induced by IL-4 as previously described, MH-S cells were seeded into plastic 6-well plates at a concentration of 1×10^5 cells/mL and incubated in serum-deprived medium for 12 h followed by treatment with IL-4 at 20 ng/ml for 48 h (Su et al., 2015). Then, the cells were harvested for further analysis.

Culture of α-SMA-Positive Cells

Primary α-SMA-positive cells of mice were isolated by the tissue digestion method and purified by differential adhesion as previously described with slight modifications (Chen et al., 2016). Briefly, lungs were removed from 6-8-week-old male BALB/c mice and pulmonary tissues were scraped off. Bronchial tissues were cut into small pieces approximately 1 × 1 × 1 mm in size and incubated in RPMI 1640 containing 1 mg/ml collagenase I at 37°C for 4 h. Thereafter, the adherent cells within 30 min which were mainly airway fibroblasts were discarded and the suspended α-SMA-positive cells were pipetted into another culture flask. Successful isolation of α-SMA-positive cells was determined by immunofluorescence staining of α-SMA (Wang et al., 2020). α-SMA-positive cells were cultured in RPMI 1640 containing 10% FBS and passaged every 6–8 days, and cells from 4 to 9 passages were used for further experiments.

Arginase Activity

To determine the polarization of alveolar macrophages, arginase assay was carried out following the manufacturer's instructions (Ndolo et al., 2010). Total proteins were extracted from MH-S cells using ice-cold RIPA buffer containing 1 mM of PMSF. The supernatants of each sample were added into two separate wells of a 96-well microplate. 5X Substrate Buffer was added into one of the two wells, leaving the other one empty as a blank control. After incubation for 2 h at 37°C, urea reagent was added into all the wells while 5X Substrate Buffer was added into the blank control well. After further incubation for 1 h at room temperature, the optical density (OD) was measured by a microplate reader (Becan, Swissland) at 430 nm. Additionally, urea standard and ddH_2O were used as standard and control, respectively. Arginase activity is calculated as $(OD_{sample}-OD_{blank})/(OD_{standard}-OD_{water}) \times 10.4$ (U/L).

Co-Culture Experiment and EdU Incorporation Assay

For the co-culture experiment, transwell assay was carried out using a 24-well transwell apparatus with 0.4 μm pore size (Corning, New York, United States). α-SMA-positive cells were added into the lower chamber and MH-S cells were added into the upper chamber to explore the effect of M2 macrophages on α-SMA-positive cells. After co-culture for 48 h, proliferation of α-SMA-positive cells were determined using EdU kit according to the manufacturer's instructions (Zhao et al., 2019). Cells were incubated with 50 μM 5-Ethynyl-2′-deoxyuridine (EdU) for 2 h followed by fixation with 4% paraformaldehyde and permeabilization with 0.5% Triton X-100. The incorporated EdU was visualized using Alexa Fluor 567 and the nuclear DNA was stained by Hoechst 33342. The images were obtained using a fluorescence microscope (Olympus, Tokyo, Japan).

Flow Cytometry

Cells from BALF and MH-S cells were examined by flow cytometry. The amount of M1 macrophages ($CD80^+$), M2 macrophages ($CD206^+$) and eosinophils ($CCR3^+$) were identified with specific antibodies and analyzed by multicolor flow cytometer (BD Celesta, New-Jersey, United States). The mean fluorescence intensity (MFI) was calculated by FlowJo software version 10 (Stanford, California, United States).

Enzyme-Linked Immunosorbent Assay

The levels of IL-4 in BALF supernatants and plasma were determined by commercial ELISA kits following the manufacturer's instructions. Briefly, samples were added into a 96-well microplate coated with capture antibody specific for murine IL-4. After incubation overnight at 4°C followed by three washes with washing buffer, detection antibody and streptavidin-peroxidase enzyme were added. After a further incubation for 1 h at room temperature and seven washes, substrate reagents were added, and the reaction was stopped by adding stop solution after 30 min. The intensity of the color was measured by a microplate reader (Tecan, Zurich, Switzerland) at 450 nm, which was subtracted by the absorbance at 570 nm. IL-4 protein levels were calculated with standard curves for each measurement.

Histological Evaluation

The left lungs were perfused with PBS, fixed in 4% paraformaldehyde, embedded in paraffin and cut into 4 μm thick slices. Sections were stained with H&E, Periodic acid-Schiff (PAS) and Masson's trichrome stain for evaluation of airway inflammation, mucus gland hyperplasia and collagen deposition, respectively. Semi-quantitative morphometric analysis was performed where the degrees of inflammation, mucus and collagen deposition were scored from 0 (absent) to 3 (severe), as modified from a previously described protocol (Stellari et al., 2015). The thickness of the airway wall was determined by morphometric analysis on transverse sections after α-SMA staining. F4/80 is a general marker for

TABLE 1 | The mRNA-specific primer sequences.

mRNA name	Forward (5′-3′)	Reverse (5′-3′)
IL-6	CCTCTGGTCTTCTGGAGTACC	ACTCCTTCTGTGACTCCAGC
IL-10	TGCCTGCTCTTACTGACTGG	CTCTAGGAGCATGTGGCTCTG
IL-12	CCCTTGCCCTCCTAAACCA	CTAAGACACCTGGCAGGTCCA
CCL5	ATATGGCTCGGACACCACTC	ACTTGGCGGTTCCTTCGAG
CCL24	CTGTCTGTCTGTCCATCTCTGG	GCTGCTGTTGAAATCCTCCGTT
iNOS	TTCACCCAGTTGTGCATCGACCTA	TCCATGGTCACCTCCAACACAAGA
FIZZ1	TGCTGGGATGACTGCTACTG	AGCTGGGTTCTCCACCTCTT
Arg1	TTGGCTTGCTTCGGAACTCA	TTCATGTGGCGCATTCACAG
GRB2	AACATCCGTGTCCAGGAACC	AAGTCTCCTCTGCGAAAGCC
β-ACTIN	GATCAGCAAGCAGGAGTACGA	CAGCTCAGTAACAGTCCGC

macrophages, and ECP-1 is a marker for eosinophils (Park et al., 2013). Sections were deparaffinized and rehydrated followed by microwave antigen retrieval in citric acid buffer (pH 6.0) and the blocking of endogenous peroxidase with 3% H_2O_2. Thereafter, sections were blocked with 5% BSA for 30 min at room temperature and incubated with the appropriate primary antibody overnight at 4°C in a humidified chamber. Staining was revealed followed by incubation with HRP-conjugated secondary antibody for 1 h at room temperature and the diaminobenzidine substrate kit for peroxidase. Counterstaining was performed using hematoxylin in 2 s.

TABLE 2 | The miRNA-specific primer sequences.

miRNA name	Sequences (5′-3′)
Universal primer	GTGCGTGTCGTGGAGTCG
miR-431-5p	AGGTGTCTTGCAGGCCGT
miR-677-3p	AAGCCAGATGCCGTTCCT
Let-7i-3p	GGCTCTGCGCAAGCTACTG
miR-3093-5p	CGCGGAGCTCACACTAAAA
miR-378a-3p	GGGCACTGGACTTGGAGTC
miR-370-5p	GGGACAGGTCACGTCTCTGC
U6-Forward	GCTTCGGCAGCACATATACTAAAAT
U6-Reverse	CGCTTCACGAATTTGCGTGTCAT

miRNA Microarray Analysis and Target Prediction

Total RNA from MH-S cells which were treated with or without 20 ng/ml of IL-4 for 48 h was isolated using TRIzol and purified with the RNeasy mini kit according to the manufacturer's instructions. The samples were labelled using the miRCURY Hy3/Hy5 Power labelling kit (Exiqon) and hybridized on the miRCURY LNA Array (v.19.0, Exiqon). The slides were then scanned using the Axon GenePix 4000B microarray scanner. Scanned images were then imported into GenePix Pro 6.0 software (Axon) for grid alignment and data extraction. Replicated miRNAs were averaged and miRNAs with intensities ≥30 Units in all samples were chosen for calculation of the normalization factor. Expression data were normalized using median normalization. After normalization, differentially expressed miRNAs between two groups were identified through relative quantity, fold change (≥2.0) and *p*-value (<0.05). Finally, hierarchical clustering was performed to demonstrate distinguishable miRNA expression profiling among samples. The miRNA target prediction tools miRDB, TargetScan7.2 and DIANA-microT were used to identify target genes of candidate miRNAs. Kyoto Encyclopedia of Genes and Genomes (KEGG) analysis of the common target genes were further performed using the DAVID 6.8 website (https://david.ncifcrf.gov/home.jsp).

Quantitative Real-Time PCR

Total RNA from MH-S cells or lungs was extracted using TRIzol according to the manufacturer's instructions. RNA was converted to cDNA with PrimeScript Master Mix for mRNA detection and with Mir-X miRNA First-Strand Synthesis Kit for miRNA evaluation. RT-qPCR was performed using the TB Green Premix Ex Taq II in a LightCycler 480 instrument (Roche, Basel, Switzerland). The fold-change of the transcript mRNA or miRNA was analyzed using the $2^{-\Delta\Delta C}T$ method. Expression of mRNA was normalized to that of β-ACTIN, and mature miRNAs were calculated using U6 as an internal control. The gene-specific primer sequences used for mRNA are listed in **Table 1** and the primers for miRNAs are listed in **Table 2**.

Fluorescence *In situ* Hybridization

Fluorescence *in situ* hybridization was performed on paraffin-embedded sections of lungs according to the manufacturer's instructions. First, the sections were deparaffinized and rehydrated. After rinsing with PBS, the slides were digested with protease K for 20 min at 37°C and then dehydrated by ethanol. The sections were prehybridized in denaturation solution for 8 min at 78°C and dehydrated by ethanol again. Then the sections were hybridized with 20 ng/μl Cy3-labelled LNA miR-378a-3p probe overnight at 37°C. After post-hybridization washes, the nuclei were counterstained with DAPI and the fluorescence images were captured by a confocal microscope (Olympus, Tokyo, Japan).

Transfection of miRNAs or siRNAs

To determine the effect of miR-378a-3p or GRB2 on polarization of alveolar macrophages or the influence of miR-378a-3p on GRB2, we used RNAi to silence miR-378a-3p or GRB2. MH-S cells were seeded into 6-well plates at a density of 1×10^5 cells/ml, and transfection was performed when cells were at 60~70%

TABLE 3 | Sequences of the specific miRNA and siRNA.

Sequence name	Forward (5′-3′)	Reverse (5′-3′)
miR-378a-3p mimic	ACUGGACUUGGAGUCAGAAGG	UUCUGACUCCAAGUCCAGUUU
miRNA mimics NC	UUCUCCGAACGUGUCACGUTT	ACGUGACACGUUCGGAGAATT
miR-378a-3p inhibitor	CCUUCUGACUCCAAGUCCAGU	–
miRNA inhibitor NC	CAGUACUUUUGUGUAGUACAA	–
si-GRB2	GGAACCAGCAGAUAUUCUUTT	AAGAAUAUCUGCUGGUUCCTT
siRNA NC	UUCUCCGAACGUGUCACGUTT	ACGUGACACGUUCGGAGAATT

confluence. 100 pmol of miR-378a-3p mimics, miR-378a-3p inhibitor, siRNA specific to GRB2 (si-GRB2) or negative control siRNA (si-NC) were mixed with 250 µl Opti-MEM, and 5 µl Lipofectamine RNAiMax was mixed with 250 µl Opti-MEM for 5 min. Then the RNA complexes and liposome complexes were mixed together, incubated for 20 min and transfected into cells. The cells were harvested 48 h later for further analysis. Sequences of miR-378a-3p inhibitor and si-GRB2 are provided in **Table 3**.

Western Blot

Protein lysates extracted from lung tissues or MH-S cells which were transfected with miR-378a-3p mimics, miR-378a-3p inhibitor, or si-GRB2 were centrifuged at 16,000 *g* for 20 min at 4°C and quantified using the BCA method. 20 µg of proteins were separated by 10% SDS-PAGE and transferred onto PVDF membranes. After blocking, blots were probed with primary antibodies against GRB2 or β-tubulin at 4°C overnight followed by incubation with HRP-conjugated secondary antibody for 1 h at room temperature. Protein bands were detected by enhanced chemiluminescence assay and the blots were visualized by Minichemi Imaging System (Beijing, China). Densitometric quantitation of band intensity was carried out with ImageJ software version 5.0 (NIH, Maryland, United States).

Dual Luciferase Reporter Assay

To identify the binding site between miR-378a-3p and GRB2, the 3′ untranslated region (UTR) of GRB2 including wild type (WT) or mutant type (MUT) of the binding site was synthesized and cloned into the SV40-firefly_Luciferase-MCS vectors (Genechem, Shanghai, China) and 293T cells were used for reporter assays. 293T cells (5×10^4 cells per well) were seeded into 24-well plates and transfected with miR-378a-3p mimics or negative control (20 pmol) for 24 h when the cells reached 60–70% confluence. Then cells were co-transfected with WT or MUT GRB2 3′ UTR vector and the control vector coding for Renilla luciferase using X-tremeGENE HP DNA transfection reagent for 48 h. Cells were harvested using 300 µl of Passive Lysis Buffer and luciferase activities were measured by a microplate reader (Zeng et al., 2019). The firefly luciferase activity was normalized to that of Renilla luciferase. Sequences of miR-378a-3p mimics and negative control are provided in **Table 3**.

Statistical Analysis

The quantitative data were presented as the mean ± SEM. For quantification analysis, each experiment was performed at least three times. Statistical analysis was conducted using GraphPad Prism software version 5.0 (GraphPad, California, United States) and SPSS software version 20.0 (SPSS, Chicago, United States). Analysis between two groups was performed using Student's t-test and multiple comparisons of continuous variables were analyzed using one-way analysis of variance. Differences were considered statistically significant when the *p*-value was less than 0.05.

RESULTS

Airway Inflammation and Remodeling Along With M2 Macrophage Polarization in OVA-Sensitized Mice With Chronic Asthma

In the present study, we have developed an OVA-sensitized mouse model (**Figure 1A**). In asthmatic mice, HE staining revealed inflammatory cell infiltration; a large number of PAS^+ goblet cells were detected by PAS staining; immunohistochemical staining of ECP-1 showed a significant increase of eosinophilic infiltration; the total amount of collagen was significantly increased as defined by Masson staining; and marked airway smooth muscle cell hyperplasia and hypertrophy have been identified by α-SMA immunohistochemical staining of the lungs (**Figure 1B**). IL-4 levels of plasma and BALF in OVA-challenged mice were significantly increased (**Figure 1C**). The results of flow cytometry analysis showed that the MFI of eosinophils in BALF was increased in OVA-challenged mice (**Figure 1D**). These data showed the airway inflammation and remodeling in OVA-sensitized mice.

A large number of $F4/80^+$ macrophages were detected around asthmatic airways in the lungs of asthmatic mice (**Figure 1E**). With OVA challenges, a significant downregulation of $CD80^+$ M1 macrophages and upregulation of $CD206^+$ M2 macrophages were detected in the BALF of asthmatic mice (**Figure 1F**). In addition, OVA challenge resulted in a significant increase in M2 markers such as FIZZ1, Arg1, and IL-10, with a decrease in M1 markers such as IL-6, IL-12, and iNOS (**Figure 1G**). These results indicated strong M2 macrophage infiltration in the BALF and lungs of asthmatic mice.

Inhibition of M2 Macrophage Polarization by 2-CA is Accompanied by Alleviation of Airway Inflammation and Remodeling

The timeline in which 2-CA was used to reduce AMs was depicted in **Figure 2A**. Treatment with 2-CA effectively reduced the number of $F4/80^+$ macrophages in asthmatic mice

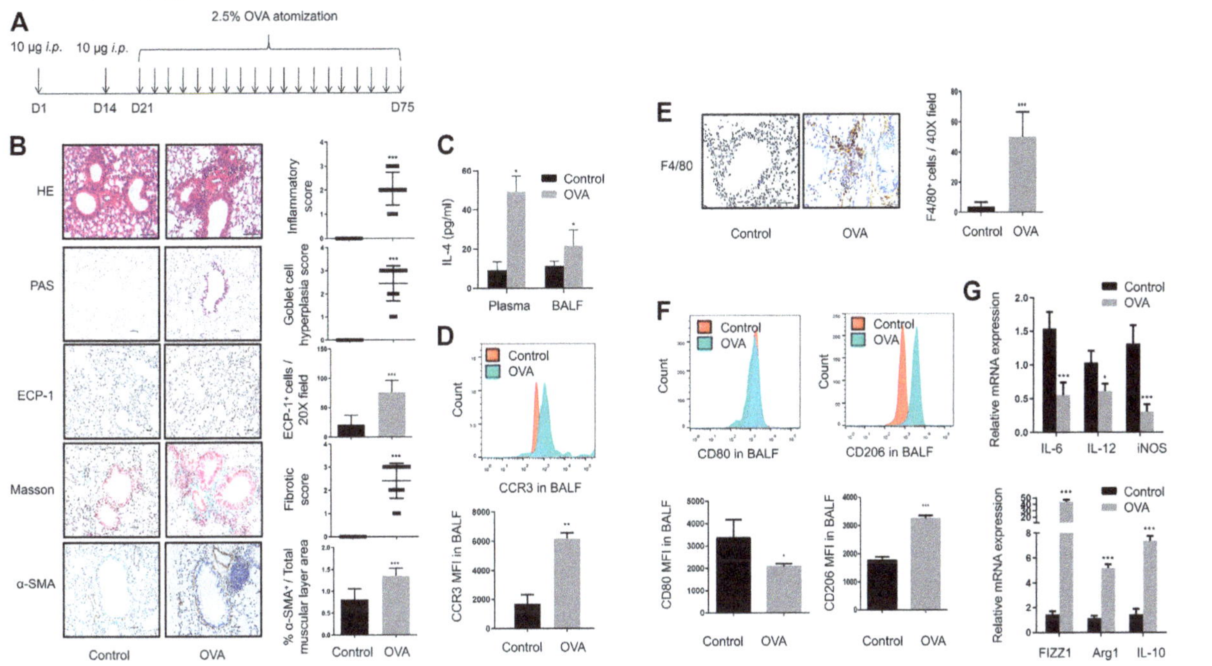

FIGURE 1 | Airway inflammation and remodeling along with M2 macrophage polarization in OVA-sensitized mice with chronic asthma **(A)**. Timeline of establishment of the chronic asthma model which was sensitized and challenged with OVA for 8 weeks **(B)**. Representative images of HE, PAS, Masson, ECP-1, and α-SMA immunohistochemistry staining of lung sections from control and OVA-sensitized mice as shown at a magnification of 20X. Scale bar: 50 μm. Bar graph represent morphometric semi-quantitative analysis of histopathological data from HE, PAS, and Masson staining. Quantification of ECP-1$^+$ cells per 20X field and percentage of α-SMA$^+$/total muscular layer area **(C)**. IL-4 levels in plasma and BALF from control and OVA-sensitized mice assessed by ELISA **(D)**. Expression of CCR3 in BALF from control and OVA-sensitized mice as determined by flow cytometry analysis. The representative histograms and quantitation of the MFI are shown **(E)**. Representative images of F4/80 immunohistochemistry staining of lung sections from control and OVA-sensitized mice as shown at a magnification of 40X. Scale bar: 50 μm. Quantification of F4/80$^+$ cells per 40X field **(F)**. Expression of CD80 and CD206 in alveolar macro-phages of BALF from control and OVA-sensitized mice as determined by flow cytometry analysis. The representative histograms and quantitation of the MFI are shown **(G)**. Expression of IL-6, IL-12, iNOS, FIZZ1, Arg1, and IL-10 in lungs from control and OVA-sensitized mice evaluated by RT-qPCR. (n = 8, $^*p < 0.05$, $^{**}p < 0.01$, $^{***}p < 0.001$ vs. control mice).

(**Figure 2B**). With 2-CA management, the downregulation of CD80$^+$ M1 macrophages and upregulation of CD206$^+$ M2 macrophages in BALF of asthmatic mice could be reversed (**Figure 2C**). In addition, 2-CA challenge within asthmatic mice resulted in a decrease in M2 markers such as FIZZ1, Arg1, and IL-10 and an increase in M1 markers such as IL-6, IL-12, and iNOS, which suggested that 2-CA could inhibit M2 polarization in asthmatic mice (**Figure 2D**). Meanwhile, the inflammatory cell infiltration, goblet cell hyperplasia, eosinophilic infiltration, subepithelial fibrosis, and smooth muscle cell hyperplasia and hypertrophy in the lungs of asthmatic mice could be alleviated by 2-CA treatment (**Figure 2E**). Consistent with this finding, the increased IL-4 levels of plasma and BALF and MFI of eosinophils in BALF in OVA-challenged mice were reduced by 2-CA (**Figures 2F,G**). The results suggested that 2-CA could attenuate airway inflammation and remodeling in parallel with the reduction of M2 macrophages in asthmatic mice.

IL-4-Induced M2 Macrophages Promote the Proliferation of α-SMA-positive Cells *in vitro*

In addition to *in vivo* experiment, macrophage polarization also affects the function of airway cells *in vitro*. After IL-4 induction, MH-S cells displayed a highly enhanced expression of CD206 and a markedly reduced expression of CD80 by flow cytometry (**Figure 3A**). Also, the mRNA expression of FIZZ1, Arg1, and CCL24 were largely increased ($p < 0.05$) while IL-6, CCL5, and iNOS were significantly reduced (**Figure 3B**). Besides, the expression of arginase was significantly increased (**Figure 3C**). To investigate the effect of M2 macrophages on α-SMA-positive cells, MH-S cells were stimulated with IL-4 and then co-cultured with α SMA-positive cells to evaluate the proliferative ability of α-SMA-positive cells. As shown in **Figure 3D**, primary α-SMA-positive cells were identified by the typical "hill and valley" growth pattern and immunofluorescent staining of α-SMA. The proliferative ability of α-SMA-positive cells was strongly enhanced when co-cultured with IL-4-induced M2 macrophages (**Figure 3E**).

MiR-378a-3p is Upregulated in IL-4-Induced M2 Macrophages

To explore the important roles of miRNAs in macrophage polarization, we identified differentially expressed miRNAs in murine alveolar macrophages (MH-S) exposed to IL-4 *via* miRNA microarray analysis. The results showed that 13

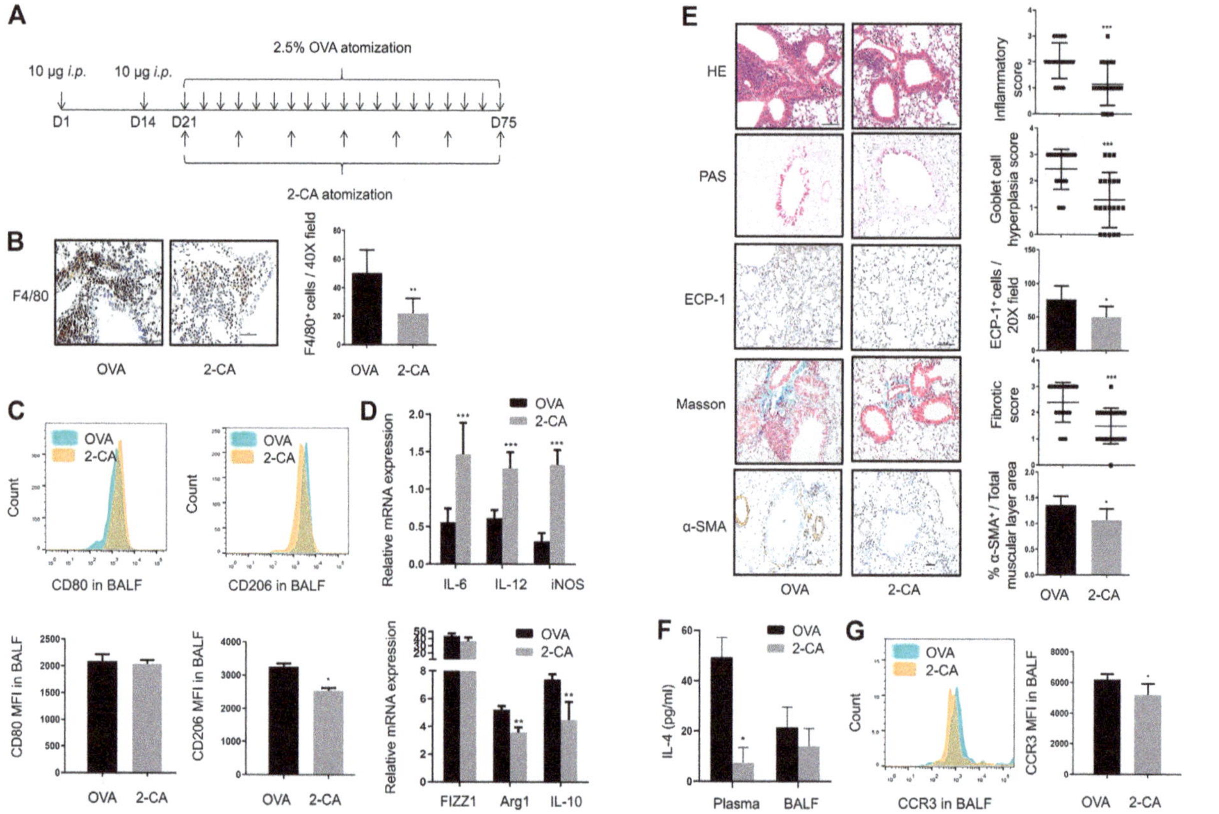

FIGURE 2 | Inhibition of M2 macrophage polarization by 2-CA is accompanied by alleviation of airway inflammation and remodeling **(A)**. Timeline of mice with chronic asthma treated with 2-CA before every subsequent three challenges of OVA **(B)**. Representative images of F4/80 immunohistochemistry staining of lung sections from OVA-sensitized and 2-CA-treated mice as shown at a magnification of 40X. Scale bar: 50 μm. Quantification of F4/80⁺ cells per 40X field **(C)**. Expression of CD80 and CD206 in alveolar macrophages of BALF from OVA-sensitized and 2-CA-treated mice as determined by flow cytometry analysis. The representative histograms and quantitation of the MFI are shown **(D)**. Expression of IL-6, IL-12, iNOS, FIZZ1, Arg1, and IL-10 in lungs from OVA-sensitized and 2-CA-treated mice evaluated by RT-qPCR **(E)**. Representative images of HE, PAS, Masson, ECP-1, and α-SMA immunohistochemistry staining of lung sections from OVA-sensitized and 2-CA-treated mice as shown at a magnification of 20X. Scale bar: 50 μm. Bar graph represent morphometric semi-quantitative analysis of histopathological data from HE, PAS and Masson staining. Quantification of ECP-1⁺ cells per 20X field and percentage of α-SMA⁺/total muscular layer area **(F)**. IL-4 levels in plasma and BALF from OVA-sensitized and 2-CA-treated mice assessed by ELISA **(G)**. Expression of CCR3 in BALF from OVA-sensitized and 2-CA-treated mice as determined by flow cytometry analysis. The representative histograms and quantitation of the MFI are shown. (n = 8, $^*p < 0.05$, $^{**}p < 0.01$, $^{***}p < 0.001$ vs. asthmatic mice).

miRNAs were upregulated, and 49 miRNAs were down-regulated between groups (**Figure 4A**). We further determined the expression of a subset of miRNAs to validate the microarray results by RT-qPCR (**Figure 4B**). Among these miRNAs, miR-677-3p, miR-3093-5p, miR-378a-3p, and miR-370a-5p were found to be significantly upregulated. The same subset of miRNAs was detected in the lungs of OVA-challenged mice by RT-qPCR (**Figure 4B**). Notably, miR-378a-3p was the most upregulated miRNA both in IL-4-induced M2 macrophages and the lungs of mice with chronic asthma, which might be involved in M2 polarization of macrophages (Vats et al., 2006; Eichner et al., 2010). In accordance with the results, FISH analysis also showed an increase of miR-378a-3p expression in the lungs of asthmatic mice (**Figure 4C**). Besides, the correlation coefficient between CD80 MFI in BALF and relative miR-378a-3p expression was negative while the correlation coefficient between CD206 MFI in BALF and relative miR-378a-3p expression was positive, though both of them didn't achieve statistical significance (**Figure 4D**).

MiR-378a-3p Directly Targets GRB2 in Murine Alveolar Macrophages

We used different target-prediction algorithms including miRDB, TargetScan7.2 and DIANA-microT to screen for mRNA targets of miR-378a-3p. 21 target genes were predicted by all three databases (**Figure 5A**). Among these target genes, KEGG_PATHWAY analysis suggested that GRB2 might participate in osteoclast differentiation and T cell receptor signaling pathway which was associated with macrophage polarization. Therefore we hypothesized that GRB2 might participate in alveolar macrophage differentiation since osteoclasts acted as a type of macrophage (**Figure 5B**). Firstly, we found two identical seed-matching sites exist between the 3′-UTR of GRB2 and miR-378a-3p (**Figure 5C**). And there is no

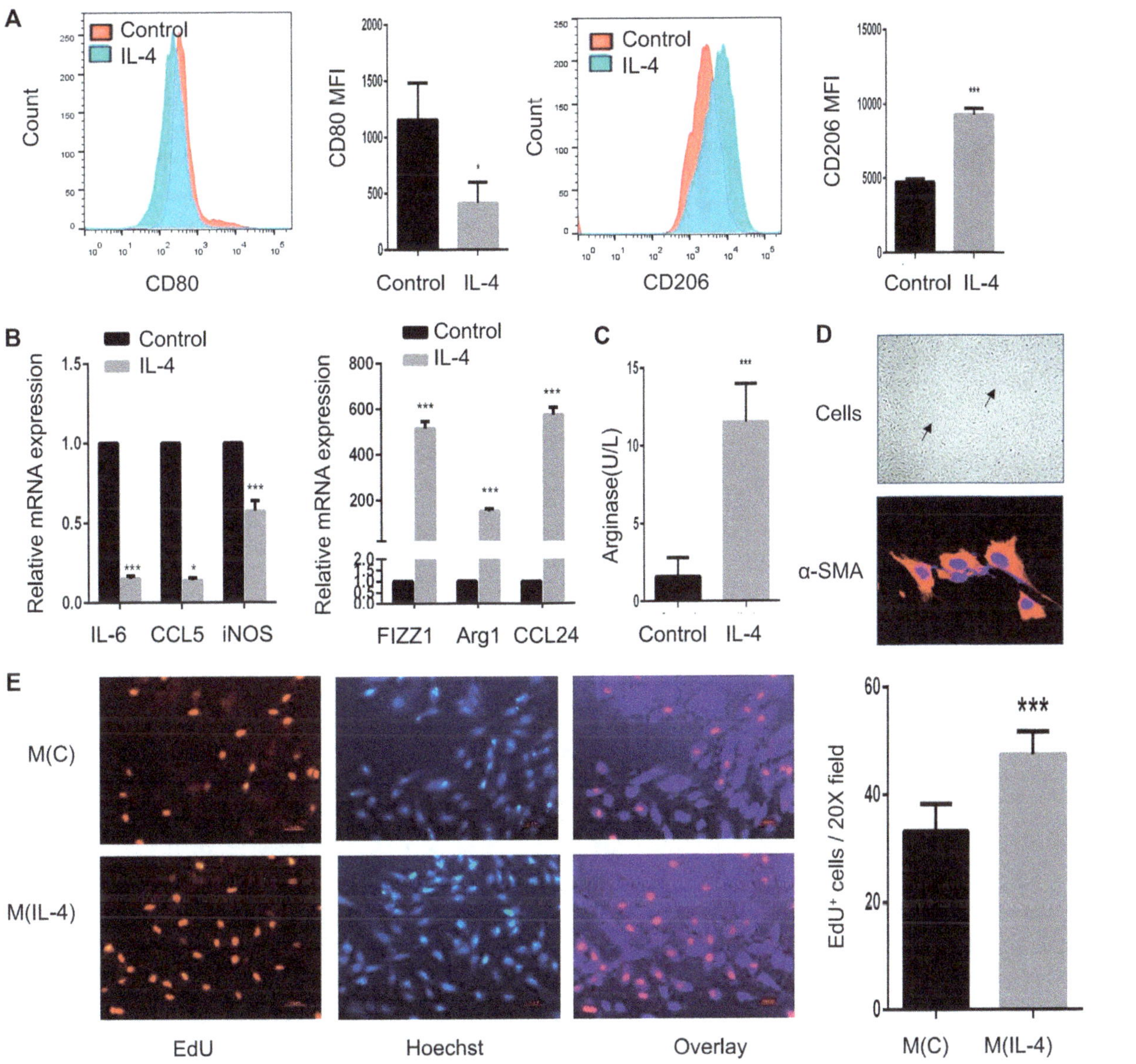

FIGURE 3 | IL-4-induced M2 macrophages promote the proliferation of α-SMA-positive cells *in vitro*. MH-S cells were treated for 48 h with 20 ng/ml IL-4, and the identification and function of IL-4-induced M2 macrophages were analyzed **(A–C)** **(A)**. Expression of CD80 and CD206 in IL-4-induced M2 macrophages evaluated by flow cytometry analysis. The representative histograms and quantitation of the MFI are shown **(B)**. Expression of IL-6, CCL5, iNOS, FIZZ1, Arg1, and CCL24 in IL-4-induced M2 macrophages evaluated by RT-qPCR **(C)**. Arginase in IL-4-induced M2 macrophages measured by the arginase assay **(D)**. Representative image of α-SMA-positive cells under light microscope and immunofluorescent staining of α-SMA as shown at a magnification of 40X. Scale bar: 50 μm. The solid arrow points to the hill and the dotted arrow points to the valley **(E)**. MH-S cells were stimulated with 20 ng/ml IL-4 for 48 h and co-cultured with primary α-SMA-positive cells for another 48 h. M(C) means MH-S cells treated without IL-4 and M(IL-4) means with IL-4. The proliferation of α-SMA-positive cells detected by EdU incorporation assay as shown at a magnification of 20X. Scale bar: 10 μm. Quantitation of percentage of EdU^+ cells per 20X field. ($^*p < 0.05$, $^{***}p < 0.001$ vs. control).

target site at the 3′UTR of GRB2 for miRNAs identified in microarray analysis besides miR-378a-3p. To validate whether GRB2 was a target gene of miR-378a-3p, we further carried out gain and loss of function analysis as well as dual luciferase reporter assay. The mRNA and protein expression of GRB2 were significantly decreased after MH-S cells were transfected with miR-378a-3p mimics and increased after transfected with miR-378a-3p inhibitor, implying that the reduced transcription and translation of GRB2 caused by miR-378a-3p was reversed by miR-378a-3p inhibitor (**Figure 5D**). Furthermore, the results of dual luciferase reporter assay showed that the luciferase activity decreased obviously in cells co-transfected with the wild-type binding site vector in the presence of miR-378a-3p. On the contrary, cells containing the mutated binding sites vector did not show such suppression (**Figure 5E**). These data confirmed that GRB2 was a specific target of miR-378a-3p.

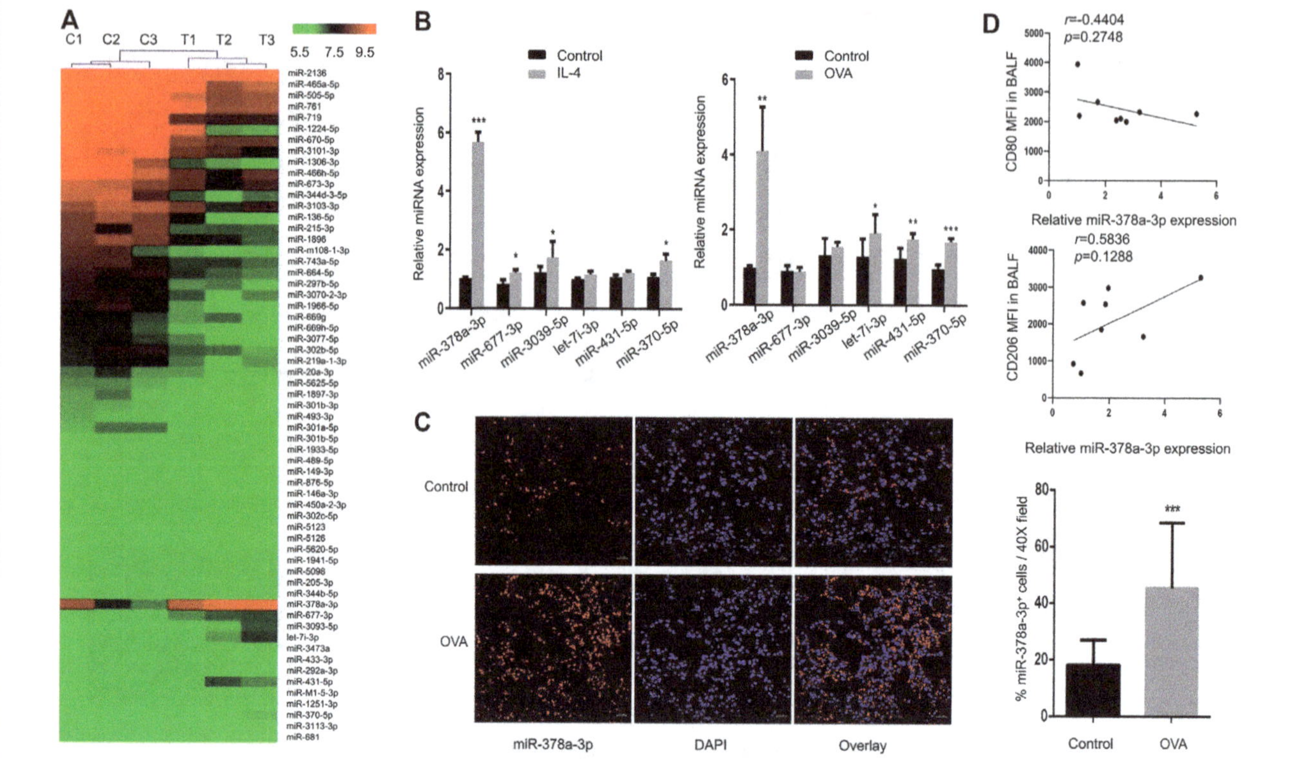

FIGURE 4 | MiR-378a-3p is upregulated in IL-4-induced M2 macrophages **(A)**. Differential expression levels of miRNAs (fold changes ≥2 and p-value < 0.05) in MH-S cells treated with or without 20 ng/ml IL-4 for 48 h were presented in a heatmap. The mean fluorescence intensity was calculated as the average for three replicates **(B)**. Expression levels of the candidate miRNAs in MH-S cells following 20 ng/ml IL-4 for 48 h treatment and in the lungs of control and OVA-sensitized mice as determined by RT-qPCR **(C)**. Representative images of FISH for miR-378a-3p in the lung tissues of control and OVA-sensitized mice as shown at a magnification of 40X. Scale bar: 20 μm. Quantitation of percentage of miR-378a-3p$^+$ cells per 40X field **(D)**. Scatter plots of CD80, CD206 MFI in BALF and relative miR-378a-3p expression from control and OVA-sensitized mice. Individual data points are shown with p value and linear regression. (n = 8, $^*p$ < 0.05, $^{**}p$ < 0.01, $^{***}p$ < 0.001 vs. control).

MiR-378a-3p Contributes to Alveolar Macrophage Polarization by Targeting GRB2

As showed in **Figure 6A**, M1 markers such as IL-6, IL-12, and iNOS were downregulated while M2 markers such as FIZZ1, Arg1, and IL-10 were upregulated in alveolar macrophages transfected with miR-378a-3p mimics. When alveolar macrophages were transfected with miR-378a-3p inhibitor, M1 markers were upregulated while M2 markers were downregulated (**Figure 6B**), suggesting that miR-378a-3p might promote M2 polarization of alveolar macrophages. The function of GRB2 in alveolar macrophage polarization was evaluated by silencing GRB2 expression with RNAi. As shown in **Figure 6C**, the mRNA and protein expression of GRB2 was significantly repressed after si-GRB2 silencing (p < 0.05). Silencing of GRB2 also resulted in a downregulation of IL-6, IL-12, and iNOS mRNA with an upregulation FIZZ1, Arg1, and IL-10 mRNA in alveolar macrophages (**Figure 6D**). These data suggested that miR-378a-3p might contribute to M2 polarization of alveolar macrophages *via* the direct downregulation of GRB2.

DISCUSSION

Since M2/M1 imbalance has been a recognized pathology in asthma, studies have been conducted to explore the therapeutic potential of repolarizing M2 to M1 macrophages. In this study, we found that M2 macrophages were the predominant phenotype in the lungs and BALF of mice with chronic asthma induced by OVA. We also observed that the predominant M2 phenotype could be repolarized to the M1 phenotype by 2-CA in mice with chronic asthma, which was accompanied by the alleviation of airway inflammation and remodeling. These data suggested that 2-CA could reduce airway inflammation and remodeling in asthmatic mice by shifting macrophages from M2 to M1.

Recently, miRNAs have been found to affect the M1/M2 macrophage polarization (Self-Fordham et al., 2017; Li et al., 2018). For example, miRNA-9, miRNA-27, miRNA-155 and miRNA-125b could promote M1 polarization while miRNA-21, miRNA-223, miRNA-34, let-7c, miRNA-146a, and miRNA-511 could promote M2 polarization in various tissues (Feketea et al., 2019). However, the role of miRNAs in M2 alveolar macrophage polarization still needs more explorations. A continuous cell line of murine alveolar macrophages, designated MH-S, has been established and been used in our experiments. In our study, we confirmed that MH-S cells displayed a M2 phenotype after IL-4 induction. Then, differentially expressed miRNAs in M2 MH-S cells were screened, and miR-378a-3p was the most significantly increased miRNA in M2 MH-S cells and the lungs of mice

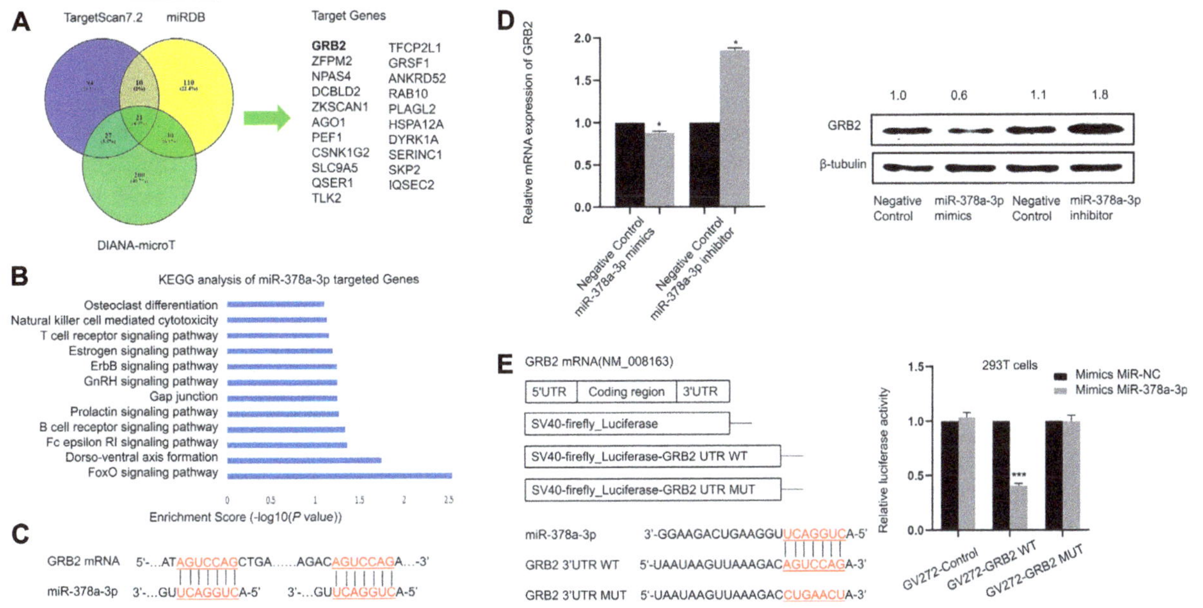

FIGURE 5 | miR-378a-3p directly targets GRB2 in murine alveolar macrophages (A). Target gene prediction of miR-378a-3p with three bioinformatics tools and the results are shown in the Venn diagram **(B)**. KEGG pathway analysis of target genes of miR-378a-3p **(C)**. The binding sites between miR-378a-3p and target gene GRB2 **(D)**. RT-qPCR and Western blotting assay of GRB2 expression in MH-S cells treated with miR-378a-3p mimics and miR-378a-3p inhibitor or control **(E)**. Diagram of the wild-type and a mutated-type of binding site between miR-378a-3p and GRB2 and luciferase reporter assays for 293T cells transfected with GV272 vectors carrying GRB2-3′ UTR *versus* GRB2-MUT-3′ UTR in the absence or presence of miR-378a-3p mimics. (*p < 0.05, **p < 0.01, ***p < 0.001 vs. control).

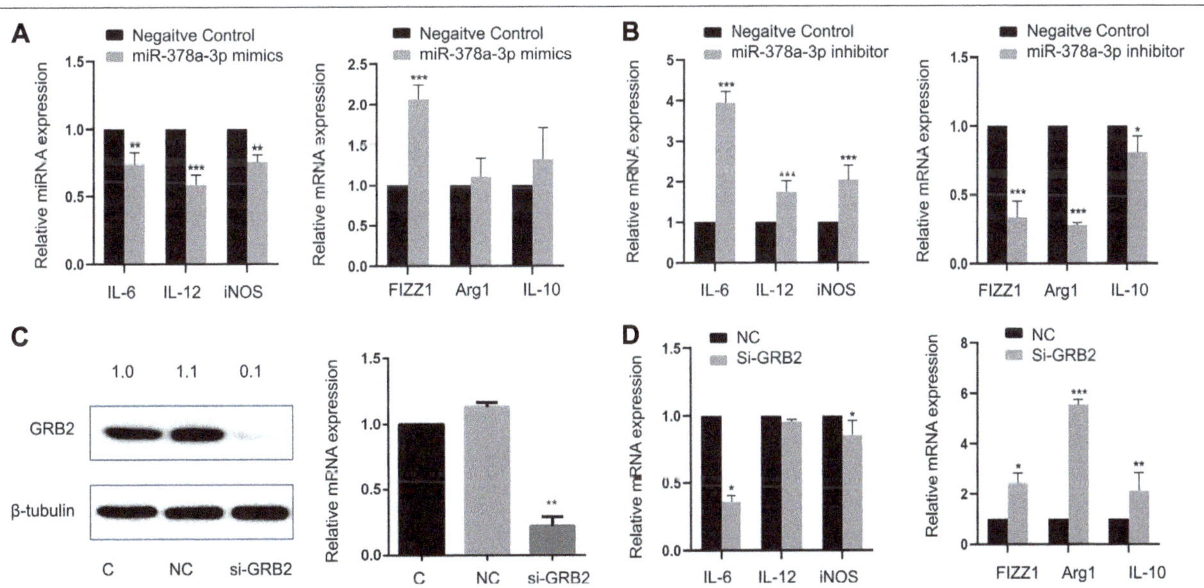

FIGURE 6 | (A) MiR-378a-3p contributes to alveolar macrophage polarization by targeting GRB2 Expression of IL-6, IL-12, iNOS, FIZZ1, Arg1, and IL-10 in MH-S cells treated with 100 pmol miR-378a-3p mimics or negative control for 48 h valuated by RT-qPCR **(B)**. Expression of IL-6, IL-12, iNOS, FIZZ1, Arg1, and IL-10 in MH-S cells treated with 100 pmol miR-378a-3p inhibitor or negative control for 48 h evaluated by RT-qPCR **(C)**. GRB2 mRNA and protein in MH-S cells treated with 100 pmol si-GRB2 for 48 h measured by RT-qPCR and Western Blot **(D)**. Expression of IL-6, IL-12, iNOS, FIZZ1, Arg1, and IL-10 in MH-S cells treated with 100 pmol si-GRB2 for 48 h evaluated by RT-qPCR. (*p < 0.05, **p < 0.01, ***p < 0.001 vs. control).

with chronic asthma. miR-378a-3p is encoded in an intronic region of PPARGC1b, a protein associated with M2 polarization of macrophages (Vats et al., 2006; Eichner et al., 2010). Li et al. reported that miR-378 was increased in the peripheral blood and lungs of asthmatic children (Li et al., 2019). Rückerl et al. reported that miR-378-3p was significantly upregulated by IL-4 in peritoneal macrophages and was involved in IL-4-driven macrophage proliferation in mice implanted with *Brugia malayi* nematodes (Ruckerl et al., 2012), which didn't mention the role of downstream gene targets. In our study, we found that miR-378a-3p inhibitor promoted a shift from the M2 to M1 phenotype of alveolar macrophages, which meant that miR-378a-3p might participate in M2 polarization of alveolar macrophages.

With online target prediction tools, we have identified GRB2 as a target of miR-378a-3p, which have been verified by gain and loss of function analysis as well as luciferase reporter assay. GRB2 is a receptor-bound protein in various cells which link signaling events initiated by tyrosine kinases to downstream pathways. It can directly bind to activated EGF receptor phosphorylated tyrosine, participate in EGF receptor mediated signal transduction, and indirectly participate in insulin receptor-mediated signal transduction by binding with SHC phosphorylated tyrosine. GRB2 can combine with SHC and SOS at the same time to form SHC-GRB2-SOS complex and activate SOS. The activated SOS can combine with Ras protein on plasma membrane, and activate it to cause signal cascade reaction. (Rao 1996). It is reported that reducing GRB2 expression by shRNA or by gene targeting slowed down the osteoclast-like differentiation of cells (Levy-Apter et al., 2014). CD206 activation mediated GRB2 recruitment to initiate phagocytosis signaling in human monocyte-derived macrophages (Rajaram et al., 2017). Several studies have shown the important effects of GRB2 in eosinophils, mast cells and T cells in allergic diseases (Ben Baruch-Morgenstern et al., 2014; Massoud et al., 2016; Lin et al., 2018). Xu et al. reported that miR-378a-3p sensitized ovarian cancer cells to cisplatin through targeting MAPK1/GRB2 (Xu et al., 2018). Yu et al. suggested that LMV induced osteogenic differentiation of BMSCs through miR-378a-3p/Grb2 pathway to improve bone mineral density and mechanical properties (Yu et al., 2020). However, whether GRB2 participated in alveolar macrophage polarization is still unknown. We demonstrated that the knockdown of GRB2 resulted in repolarization of alveolar macrophages from the M1 to M2 phenotype. Taken together, these findings indicated that the miR-378a-3p/GRB2 axis might act as a mediator of M2 polarization of alveolar macrophages. However, whether other miRNAs or target genes participate in functions of macrophage deserves further experiments.

In conclusion, our study has provided evidences that miR-378a-3p is upregulated in M2 alveolar macrophages which aggravate airway inflammation and remodeling in asthmatic mice. Persistent elevation of miR-378a-3p levels in alveolar macrophages promotes the switch towards the M2 phenotype by suppressing the expression of GRB2. Our results provide the possibility that the inhibition of miR-378a-3p may serve as a promising therapeutic strategy for chronic asthma which deserves further *in vivo* experiments.

BIOSECURITY STATEMENT

All the experiments were performed in Guangdong Provincial Key Laboratory of Malignant Tumor Epigenetics and Gene Regulation, Medical Research Center, Sun Yat-Sen Memorial Hospital and in the Laboratory Animal Center of Sun Yat-sen University, which strictly adhered to standard biosecurity and institutional safety procedures.

AUTHOR CONTRIBUTIONS

SJ and XY conceived the study. QW and JS designed the experiments. QW, LuH, YG, XL, and TT performed the experiments, collected the data and contributed to the statistical analysis. LiH, MC, XY, and SJ interpreted the data. QW drafted the manuscript. QW, XY, and SJ reviewed and edited the manuscript. SJ acquired funding.

ACKNOWLEDGMENTS

The authors would like to thank KC Biotech Co. Ltd. (Shanghai, China) for the library construction and data analysis of miRNA microarray.

REFERENCES

Anderson, G. P. (2008). Endotyping Asthma: New Insights Into Key Pathogenic Mechanisms in a Complex, Heterogeneous Disease. *The Lancet.* 372 (9643), 1107–1119. doi:10.1016/s0140-6736(08)61452-x

Ben Baruch-Morgenstern, N., Shik, D., Moshkovits, I., Itan, M., Karo-Atar, D., Bouffi, C., et al. (2014). Paired Immunoglobulin-Like Receptor A Is an Intrinsic, Self-Limiting Suppressor of IL-5-induced Eosinophil Development. *Nat. Immunol.* 15 (1), 36–44. doi:10.1038/ni.2757

Brightling, C. E., Gupta, S., Gonem, S., and Siddiqui, S. (2012). Lung Damage and Airway Remodelling in Severe Asthma. *Clin. Exp. Allergy.* 42 (5), 638–649. doi:10.1111/j.1365-2222.2011.03917.x

Byrne, A. J., Mathie, S. A., Gregory, L. G., and Lloyd, C. M. (2015). Pulmonary Macrophages: Key Players in the Innate Defence of the Airways. *Thorax.* 70 (12), 1189–1196. doi:10.1136/thoraxjnl-2015-207020

Chen, M., Huang, L., Zhang, W., Shi, J., Lin, X., Lv, Z., et al. (2016). MiR-23b Controls TGF-B1 Induced Airway Smooth Muscle Cell Proliferation *via* TGFβR2/p-Smad3 Signals. *Mol. Immunol.* 70, 84–93. doi:10.1016/j.molimm.2015.12.012

Chen, M., Lv, Z., and Jiang, S. (2011). The Effects of Triptolide on Airway Remodelling and Transforming Growth Factor-β1/Smad Signalling Pathway in Ovalbumin-Sensitized Mice. *Immunology.* 132 (3), 376–384. doi:10.1111/j.1365-2567.2010.03392.x

Collaborators, G. B. D. C. R. D. (2017). Global, Regional, and National Deaths, Prevalence, Disability-Adjusted Life Years, and Years Lived With Disability for Chronic Obstructive Pulmonary Disease and Asthma, 1990-2015: a Systematic Analysis for the Global Burden of Disease Study 2015. *Lancet Respir. Med.* 5 (9), 691–706. doi:10.1016/S2213-2600(17)30293-X

Eichner, L. J., Perry, M.-C., Dufour, C. R., Bertos, N., Park, M., St-Pierre, J., et al. (2010). miR-378 ∗ Mediates Metabolic Shift in Breast Cancer Cells *via* the PGC-1β/ERRγ Transcriptional Pathway. *Cel Metab.* 12 (4), 352–361. doi:10.1016/j.cmet.2010.09.002

Fehrenbach, H., Wagner, C., and Wegmann, M. (2017). Airway Remodeling in Asthma: What Really Matters. *Cell Tissue Res.* 367 (3), 551–569. doi:10.1007/s00441-016-2566-8

Feketea, G., Bocsan, C. I., Popescu, C., Gaman, M., Stanciu, L. A., and Zdrenghea, M. T. (2019). A Review of Macrophage MicroRNAs' Role in Human Asthma. *Cells.* 8 (5), 420. doi:10.3390/cells8050420

Gordon, S., and Martinez, F. O. (2010). Alternative Activation of Macrophages: Mechanism and Functions. *Immunity.* 32 (5), 593–604. doi:10.1016/j.immuni.2010.05.007

Hadjigol, S., Netto, K. G., Maltby, S., Tay, H. L., Nguyen, T. H., Hansbro, N. G., et al. (2020). Lipopolysaccharide Induces Steroid-Resistant Exacerbations in a Mouse Model of Allergic Airway Disease Collectively Through IL-13 and Pulmonary Macrophage Activation. *Clin. Exp. Allergy.* 50, 82. doi:10.1111/cea.13505

Holgate, S. T. (2012). Innate and Adaptive Immune Responses in Asthma. *Nat. Med.* 18 (5), 673–683. doi:10.1038/nm.2731

Holtzman, M. J. (2012). Asthma as a Chronic Disease of the Innate and Adaptive Immune Systems Responding to Viruses and Allergens. *J. Clin. Invest.* 122 (8), 2741–2748. doi:10.1172/jci60325

James, A. L., Elliot, J. G., Jones, R. L., Carroll, M. L., Mauad, T., Bai, T. R., et al. (2012). Airway Smooth Muscle Hypertrophy and Hyperplasia in Asthma. *Am. J. Respir. Crit. Care Med.* 185 (10), 1058–1064. doi:10.1164/rccm.201110-1849oc

Kubota, Y., Iwasaki, Y., Harada, H., Yokomura, I., Ueda, M., Hashimoto, S., et al. (1999). Depletion of Alveolar Macrophages by Treatment With 2-Chloroadenosine Aerosol. *Clin. Diagn. Lab. Immunol.* 6 (4), 452–456. doi:10.1128/cdli.6.4.452-456.1999

Lee, Y. G., Jeong, J. J., Nyenhuis, S., Berdyshev, E., Chung, S., Ranjan, R., et al. (2015). Recruited Alveolar Macrophages, in Response to Airway Epithelial-Derived Monocyte Chemoattractant Protein 1/CCl2, Regulate Airway Inflammation and Remodeling in Allergic Asthma. *Am. J. Respir. Cel Mol Biol.* 52 (6), 772–784. doi:10.1165/rcmb.2014-0255oc

Levy-Apter, E., Finkelshtein, E., Vemulapalli, V., Li, S. S.-C., Bedford, M. T., and Elson, A. (2014). Adaptor Protein GRB2 Promotes Src Tyrosine Kinase Activation and Podosomal Organization by Protein-Tyrosine Phosphatase ϵ in Osteoclasts. *J. Biol. Chem.* 289 (52), 36048–36058. doi:10.1074/jbc.m114.603548

Li, H., Jiang, T., Li, M.-Q., Zheng, X.-L., and Zhao, G.-J. (2018). Transcriptional Regulation of Macrophages Polarization by MicroRNAs. *Front. Immunol.* 9, 1175. doi:10.3389/fimmu.2018.01175

Li, P., Lang, X., and Xia, S. (2019). Elevated Expression of MicroRNA-378 in Children With Asthma Aggravates Airway Remodeling by Promoting the Proliferation and Apoptosis Resistance of Airway Smooth Muscle Cells. *Exp. Ther. Med* 17 (3), 1529–1536. doi:10.3892/etm.2018.7141

Lin, W., Su, F., Gautam, R., Wang, N., Zhang, Y., and Wang, X. (2018). Raf Kinase Inhibitor Protein Negatively Regulates FcεRI-Mediated Mast Cell Activation and Allergic Response. *Proc. Natl. Acad. Sci. USA.* 115 (42), E9859–E9868. doi:10.1073/pnas.1805474115

Liu, G., and Yang, H. (2013). Modulation of Macrophage Activation and Programming in Immunity. *J. Cel. Physiol.* 228 (3), 502–512. doi:10.1002/jcp.24157

Massoud, A. H., Charbonnier, L.-M., Lopez, D., Pellegrini, M., Phipatanakul, W., and Chatila, T. A. (2016). An Asthma-Associated IL4R Variant Exacerbates Airway Inflammation by Promoting Conversion of Regulatory T Cells to TH17-Like Cells. *Nat. Med.* 22 (9), 1013–1022. doi:10.1038/nm.4147

Murray, P. J., and Wynn, T. A. (2011). Protective and Pathogenic Functions of Macrophage Subsets. *Nat. Rev. Immunol.* 11 (11), 723–737. doi:10.1038/nri3073

Ndolo, R. A., Forrest, M. L., and Krise, J. P. (2010). The Role of Lysosomes in Limiting Drug Toxicity in Mice. *J. Pharmacol. Exp. Ther.* 333 (1), 120–128. doi:10.1124/jpet.109.160226

Ohtani, A., Kumazawa, Y., Fujisawa, H., and Nishimura, C. (1982). Inhibition of Macrophage Function by 2-Chloroadenosine. *J. Reticuloendothel Soc.* 32 (3), 189–200.

Park, S. Y., Jing, X., Gupta, D., and Dziarski, R. (2013). Peptidoglycan Recognition Protein 1 Enhances Experimental Asthma by Promoting Th2 and Th17 and Limiting Regulatory T Cell and Plasmacytoid Dendritic Cell Responses. *J.I.* 190 (7), 3480–3492. doi:10.4049/jimmunol.1202675

Rajaram, M. V. S., Arnett, E., Azad, A. K., Guirado, E., Ni, B., Gerberick, A. D., et al. (2017). *M. tuberculosis* -Initiated Human Mannose Receptor Signaling Regulates Macrophage Recognition and Vesicle Trafficking by FcRγ-Chain, Grb2, and SHP-1. *Cel Rep.* 21 (1), 126–140. doi:10.1016/j.celrep.2017.09.034

Rao, G. N. (1996). Hydrogen Peroxide Induces Complex Formation of SHC-Grb2-SOS With Receptor Tyrosine Kinase and Activates Ras and Extracellular Signal-Regulated Protein Kinases Group of Mitogen-Activated Protein Kinases. *Oncogene.* 13 (4), 713–719.

Rückerl, D., Jenkins, S. J., Laqtom, N. N., Gallagher, I. J., Sutherland, T. E., Duncan, S., et al. (2012). Induction of IL-4Rα-Dependent MicroRNAs Identifies PI3K/Akt Signaling as Essential for IL-4-driven Murine Macrophage Proliferation *In Vivo. Blood.* 120 (11), 2307–2316. doi:10.1182/blood-2012-02-408252

Saito, T., and Yamaguchi, J. (1985). 2-Chloroadenosine: a Selective Lethal Effect to Mouse Macrophages and its Mechanism. *J. Immunol.* 134 (3), 1815–1822.

Self-Fordham, J. B., Naqvi, A. R., Uttamani, J. R., Kulkarni, V., and Nares, S. (2017). MicroRNA: Dynamic Regulators of Macrophage Polarization and Plasticity. *Front. Immunol.* 8, 1062. doi:10.3389/fimmu.2017.01062

Shenoy, A., and Blelloch, R. H. (2014). Regulation of MicroRNA Function in Somatic Stem Cell Proliferation and Differentiation. *Nat. Rev. Mol. Cel Biol.* 15 (9), 565–576. doi:10.1038/nrm3854

Stellari, F., Sala, A., Ruscitti, F., Carnini, C., Mirandola, P., Vitale, M., et al. (2015). Monitoring Inflammation and Airway Remodeling by Fluorescence Molecular Tomography in a Chronic Asthma Model. *J. Transl Med.* 13, 336. doi:10.1186/s12967-015-0696-5

Su, S., Zhao, Q., He, C., Huang, D., Liu, J., Chen, F., et al. (2015). miR-142-5p and miR-130a-3p Are Regulated by IL-4 and IL-13 and Control Profibrogenic Macrophage Program. *Nat. Commun.* 6, 8523. doi:10.1038/ncomms9523

Van Dyken, S. J., and Locksley, R. M. (2013). Interleukin-4- and Interleukin-13-Mediated Alternatively Activated Macrophages: Roles in Homeostasis and Disease. *Annu. Rev. Immunol.* 31, 317–343. doi:10.1146/annurev-immunol-032712-095906

Vats, D., Mukundan, L., Odegaard, J. I., Zhang, L., Smith, K. L., Morel, C. R., et al. (2006). Oxidative Metabolism and PGC-1β Attenuate Macrophage-Mediated Inflammation. *Cel Metab.* 4 (1), 13–24. doi:10.1016/j.cmet.2006.05.011

Wang, X., Zhang, D., Higham, A., Wolosianka, S., Gai, X., Zhou, L., et al. (2020). ADAM15 Expression Is Increased in Lung CD8+ T Cells, Macrophages, and Bronchial Epithelial Cells in Patients With COPD and Is Inversely Related to Airflow Obstruction. *Respir. Res.* 21 (1), 188. doi:10.1186/s12931-020-01446-5

Xu, Z.-h., Yao, T.-z., and Liu, W. (2018). miR-378a-3p Sensitizes Ovarian Cancer Cells to Cisplatin Through Targeting MAPK1/GRB2. *Biomed. Pharmacother.* 107, 1410–1417. doi:10.1016/j.biopha.2018.08.132

Yang, M., Kumar, R. K., Hansbro, P. M., and Foster, P. S. (2012). Emerging Roles of Pulmonary Macrophages in Driving the Development of Severe Asthma. *J. Leukoc. Biol.* 91 (4), 557–569. doi:10.1189/jlb.0711357

Yu, X., Zeng, Y., Bao, M., Wen, J., Zhu, G., Cao, C., et al. (2020). Low-Magnitude Vibration Induces Osteogenic Differentiation of Bone Marrow Mesenchymal Stem Cells *via* miR-378a-3p/Grb2 Pathway to Promote Bone Formation in a Rat Model of Age-related Bone Loss. *FASEB j.* 34 (9), 11754–11771. doi:10.1096/fj.201902830rrr

Zeng, T., Wang, X., Wang, W., Feng, Q., Lao, G., Liang, Y., et al. (2019). Endothelial Cell-Derived Small Extracellular Vesicles Suppress Cutaneous Wound Healing Through Regulating Fibroblasts Autophagy. *Clin. Sci. (Lond).* 133 (9), CS20190008. doi:10.1042/CS20190008

Zhao, Y., Tang, X., Huang, Y., Tang, Q., Ma, C., Zheng, F., et al. (2019). Interaction of C-Jun and HOTAIR- Increased Expression of P21 Converge in Polyphyllin I-Inhibited Growth of Human Lung Cancer Cells. *Onco Targets Ther.* Vol. 12, 10115–10127. doi:10.2147/ott.s226830

5

STAT3 and IL-6 Contribute to Corticosteroid Resistance in an OVA and Ozone-Induced Asthma Model with Neutrophil Infiltration

*Yishu Xue†, Yan Zhou†, Wuping Bao†, Qiang Fu, Huijuan Hao, Lei Han, Xue Zhang, Xue Tian and Min Zhang**

Department of Respiratory and Critical Care Medicine, Shanghai General Hospital, Shanghai Jiao Tong University School of Medicine, Shanghai, China

Correspondence:
Min Zhang
maggie_zhangmin@163.com

†These authors have contributed equally to this work and share first authorship

Exposure to high levels of ozone contributes to insensitivity to glucocorticoids in asthma treatment, but the underlying mechanisms are not known. We built two asthma models: a "T2-high" asthma model was established by ovalbumin (OVA) sensitization/challenge and OVA sensitization/challenge combined with ozone exposure (OVA + ozone) was used to induce airway inflammation with increased numbers of neutrophils to simulate "T2-low" asthma. The expression of T-helper (Th)1/2/17-related cytokines was measured by cytokine antibody arrays. Bronchial provocation tests were carried out to evaluate the lung resistance of mice. Hematoxylin and eosin staining, periodic acid-Schiff staining, and immunohistochemical (IHC) analyses of alpha-smooth muscle actin were undertaken to observe morphology changes in lungs. The expression of glucocorticoid receptors (GRs) and phosphorylated-GR (p-GR) was measured by western blotting. *Nr3c1* mRNA was quantified by RT-qPCR. Protein expression of proinflammatory cytokines, signal transducer and activator of transcription 3 (STAT3), suppressor of cytokine signaling 3 (SOCS3), and CXCL1 was measured through ELISAs, western blotting, or IHC analyses. Resected lung tissue from seven asthma patients and 10 healthy controls undergoing thoracotomy for pulmonary nodules was evaluated by IHC analyses and ELISAs. In both asthma models, mucus hypersecretion, as well as inflammation, hyperresponsiveness, and remodeling of the airways, was present compared with the control group, whereas the OVA + ozone group showed severe neutrophil infiltration. The expression of Th17-related cytokines (interleukin (IL)-6, IL-17A, IL-21), GR protein, and CXCL1 increased in the OVA + ozone group, whereas the expression of p-GR decreased. Dexamethasone (Dex) could not totally reverse the expression of p-GR and histone deacetylase-2 in the OVA + ozone group. STAT3 expression increased in the OVA + ozone group and could not be

Abbreviations: ACh, acetylcholine chloride; α-SMA, α-smooth muscle actin; BALF, bronchoalveolar lavage fluid; CXCL1, chemokine (C-X-C motif) ligand 1; CXCR2, chemokine (C-X-C motif) receptor 2; Dex, dexamethasone; ELISA, enzyme-linked immunosorbent assay; FEV1, forced expiratory volume in one second; FVC, forced vital capacity; GR, glucocorticoid receptor; HDAC2, histone deacetylase 2; H&E, hematoxylin and eosin; IHC, immunohistochemical; OVA, ovalbumin; PAS, periodic acid-Schiff; PC100, the ACh concentration required to increase R_L by 100% from baseline; p-GR, phosphorylated-GR; p-STAT3, phosphorylated-STAT3; R_L, lung resistance; SOCS3, suppressor of cytokine signaling 3; STAT3, signal transducer and activator of transcription 3.

completely reversed by Dex, and nor could IL-6 expression. A positive correlation between IL-6 or IL-17A and STAT3 and negative correlation between SOCS3 and STAT3 were shown, suggesting that the IL-6/STAT3 pathway may be involved in OVA + ozone–induced corticosteroid-resistant airway inflammation. In clinical samples, IL-17A expression in lung tissue was positively correlated with percent STAT3-positive area and negatively correlated with SOCS3 expression. The IL-6/STAT3 pathway may contribute to corticosteroid insensitivity in OVA + ozone–induced neutrophilic airway inflammation through regulation of Th17 cells and could provide new targets for individual treatment of corticosteroid resistance in asthma.

Keywords: T2-low asthma, STAT3, IL-6, SOCS3, steroid resistance, ozone

INTRODUCTION

In 2009, Wenzel et al. (1999) defined two distinct inflammatory endotypes of asthma: T-helper type 2 (T2)-high and T2-low. They have remained the most well-recognized and described endotypes of asthma (Svenningsen S and Nair P, 2017).

T2-high asthma is characterized by eosinophilic airway inflammation. It presents with an immune response involving mainly T-helper type 2 (Th2)-related cytokines and, in general, is sensitive to corticosteroid therapy. T2-low asthma is usually characterized by neutrophilic airway inflammation and often exhibits an immune response mediated by interleukin (IL)-17 and Th17 cells (Chung, 2016).

Glucocorticoids are the main choice of asthma treatment due to their significant anti-inflammatory, immunosuppressive, and immunomodulatory effects (Alangari, 2014; Barnes, 2017). However, ≤10% of asthma patients do not respond to glucocorticoids even at high doses or in combination with oral corticosteroids (Chung, 2016). This absence of response makes asthma difficult to control and consumes considerable medical resources.

It has been revealed that proinflammatory cytokines can contribute to corticosteroid resistance in severe asthma and chronic obstructive pulmonary disease. Proinflammatory cytokines (e.g., IL-17A) together with allergens, pathogens, and cigarette smoke can modulate multiple signaling pathways, including nuclear factor, erythroid 2-like 2/histone deacetylase 2/c-Jun (Nrf2/HDAC/c-Jun), and a heightened glucocorticoid receptor (GR) ratio to induce corticosteroid insensitivity (Mei et al., 2019). Neutrophils are involved in corticosteroid insensitivity in asthma and may be regulated by Th17 cells (Chung, 2016; Panettieri, 2018).

An important pathway of initial differentiation of mouse Th17 cells requires IL-6 and signal transducer and activator of transcription 3 (STAT3). Murine and human Th17 cells express IL-17A, IL-17F, IL-21, IL-22, granulocyte-macrophage colony-stimulating factor, and IL-23R (Miossec and Kolls, 2012). STAT3 phosphorylation promotes the transformation of Th0 cells to Th17 cells (Cosmi et al., 2011). Suppressor of cytokine signaling 3 (SOCS3) is a negative regulator of Th17, which usually regulates Th17 cells through the interaction with STAT3 (Rottenberg and Carow, 2014).

STAT3–SOCS3 is an important pathway involved in inflammation modulation (Rottenberg and Carow, 2014). The role of STAT3 and SOCS3 was investigated in some models of allergic airway inflammation (Santana et al., 2019; Pinheiro et al., 2020), but the results were controversial. Their roles in asthma, especially T2-low asthma, are not clear.

Here, an asthma model with a mixed Th2/Th17 response was constructed by ovalbumin (OVA) sensitization/challenge combined with ozone exposure (OVA + ozone) to simulate some types of T2-low asthma in patients (Last et al., 2004; Zhang J.-h. et al., 2019; Zhang Y. et al., 2019) and show the features of corticosteroid resistance. The expression of total STAT3 was increased in both asthma models, and phosphorylated-STAT3 (p-STAT3) expression increased in the OVA + ozone group, whereas SOCS3 expression was reduced. The expression of STAT3 protein and IL-6 protein in lung tissue did not show an obvious response to corticosteroid intervention. We discovered higher STAT3 expression and lower SOCS3 expression in the lung tissue of asthma patients compared with that of healthy controls (HCs) and observed a correlation between STAT3 expression or SOCS3 expression and the expression of IL-17A protein. The findings from human tissue and mouse models suggested that, by regulating the expression of Th17 cytokines and related cytokines, STAT3 and IL-6 may contribute to corticosteroid insensitivity in an asthma model with a mixed Th2/Th17 response and may become a potential target for treatment of T2-low asthma.

MATERIALS AND METHODS

Animals

Male C57BL/6 mice (specific-pathogen-free; 6 weeks) were purchased from SLRC Laboratory (Shanghai, China). They were housed in controlled conditions of temperature (21–25°C) and humidity (40–60%) and had free access to water and food (free from OVA). Mice were acclimatized for 7 days before experimentation and exposed to a 12 h light–dark cycle.

Induction of Allergic Airway Inflammation and Ozone Exposure

Mice were divided randomly into four groups of eight. OVA sensitization was initiated on day 0 and day 7. OVA sensitization was achieved by intraperitoneal injection of 20 μg of OVA (grade V; Sigma-Aldrich, Saint Louis, MO, United States) dissolved in 0.2 ml of phosphate-buffered saline (PBS) emulsified in aluminum hydroxide (2 mg; Sigma-Aldrich) as an adjuvant. OVA challenge was undertaken on days 14, 16, 18, 20, and 22, with exposure to 5% aerosolized OVA (20 ml; grade II, Sigma-Aldrich) in a plastic box linked to an ultrasonic nebulizer (Clenny 2 Aerosol; Medel, San Polo di Torrile, Italy) for 30 min. Mice in the control group were sensitized and challenged with an identical volume (0.2 ml for sensitization and 20 ml for challenge) of PBS as a vehicle.

Mice were exposed to ozone (2 ppm) or air in a Perspex™ container 30 min after each OVA/PBS challenge on days 14, 16, 18, 20, and 22. Ozone was produced by an ozonizer (300 series; Aqua Medic, Bissendorf, Germany). Each exposure lasted for 2 h. The ozone concentration was controlled and adjusted by an OS-4 Ozone Switch (Ecosensor; KWJ Engineering, Newark, CA, United States) continuously. Mice in the control group were exposed to air during this time.

In the dexamethasone (Dex)-treated group (OVA + ozone + Dex), mice were injected (i.p.) with Dex (5 mg/kg; Solarbio, Beijing, China) each time before OVA challenge on days 14, 16, 18, 20, and 22.

Airway Responsiveness

24 h after the last challenge, mice were anesthetized with Zoletil 50 (tiletamine hydrochloride and zolazepam hydrochloride, 25 mg/kg, Virbac S.A., France) and xylazine hydrochloride (10 mg/kg, Chang Sha Best Biological Technology Institute Co., Ltd., China) via IP injection. Mice under anesthesia were then ventilated (MiniVent™; Hugo Sachs Elektronik, March, Germany) at 180 breaths/min and a tidal volume of 210 μl in a whole-body plethysmograph with a pneumotachograph connected to a transducer (Electro-Medical Measurement Systems, Bordon, United Kingdom), as described previously (Bao et al., 2018). Pulmonary airway resistance (R_L) was recorded during a 3 min period after increasing concentrations (4–256 mg/ml; 10 μl each time) of acetylcholine chloride (ACh; Sigma-Aldrich). R_L was expressed as percentage change from baseline R_L (measured following nebulization with PBS). The ACh concentration required to increase R_L by 100% from baseline (PC100) was calculated.

Blood Collection, Bronchoalveolar Lavage, and Protein Isolation From Lung Tissue

After lung-function tests, mice were killed and blood was obtained from the right ventricle. Then, the trachea was exposed, and three aliquots of sterilized saline (0.6 ml each time) were instilled through a PE-60 tube. Bronchoalveolar lavage fluid (BALF) was retrieved (Bao et al., 2020), and the return volume was consistently ≥70% of the instilled volume. Samples of blood and BALF were centrifuged at 3,000 rpm for 10 min at 4°C, and the supernatants were used for measurements.

Lung tissues [for enzyme-linked immunosorbent assays (ELISAs)] were flushed with PBS before freezing. They were homogenized in lysis buffer containing protease and phosphatase inhibitors and then centrifuged for ELISAs, real-time reverse transcription–quantitative polymerase chain reaction (RT-qPCR), and western blotting.

ELISAs

ELISAs of serum, BALF, and lung-tissue homogenates were conducted using commercial kits for IgE (Crystal Chem, Chicago, IL, United States), IL-6 and IL-17A (Anogen, Mississauga, Canada), IL-21, p-STAT3 (Tyr705), and total STAT3 (RayBiotech, Peachtree Corners, GA, United States), HDAC2 (EpiGentek, Farmingdale, NY, United States), and hypoxia inducible factor (HIF)-1α (Cell Biolabs, San Diego, CA, United States) according to the manufacturer's instructions.

Gene Expression

Nr3c1 is the gene of GRs. Total RNA was isolated from lung tissue by TRIzol™ Reagent (Invitrogen, Carlsbad, CA, United States) and was translated into complementary DNA using the cDNA Reverse Transcription Kit (Applied Biosystems, Foster City, CA, United States) in a PTC-200 Peltier Thermal Cycler (MJ Research, Hercules, CA, United States). Real-time RT-qPCR was undertaken using the ViiA™ 7 Real-Time PCR System (Thermo Fisher, Waltham, MA, United States), as described previously (Bao et al., 2018). The mean fluorescence intensity of the internal reference gene (β-actin) and target gene (*Nr3c1*) was measured. The relative expression of target genes was calculated by the $2^{-\Delta\Delta Ct}$ method.

The primer sequences (forward and reverse, respectively) used for PCR were 5′-GAA GCA GAT GAG CCA TCA CTT-3′ and 5′-CGG TCC TTC TCT GAT AGT GGA-3′ for *Nr3c1* and 5′-CCT CTA TGC CAA CAC AGT-3′ and 5′-AGC CAC CAA TCC ACA CAG-3′ for β-actin.

Measurement of Cytokine Levels in Serum

Levels of Th1-, Th2-, and Th17-related cytokines in the serum of mice were measured through cytokine antibody arrays (Mouse TH17 Array 1; RayBiotech), as described previously (Zhu et al., 2020), following the manufacturer's instructions.

Western Blotting

Total protein from lung tissues was extracted using RIPA lysis buffer (Beyotime Biotechnology, Shanghai, China). Extracted proteins were separated by sodium dodecyl sulfate–polyacrylamide gel electrophoresis and transferred to polyvinylidene difluoride (PVDF) membranes. The relative expression of proteins was determined using an ECL detection system (Li et al., 2021). The primary antibodies were those against GR (Cell Signaling Technology, Danvers, MA, United States), p-GR (Ser211; Cell Signaling Technology), SOCS3 (Thermo Scientific), and STAT3 (124H6; Cell Signaling Technology).

Histology and Morphology

Mouse lungs were dissected out. The left lung was inflated by injecting 4% paraformaldehyde to provide 20 cm of water pressure. Then, it was immersed overnight in paraformaldehyde, embedded in paraffin, and sectioned for staining. Morphologic changes in the epithelia of lungs and airways were assessed by staining with hematoxylin and eosin (H&E) and periodic acid-Schiff (PAS).

Neutrophils, eosinophils, and lymphocytes located along lobar bronchi and segmental bronchi were counted (magnification = 400×) in a double-blinded manner by two investigators independently, as described previously (Bao et al., 2018). The mean width of the observed area was 100 μm. Peribronchiolar and perivascular inflammation observed in H&E-stained lung slices was scored from 0 to 3, as described previously (Bao et al., 2018).

Blue/purple-stained cells were identified as being PAS-positive. The percent PAS-positive area in the total epithelial area was calculated using ImageJ (National Institutes of Health, Bethesda, MD, United States).

Immunohistochemical Analyses

IHC staining for α-smooth muscle actin (α-SMA), STAT3, and SOCS3 in lung-tissue sections with mouse α-SMA antibody (Proteintech, Chicago, IL, United States), SOCS3 antibody (Thermo Scientific), STAT3 antibody (124H6; Cell Signaling Technology), chemokine (C-X-C motif) ligand 1 (CXCL1), chemokine (C-X-C motif) receptor 2 (CXCR2) antibody (Proteintech, Chicago, IL, United States), and CXCR2 antibody (Servicebio, Wuhan, China) was done, as described previously (Zhang et al., 2018). The area of positive expression was identified in a double-blinded and independent fashion by two investigators using ImageJ.

Patient Cohort

Inclusion Criteria

The inclusion criteria were patients 1) aged 16–75 years; 2) who accepted pneumectomy for lung nodules; 3) who completed spirometry before surgery; 4) had percent forced expiratory volume in one second (FEV_1%) ≥80% predicted; 5) with FEV_1/ forced vital capacity (FVC) > 0.7 after salbutamol administration; and 6) with the diameter of pulmonary nodules <3 cm.

Exclusion Criteria

The exclusion criteria were patients 1) who had suffered a respiratory infection in the 8 weeks before screening; 2) who were pregnant; 3) who had concomitant systemic respiratory disease (including chronic obstructive pulmonary disease); and 4) who had other significant medical problems as determined by the principal investigator.

Grouping

Individuals with a history of asthma, confirmed to have variable symptoms (chronic recurrent wheezing, dyspnea, chest tightness, and/or cough) and variable airflow restriction (positive bronchodilation test or bronchial provocation test), were classified as the "asthma" group. Patients with no symptoms or other pulmonary diseases were classified as the "control" group.

Statistical Analyses

Statistical analyses and graph creation were undertaken using Prism 8.0 (GraphPad, San Diego, CA, United States). However, the Spearman correlation coefficient matrix and Spearman rank correlation tests were undertaken using R 3.6.1 (R Institute for Statistical Computing, Vienna, Austria). Data are expressed as mean ± SD unless indicated otherwise. The Kruskal–Wallis one-way analysis of variance with Bonferroni's *post hoc* test (for equal variance) or Dunnett's T3 *post hoc* test (for unequal variance) was used to evaluate differences in variances between multiple groups. A post-test Mann–Whitney analysis was conducted to evaluate differences in variances between two groups. $p < 0.05$ was considered significant.

RESULTS

Expression of Th17-Related Cytokines Increased in the OVA Group, but Expression of Th2-Related Cytokines Increased in the OVA + Ozone Group

Cytokine antibody arrays were used to measure the expression of Th1-, Th2-, and Th17-related cytokines in the serum of each group (**Figure 1A**). The expression of Th1-related cytokines (IFN-γ, IL-2, and TNF-α) showed no significant difference among the two asthma models and control group. The expression of Th2-related cytokines (IL-4, IL-5, and IL-13) increased in the OVA group compared with the control group. IL-13 increased in the OVA + ozone group as well (**Supplementary Figure S2**). The expression of IL-10 (a cytokine associated with T regulatory cells) in mouse serum was higher in the OVA group. The expression of Th17-related cytokines (IL-17A and IL-21) was significantly higher in the serum of mice in the OVA + ozone group than that in the control group (**Figure 1B**). IL-6 expression was also increased in the OVA + ozone group. Although often classified as a Th2-related cytokine, IL-6 has an important role in a pathway of the initial differentiation of mouse Th17 cells (Miossec and Kolls, 2012).

Subsequently, the expression of Th17-related cytokines was measured in the BALF and lung-tissue homogenates of mice. Protein expression of IL-6, IL-17A, and IL-21 in the lungs of mice in the OVA + ozone group was significantly higher than that in the control group (**Figure 1C**). Protein expression of Th17-related cytokines in BALF was similar to that in serum. The expression of IL-6, IL-17A, and IL-21 in the lungs of mice in the OVA + ozone group was significantly higher than that in the control group. The expression of IL-6 and IL-17A in the lungs of mice in the OVA + ozone group was significantly higher than that in the OVA group (**Figure 1D**). These data suggested that Th17-related cytokines, rather than Th1- or Th2-related cytokines, may have important roles in our OVA + ozone mouse model.

The OVA + Ozone Group Showed Severe Airway Inflammation, Hypersecretion, and Airway Hyperresponsiveness Compared With Those in the OVA Group

Compared with the control group, the OVA group and OVA + ozone group showed significant airway inflammation (as reflected in airway thickening) as well as infiltration of inflammatory cells (e.g., eosinophils, neutrophils, and lymphocytes) around the

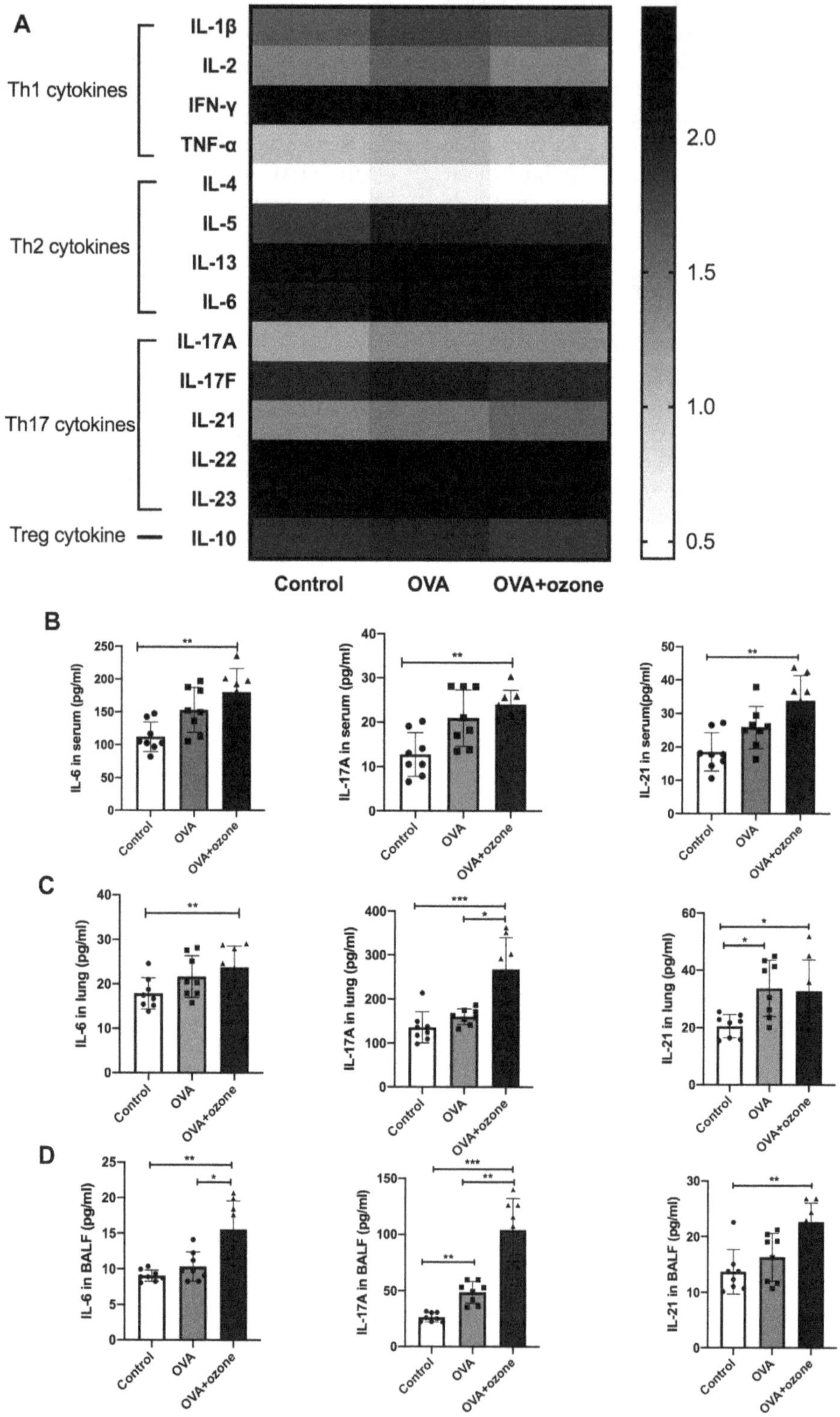

FIGURE 1 | Expression of Th1-, Th2-, and Th17-related cytokines in the serum of mice and expression of Th17-related cytokines in the lung tissue and BALF of mice. The expression of cytokines in serum was measured by cytokine antibody arrays. The expression of Th17-related cytokines in BALF and lung tissue was measured through ELISAs. **(A)** Expression of different types of cytokines in serum (statistical analysis of cytokines is shown in **Supplementary Figure S1**). **(B)** Expression of Th17-related cytokines in serum. **(C)** Expression of Th17-related cytokines in lung tissue. **(D)** Expression of Th17-related cytokines in BALF. To reduce the difference in expression among different cytokines, the values in panel **(A)** are shown in logarithmic form, whereas the original values of measured protein concentration are used for the remainder of the plates. *$p < 0.05$; **$p < 0.01$; ***$p < 0.001$.

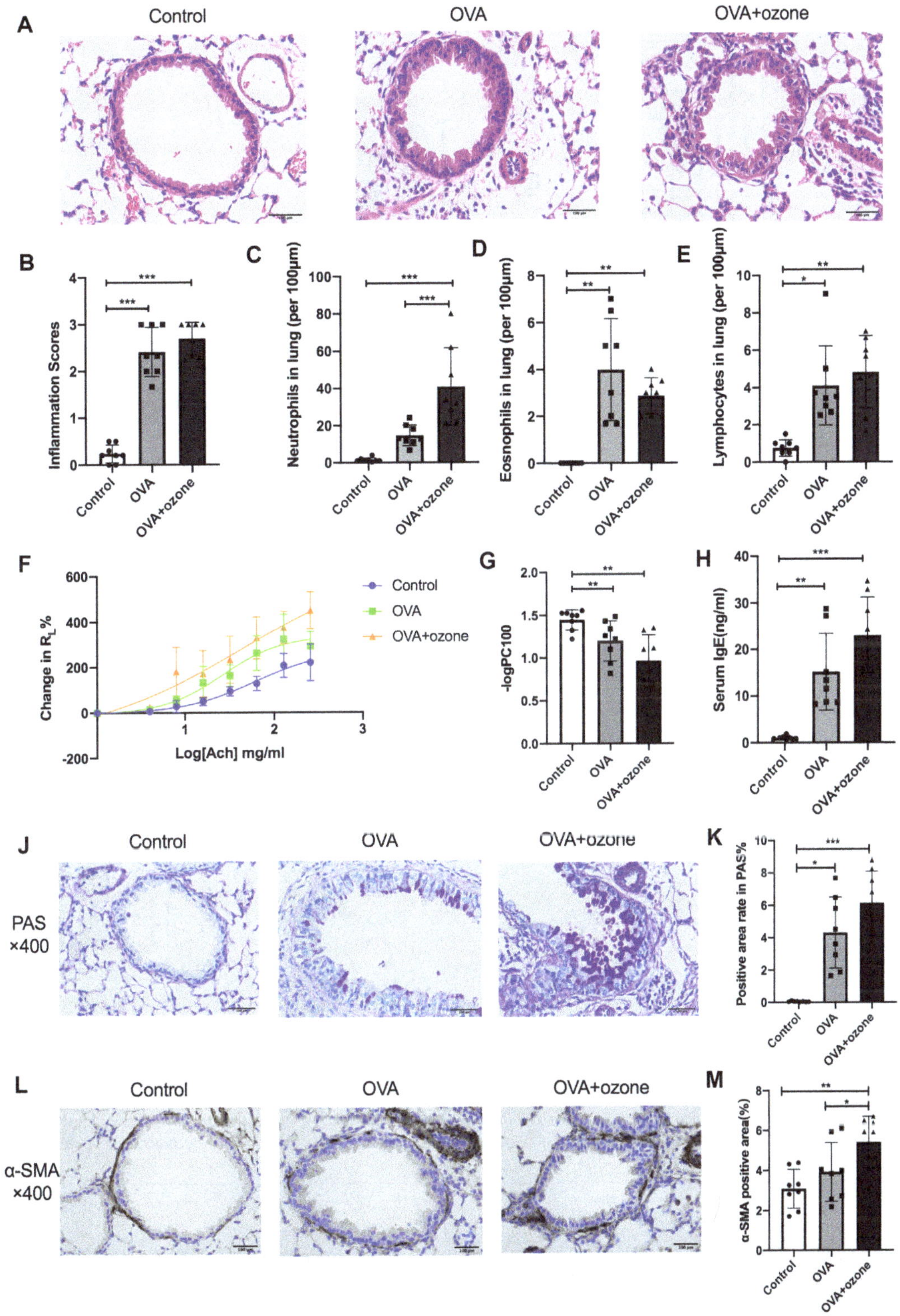

FIGURE 2 | Mucus secretion, inflammation, responsiveness, and remodeling of the airways and IgE level of serum in T2-high and T2-low asthma models. Airway inflammation was evaluated through H&E staining. The IgE level in serum was analyzed by ELISAs. R_L (to acetylcholine chloride) was measured by a commercial setup from Electro-Medical Measurement Systems. **(A)** Representative photomicrographs of the lung with inflammatory-cell infiltration and hyperemia in hematoxylin and eosin–stained sections. **(B)** Airway inflammation scores. **(C)** Density of neutrophil infiltration. **(D)** Density of eosinophil infiltration. **(E)** Density of lymphocyte infiltration. **(F)** Mean percent increase in R_L in response to increasing concentrations of ACh. **(G)** –logPC100 (the ACh concentration required to increase R_L by 100% from baseline). **(H)** IgE level in serum. **(J)** Representative photomicrographs of the lung with airway mucus production and goblet-cell hyperplasia. **(K)** PAS-positive area. **(L)** Representative photomicrographs of immunohistochemistry of α-SMA in lung-tissue slices. **(M)** Percent SMA-positive area around airways. ACh, acetylcholine chloride; R_L, lung resistance; α-SMA, α-smooth muscle actin. $^{*}p < 0.05$; $^{**}p < 0.01$; $^{***}p < 0.001$. Scale bar = 100 μm.

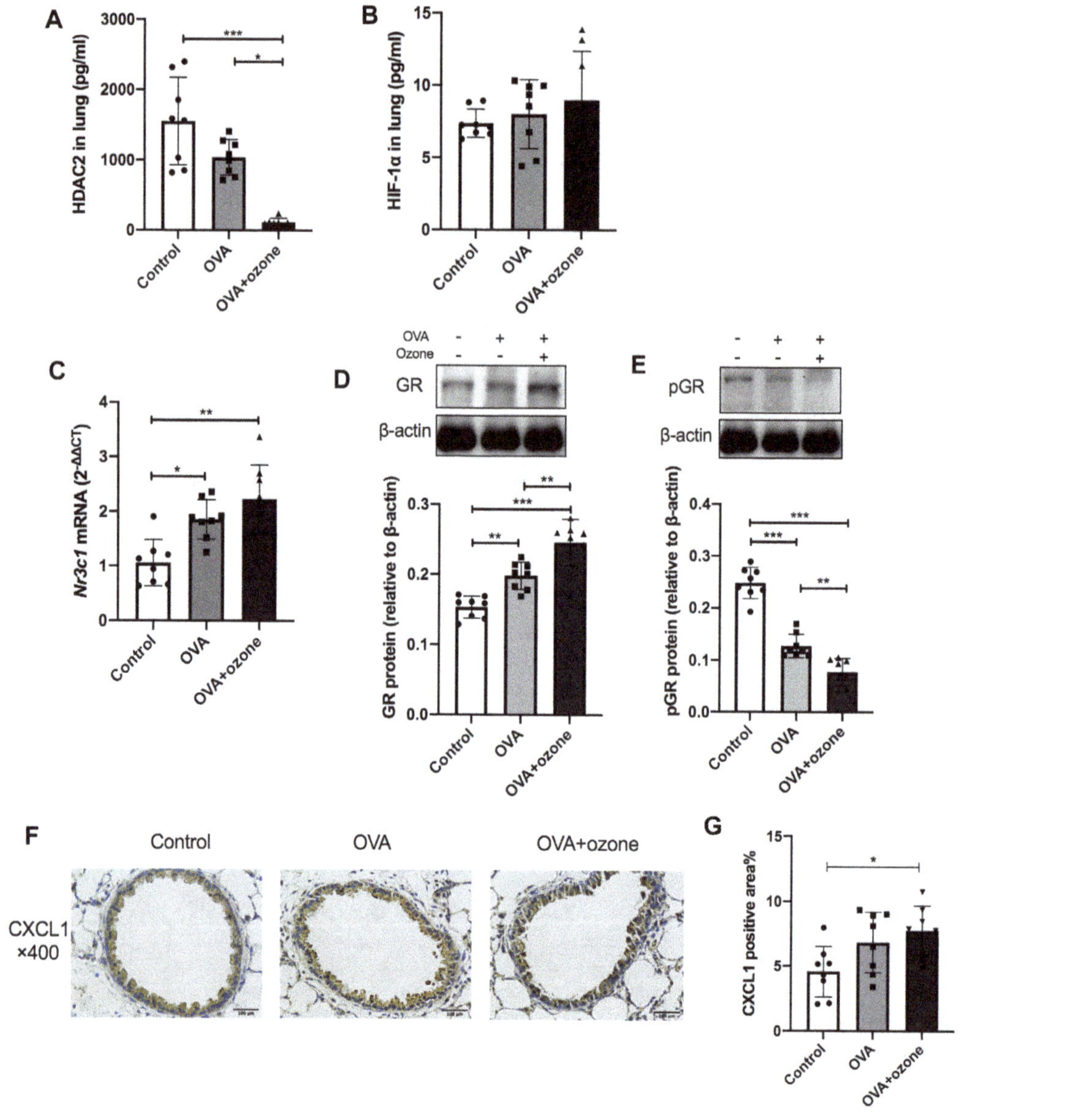

FIGURE 3 | Expression of cytokines and receptors related to corticosteroid resistance in the lung tissue of mice suffering from asthma. The expression of HDAC2 and HIF-1α in the lung tissue of mice was measured by ELISAs. *Nr3c1* (gene of GRs) mRNA was detected by RT-qPCR. The expression of GR protein and p-GR protein was measured by western blotting. **(A)** HDAC2 expression in lung tissue. **(B)** HIF-1α expression in lung tissue. **(C)** Expression of *Nr3c1* mRNA in lung tissue. **(D)** Expression of GR protein in lung tissue. **(E)** Expression of p-GR protein in lung tissue. **(F)** Representative photomicrographs of immunohistochemistry of CXCL1 in lung-tissue slices. **(G)** Percent CXCL1-positive area around airways. CXCL1, chemokine (C-X-C motif) ligand 1; GR, glucocorticoid receptor; HDAC2, histone deacetylase 2; p-GR, phosphorylated-GR. $^{*}p < 0.05$; $^{**}p < 0.01$; $^{***}p < 0.001$.

trachea and blood vessels (**Figures 2A–E**). The OVA + ozone group showed more neutrophil infiltration than that in the OVA group (**Figure 2C**). Airway hyperresponsiveness (**Figures 2F,G**) and increased levels of IgE in serum (**Figure 2H**) were observed in both endotypes of asthma models. The ozone group showed neutrophilic infiltration (**Supplementary Figures S4A,B,D**) and airway hyperactivity (**Supplementary Figures S4E,F**) compared to the control group, while its eosinophilic infiltration around the trachea and blood vessels showed no statistical differences from that in the control group (**Supplementary Figure S4C**).

Airway hypersecretion was observed in mice of both asthma-model groups (**Figure 2J**). The percent positive PAS-stained area demonstrated that increased mucus secretion occurred in the OVA group and OVA + ozone group compared with that in the control group (**Figure 2K**).

Airway smooth muscle (ASM) mass (as indicated by the amount of α-SMA around the airways) increased in lung slices from mice treated with OVA + ozone compared with that in the control group (**Figures 2L,M**). The OVA group had a slightly (but not significantly) thicker ASM mass than control mice. The ASM

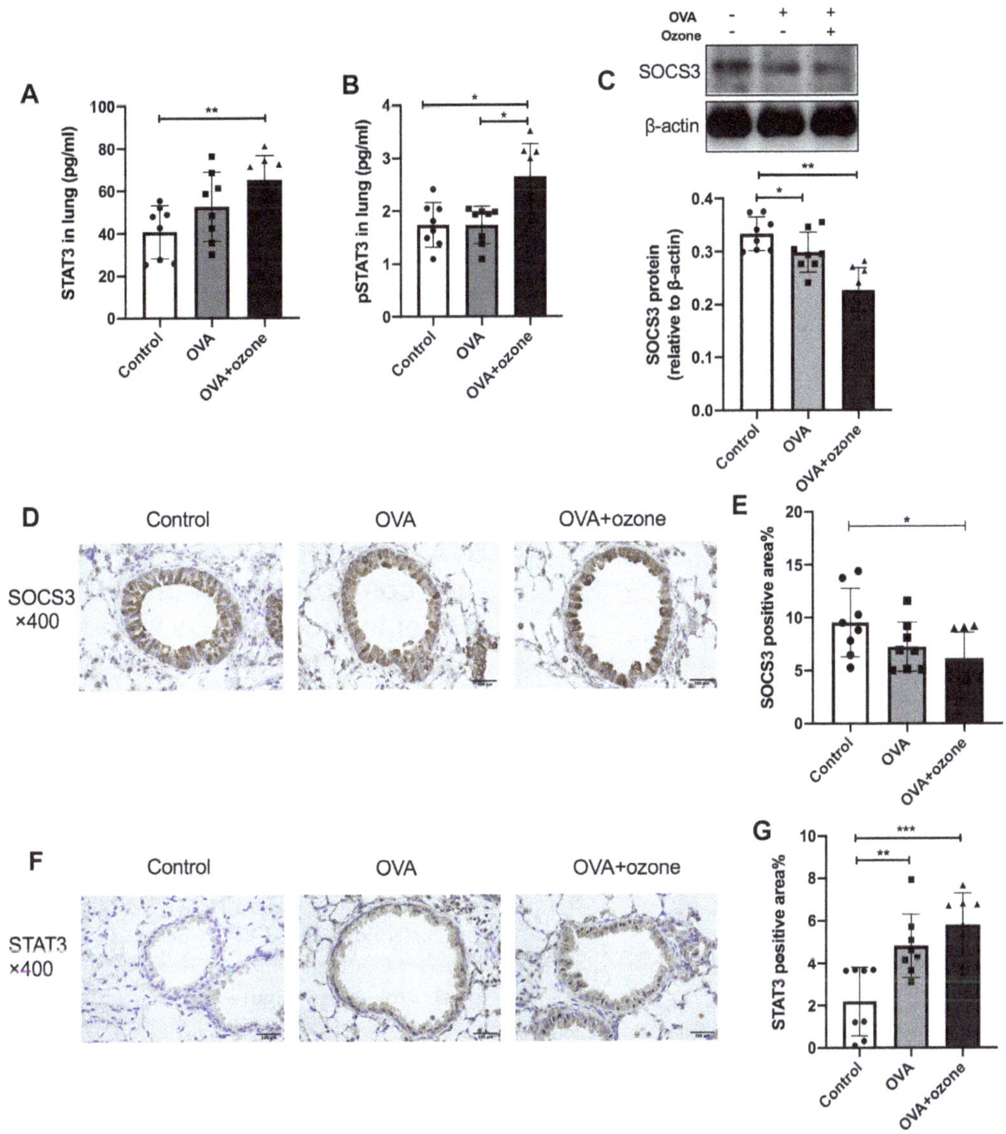

FIGURE 4 | Expression of STAT3 and SOCS3 in the lung tissue of mice suffering from asthma. The expression of STAT3 and p-STAT3 in the lung tissue of mice was measured by ELISAs. The expression of SOCS3 protein in the lung tissue of mice was measured by western blotting, and protein expression of STAT3 and SOCS3 in the lung tissue of mice was evaluated by immunohistochemistry. **(A)** Expression of STAT3 protein in lung tissue. **(B)** Expression of p-STAT3 protein in lung tissue. **(C)** Expression of SOCS3 protein in lung tissue. **(D)** Representative photomicrographs of immunohistochemistry of SOCS3 in lung-tissue slices. **(E)** Percent SOCS3-positive area around airways. **(F)** Representative photomicrographs of immunohistochemistry of STAT3 in lung-tissue slices. **(G)** Percent STAT3-positive area around airways. SOCS3, suppressor of cytokine signaling 3; STAT3, signal transducer and activator of transcription 3; p-STAT3, phosphorylated-STAT3. $^{*}p < 0.05$; $^{**}p < 0.01$; $^{***}p < 0.001$. Scale bar = 100 μm.

mass in the lung slices of mice of the OVA + ozone group increased more than that of the OVA group (**Figure 2M**), which indicated severe airway remodeling in the OVA + ozone group.

The OVA + Ozone Group Showed Features of Corticosteroid Resistance

As mentioned above, the number of neutrophils and expression of Th17-related cytokines were increased in the OVA + ozone group, which could lead to corticosteroid resistance. Protein expression of HDAC2 (which is related to corticosteroid resistance) decreased in the lung tissues of mice in the OVA + ozone group (**Figure 3A**). As a model involving neutrophil infiltration induced by oxidative stress, the OVA + ozone group showed a trend of increased HIF-1α expression, but there was no significant difference between the OVA + ozone group and the control group (**Figure 3B**). Compared with that in the control group, the expression of *Nr3c1* mRNA in the lung tissue of mice in the OVA + ozone group increased (**Figure 3C**). Correspondingly, the expression of GR protein increased significantly in the OVA + ozone group (**Figure 3D**). However, the expression of p-GR in the lung tissue of the OVA

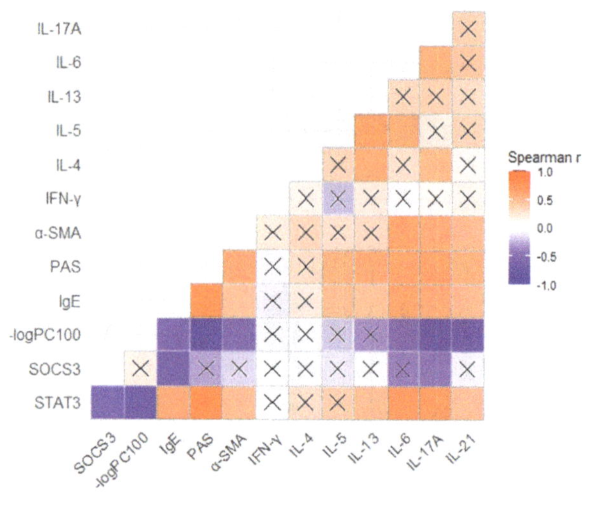

FIGURE 5 | Correlation between the expression of STAT3 or SOCS3 and mucus secretion as well as inflammation, responsiveness, and remodeling of the airways in different asthma models. Spearman's correlation coefficient matrix and Spearman's rank correlation tests were conducted. The expression of STAT3, SOCS3, and α-SMA was discovered from the results of immunohistochemical analyses. The expression of IgE and Th1/Th2/Th17-related cytokines was obtained using ELISAs of serum. A cross indicates no significance. *p*-Values are shown in **Supplementary Table S1**. SOCS3, suppressor of cytokine signaling 3; STAT3, signal transducer and activator of transcription 3; α-SMA, α-smooth muscle actin.

+ ozone group decreased more than that in the OVA group (**Figure 3E**). GR phosphorylation may have been involved in corticosteroid resistance observed in the OVA + ozone group.

CXCL1 significantly increased in the lung of the OVA + ozone group compared to the control group (**Figures 3F,G**), while the positive area percentage of CXCR2 showed no statistical difference among the three groups (**Supplementary Figure S2**).

STAT3 Expression Increased and SOCS3 Expression Decreased in the OVA + Ozone Group

The expression of total STAT3 and p-STAT3 (phosphorylated at Y705) in the lung tissues of mice in the OVA + ozone group increased, and the expression of p-STAT3 showed a significant increase compared with that in the OVA group (**Figures 4A,B**). Simultaneously, the expression of SOCS3 protein decreased in both mouse models of asthma compared with that in the control group (**Figure 4C**). Similar to the results of protein levels, the percent STAT3-positive area in the lung tissues of the OVA group and OVA + ozone group increased compared with that in the control group (**Figures 4F,G**), whereas the percent SOCS3-positive area decreased in the OVA + ozone group (**Figures 4D,E**). Single ozone exposure showed no significant statistical difference from the control group (**Supplementary Figure S5**).

Expression of STAT3 and SOCS3 Was Correlated With Expression of Th17-Related Cytokines

Correlation was evaluated using Spearman's rank analysis. STAT3 expression and SOCS3 expression showed a strong correlation with each other ($r = -0.53$). The expression of STAT3 and SOCS3 was correlated with the expression of IgE and IL-17A in mouse serum ($r = 0.57$ and 0.67 with STAT3 and -0.53 and -0.43 with SOCS3, respectively) (**Figure 5**). STAT3 expression showed a stronger correlation with the expression of Th17-related cytokines (IL-6, IL-17A, and IL-21) than Th2-related cytokines, in serum. STAT3 expression correlated with the percent stained areas of PAS and α-SMA ($r = 0.75$ and 0.46, respectively) and −logPC100 ($r = -0.62$) (**Figure 5**). Hence, STAT3 may be involved in the hypersecretion, remodeling, and hyperresponsiveness of airways observed in asthma.

STAT3 and IL-6 Are Involved in the Corticosteroid Resistance of an Asthma Model Induced by OVA and Ozone

The expression of HDAC2 and p-GR protein in the OVA + ozone group could not be restored completely by Dex treatment (**Figures 6A,B**). Protein expression of total STAT3 and p-STAT3 could not be reversed completely by Dex treatment (**Figures 6C,D**). IL-6 (which is important for the differentiation of Th17 cells and may be upstream of STAT3) expression appeared to be corticosteroid-insensitive in mice in the OVA + ozone group (**Figure 6E**). Protein expression of IL-13 (Th2-related cytokine) showed an evident response to this corticosteroid (**Figure 6F**), whereas IL-17A seemed to decline after Dex treatment, but continued to remain higher than that in the control group (**Figure 6G**).

Expression of STAT3 and SOCS3 Was Altered in the Lung Tissue of Asthma Patients and Showed Correlation With Expression of IL-17A Protein

The normal lung tissues of seven asthma patients and 10 HCs who underwent thoracotomy were evaluated through IHC staining and ELISAs. The STAT3-positive area increased in the lung tissue of asthma patients compared with that in HCs (**Figures 7A,B**), whereas SOCS3 expression decreased in the lung tissue of asthma patients (**Figures 7C,D**). The expression of STAT3 and SOCS3 showed a strong correlation with the expression of IL-17A protein in the lung tissue of patients ($r = 0.5624$ and -0.6553, respectively) (**Figures 7E,F**). The characteristics of these patients at baseline are shown in **Supplementary Table S2**.

DISCUSSION

We established a T2-high asthma model with eosinophil infiltration and increased expression of Th2-related cytokines

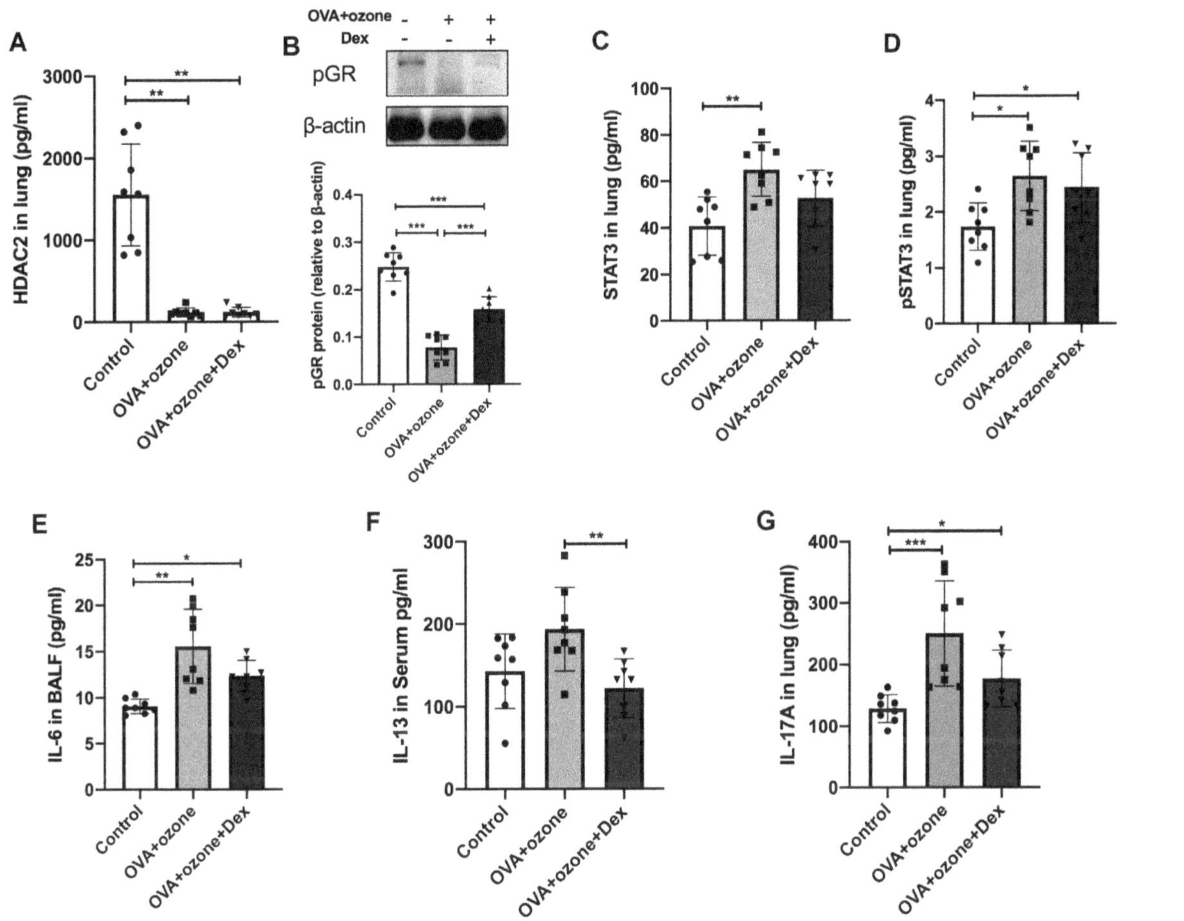

FIGURE 6 | Changes in the expression of cytokines and transcription factors after intervention by dexamethasone. The expression of HDAC2, IL-6, IL-13, and IL-17A was measured by ELISAs. The expression of p-GR protein was analyzed by western blotting. **(A)** Expression of HDAC2 protein in lung tissue after Dex treatment. **(B)** Expression of p-GR protein in lung tissue after Dex treatment. **(C)** Expression of STAT3 protein in lung tissue after Dex treatment. **(D)** Expression of p-STAT3 protein in lung tissue after Dex treatment. **(E)** Expression of IL-6 protein in BALF after Dex treatment. **(F)** Expression of IL-13 protein after Dex treatment. **(G)** Expression of IL-17A protein after Dex treatment. Dex, dexamethasone; HDAC2, histone deacetylase 2; p-GR, phosphorylated-GR; STAT3, signal transducer and activator of transcription 3.*$p < 0.05$; **$p < 0.01$; ***$p < 0.001$.

through OVA sensitization/challenge. We constructed a mixed Th2/Th17 response model with neutrophil infiltration and increased expression of Th17-related cytokines through OVA sensitization/challenge combined with ozone exposure.

The OVA + ozone group showed more severe airway inflammation, airway hyperresponsiveness, and severe airway remodeling than those in the OVA group. Th17-related cytokines have important roles in T2-low asthma (Chung, 2016; Svenningsen and Nair, 2017). To ascertain the differences in endotypes of our mouse models, we adopted cytokine antibody arrays for simultaneous and accurate detection of multiple cytokines.

After establishing models of T2-high asthma or a mixed Th2/Th17 response with neutrophil infiltration–based airway inflammation, we discovered the characteristics of corticosteroid resistance in the OVA + ozone group. Studies using mouse models of asthma and human type II alveolar epithelial cells have shown that exposure to high ozone levels can reduce the response of asthma patients to glucocorticoid therapy during acute exacerbations (Flayer et al., 2019). In our previous study, a mouse model induced by OVA and ozone showed the traits of corticosteroid resistance (Zhang J.-h. et al., 2019). In the present study, we demonstrated that the expression of HDAC2 and p-GR decreased in the OVA + ozone group, which is a characteristic of corticosteroid resistance. The development of corticosteroid resistance is closely related to the expression and phosphorylation of GRs. Reduced phosphorylation of GRs leads to reduced nuclear translocation, which results in corticosteroid resistance (Irusen et al., 2002). The anti-inflammatory effect of GRs is promoted by HDAC2, and studies have revealed that HDAC2 expression is decreased in patients with severe asthma and may be involved in the development of glucocorticoid resistance (Irvin et al., 2014). The expression of *Nr3c1* (the gene of GRs) (Farrell et al., 2018) was found to be increased, and synchronously, the expression of GR protein increased, in the OVA + ozone

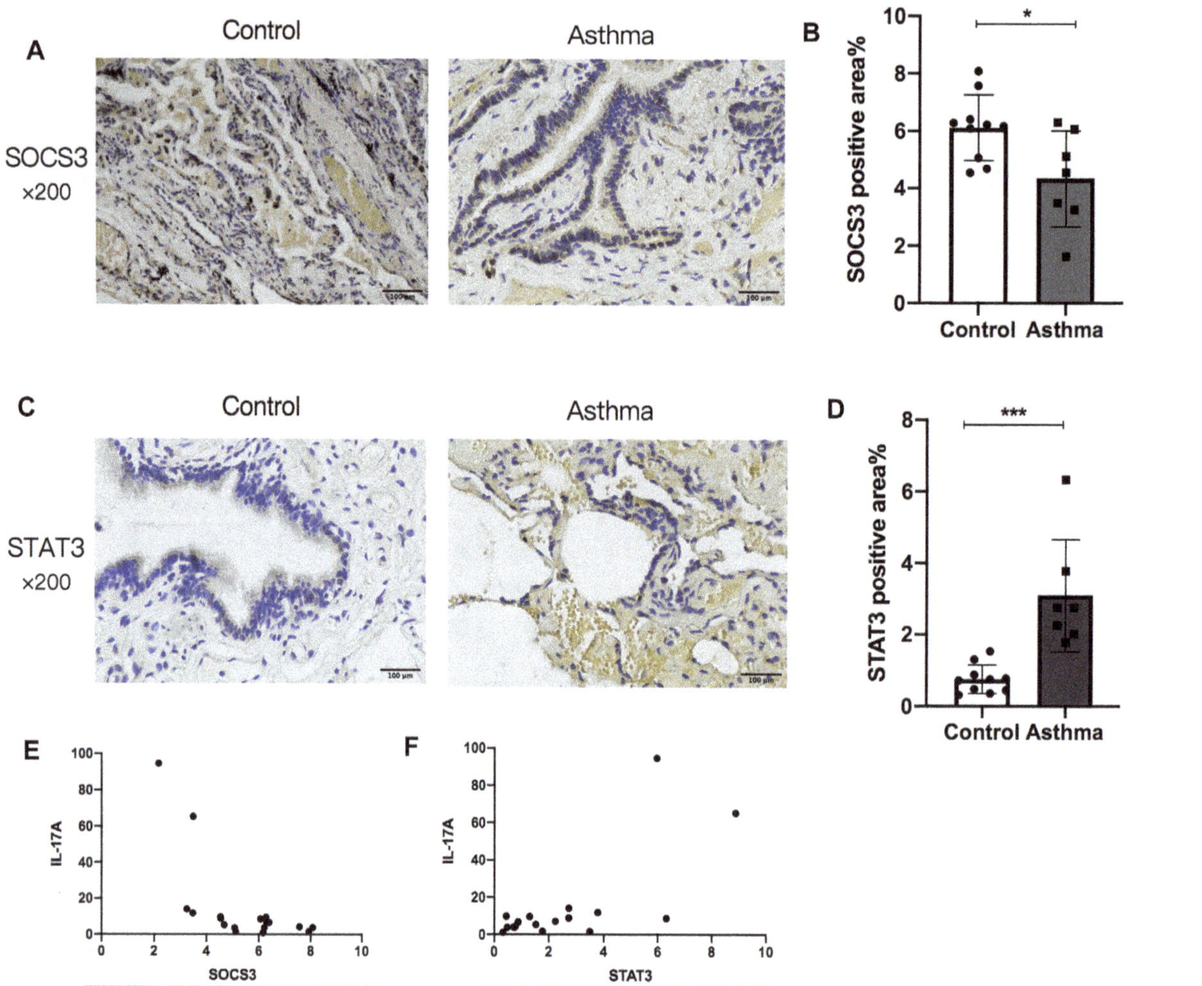

	SOCS3 vs. IL-17A
Spearman r	
r	-0.6553
95% confidence interval	-0.8632 to -0.2576
P value	
P (two-tailed)	0.0032

	STAT3 vs. IL-17A
Spearman r	
r	0.5624
95% confidence interval	0.1149 to 0.8202
P value	
P (two-tailed)	0.0151

FIGURE 7 | Comparison of SOCS3 expression and STAT3 expression in normal lung tissue between asthma patients and healthy controls and their correlation with IL-17A expression in the lung. The expression of STAT3 and SOCS3 in lung tissues of 17 patients undergoing thoracotomy for pulmonary nodules was analyzed by immunohistochemistry. **(A)** Representative photomicrographs of immunohistochemistry of SOCS3 in lung-tissue slices of the asthma group and control group. **(B)** Percent SOCS3-positive area around airways. **(C)** Representative photomicrographs of immunohistochemistry of STAT3 in lung-tissue slices of asthma and control groups. **(D)** Percent STAT3-positive area around airways. **(E)** Correlation between the percent STAT3-positive area and the expression of IL-17A protein in human lung tissue. **(F)** Correlation between the percent SOCS3-positive area and the expression of IL-17A protein in human lung tissue. SOCS3, suppressor of cytokine signaling 3; STAT3, signal transducer and activator of transcription 3. $^{*}p < 0.05$; $^{**}p < 0.01$; $^{***}p < 0.001$. Scale bar = 100 μm.

group. However, a reduction of expression of the active form of GR (p-GR), which may be facilitated by HDAC2, could have led directly to corticosteroid resistance in the OVA + ozone group.

As important pathophysiological features of severe asthma, neutrophil infiltration and activation in the lung are mostly mediated by CXCL8 and CXCL1 via CXCR1 and CXCR2 (Planagumà et al., 2015). Bao, A. et al. once found increased CXCL1 mRNA expression in an ozone-exposed ovalbumin mouse model (Bao et al., 2017). Johnston, R. A. and others showed an essential role of CXCR2 in maximal neutrophil recruitment after an acute O(3) exposure (Johnston et al., 2005). The ligand CXCL1 increased in our OVA + ozone-induced mouse model with neutrophil infiltration, indicating a role of chemoattractant for neutrophils in the steroid resistance of this model. The receptor CXCR2 showed a trend of increase compared with that in the control group while having no statistical difference. The difference in the mouse model and concentration or duration of ozone exposure may lead to the discrepancy of our results and Johnston, R. A. and others'. Further quantitative research should be conducted to determine the change of chemoattractant for neutrophils in the OVA + ozone mouse model.

Ozone can induce tissue injury due to oxidative stress. Some studies have shown that the hypoxia inducer HIF-1α is associated with oxidative stress and may affect asthma pathogenesis (Saini et al., 2010). HIF-1α expression in the OVA + ozone group showed an increasing trend compared with that in the control group, but the difference was not significant, which may have been related to the low ozone concentration (2 ppm) used in our modeling process. This finding suggested that oxidative-stress injury may not have been the leading cause of corticosteroid insensitivity in the OVA + ozone group.

Because of high expression of Th17-related cytokines (IL-6, IL-17A, and IL-21) in the OVA + ozone group, the expression of STAT3 and SOCS3 (which are important transcription factors of Th17) was evaluated further. The role of STAT3 and SOCS3 in asthma has been discussed in relation to the T2-mediated allergic response (Seki et al., 2003; Gao and Ward, 2007). Several studies have shown that short-term ozone exposure increased levels of STAT3 or p-STAT3 (Lang et al., 2008; Mishra et al., 2016a), while our study showed an increasing trend but no statistical difference between the ozone group and the control group. Maybe, the difference in methods and the duration of ozone exposure led to this discrepancy. There is still lack of study in effects of ozone exposure on SOCS3, and few scholars have focused on the role of STAT3 and SOCS3 in the mechanism of action of T2-low asthma and corticosteroid resistance. Inhibition of STAT3 expression by C188-9 was shown to reduce airway inflammation and airway remodeling in a house dust mite–induced asthma model created by Gavino and coworkers (Gavino et al., 2016). They adopted a different type of modeling compared with our model. However, studies have demonstrated the ability of house dust mites to induce the production of Th2 cells and Th17 cells simultaneously (Lan et al., 2011), which is similar to the model induced by OVA + ozone in our study. STAT3 expression increased in the OVA + ozone group. p-STAT3 expression increased in the OVA + ozone group more than that in the OVA group. Therefore, STAT3 activated after phosphorylation may have an important role in T2-low asthma and be involved in the development of corticosteroid resistance.

The transcription suppressor SOCS3 showed an opposite trend to that of STAT3 in the OVA + ozone group. This trend has been documented in other studies related to airway inflammation. Sun and others demonstrated the inhibitory effect of SOCS3 on differentiation of Th17 cells in an asthma model (Sun et al., 2018). However, Mishra and coworkers discovered different results: the expression of SOCS3 and STAT3 increased synchronously in allergic airway inflammation (Mishra et al., 2016b). The reason for this disparity may be related to differences in the mouse model employed. Those controversial results further demonstrate the complex regulatory role of SOCS3 in asthma pathogenesis. Some studies have discussed the role of STAT3 in corticosteroid resistance (Banuelos et al., 2016; Halwani et al., 2016). However, few studies have paid attention to the potential role of SOCS3 in corticosteroid resistance in an asthma model closely related to Th17 cells.

We showed that the expression of IL-6 and IL-17A was correlated with that of STAT3 and SOCS3. STAT3 showed a stronger correlation with the expression of Th17-related cytokines in serum (e.g., IL-6 and IL-17A) than the expression of Th2-related cytokines, which indicates its interaction with Th17 cells. The correlation between the expression of STAT3 or SOCS3 and airway inflammation indicated that STAT3 and SOCS3 are involved in asthma. A strong correlation between SOCS3 expression and asthma severity and serum IgE levels in allergic patients has been reported (Gao and Ward, 2007), which is in accordance with our findings in mouse models. Gavino and others found that blockade of Th2 and Th17 pathways by STAT3 inhibitors in a mouse model of asthma was effective in reducing lung inflammation compared with that employing blockade of one pathway alone (Gavino et al., 2016), which conformed to the correlation between STAT3 expression and IL-13 and IL-17A expressions in our study. However, we speculate that STAT3 expression may be correlated more closely with Th17 pathways than Th2 pathways in the present study due to its stronger correlation with Th17-related cytokines rather than Th2-related cytokines.

As demonstrated above, STAT3 expression is correlated with mucus secretion as well as inflammation, responsiveness, and remodeling of the airways, which suggests an important role of STAT3 in asthma pathogenesis. We found that STAT3 phosphorylation as well as the expression of IL-6 and IL-17A could not be reversed by Dex treatment, which indicates their involvement in corticosteroid resistance of OVA- and ozone-induced asthma. In an animal study, Banuelos and collaborators showed that IL-17A production was not suppressed by glucocorticoids (Banuelos et al., 2016). Previously, we found that treatment with the IL-17A monoclonal antibody reduced corticosteroid insensitivity in a mouse model of asthma (Zhang Y. et al., 2019). Here, we paid more attention to p-STAT3. It has been reported that STAT3 phosphorylation in Th17 cells is insensitive to glucocorticoid inhibition (Banuelos et al., 2016). IL-6 is involved in STAT3-regulated inflammation and may interact with STAT3 (Rottenberg and Carow, 2014). Dex and budesonide help protect human type II alveolar epithelial cells by epithelium-derived surfactant protein D in a manner that is dependent on GRs and STAT3 (an IL-6–responsive transcription factor) (Flayer et al., 2019). Thus, IL-6 and STAT3 may have important roles in an OVA- and ozone-induced corticosteroid-resistant asthma model. Our analyses in the human lung tissue of the expression of STAT3 and SOCS3 further convinced us that STAT3 and SOCS3 are involved in asthma. We analyzed the correlation between the expression of STAT3 or SOCS3 and IL-17A. The expression of IL-17A in the lung tissue of asthma patients and HCs showed a strong correlation with the expression of STAT3 and SOCS3. These findings further indicated the possible role of interaction between STAT3 or SOCS3 and Th17 cells in asthma. The expression of SOCS3 and STAT3 has been evaluated in airway inflammation in some animal models (Gao and

Ward, 2007; Santana et al., 2019; Pinheiro et al., 2020), but we are the first to observe their changes in the lung tissue of asthma patients. Though we failed to divide asthma patients to T2-high or -low endotypes, eosinophil counts in blood were <150/μl in the asthma group and did not show a significant difference from that in the control group (**Supplementary Table S2**).

However, there are several limitations of the current study. Firstly, increasing studies have demonstrated non-HLA antibodies such as Col-V and EGFR involved in the IL-17–related pathways in different pulmonary diseases (and may contribute to severe asthma). More attention should be paid to these pathways but not the conventional pathway. We will try to involve these non-HLA antibodies in our studies of IL-17 and its pathways. Secondly, further studies on the intervention of STAT3 and SOCS3, as well as the discussion of the mechanisms of their regulation in Th17 cells and corticosteroid resistance, should be conducted.

CONCLUSION

We established an asthma model with neutrophil infiltration and increased expression of Th17-related cytokines by OVA sensitization/challenge and ozone exposure. The OVA + ozone group showed corticosteroid resistance with reduction of expression of HDAC2 and p-GR. STAT3 and SOCS3 appeared to be involved in asthma pathogenesis in mouse models and asthma patients. IL-6 and STAT3 may have contributed to corticosteroid resistance in the OVA + ozone group through regulation of Th17 cells. SOCS3 (a negative transcription factor) may interact with STAT3 and be involved in the corticosteroid insensitivity of the T2-low asthma model.

ETHICS STATEMENT

The studies involving human participants were reviewed and approved by the Institutional Review Board at Shanghai General Hospital (No. 2018KY186) and registered on chictr.org.cn (No. ChiCTR2000029065). The patients/participants provided their written informed consent to participate in this study. The animal study was reviewed and approved by the Ethics Committee for Animal Studies at Shanghai General Hospital, China (IACUC: 2019-A011-01).

AUTHOR CONTRIBUTIONS

MZ designed the experiments. YX, HH, QF, LH, XZ, and XT performed the experiments. YX, WB, YZ, and MZ analyzed and interpreted the data, drafted the article, and supervised the work. All authors read and approved the final article.

REFERENCES

Alangari, A. (2014). Corticosteroids in the Treatment of Acute Asthma. *Ann. Thorac. Med.* 9, 187–192. doi:10.4103/1817-1737.140120

Banuelos, J., Shin, S., Cao, Y., Bochner, B. S., Morales-Nebreda, L., Budinger, G. R. S., et al. (2016). BCL-2 Protects Human and Mouse Th17 Cells from Glucocorticoid-Induced Apoptosis. *Allergy* 71 (5), 640–650. doi:10.1111/all.12840

Bao, A., Ma, A., Zhang, H., Qiao, L., Ben, S., Zhou, X., et al. (2020). Inducible Expression of Heat Shock Protein 20 Protects Airway Epithelial Cells against Oxidative Injury Involving the Nrf2-NQO-1 Pathway. *Cell Biosci.* 10, 120. doi:10.1186/s13578-020-00483-3

Bao, A., Yang, H., Ji, J., Chen, Y., Bao, W., Li, F., et al. (2017). Involvements of P38 MAPK and Oxidative Stress in the Ozone-Induced Enhancement of AHR and Pulmonary Inflammation in an Allergic Asthma Model. *Respir. Res.* 18 (1), 216. doi:10.1186/s12931-017-0697-4

Bao, W., Zhang, Y., Zhang, M., Bao, A., Fei, X., Zhang, X., et al. (2018). Effects of Ozone Repeated Short Exposures on the Airway/lung Inflammation, Airway Hyperresponsiveness and Mucus Production in a Mouse Model of Ovalbumin-Induced Asthma. *Biomed. Pharmacother.* 101, 293–303. doi:10.1016/j.biopha.2018.02.079

Barnes, P. J. (2016). Glucocorticosteroids. *Handb Exp. Pharmacol.* 237, 93–115. doi:10.1007/164_2016_62

Bobadilla, J. L., Love, R. B., Jankowska-Gan, E., Xu, Q., Haynes, L. D., Braun, R. K., et al. (2008). Th-17, Monokines, Collagen Type V, and Primary Graft Dysfunction in Lung Transplantation. *Am. J. Respir. Crit. Care Med.* 177 (6), 660–668. doi:10.1164/rccm.200612-1901OC

Chung, K. F. (2016). Asthma Phenotyping: a Necessity for Improved Therapeutic Precision and New Targeted Therapies. *J. Intern. Med.* 279 (2), 192–204. doi:10.1111/joim.12382

Cosmi, L., Liotta, F., Maggi, E., Romagnani, S., and Annunziato, F. (2011). Th17 Cells: New Players in Asthma Pathogenesis. *Allergy* 66 (8), 989–998. doi:10.1111/j.1398-9995.2011.02576.x

Farrell, A. K., Slatcher, R. B., Tobin, E. T., Imami, L., Wildman, D. E., Luca, F., et al. (2018). Socioeconomic Status, Family Negative Emotional Climate, and Anti-inflammatory Gene Expression Among Youth with Asthma. *Psychoneuroendocrinology* 91, 62–67. doi:10.1016/j.psyneuen.2018.02.011

Flayer, C. H., Ge, M. Q., Hwang, J. W., Kokalari, B., Redai, I. G., Jiang, Z., et al. (2019). Ozone Inhalation Attenuated the Effects of Budesonide on Aspergillus Fumigatus-Induced Airway Inflammation and Hyperreactivity in Mice. *Front. Immunol.* 10, 2173. doi:10.3389/fimmu.2019.02173

Gao, H., and Ward, P. A. (2007). STAT3 and Suppressor of Cytokine Signaling 3: Potential Targets in Lung Inflammatory Responses. *Expert Opin. Ther. Targets* 11 (7), 869–880. doi:10.1517/14728222.11.7.869

Gavino, A. C., Nahmod, K., Bharadwaj, U., Makedonas, G., and Tweardy, D. J. (2016). STAT3 Inhibition Prevents Lung Inflammation, Remodeling, and Accumulation of Th2 and Th17 Cells in a Murine Asthma Model. *Allergy* 71 (12), 1684–1692. doi:10.1111/all.12937

Halwani, R., Sultana, A., Al-Kufaidy, R., Jamhawi, A., Vazquez-Tello, A., and Al-Muhsen, S. (2016). Th-17 Regulatory Cytokines Inhibit Corticosteroid Induced Airway Structural Cells Apoptosis. *Respir. Res.* 17, 6. doi:10.1186/s12931-015-0307-2

Irusen, E., Matthews, J. G., Takahashi, A., Barnes, P. J., Chung, K. F., and Adcock, I. M. (2002). p38 Mitogen-Activated Protein Kinase-Induced Glucocorticoid Receptor Phosphorylation Reduces its Activity: Role in Steroid-Insensitive Asthma. *J. Allergy Clin. Immunol.* 109 (4), 649–657. doi:10.1067/mai.2002.122465

Irvin, C., Zafar, I., Good, J., Rollins, D., Christianson, C., Gorska, M. M., et al. (2014). Increased Frequency of Dual-Positive TH2/TH17 Cells in Bronchoalveolar Lavage Fluid Characterizes a Population of Patients with Severe Asthma. *J. Allergy Clin. Immunol.* 134 (5), 1175–1186. e7. doi:10.1016/j.jaci.2014.05.038

Johnston, R. A., Mizgerd, J. P., and Shore, S. A. (2005). CXCR2 Is Essential for Maximal Neutrophil Recruitment and Methacholine Responsiveness after

Ozone Exposure. *Am. J. Physiology-Lung Cell Mol. Physiol.* 288 (1), L61–L67. doi:10.1152/ajplung.00101.2004

Lan, F., Liu, K., Zhang, J., Qi, Y., Li, K., and Lin, P. (2011). Th17 Response Is Augmented in OVA-Induced Asthmatic Mice Exposed to HDM. *Med. Sci. Monit.* 17 (5), BR132–BR138. doi:10.12659/msm.881759

Lang, J. E., Williams, E. S., Mizgerd, J. P., and Shore, S. A. (2008). Effect of Obesity on Pulmonary Inflammation Induced by Acute Ozone Exposure: Role of Interleukin-6. *Am. J. Physiology-Lung Cell Mol. PhysiologyLung Cell. Mol. Physiol.* 294 (5), L1013–L1020. doi:10.1152/ajplung.00122.2007

Last, J. A., Ward, R., Temple, L., and Kenyon, N. J. (2004). Ovalbumin-induced Airway Inflammation and Fibrosis in Mice Also Exposed to Ozone. *Inhalation Toxicol.* 16 (1), 33–43. doi:10.1080/08958370490258237

Lee, K.-L., Lai, T.-C., Wang, Y.-C., Shih, P.-C., Yang, Y.-C., Tsao, T. C.-Y., et al. (2021). Potential Impacts of Interleukin-17A Promoter Polymorphisms on the EGFR Mutation Status and Progression of Non-small Cell Lung Cancer in Taiwan. *Genes* 12 (3), 427. doi:10.3390/genes12030427

Li, Z., Fan, H., Chen, W., Xiao, J., Ma, X., Ni, P., et al. (2021). MicroRNA-653-5p Promotes Gastric Cancer Proliferation and Metastasis by Targeting the SOCS6-STAT3 Pathway. *Front. Mol. Biosci.* 8, 655580. doi:10.3389/fmolb.2021.655580

Mei, D., Tan, W. S. D., and Wong, W. S. F. (2019). Pharmacological Strategies to Regain Steroid Sensitivity in Severe Asthma and COPD. *Curr. Opin. Pharmacol.* 46, 73–81. doi:10.1016/j.coph.2019.04.010

Miossec, P., and Kolls, J. K. (2012). Targeting IL-17 and TH17 Cells in Chronic Inflammation. *Nat. Rev. Drug Discov.* 11 (10), 763–776. doi:10.1038/nrd3794

Mishra, V., Baranwal, V., Mishra, R. K., Sharma, S., Paul, B., and Pandey, A. C. (2016a). Titanium Dioxide Nanoparticles Augment Allergic Airway Inflammation and Socs3 Expression via NF-Kb Pathway in Murine Model of Asthma. *Biomaterials* 92, 90–102. doi:10.1016/j.biomaterials.2016.03.016

Mishra, V., DiAngelo, S. L., and Silveyra, P. (2016b). Sex-specific IL-6-associated Signaling Activation in Ozone-Induced Lung Inflammation. *Biol. Sex. Differ.* 7, 16. doi:10.1186/s13293-016-0069-7

Panettieri, R. A., Jr (2018). The Role of Neutrophils in Asthma. *Immunol. Allergy Clin. North America* 38 (4), 629–638. doi:10.1016/j.iac.2018.06.005

Pinheiro, N. M., Miranda, C. J. C. P., Santana, F. R., Bittencourt-Mernak, M., Arantes-Costa, F. M., Olivo, C., et al. (2020). Effects of VAChT Reduction and α7nAChR Stimulation by PNU-282987 in Lung Inflammation in a Model of Chronic Allergic Airway Inflammation. *Eur. J. Pharmacol.* 882, 173239. doi:10.1016/j.ejphar.2020.173239

Planagumà, A., Domènech, T., Pont, M., Calama, E., García-González, V., López, R., et al. (2015). Combined Anti CXC Receptors 1 and 2 Therapy Is a Promising Anti-inflammatory Treatment for Respiratory Diseases by Reducing Neutrophil Migration and Activation. *Pulm. Pharmacol. Ther.* 34, 37–45. doi:10.1016/j.pupt.2015.08.002

Rottenberg, M. E., and Carow, B. (2014). SOCS3 and STAT3, Major Controllers of the Outcome of Infection with *Mycobacterium tuberculosis*. *Semin. Immunol.* 26 (6), 518–532. doi:10.1016/j.smim.2014.10.004

Saini, Y., Kim, K. Y., Lewandowski, R., Bramble, L. A., Harkema, J. R., and Lapres, J. J. (2010). Role of Hypoxia-Inducible Factor 1α in Modulating Cobalt-Induced Lung Inflammation. *Am. J. Physiology-Lung Cell Mol. PhysiologyLung Cell. Mol. Physiol.* 298 (2), L139–L147. doi:10.1152/ajplung.00252.2009

Santana, F. P. R., da Silva, R. C., Grecco, S. d. S., Pinheiro, A. J. M. C. R., Caperuto, L. C., Arantes-Costa, F. M., et al. (2019). Inhibition of MAPK and STAT3-SOCS3 by Sakuranetin Attenuated Chronic Allergic Airway Inflammation in Mice. *Mediators Inflamm.* 2019, 1–14. doi:10.1155/2019/1356356

Seki, Y.-i., Inoue, H., Nagata, N., Hayashi, K., Fukuyama, S., Matsumoto, K., et al. (2003). SOCS-3 Regulates Onset and Maintenance of TH2-Mediated Allergic Responses. *Nat. Med.* 9 (8), 1047–1054. doi:10.1038/nm896

Sun, W., Xiao, B., Jia, A., Qiu, L., Zeng, Q., Liu, D., et al. (2018). MBD2-mediated Th17 Differentiation in Severe Asthma Is Associated with Impaired SOCS3 Expression. *Exp. Cel. Res.* 371 (1), 196–204. doi:10.1016/j.yexcr.2018.08.010

Svenningsen, S., and Nair, P. (2017). Asthma Endotypes and an Overview of Targeted Therapy for Asthma. *Front. Med.* 4, 158. doi:10.3389/fmed.2017.00158

Wenzel, S. E., Schwartz, L. B., Langmack, E. L., Halliday, J. L., Trudeau, J. B., Gibbs, R. L., et al. (1999). Evidence that Severe Asthma Can Be Divided Pathologically into Two Inflammatory Subtypes with Distinct Physiologic and Clinical Characteristics. *Am. J. Respir. Crit. Care Med.* 160 (3), 1001–1008. doi:10.1164/ajrccm.160.3.9812110

Zhang, J.-h., Yang, X., Chen, Y.-p., Zhang, J.-f., and Li, C.-q. (2019a). Nrf2 Activator RTA-408 Protects against Ozone-Induced Acute Asthma Exacerbation by Suppressing ROS and γδT17 Cells. *Inflammation* 42 (5), 1843–1856. doi:10.1007/s10753-019-01046-6

Zhang, X., Bao, W., Fei, X., Zhang, Y., Zhang, G., Zhou, X., et al. (2018). Progesterone Attenuates Airway Remodeling and Glucocorticoid Resistance in a Murine Model of Exposing to Ozone. *Mol. Immunol.* 96, 69–77. doi:10.1016/j.molimm.2018.02.009

Zhang, Y., Li, X., He, M., Zhang, G., Bao, W., Fei, X., et al. (2019b). The Effects of Neutralizing Anti-murine interleukin-17A Monoclonal Antibody on Ozone-Induced Inflammation and Glucocorticoids Insensitivity in a Murine Model of Asthma. *Biomed. Pharmacother.* 114, 108786. doi:10.1016/j.biopha.2019.108786

Zhu, S.-q., Zhou, B.-h., Tan, P.-p., Chai, J., Yu, Y.-m., and Wang, H.-w. (2020). Based on G-Series Mouse TH17 Array Study the Effect of Fluoride on C2C12 Cells Cytokines Expression. *Biol. Trace Elem. Res.* doi:10.1007/s12011-020-02464-6

6

Multi-Dimensional Display of Wang's Lymph Node Map using Virtual Bronchoscopic Navigation System

Fen Lan[1†], Yaling Yue[2†], Hong Shen[3†], Hui Shen[1,4†], Qiyuan Wang[5†], Xiujing Yu[6], Laijuan Chen[6], Qin Li[1], Kopen Wang[7], Qinghua Liu[8] and Yang Xia[1]**

[1]Key Laboratory of Respiratory Disease of Zhejiang Province, Department of Respiratory and Critical Care Medicine, Second Affiliated Hospital of Zhejiang University School of Medicine, Hangzhou, China, [2]Department of Medical Oncology, Handan Central Hospital, Handan, China, [3]Department of Respiratory and Critical Care Medicine, Second Affiliated Hospital of Nanjing Medical University, Nanjing, China, [4]Department of Respiratory and Critical Care Medicine, Huzhou Central Hospital, Huzhou, China, [5]Department of Radiology, Second Affiliated Hospital of Zhejiang University School of Medicine, Hangzhou, China, [6]Department of Endoscopic Center, Second Affiliated Hospital of Zhejiang University School of Medicine, Hangzhou, China, [7]Division of Pulmonary and Critical Care Medicine, Johns Hopkins University School of Medicine, Baltimore, MD, United States, [8]Department of Respiratory and Critical Care Medicine, Shanghai East Hospital, Tongji University, Shanghai, China

***Correspondence:**
Yang Xia
yxia@zju.edu.cn
Qinghua Liu
lzlqhlz@163.com

†These authors share first authorship

Background: Transbronchial needle aspiration (TBNA) is a classical technique for diagnosing mediastinal-hilar lymph node enlargement. However, the diagnostic value of conventional TBNA (cTBNA) is limited in small lymph nodes.

Methods: Here, we generated an innovative multi-dimensional virtual lymph node map on top of Wang's lymph node map using a Lungpoint Virtual Bronchoscopic Navigation System.

Results: The virtual bronchoscopic navigation (VBN) system was combined with computed tomography (CT) images to generate extrabronchial, endobronchial, sagittal, coronal as well as horizontal views of the 11 intrathoracic lymph node stations and their adjacent tissues and blood vessels. We displayed the specific puncture site of each lymph node station. The 11 stations were divided into four groups: right mediastinal stations, left mediastinal stations, central mediastinal stations and hilar stations.

Conclusion: The VBN system provides a precise view of the intrabronchial landmarks, which may increase the diagnostic accuracy of intrathoracic lymph node adenopathy and assist bronchoscopists with practicing TBNA.

Keywords: lymph node map, TBNA, mediastinal-hilar lymph node, virtual navigation system, bronchoscopy

INTRODUCTION

Transbronchial needle aspiration (TBNA) is a classical bronchoscopic technique for diagnosing benign and malignant mediastinal-hilar lymph node enlargement. With technological progress, endobronchial ultrasound-guided TBNA (EBUS-TBNA) provides real-time ultrasound imaging, resulting in a higher diagnostic yield than conventional TBNA (cTBNA) and has been widely practiced in clinical settings worldwide (Herth et al., 2004; Bonifazi et al., 2017; Madan et al., 2017). However, even with ultrasound guidance, the diagnostic yield of TBNA varies, largely due to the skill and experience of the operator (Rodriguez de Castro et al., 1997; Hsu et al., 2004). Therefore, whether the operator can accurately locate the target lymph nodes is of great importance, and requires a comprehensive understanding of the anatomy of mediastinal-hilar lymph nodes.

The International Association for the Study of Lung Cancer (IASLC) lymph node map and Wang's lymph node map are the two most commonly used lymph node maps (Wang, 1994; Rusch et al., 2009). The eighth edition of the IASLC map was introduced in 2009 and most of the lymph node stations are defined according to the positions of blood vessels (El-Sherief et al., 2014). Without ultrasound, it is challenging to identify the blood vessels under bronchoscopy. Wang's map was proposed in 1994 and the targeted lymph nodes are located by airway landmarks under endoscopic view, which is more practical for practitioners (Wang, 1994).

Electromagnetic navigation bronchoscopy (ENB) was first applied in human subjects in 2006 (Schwarz et al., 2006). Compared with traditional bronchoscopy, ENB improved the diagnostic accuracy for peripheral pulmonary lesions (PPLs) and mediastinal lymph nodes (Gildea et al., 2006). However, the EBN process requires expensive equipment and special training for operators, and therefore it can only be applied in qualified medical centers. On the other hand, virtual bronchoscopy can simulate a three-dimensional view of the bronchi and adjacent structures using. The reported diagnostic yield of virtual bronchoscopic navigation (VBN) system for peripheral pulmonary lesions was 70.9%–76.8% for peripheral pulmonary lesions, that of thin bronchoscopy combined with computed tomography (CT) and VBN was 65.4%–81.6% and that of X-ray fluoroscopy plus VBN was 62.5%–78.7% (Asano et al., 2014). Electromagnetic navigation and virtual navigation could also be used as advanced lymph node localisation systems. Previously, we reported the intrabronchial display of hilar-mediastinal lymph nodes by the SPiN Thoracic Navigation System (Wu et al., 2018). However, only an endobronchial map of mediastinal-hilar lymph nodes was generated, without demonstration of the extrabronchial anatomical position of each lymph node. Here, we further devised a virtual extrabronchial and endobronchial map together with horizontal, coronal and sagittal views on chest CT for each mediastinal and hilar lymph node using the Lungpoint Virtual Bronchoscopic Navigation System, in accordance with the recommended lymph node puncture site in Wang's map. Therefore, clinicians can gain an overall impression of the three-dimensional (3D) spatial structure of the most frequently punctured lymph nodes, thus improving the accuracy and safety of TBNA.

METHODS

CT images 1 mm thick were acquired and transferred to a workstation where the Lungpoint Virtual Bronchoscopic Navigation System (Broncus Technologies, Inc., Mountain View, CA, United States) automatically generated a 3D model of the airway. We set up 3D markers of the locations of intrathoracic lymph nodes. The extrabronchial anatomical positions of each target lymph node were shown as green spheres. The positions and borders of 11 target lymph nodes were described according to Wang's lymph node map.

RESULTS

We generated an overall view of 11 lymph node stations in Wang' map under 3D reconstruction (**Figure 1**). Next, we collected the horizontal, coronal and sagittal views of chest CT, labeled extrabronchial 3D anatomical locations of the 11 nodal stations in terms of Wang's lymph node map and generated a virtual view from an extrabronchial perspective. We classified the 11 stations into four groups: right mediastinal stations (**Figure 2**), left mediastinal stations (**Figure 3**), central mediastinal stations (**Figure 4**) and hilar stations (**Figure 5**). The recommended TBNA puncture sites of particular lymph nodes were also described in detail (Wang, 1994; Wang, 1995; Xia and Wang, 2013) (see **Supplementary Table S1**).

W1 station, anterior carina (correlated with IASLC 4R).
Location: In front and between the proximal portions of the right and left main bronchi.
Posterior border: The carina of the trachea.
Puncture point: The first trachea cartilage ring gap at 12–1 o'clock.
W2 station, posterior carina (correlated with IASLC-7).
Location: Behind and between the proximal portions of the right and left main bronchi or directly behind the right main bronchus.
Upper border: tip of the carina.
Lower border: The superior portion of the opening of the right upper lobe bronchus.
Puncture point: The opposite side of W1, 5–6 o'clock at the posterior wall of the carina.
W3 station, right paratracheal (correlated with IASLC-4R).
Location: Behind the superior vena cava and in front of the anterolateral aspect of the lower trachea near the azygous arch.
Upper border: The inferior margin of the brachiocephalic vein or superior margin of the aortic arch.
Lower border: The superior margin of the azygous arch.
Puncture point: Second to fourth trachea cartilage ring gaps at 1–2 o'clock.
W4 station, left paratracheal (A-P window, correlated with IASLC-4L).
Location: Lateral to trachea near the tracheobronchial angulation, below the aortic arch and above the left main pulmonary artery.
The W4 lymph nodes are divided into interior, middle and exterior windows.
Puncture point: First or second cartilage ring gap from the distal trachea at 9 o'clock or one trachea cartilage ring distal or proximal from the tracheobronchial angle.
W5 station, right main bronchus (distal W5 correlated with IASLC-10R, proximal W5 correlated with IASLC-4R).
Location: In front of the proximal proportion of the right main bronchus.

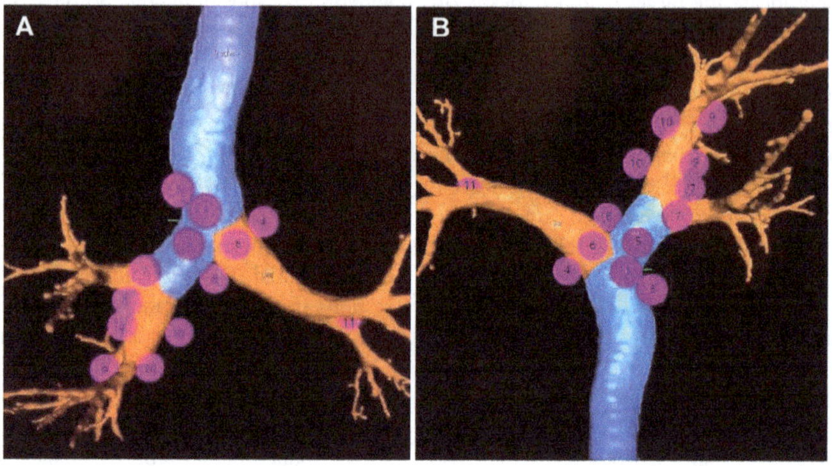

FIGURE 1 | Note: The overall view of eleven lymph node stations of Wang' map in a 3D reconstructed imaging.

Puncture point: The first or second trachea cartilage ring gap of the right main bronchus at 12 o'clock.

W6 station, left main bronchus (correlated with IASLC-10L).

Location: In front of the proximal proportion of the left main bronchus. The W6 lymph node is a mediastinal lymph node.

Puncture point: The first or second trachea cartilage ring gap of the left main bronchus at 12 o'clock.

W7 station, right upper hilar (correlated with IASLC-11Rs).

Location: In front and between the right upper lobe bronchus and bronchus intermedius.

Puncture point: Anterolateral direction of the right upper lobe crest.

W8 station, subcarina (correlated with IASLC-7).

Location: Between the right and left main bronchi, at or near the level of the right upper lobe bronchus.

Upper border: The superior margin of the opening of the right upper lobe bronchus.

Lower border: The opening of the right intermediate bronchus.

Puncture point: Right main bronchus at the level of the opening of the right upper lobe bronchus, at 9 o'clock.

W9 station, right lower hilar (correlated with IASLC-11Ri).

Location: Lateral or in front of the bronchus intermedius, at or near the level of the right middle lobe bronchus. The W9 lymph nodes consist of lymph nodes at the right lateral side of the right intermediate bronchus and near the ridge of the right middle and lower lobe bronchi.

Puncture point: Lateral side of the right intermediate bronchus.

W10 station, subsubcarina (correlated with the lower part of IASLC-7).

Location: Between the bronchus intermedius and the left main bronchus, at or near the level of the right middle lobe bronchus.

Upper border: The opening of the right intermediate bronchus.

Lower border: The distal end of the right intermediate bronchus, extending to the inferior side of the opening of the right middle lobe.

Puncture point: Right intermediate bronchus at 9 o'clock.

W11 station, left hilar (correlated with IASLC-11L).

Location: Between the left upper lobe and the left lower lobe bronchus.

Puncture point: The opening of the dorsal segment of the left lower lobe at 9 o'clock.

DISCUSSION

In the present study, we introduced a virtual map of lymph node landmarks under the assistance of a VBN system. Our map displays the intrabronchial and extrabronchial spatial relationships of 11 lymph node stations and their recommended puncture sites corresponding to Wang's map.

The VBN system in combination with CT of the 11 mediastinal and hilar lymph nodes and their surrounding structures from extrabronchial and endobronchial, sagittal, coronal as well as horizontal views provided a full understanding of the thoracic lymph nodes and their intrabronchial and extrabronchial relationships with adjacent tissues and blood vessels. A detailed view of the lymph nodes and their adjacent tissues can reinforce the understanding of the anatomy and assist in training of operators for TBNA.

There are two major differences between Wang's map and the IASLC map (Xia et al., 2015). First, stations five and six in Wang's map are located in front of the proximal proportion of the right and left main bronchi, respectively. Both W5 and W6 stations are defined as mediastinal lymph nodes. Second, W5 covers two IASLC lymph nodal stations: the distal end of

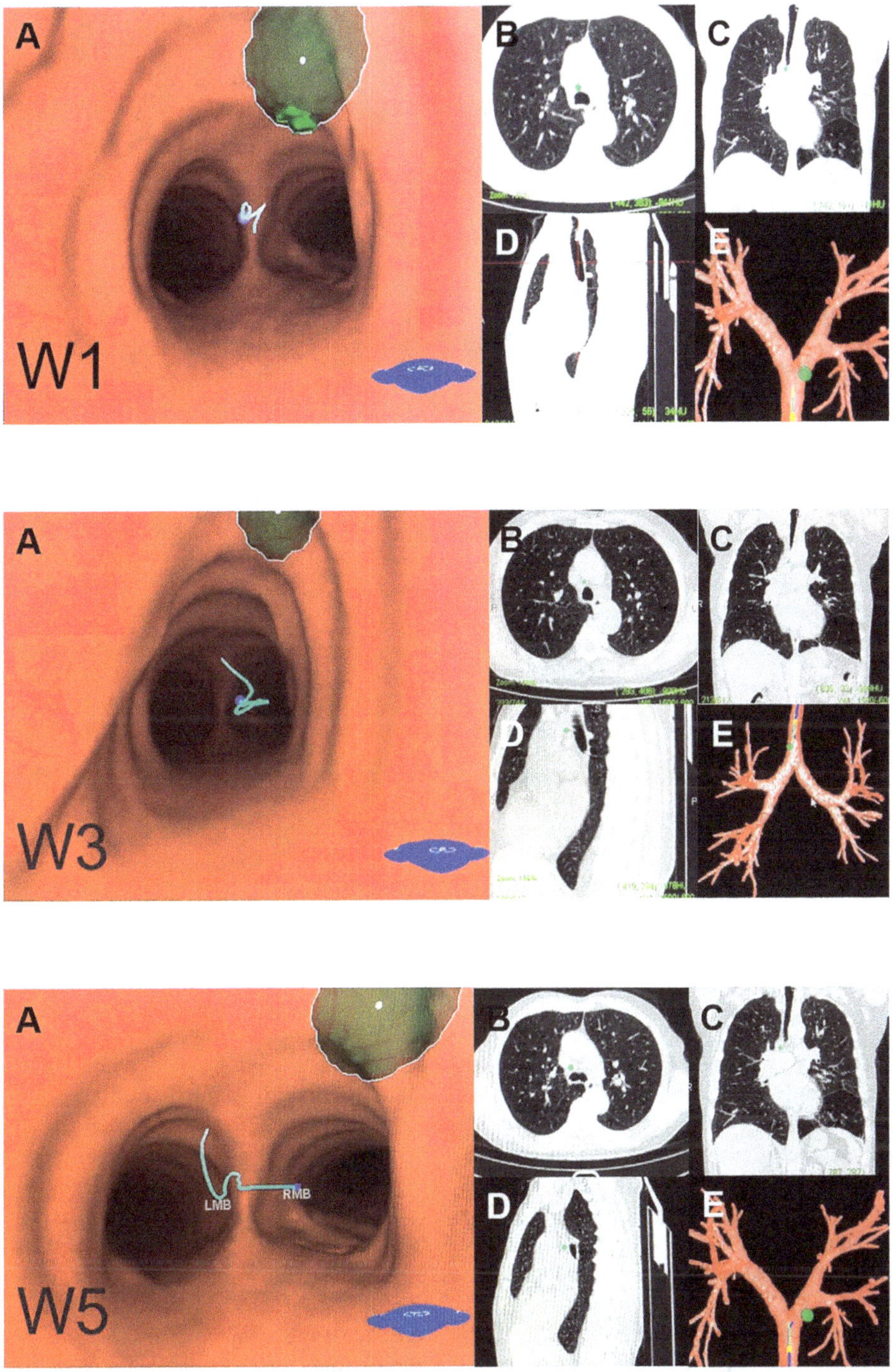

FIGURE 2 | Right mediastinal lymph node (N2) Note: (W1) anterior carina lymph nodes. (W3) right paratracheal lymph nodes. (W5) right main bronchus lymph nodes. **(A)** Intraluminal view and puncture sight (green). **(B)** Axial view. **(C)** Coronal view. **(D)** Sagittal view. **(E)** Reconstruction image.

4R as well as 10R station. Third, compared with the previous edition of the IASLC lymph node map, the lower border is extended to the azygos vein on the right, which fits the principle of Wang's map that 4R is correlated with station W1 and W3 as well as proximal W5 station. Similarly, the lower border of station seven in the IASLC map is extended to the upper border of the lower lobe bronchus on the left and the lower border of the bronchus intermedius on the right. This changed definition is also correlated with the definitions of W8 and W10.

VBN is generally conducted for guidance in treatment of PPLs. PPLs cannot be accessed easily by cTBNA because they are

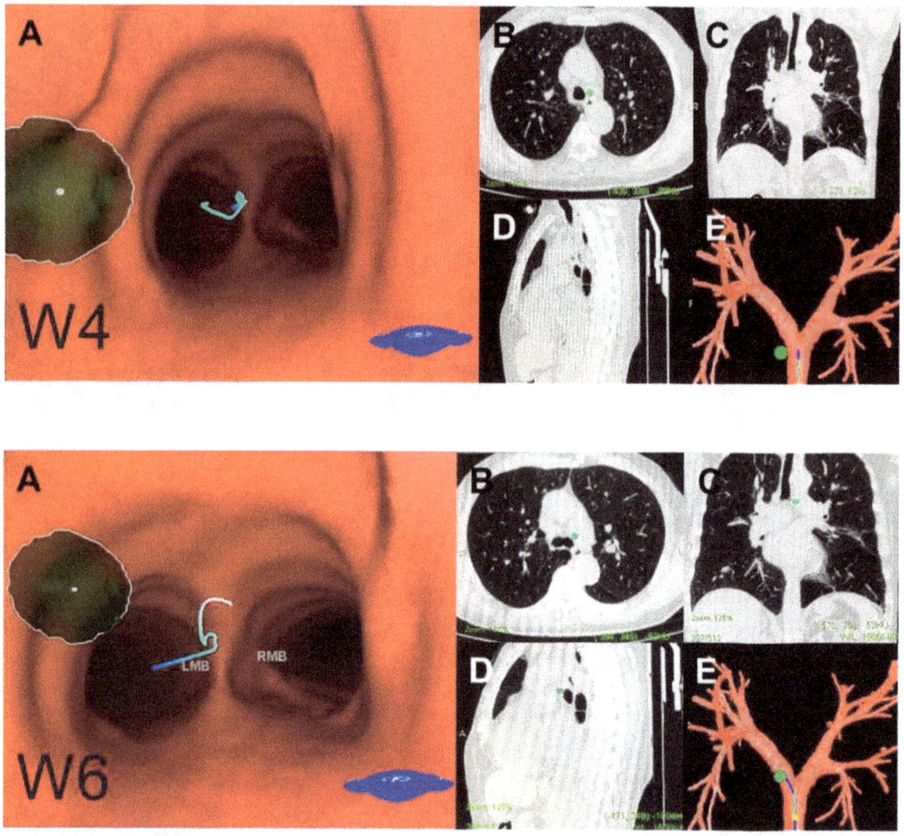

FIGURE 3 | Left mediastinal lymph node (N2). Note: (W4) left paratracheal lymph nodes or aortic pulmonary (A-P) window lymph nodes. (W6) left main bronchus lymph nodes. **(A)** Intraluminal view and puncture sight (green). **(B)** Axial view. **(C)** Coronal view. **(D)** Sagittal view. **(E)** Reconstruction image.

distinct from the trachea and central bronchus. The development of image-guided bronchoscopy techniques significantly enhances the diagnostic accuracy of PPLs. The VBN system was designed to reach and guide aspiration of PPLs with a diagnostic value of 72.0%–73.8% (Wang Memoli et al., 2012; Asano et al., 2014), and the diagnostic value reached 67.4% for lesions <2 cm in diameter (Asano et al., 2014). In combination with CT-guided ultrathin bronchoscopy, the diagnostic value of VBN increases to 65.4%–81.6% (Asano et al., 2014). On the other hand, the VBN system has also been applied in diagnosis of thoracic lymph node adenopathy. The sensitivity and diagnostic accuracy are both significantly increased for mediastinal lymph nodes by VBN (McAdams et al., 1998; Fiorelli et al., 2017), suggesting that the VBN system is also valuable in cases of mediastinal lymph node enlargement.

Aside from the advantages of the VBN system, the bronchoscopist still has to perform cTBNA blindly in clinical practice, as the exact puncture site cannot be confirmed in real-time. In general, the main purpose of generating our multi-dimensional virtual Wang's lymph node map is for training junior interventional pulmonology fellows or bronchoscopists. Compared with EBUS-TBNA, our approach does not require the use of a regular scope for the airway survey. In addition, although EBUS-TBNA allows real-time visualisation of a punctured lymph node, the operator cannot precisely identify the puncture site. In contrast, our system probes the 3D anatomy of each lymph node station with the puncture site. We expect that our multi-dimensional virtual Wang's lymph node map would allow precise targeting of lymph nodes 1–2 cm in diameter. Hence, the two methods are not competitive but complementary for bronchoscopists within the learning curve. The diagnostic yield is satisfactory upon combining virtual endobronchial ultrasound with EBUS-TBNA bronchoscopy when diagnosing mediastinal-hilar lymph node enlargement (Sato et al., 2013), but its necessity is doubtful. In addition, rapid on-site evaluation (ROSE) may be a good alternative to EBUS for combination with the VBN system. In addition, we recommend a probe designed to determine whether the needle is aligned in the

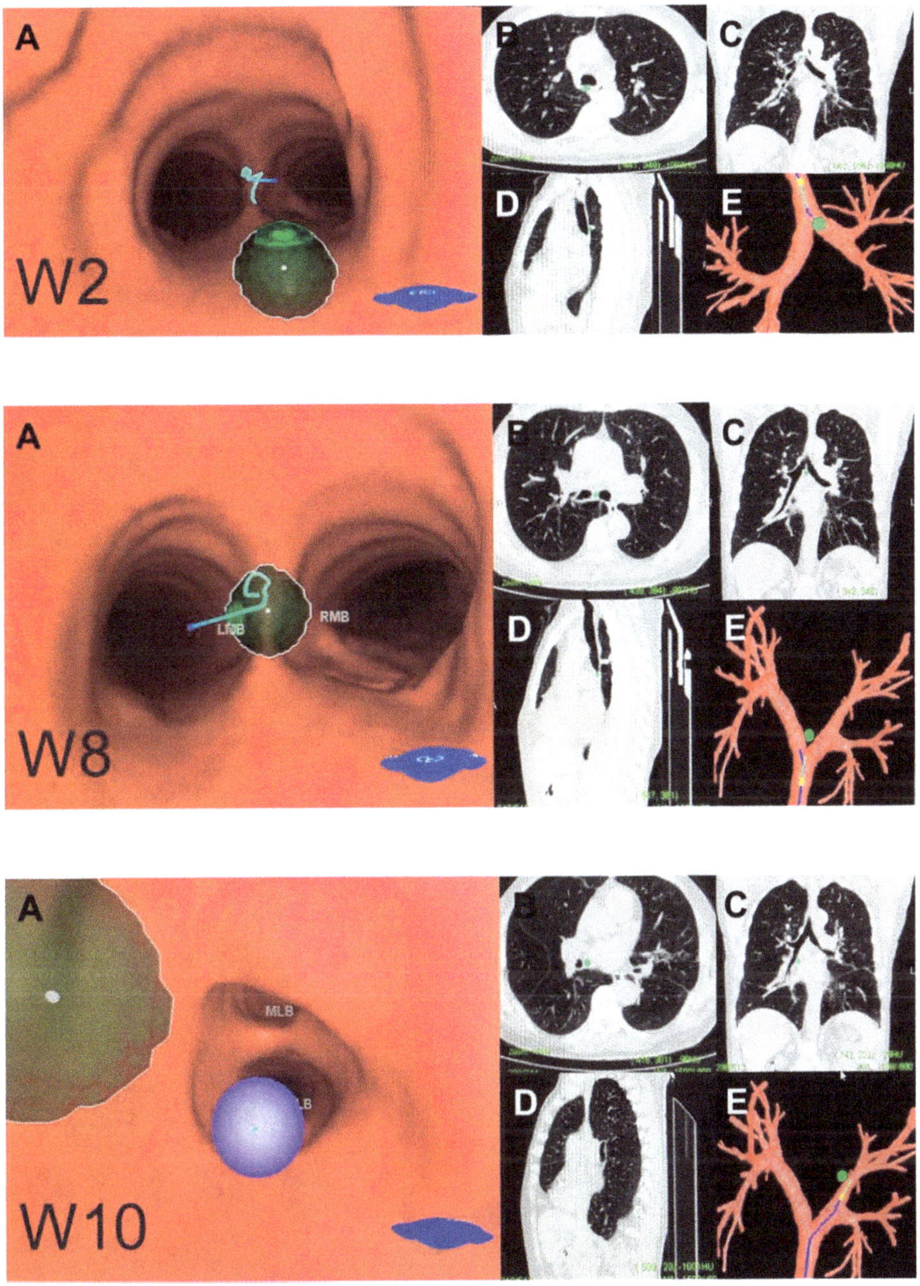

FIGURE 4 | Central mediastinal lymph node (N2). Note: (W2) posterior carina lymph nodes. (W8) subcarinal lymph nodes. (W10) subsubcarinal lymph nodes. **(A)** Intraluminal view and puncture sight (green). **(B)** Axial view. **(C)** Coronal view. **(D)** Sagittal view. **(E)** Reconstruction image.

puncture site. When it is aligned properly, the inducer could turn from green to red to alert the practitioner of puncture. Such a device may further improve the diagnostic value of VBN-guided TBNA.

There was a significant limitation of this study in that the diagnostic yield of this particular VBN-assisted TBNA has not yet been verified. A clinical trial is required to examine the validity of this VBN plus TBNA system. In addition, the quality of the CT image can also affect the accuracy of the derived 3D images.

Overall, we have proposed a virtual map for intra- and extrabronchial landmarks of hilar and mediastinal lymph nodes based on the Lungpoint VBN system. This map can help in training bronchoscopists as well as enhancing the

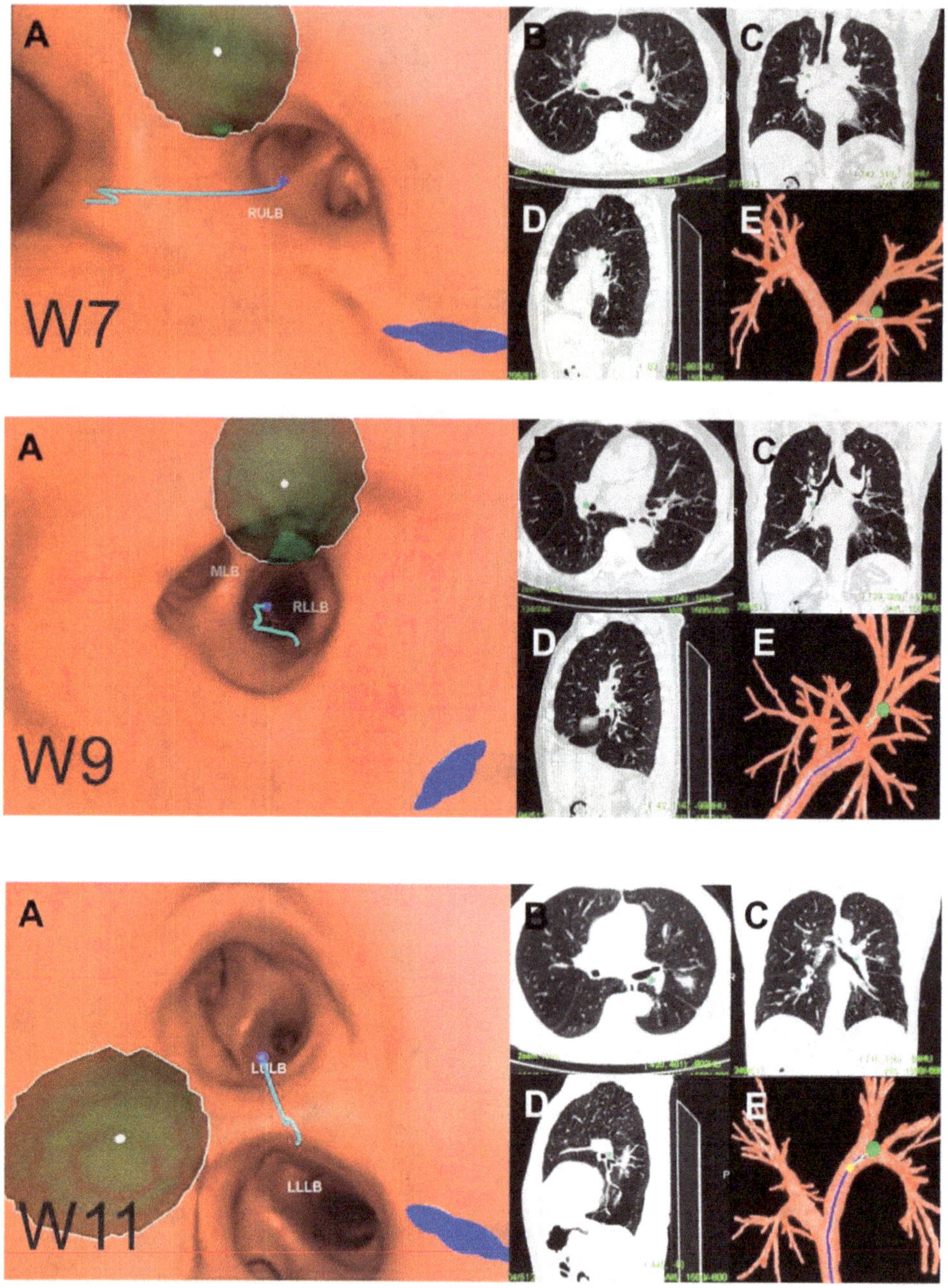

FIGURE 5 | Hilar lymph node (N1). Note: (W7) right upper hilar lymph nodes. (W9) right lower hilar lymph nodes. (W11) left hilar lymph nodes. **(A)** Intraluminal view and puncture sight (green). **(B)** Axial view. **(C)** Coronal view. **(D)** Sagittal view. **(E)** Reconstruction image.

diagnostic value of the VBN system. Further clinical trials are required to determine the efficacy of this strategy.

AUTHOR CONTRIBUTIONS

KW, QLiu, HoS, and YX contributed to study conception and design. FL, YY, HuS, QW, XY, QLi, LC, and YX conducted data collection and data analysis. QLiu, HoS, HuS, KW, YY, FL, and YX drafted the manuscript. All authors contributed to revision of the manuscript, and confirmed the final approval of manuscript.

REFERENCES

Asano, F., Eberhardt, R., and Herth, F. J. F. (2014). Virtual bronchoscopic navigation for peripheral pulmonary lesions. *Respiration* 88 (5), 430–440. doi:10.1159/000367900

Bonifazi, M., Tramacere, I., Zuccatosta, L., Mei, F., Sediari, M., Paonessa, M.C., et al. (2017). Conventional versus Ultrasound-Guided Transbronchial Needle Aspiration for the Diagnosis of Hilar/Mediastinal Lymph Adenopathies: A Randomized Controlled Trial. *Respiration.* 94 (2), 216–223. doi:10.1159/000475843

El-Sherief, A. H., Lau, C. T., Wu, C. C., Drake, R. L., Abbott, G. F., and Rice, T. W. (2014). International association for the study of lung cancer (IASLC) lymph node map: radiologic review with CT illustration. *Radiographics* 34 (6), 1680–1691. doi:10.1148/rg.346130097

Fiorelli, A., Raucci, A., Cascone, R., Reginelli, A., Di Natale, D., Santoriello, C., et al. (2017). Three-dimensional virtual bronchoscopy using a tablet computer to guide real-time transbronchial needle aspiration. *Interact Cardiovasc Thorac Surg* 24 (4), ivw404–575. doi:10.1093/icvts/ivw404

Gildea, T. R., Mazzone, P. J., Karnak, D., Meziane, M., and Mehta, A. C. (2006). Electromagnetic Navigation Diagnostic Bronchoscopy. *Am J Respir Crit Care Med* 174 (9), 982–989. doi:10.1164/rccm.200603-344OC

Herth, F., Becker, H. D., and Ernst, A. (2004). Conventional vs Endobronchial Ultrasound-Guided Transbronchial Needle Aspiration. *Chest* 125 (1), 322–325. doi:10.1378/chest.125.1.322

Hsu, L.-H., Liu, C.-C., and Ko, J.-S. (2004). Education and Experience Improve the Performance of Transbronchial Needle Aspiration. *Chest* 125 (2), 532–540. doi:10.1378/chest.125.2.532

Madan, K., Dhungana, A., Mohan, A., Hadda, V., Jain, D., Arava, S., et al. (2017). Conventional Transbronchial Needle Aspiration Versus Endobronchial Ultrasound-guided Transbronchial Needle Aspiration, With or Without Rapid On-Site Evaluation, for the Diagnosis of Sarcoidosis: A Randomized Controlled Trial. *J Bronchology Interv Pulmonol* 24 (1), 48–58. doi:10.1097/LBR.0000000000000339

McAdams, H. P., Goodman, P. C., and Kussin, P. (1998). Virtual bronchoscopy for directing transbronchial needle aspiration of hilar and mediastinal lymph nodes: a pilot study. *American Journal of Roentgenology* 170 (5), 1361–1364. doi:10.2214/ajr.170.5.9574616

Rodríguez de Castro, F., López, F. D., Serdá, G. J., Navarro, P. C., López, A. R., and Gilart, J. F. (1997). Relevance of training in transbronchial fine-needle aspiration technique. *Chest* 111 (1), 103–105. doi:10.1378/chest.111.1.103

Rusch, V. W., Asamura, H., Watanabe, H., Giroux, D. J., Rami-Porta, R., Goldstraw, P., et al. (2009). The IASLC lung cancer staging project: a proposal for a new international lymph node map in the forthcoming seventh edition of the TNM classification for lung cancer. *Journal of Thoracic Oncology* 4 (5), 568–577. doi:10.1097/JTO.0b013e3181a0d82e

Sato, M., Chen, F., Aoyama, A., Yamada, T., Ikeda, M., Bando, T., et al. (2013). Virtual endobronchial ultrasound for transbronchial needle aspiration. *The Journal of Thoracic and Cardiovascular Surgery* 146 (5), 1204–1212. doi:10.1016/j.jtcvs.2013.01.019

Schwarz, Y., Greif, J., Becker, H. D., Ernst, A., and Mehta, A. (2006). Real-Time Electromagnetic Navigation Bronchoscopy to Peripheral Lung Lesions Using Overlaid CT Images. *Chest* 129 (4), 988–994. doi:10.1378/chest.129.4.988

Wang, K.-P. (1994). Staging of bronchogenic carcinoma by bronchoscopy. *Chest* 106 (2), 588–593. doi:10.1378/chest.106.2.588

Wang, KP (1995). Transbronchial needle aspiration and percutaneous needle aspiration for staging and diagnosis of lung cancer. *Clin Chest Med* 16 (3), 535–52.

Wang Memoli, J. S., Nietert, P. J., and Silvestri, G. A. (2012). Meta-analysis of guided bronchoscopy for the evaluation of the pulmonary nodule. *Chest* 142 (2), 385–393. doi:10.1378/chest.11-1764

Wu, X., Shi, L., Xia, Y., Wang, K.-p., and Li, Q. (2018). Intrabronchial display of hilar-mediastinal lymph nodes by virtual bronchoscopic navigation system. *Thorac Cancer* 9 (3), 415–419. doi:10.1111/1759-7714.12555

Xia, Y., Ma, Y., Arias, S., Lee, H., and Wang, K.-P. (2015). Utilization of the International Association for the Study of Lung Cancer and Wang's nodal map for the identification of mediastinum and hilar lymph nodes. *Thoracic Cancer* 6 (4), 464–468. doi:10.1111/1759-7714.12206

Xia, Y, and Wang, KP (2013). Transbronchial needle aspiration: where are we now? *J Thorac Dis* 5 (5), 678–82. doi:10.3978/j.issn.2072-1439.2013.09.11

7

Expression and Gene Regulation Network of Adenosine Receptor A2B in Lung Adenocarcinoma: A Potential Diagnostic and Prognostic Biomarker

Yutong Sui[1†], Jiayin Liu[2†], Jing Zhang[1], Zena Zheng[1], Ziwei Wang[1], Zhenghu Jia[3] and Ziyu Meng[4*]*

[1]Shenzhen Hospital, Southern Medical University, Shenzhen, China, [2]Department of Radiation Oncology, Harbin Medical University Cancer Hospital, Harbin, China, [3]The First Affiliated Hospital, Biomedical Translational Research Institute and Guangdong Province Key Laboratory of Molecular Immunology and Antibody Engineering, Jinan University, Guangzhou, China, [4]NHC Key Laboratory of Hormones and Development, Tianjin Key Laboratory of Metabolic Diseases, Chu Hsien-I Memorial Hospital and Tianjin Institute of Endocrinology, Tianjin Medical University, Tianjin, China

***Correspondence:**
Zhenghu Jia
jiazhenghu86@163.com
Ziyu Meng
mengziyu@tmu.edu.cn

†These authors have contributed equally to this work

Adenosine receptor A2B (*ADORA2B*) encodes a protein belonging to the G protein–coupled receptor superfamily. Abnormal expression of *ADORA2B* may play a pathophysiological role in some human cancers. We investigated whether ADORA2B is a potential diagnostic and prognostic biomarker for lung adenocarcinoma (LUAD). The expression, various mutations, copy number variations, mRNA expression levels, and related network signaling pathways of *ADORA2B* were analyzed using bioinformatics-related websites, including Oncomine, UALCAN, cBioPortal, GeneMANIA, LinkedOmics, KM Plotter, and TIMER. We found that *ADORA2B* was overexpressed and amplified in LUAD, and a high *ADORA2B* expression predicted a poor prognosis for LUAD patients. Pathway analyses of *ADORA2B* in LUAD revealed *ADORA2B*-correlated signaling pathways, and the expression level of *ADORA2B* was associated with immune cell infiltration. Furthermore, *ADORA2B* mRNA and protein levels were significantly higher in human LUAD cell lines (A549 cells and NCI-H1299 cells) than in normal human bronchial epithelial (HBE) cells, and the transcript levels of genes positively or negatively correlated with *ADORA2B* were consistent and statistically significant. siRNA transfection experiments and functional experiments further confirmed these results. *In vitro* results were also consistent with those of bioinformatics analysis. Our findings provide a foundation for studying the role of *ADORA2B* in tumorigenesis and support the development of new drug targets for LUAD.

Keywords: *ADORA2B*, lung adenocarcinoma, mRNA expression, functional network analysis, verification experiment

---

Abbreviations: AAMP, angio-associated migratory cell protein; ADORA2B, adenosine receptor A2B; ALK, anaplastic lymphoma kinase; ANXA1, annexin A1; CBFA2T2, CBFA2/RUNX1 partner transcriptional co-repressor 2; BRAF, V-raf murine sarcoma viral oncogene homolog B1; DCC, netrin 1 receptor; DPH, diphthamide biosynthesis 1; EGFR, epidermal growth factor receptor; GEO, Gene Expression Omnibus; HER2, human epidermal growth factor receptor 2; ITGA3, integrin subunit alpha 3; KCNJ3, potassium inwardly rectifying channel subfamily J member 3; KDM2B, lysine demethylase 2B; KRAS, Kirsten rat sarcoma viral oncogene; LUAD, lung adenocarcinoma; NEB, nebulin; OS, overall survival; PEX6, peroxisomal biogenesis factor 6; RET, rearranged during transfection; ROS1, ROS proto-oncogene 1; SLC29A2, solute carrier family 29 member 2; SLC9A3R2, solute carrier family 9 member A3 regulator 2; S100A6, S100 calcium binding protein A6; TCGA, The Cancer Genome Atlas; TPD52L2, tumor protein D52-like 2; ZNF267, zinc finger protein 267.

INTRODUCTION

Lung adenocarcinoma (LUAD) is a common pathological form of lung cancer and is associated with high mortality, leading to more than one million deaths worldwide every year (TCGA, 2018). LUAD is characterized by the presence of heterogeneous tumors that originate in the small airway and spread to the surrounding lung tissue (Yu et al., 2010; Russell et al., 2011). Multiple organ metastasis is the leading cause of death in LUAD patients. Within a few months after diagnosis, metastasis to different organs can occur rapidly. Traditional modalities, such as radiotherapy and chemotherapy, are ineffective for LUAD (Zagryazhskaya et al., 2015), and targeted gene therapy holds potential for the clinical management of LUAD. Epidermal growth factor receptor (*EGFR*) mutation and anaplastic lymphoma kinase (*ALK*) fusion are the common gene abnormalities reported in LUAD. Personalized therapy targeting these genes has become a well-designed standard treatment, with erlotinib and gefitinib being the main drugs for LUAD treatment (Yu et al., 2013). Furthermore, mutations in Kirsten rat sarcoma viral oncogene (*KRAS*), human epidermal growth factor receptor 2 (*HER2*), and *V-raf* murine sarcoma viral oncogene homolog B1 (*BRAF*) as well as other fusions of driver genes, such as rearranged during transfection (*RET*) and ROS proto-oncogene 1 (*ROS1*), have been reported in LUAD (Roman et al., 2018; Pillai et al., 2017; Mazieres et al., 2020; Drilon, et al., 2020; Shaw, et al., 2017). These driver genes vary depending on race, sex, and smoking status. The pathogenesis of LUAD is complex and mainly involves cell cycle regulation and signal transduction, reflected in altered gene function at different developmental stages of the disease. New drug targets for LUAD should be identified by screening gene networks associated with tumor formation and progression.

Most of the extracellular adenosine is released from adenine nucleotides in response to various stimuli, including mechanical stress, osmotic stimulation, inflammation, and tissue damage (Borea et al., 2016; Covarrubias et al., 2016; Hamidzadeh and Mosser, 2016). Extracellular adenosine binds to four adenosine receptor subtypes, namely, A1, A2A, A2B, and A3, each of which exhibits unique pharmacological and coupling effects and tissue distribution characteristics. Adenosine receptor A2B (*ADORA2B*) encodes an adenosine receptor belonging to the G protein–coupled receptor superfamily and is highly expressed in various carcinomas, which leads to the promotion of carcinoma cell proliferation and metastasis (Kasama et al., 2015; Vecchio et al., 2016). *ADORA2B* also regulates the tumor microenvironment and is involved in peripheral vascular growth, inflammatory cell infiltration, fibroblast proliferation, and extracellular matrix accumulation (Csoka et al., 2012). Therefore, *ADORA2B* regulates tumor progression and metastasis and could serve as a useful target for cancer therapy or combination therapy.

Recent studies have suggested that ADORA2B is an indispensable target in the regulation of both acute and chronic pulmonary diseases, such as pulmonary hypertension, chronic obstructive pulmonary disease, and pulmonary fibrosis (Karmouty-Quintana et al., 2013; Philip et al., 2017; Mertens et al., 2018; Tian et al., 2021). LUAD is one of the most lethal pulmonary diseases, with the highest mortality rate; however, the role of *ADORA2B* in LUAD is still unknown. In this study, we analyzed the expression and mutations of *ADORA2B* in patients with LUAD using data obtained from various public databases. We also analyzed the genomic variations, survival rates, and functional networks associated with *ADORA2B* in LUAD. Additionally, human LUAD and normal bronchial epithelial cell lines were used to confirm the role of *ADORA2B* in LUAD. siRNA transfection experiments and functional experiments further confirmed the obtained results. Therefore, we used bioinformatics analysis in combination with *in vitro* experiments to comprehensively investigate the role of *ADORA2B* in LUAD.

MATERIALS AND METHODS

Oncomine Analysis

The mRNA expression of *ADORA2B* in LUAD was analyzed using the Oncomine database (www.oncomine.org). LUAD-based databases established from the Okayama Lung, Landi Lung, Selamat Lung, Stearman Lung, Beer Lung, Su Lung, Bhattacharjee Lung, and Garber Lung datasets were used for this analysis (Bhattacharjee et al., 2001; Garber et al., 2001; Beer et al., 2002; Stearman et al., 2005; Su et al., 2007; Landi et al., 2008; Okayama et al., 2012; Selamat et al., 2012). The difference in the expression of *ADORA2B* between LUAD tissues and para-carcinoma tissues was considered statistically significant at $p < 0.01$.

UALCAN Analysis

Multiple clinical and pathological features related to the mRNA expression of *ADORA2B* in LUAD were analyzed by UALCAN (http://ualcan.path.uab.edu). *ADORA2B* expression was analyzed by TCGA Level 3 RNA sequencing in UALCAN, and the clinical data were analyzed to determine *ADORA2B* expression levels in different tumor subgroups (Chandrashekar et al., 2017).

cBioPortal Analysis

cBioPortal (http://cbioportal.org) was used to analyze *ADORA2B* alterations observed in The Cancer Genome Atlas (TCGA) LUAD samples. By analyzing various types of mutations, copy number variations, and mRNA expression levels, the tab OncoPrint displayed an overview of the genetic changes in each sample as gene mutations and heat maps of *ADORA2B* expression. The tab plots displayed an overview of the data type of clinical attributes and mutations, including clinical attributes and group mutations by mutation type.

GeneMANIA Analysis

GeneMANIA (http://genemania.org/) is a web interface that uses large sets of functional association data to identify single genes related to a set of input genes, generating hypotheses on gene function, analyzing gene lists, and prioritizing genes for functional assays. GeneMANIA was used to construct the *ADORA2B* software for the analysis (Warde-Farley et al., 2010).

LinkedOmics Analysis

The LinkFinder module of LinkedOmics (http://www.linkedomics.org/login.php) was used to identify differentially expressed genes related to *ADORA2B* (n = 515) in the TCGA LUAD section. The search and target datasets were obtained by RNA-seq, and the results were analyzed with the Pearson correlation coefficient. The data from the LinkFinder results were labeled and sorted before enrichment analysis was performed for Gene Ontology, KEGG, PANTHER, and Reactome pathway analyses.

Survival Analysis

We used the Kaplan–Meier (KM) Plotter (http://kmplot.com), an online database that contains gene expression data and survival information of 865 LUAD patients, to analyze the prognostic value of ADORA2B in LUAD. The patient samples were separated into two groups by median expression (high expression and low expression) to analyze the overall survival (OS) with hazard ratios (HRs) with 95% confidence intervals and log-rank p-values.

Immune Infiltration Analysis

Tumor Immune Estimation Resource (TIMER, https://cistrome.shinyapps.io/timer/) is a web resource for systematic analysis of the infiltration levels of different subsets of immune cells in different types of cancers. We analyzed the expression of *ADORA2B* in LUAD in relation to tumor purity and the abundance of immune infiltrating cells including B cells, $CD8^+$ T cells, $CD4^+$ T cells, macrophages, neutrophils, and dendritic cells. We also analyzed the relationship between the gene copy number variation and the abundance of immune infiltrating cells.

Cell Culture

A549 cells (human LUAD, ATCC®CCL-185™), NCl-H1299 cells (human LUAD, ATCC®CRL-5803™), and HBE cells (human bronchial epithelial cells, ATCC®CRL-2741™) were obtained from ATCC (Manassas, VA, United States). A549 cells were cultured in Dulbecco's modified Eagle's medium (DMEM, Gibco, Grand Island, NY, United States) containing 10% fetal bovine serum (FBS, Gibco), whereas the culture medium for HBE cells contained 20% FBS. NCl-H1299 cells were cultured in RPMI-1640 medium (Gibco, Grand Island, NY, United States) containing 10% FBS. All the cells were incubated in a humidified incubator at 5% CO_2 and 37°C. The cells that passaged less than five with >70% confluency were used for experiments.

RNA Extraction and Quantitative Real-time PCR (qRT-PCR)

RNA from A549, NCl-H1299, and HBE cells was isolated using TRIzol Reagent (Invitrogen, Carlsbad, CA, United States) according to the manufacturer's instructions. cDNA synthesis was performed using a cDNA First Strand Synthesis Kit (ABclonal, Wuhan, China), and mRNA expression was quantified by qRT-PCR using the SYBR Green Fast qPCR Mix (ABclonal). Relative mRNA expression levels were normalized to those of β-actin and measured by the comparative Ct ($2^{-\Delta\Delta Ct}$) method (n = 6 samples/group). Primer sequences used in this study are listed in **Supplementary Table S1**.

siRNA Transfection

ADORA2B siRNAs and negative control siRNA (50 nM) were obtained from GenePharma (Shanghai, China). The siRNAs were transfected with Lipofectamine 2000 (Invitrogen) for 4 h, following the manufacturer's protocol. *ADORA2B* knockdown efficiencies were verified by RT-PCR. The siRNA sequences are listed in **Supplementary Table S1**.

Western Blotting

A549, NCl-H1299, and HBE cells were cultured as previously described (*Cell Culture*). Total protein was extracted using RIPA buffer (Solarbio, Beijing, China). Protein concentrations were measured using a BCA protein assay kit (Solarbio). Protein extracts (50 μg/well) were separated by 10% sodium dodecyl sulfate polyacrylamide gel electrophoresis and transferred onto polyvinylidene fluoride membranes. The membranes were blocked with 5% skim milk for 2 h and incubated with anti-β-actin (Bioss, bs-0061R, Beijing, China), anti-*ADORA2B* (Bioss, bs-5900R), anti-cyclin D1 (ABclonal, A2708), anti-PCNA (Proteintech, 10205-2-AP, Wuhan, China), anti-N-cadherin (ABclonal, A0433), and anti-vimentin (ABclonal, A2584) antibodies overnight. The next day, the membranes were incubated with a HRP-conjugated secondary antibody and goat anti-rabbit IgG antibody (ABclonal) for 1 h. A western blot detection ECL kit (Advansta, Menlo Park, United States) was used to detect protein bands. Fold-changes in *ADORA2B* protein expression were normalized to those of β-actin.

Cell Proliferation Assay

Cell proliferation was measured using cell counting kit-8 (CCK-8, Beyotime, Beijing, China). A549 cells (3000 cells/well) were plated in a 96-well plate and transfected with *ADORA2B* siRNA-2 and negative control siRNA as previously described (*siRNA Transfection*). The cell proliferation rate was detected with CCK-8 at 24, 48, and 72 h. The absorbance at 450 nm was measured using a microplate reader.

Cell Migration Assay

The cells were transfected with *ADORA2B* siRNA-2 and negative control siRNA using Lipofectamine 2000 as previously described. Transfected cells were grown to 100% confluence, and then wounds were created using pipette tips. Serum-free medium was used instead of complete medium to eliminate the effects of cell proliferation. Images were captured at 0 and 48 h using a microscope. The cell migration rate was calculated by ImageJ software.

Statistical Analysis

Data are presented as the mean ± standard error of the replicates. Comparisons between two groups were performed using Student's t-test. GraphPad Prism 8.0 software (GraphPad, Inc., La Jolla, CA, United States) was used for statistical analysis.

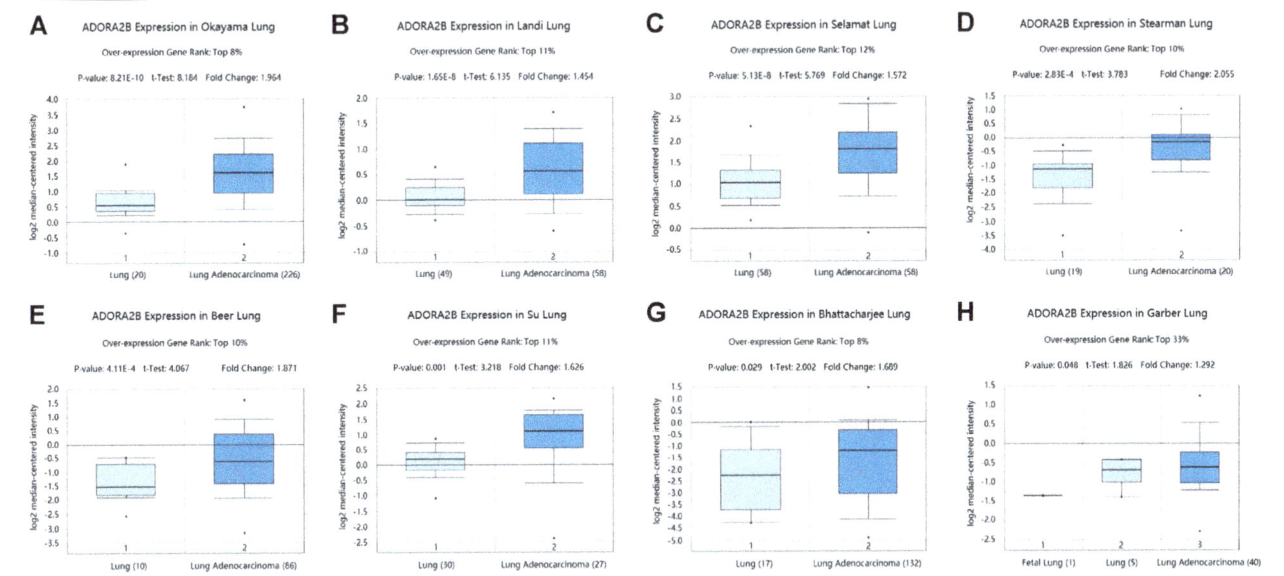

FIGURE 1 | *ADORA2B* transcription in LUAD. *ADORA2B* mRNA copy numbers were significantly higher in LUAD in **(A)** Okayama Lung, **(B)** Landi Lung, **(C)** Selamat Lung, **(D)** Stearman Lung, **(E)** Beer Lung, **(F)** Su Lung, **(G)** Bhattacharjee Lung, and **(H)** Garber Lung datasets than in para-carcinoma tissues.

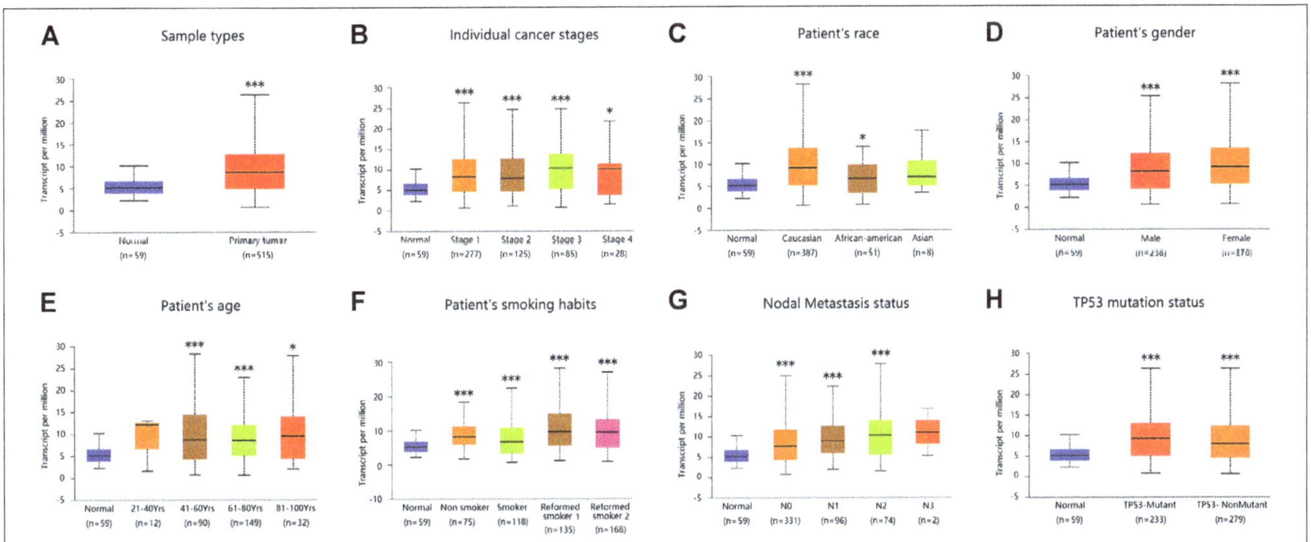

FIGURE 2 | *ADORA2B* expression level in subgroups of patients with LUAD. Relative expression of ADORA2B in normal and different classifications of LUAD tissues. **(A)** Sample types, **(B)** individual cancer stages, **(C)** patient's race, **(D)** patient's gender, **(E)** patient's age, **(F)** patient's smoking habits, **(G)** nodal metastasis status, and **(H)** TP53 mutation status. $^*p < 0.05$ and $^{***}p < 0.001$ are statistically significant.

Results with $p < 0.05$ were considered statistically significant ($^*p < 0.05$; $^{**}p < 0.01$; $^{***}p < 0.001$).

RESULTS

Expression of *ADORA2B* in LUAD

We determined *ADORA2B* transcript levels in LUAD patients using data obtained from TCGA and Gene Expression Omnibus (GEO). Data from the Oncomine database showed that the expression of *ADORA2B* mRNA was significantly upregulated in LUAD tissues when compared with that in para-carcinoma tissues ($p < 0.01$). *ADORA2B* ranked in the top 33% of genes with high mRNA expression, with fold-difference values <2 (**Figures 1A–H**).

Similarly, analysis of multiple clinical and pathological features of LUAD patients from the TCGA database revealed elevated *ADORA2B* mRNA expression. Moreover, *ADORA2B* mRNA expression was significantly higher in LUAD tissues than in para-carcinoma tissues in subgroup analyses based on

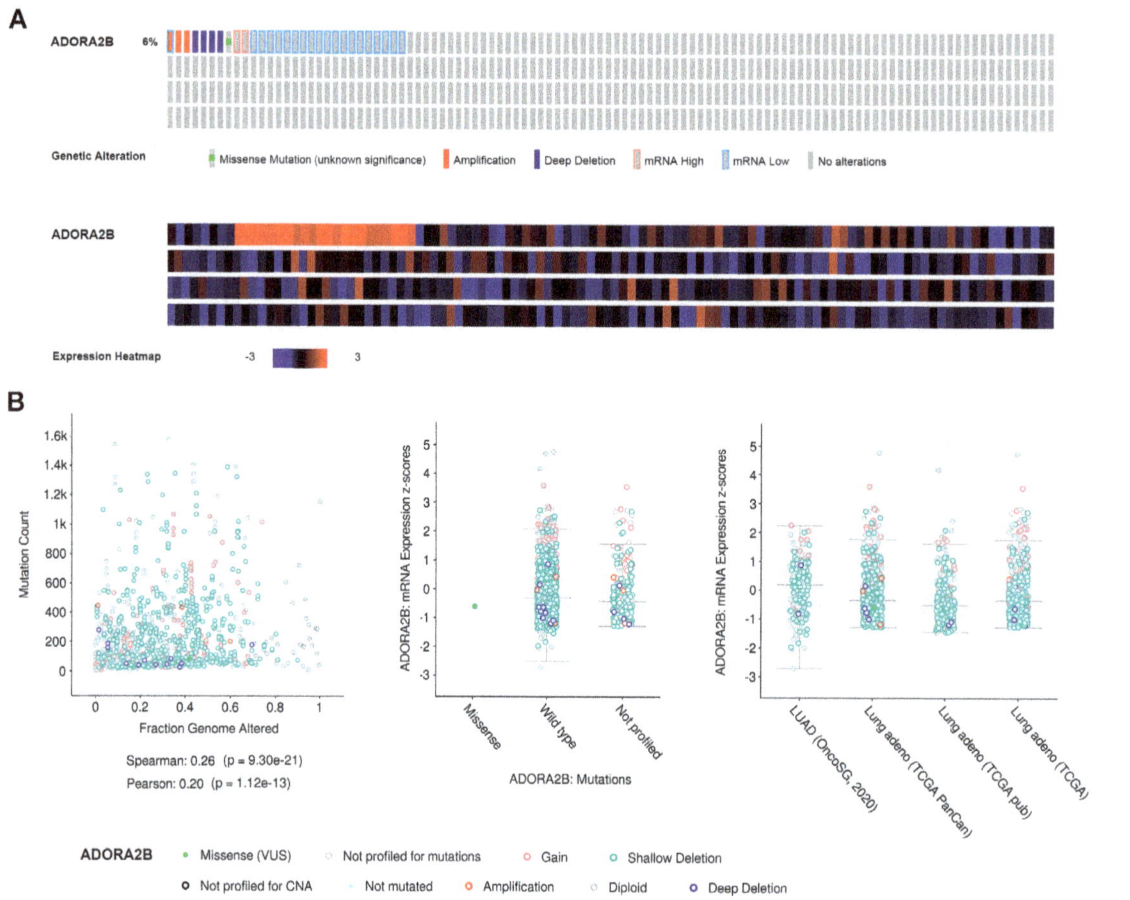

FIGURE 3 | Frequency and type of *ADORA2B* alterations in LUAD. **(A)** OncoPrint of *ADORA2B* alterations in LUAD (cBioPortal) and **(B)** plots of *ADORA2B* alterations in LUAD with clinical attributes and mutations (cBioPortal).

sample type, individual cancer stage, ethnicity, gender, age, smoking habits, nodal metastasis status, and TP53 mutation status (**Figures 2A–H**).

Frequency and Type of ADORA2B Alterations in LUAD

Next, we used the cBioPortal database to evaluate the types and frequencies of *ADORA2B* alterations in LUAD tissues based on sequencing data from patients with LUAD obtained from TCGA's Pan-Cancer Atlas database. *ADORA2B* was altered in 30 out of 503 (6%) patients with LUAD (**Figure 3A**). These genetic alterations included missense mutations (1, 0.2%), amplification (3, 0.6%), deep deletion (4, 0.8%), mRNA high (2, 0.4%), and mRNA low (20, 4%). The patient order in OncoPrint is shown in **Supplementary Table S2**. Analysis included the type of clinical attribute and mutation, fraction of genome altered, and mutation type, including missense (VUS), not mutated, not profiled for mutations, amplification, gain, diploid, shallow deletion, deep deletion, and not profiled for CNA (**Figure 3B**). mRNA low, shallow deletion, and diploid were the most common types of *ADORA2B* genetic alterations found in LUAD.

Expression of *ADORA2B* Is Associated With the Survival of LUAD Patients

Previous studies have demonstrated that *ADORA2B* participates in the proliferation and metastasis of carcinomas (Kasama et al., 2015; Vecchio et al., 2016). Thus, we further examined the prognostic value of ADORA2B in LUAD patients. LUAD patients with a higher expression of *ADORA2B* exhibited poor OS according to the KM Plotter database. Survival analysis showed that the mean OS time in the low *ADORA2B* expression group was longer than that in the high *ADORA2B* expression group ($p = 0.034$) (**Figure 4A**). The mean OS times for 12 (1 year), 36 (3 years), and 60 months (5 years) in the low *ADORA2B* expression group were significantly longer than those in the high expression group (**Figures 4B–D**). These results indicated that *ADORA2B* was significantly associated with the prognosis of LUAD patients and that a high *ADORA2B* expression predicted a poor prognosis in LUAD patients.

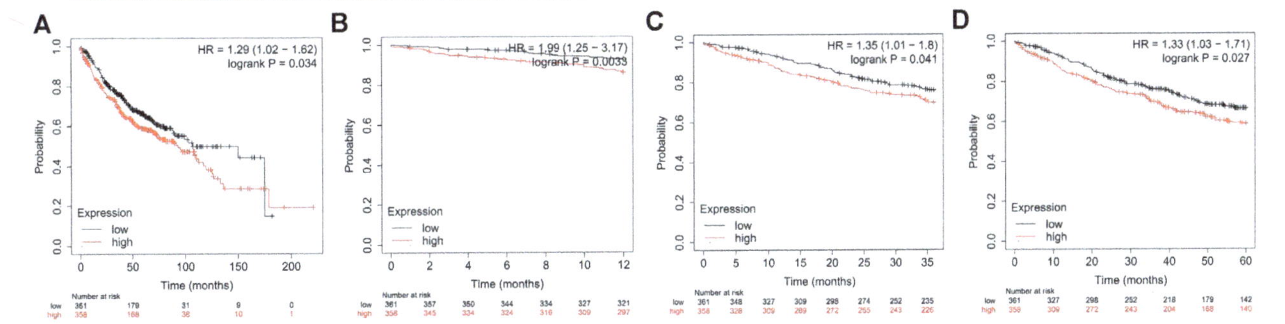

FIGURE 4 | The expression of *ADORA2B* is associated with LUAD patient survival. **(A)** Mean OS analysis of LUAD patients with high and low *ADORA2B* expression OS analysis of LUAD patients with high and low ADORA2B expressions for **(B)** 12 months (1 year), **(C)** 36 months (3 years), and **(D)** 60 months (5 years).

Interaction Network of *ADORA2B*

An *ADORA2B* correlation network was constructed to determine the potential mutual effects between *ADORA2B* and cancer-related targets. The results indicated that *ADORA2B* could interact with netrin 1 receptor (*DCC*), solute carrier family 9 member A3 regulator 2 (*SLC9A3R2*), zinc finger protein 267 (*ZNF267*), and tumor protein D52-like 2 (*TPD52L2*); *ADORA2B* was co-expressed with potassium inwardly rectifying channel subfamily J member 3 (*KCNJ3*), angio-associated migratory cell protein (*AAMP*), *TPD52L2*, and solute carrier family 29 member 2 (*SLC29A2*); and *ADORA2B* was co-located with *AAMP*, peroxisomal biogenesis factor 6 (*PEX6*), *SLC29A2*, *ADORA2A*, and diphthamide biosynthesis 1 (*DPH1*). *ADORA2B* was identified to interact with *DCC* and shared protein domains with its isoform *ADORA2A* (**Figure 5A**).

The LinkedOmics database was used to identify RNA-seq genes co-expressed with *ADORA2B* in LUAD. A volcano plot indicated that the expression of 5,246 genes was negatively correlated with *ADORA2B* expression, whereas the expression of 3,447 genes was positively correlated with *ADORA2B* expression. We confirmed the top 50 genes that negatively or positively interacted with *ADORA2B* (**Figure 5B** and **Supplementary Table S3**). The results revealed that multiple differentially expressed genes were correlated with *ADORA2B* expression.

Pearson's correlation coefficient analysis revealed a positive correlation between *ADORA2B* expression levels and those of annexin A1 (*ANXA1*), integrin subunit alpha 3 (*ITGA3*), and S100 calcium binding protein A6 (*S100A6*) and a negative correlation between the expression of *ADORA2B* and that of lysine demethylase 2B (*KDM2B*), nebulin (*NEB*), and *CBFA2/RUNX1* partner transcriptional co-repressor 2 (*CBFA2T2*) (**Figure 5C**).

Enrichment Analysis of *ADORA2B* Functional Networks in LUAD

Three independent ontologies (biological process, cellular component, and molecular function) were analyzed by gene set enrichment analysis (GSEA). The results indicated that *ADORA2B*-associated differentially expressed genes were involved in several biological processes (protein targeting, neutrophil mediated immunity, response to IFN-γ, etc.), cellular components (ribosome, cell-substrate junction, secretory granule membrane, etc.), and molecular functions (structural constituent of ribosome, cell adhesion molecule binding, enzyme inhibitor activity, etc.) (**Figure 6A**).

The differentially expressed genes associated with *ADORA2B* were then evaluated for potential functional pathways using KEGG (ribosome, proteoglycans in cancer, fluid shear stress, and atherosclerosis, etc.), PANTHER (FAS, EGF receptor, apoptosis, etc.), and Reactome (influenza infection, major pathway of rRNA processing in the nucleolus and cytosol, cell cycle, etc.) pathway analyses (**Figure 6B**).

Relationship Between *ADORA2B* Expression and Infiltrating Immune Cells in LUAD

The tumor microenvironment is a very complex system composed of a variety of cells, enzymes, cytokines, and metabolites and is characterized by low oxygen, low pH, and high pressure. An important immunosuppressive mechanism is mediated by the CD73–adenosine receptor metabolic signaling pathway (Chen et al., 2020). To comprehensively investigate the role of *ADORA2B* in LUAD, we selected the TIMER database to analyze the association of *ADORA2B* expression levels with subsets of infiltrating immune cells. The expression of *ADORA2B* was significantly correlated with the infiltration of B cells, macrophages, neutrophils, and dendritic cells (**Figure 7A**). In addition, the copy number variation (CNV) of *ADORA2B* was significantly correlated with the infiltration levels of macrophages (**Figure 7B**).

Expression Levels of *ADORA2B* and Correlated Genes in Human LUAD Cells

We found that compared with that in normal lung tissues, the expression level of *ADORA2B* was significantly elevated in tumor tissues of LUAD patients with higher morbidity. To confirm that *ADORA2B* expression is related to LUAD, we investigated the *ADORA2B* gene and protein expression in human LUAD (A549

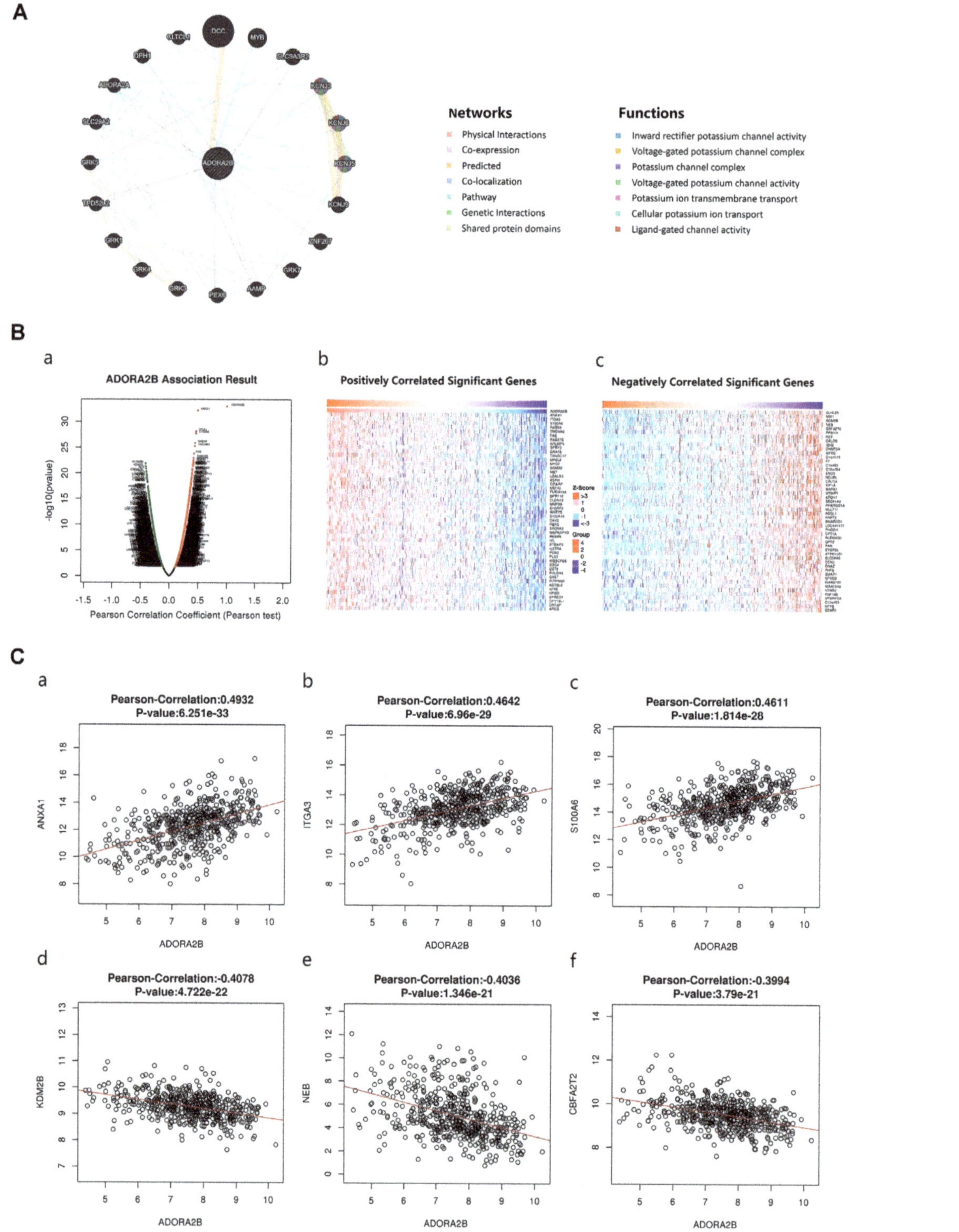

FIGURE 5 | Genes associated with *ADORA2B* expression. **(A)** Biological interaction network of *ADORA2B*. **(B)** Differentially expressed genes correlated with *ADORA2B* (LinkedOmics). (a) Correlations between *ADORA2B* and differentially expressed genes in LUAD were analyzed with Pearson's correlation coefficient. (b) Heat map of genes positively correlated with *ADORA2B* in LUAD. (c) Heat map of genes negatively correlated with *ADORA2B* in LUAD. **(C)** Gene expression correlation analysis of *ADORA2B* and *ADORA2B*-correlated genes (LinkedOmics). Pearson correlation of *ADORA2B* expression with that of (a) *ANXA1*, (b) *ITGA3*, (c) *S100A6*, (d) *KDM2B*, (e) *NEB*, and (f) *CBFA2T2* (n = 515).

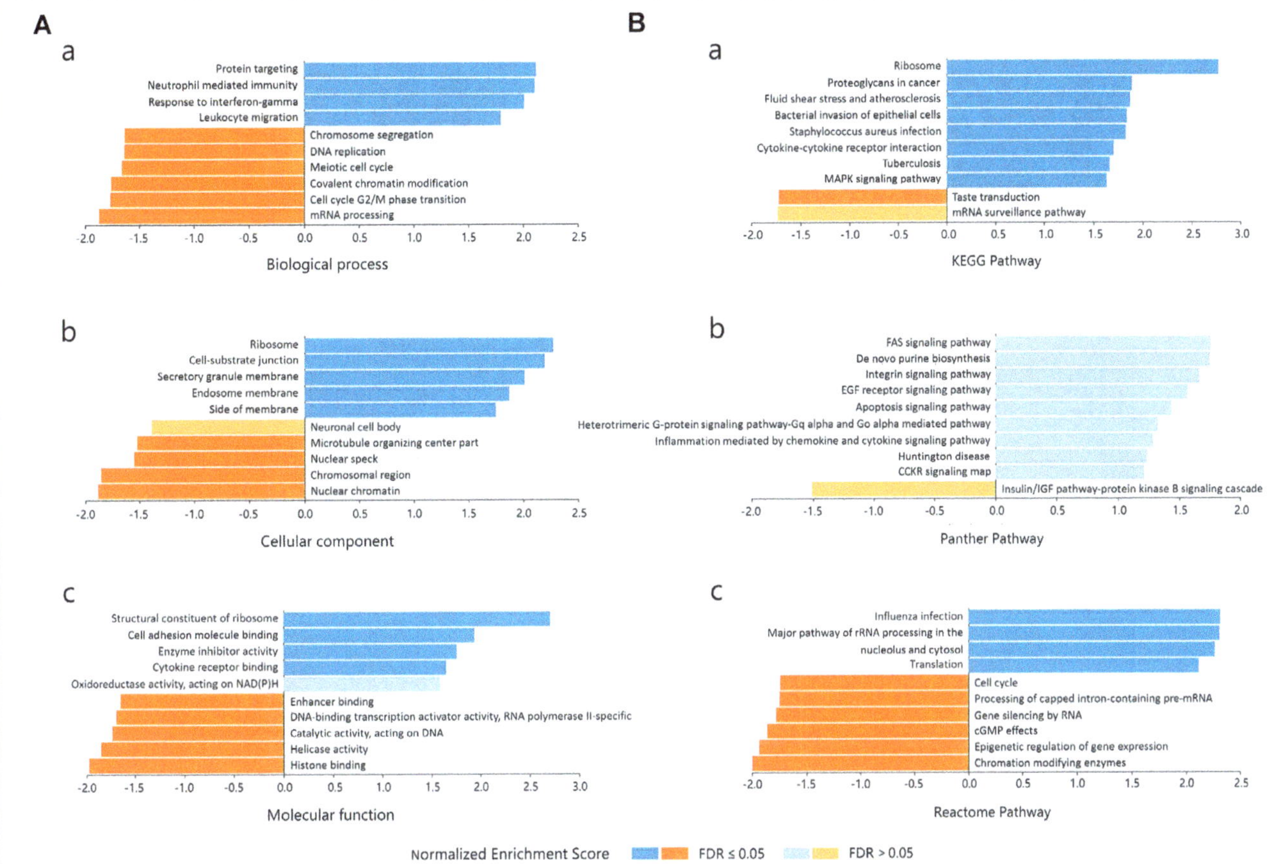

FIGURE 6 | Enrichment analysis of ADORA2B functional networks in LUAD. **(A)** Enriched Gene Ontology annotations of *ADORA2B*-correlated genes in LUAD (LinkedOmics). (a) Biological process. (b) Cellular component. (c) Molecular function. **(B)** Enrichment pathway analysis of *ADORA2B*-correlated genes in LUAD (LinkedOmics). (a) KEGG pathway. (b) PANTHER pathway. (c) Reactome pathway.

and NCl-H1299) and normal human bronchial epithelial (HBE) cell lines. Western blotting analysis indicated that the relative ADORA2B protein expression levels in A549 cells and NCl-H1299 cells were significantly higher than those in HBE cells (**Figures 8A,B**). Next, we examined the mRNA expression level of *ADORA2B* by qRT-PCR and found that the relative *ADORA2B* mRNA expression level was consistent with the protein expression level in the three cell lines (**Figure 8C**).

As shown in **Figure 5C**, LinkedOmics was used to identify the differentially expressed genes related to *ADORA2B*. The expression levels of *ADORA2B*-associated genes were positively (*ANXA1*, *ITGA3*, and *S100A6*) or negatively (*KDM2B*, *NEB*, and *CBFA2T2*) correlated with *ADORA2B* expression in LUAD. To verify these results, we measured the mRNA expression levels of these genes. The expression levels of *ANXA1*, *ITGA3*, and *S100A6* were significantly higher in A549 cells than in HBE cells and were positively correlated with *ADORA2B* expression levels (**Figure 8D**). In contrast, the expression levels of *KDM2B*, *NEB*, and *CBFA2T2* were significantly lower in A549 cells than in HBE cells and negatively correlated with *ADORA2B* expression (**Figure 8E**). These results were consistent with those from our bioinformatics analyses.

To further confirm these findings, specific ADORA2B siRNAs were transfected into A549 cells to inhibit *ADORA2B* expression. First, we verified the knockdown efficiencies of ADORA2B by qRT-PCR and then selected siRNA-2, which had the highest knockdown efficiency, for subsequent experiments (**Figure 8F**). Then, we measured the mRNA expression levels of genes that were positively or negatively correlated with *ADORA2B* expression. The expression levels of *ANXA1*, *ITGA3*, and *S100A6* were significantly lower in the *ADORA2B* siRNA group than in the control siRNA group and positively correlated with *ADORA2B* expression (**Figure 8G**). The expression levels of *KDM2B*, *NEB*, and *CBFA2T2* were significantly higher in the *ADORA2B* siRNA group than in the control siRNA group and negatively correlated with *ADORA2B* expression (**Figure 8H**). Taken together, *ADORA2B* was highly expressed in human LUAD A549 cells and the expression levels of *ANXA1*, *ITGA3*, and *S100A6* were positively correlated with *ADORA2B* expression, while those of *KDM2B*, *NEB*, and *CBFA2T2* were negatively correlated with *ADORA2B* expression. *In vitro* experimental results were consistent with those of the bioinformatics analyses.

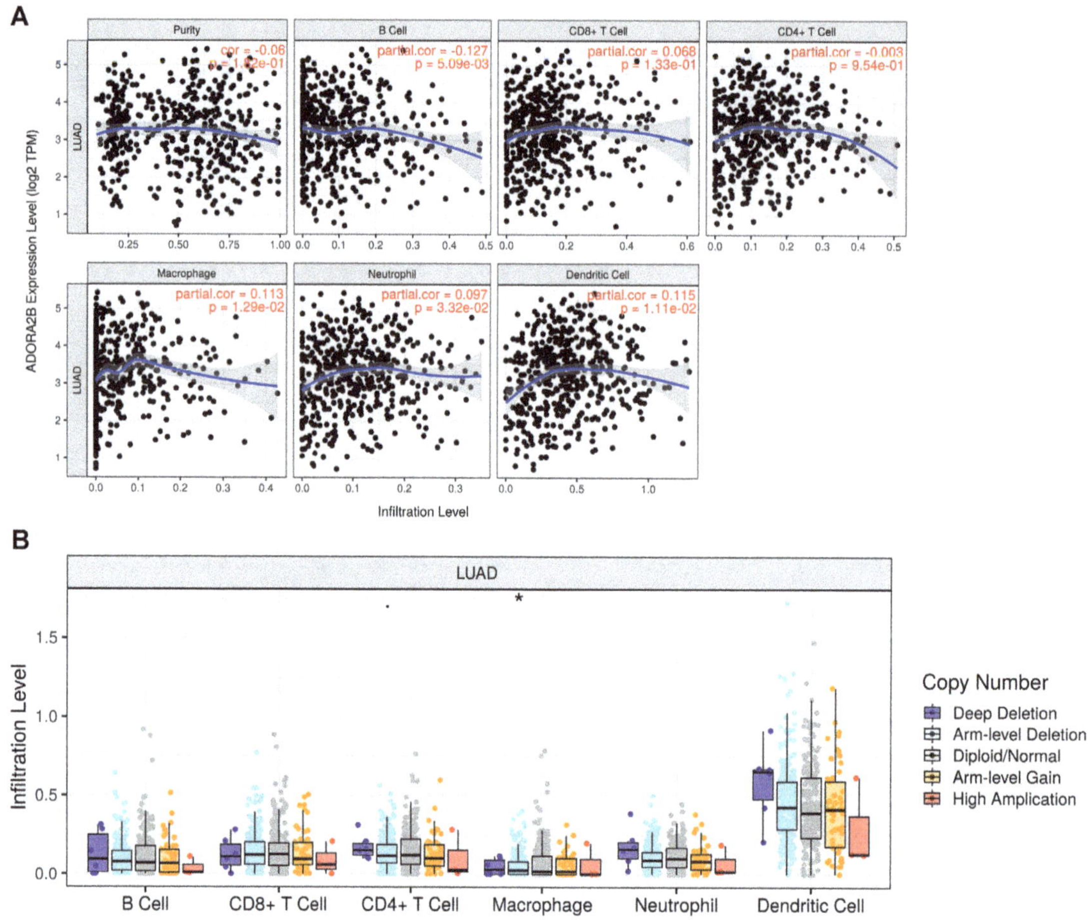

FIGURE 7 | Correlation of *ADORA2B* expression with immune cell infiltration in LUAD. **(A)** Correlation of *ADORA2B* with tumor purity and infiltration of different subsets of immune cells. **(B)** Effect of copy number variation of *ADORA2B* on the distribution of various immune cells. $^{*}p < 0.05$ is statistically significant.

Knockdown of *ADORA2B* Inhibited the Proliferation and Metastasis of LUAD Cells

Previous studies have demonstrated that *ADORA2B* participates in the proliferation and metastasis of carcinomas, such as prostate and oral cancers (Kasama et al., 2015; Vecchio et al., 2016). To further clarify the role of *ADORA2B* in the progression of LUAD, we performed related functional experiments to verify the function of *ADORA2B*. First, cell proliferation was measured using CCK-8. Compared with that of the control siRNA group, the cell viability of the *ADORA2B* siRNA group was significantly decreased at 24, 48, and 72 h after transfection (**Figure 9A**). Second, the cell migration rate was evaluated by the wound healing assay, the results of which showed that knockdown of *ADORA2B* reduced the migration capacity of A549 cells after 48 h of induction, partially supporting the role of ADORA2B in promoting metastasis in LUAD (**Figure 9B**). We further examined the protein expression levels of markers of carcinoma cell proliferation and metastasis after *ADORA2B* knockdown. Western blotting analysis indicated that the relative protein expression levels of proliferative (cyclin D1 and PCNA) and metastatic (N-cadherin and vimentin) markers in the *ADORA2B* siRNA group were significantly lower than those in the control siRNA group (**Figures 9C,D**). These results demonstrated that knockdown of *ADORA2B* inhibited the proliferation and metastasis of LUAD cells and that *ADORA2B* might participate in the proliferation and metastasis of LUAD cells.

DISCUSSION

Adenosine is a purinergic molecule that regulates tissue damage and repair. Adenosine receptors belong to the G-protein–coupled receptor superfamily and include A1, A2A, A2B, and A3, which are widely distributed in different human tissues. The expression levels and affinities of adenosine receptors can vary across different tissues and cell types. In addition, these adenosine receptors have different phosphorylation abilities and sensitivities to the G-proteins with which they are conjugated. The A1 receptor is conjugated with the Gi/G0 protein, while the A3 receptor is conjugated with the Gi protein to inhibit the activity of adenylate cyclase and reduce the level of cAMP. In contrast, A2A and A2B receptors are conjugated with Gs proteins

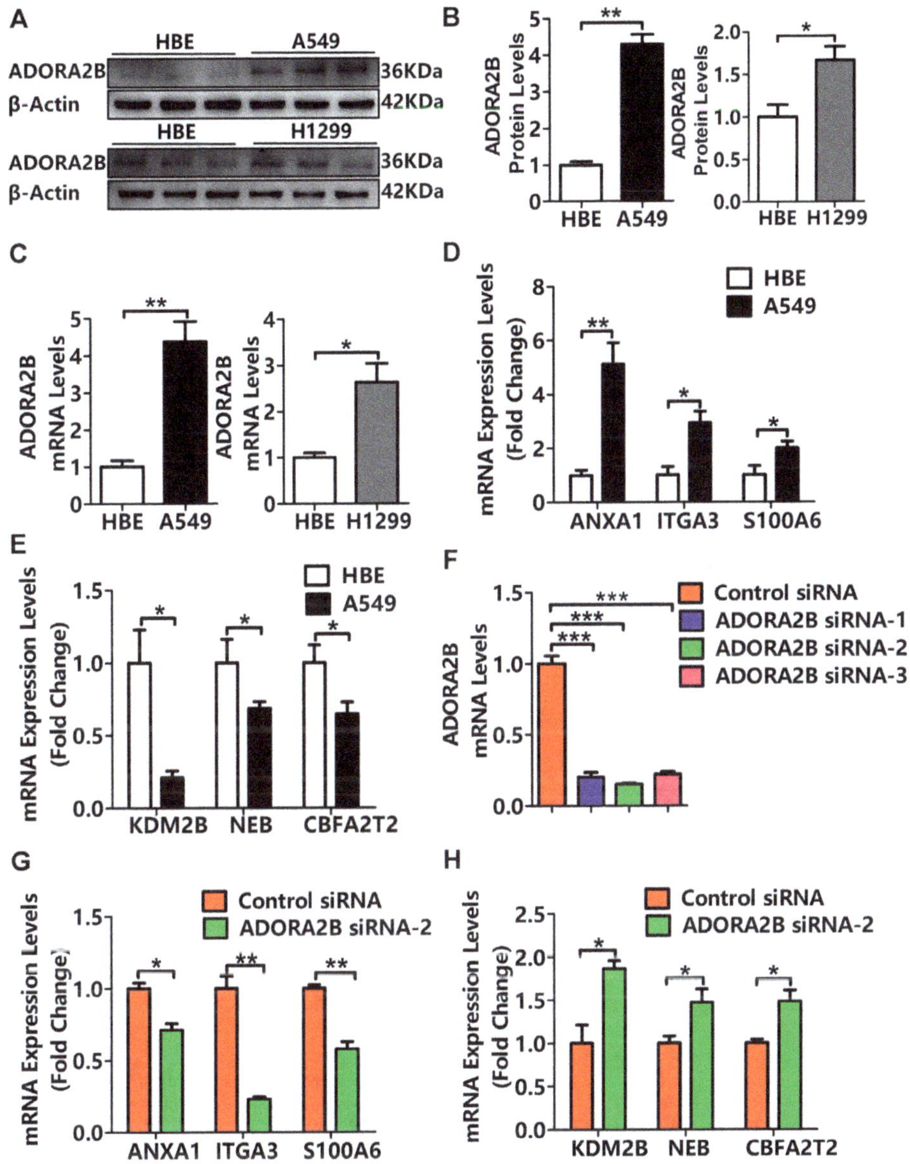

FIGURE 8 | Expression levels of *ADORA2B* and correlated genes in human LUAD cells. **(A)** Relative protein expression of ADORA2B was determined by western blotting. **(B)** Protein quantitative statistics. **(C)** Relative mRNA expression of *ADORA2B* was determined by qRT-PCR. mRNA expression levels of genes **(D)** positively and **(E)** negatively correlated with *ADORA2B*. **(F)** mRNA expression levels of *ADORA2B* after siRNA transfection. mRNA expression levels of genes **(G)** positively and **(H)** negatively correlated with *ADORA2B* after siRNA transfection. $^*p < 0.05$, $^{**}p < 0.01$, and $^{***}p < 0.001$ are statistically significant.

to activate the activity of adenylate cyclase and increase the level of cAMP. Low concentrations usually activate the A2A receptor, while higher concentrations of adenosine activate the A2B receptor, which suggests that the basal level of adenosine mainly activates the A2A receptor in a physiological state and that the A2B receptor is activated only when the adenosine level rises above physiological levels or reaches a pathological level (Vecchio et al., 2018; Fenouillet et al., 2019).

Increasing evidence suggests that adenosine receptors are potential diagnostic biomarkers for some diseases, inflammation, and certain types of cancers (Feoktistov and Biaggioni, 2011; Koeppen et al., 2011; Fishman et al., 2012). Additionally, adenosine receptors are upregulated in various tumors (Fishman et al., 2009). *ADORA2B* plays an important role in the occurrence, development, and metastasis of human tumors and is expressed in a variety of tumor cells. In the present study, to observe the functional network of *ADORA2B* in LUAD, we performed bioinformatics analyses to analyze transcriptional sequencing data from clinical sample data obtained from the Gene Expression Omnibus (GEO) and TCGA databases. To determine the role of *ADORA2B* in LUAD, we evaluated the expression pattern of several genes expressed in the disease. The analysis of the Oncomine database revealed fold-changes in gene expression levels that were similar

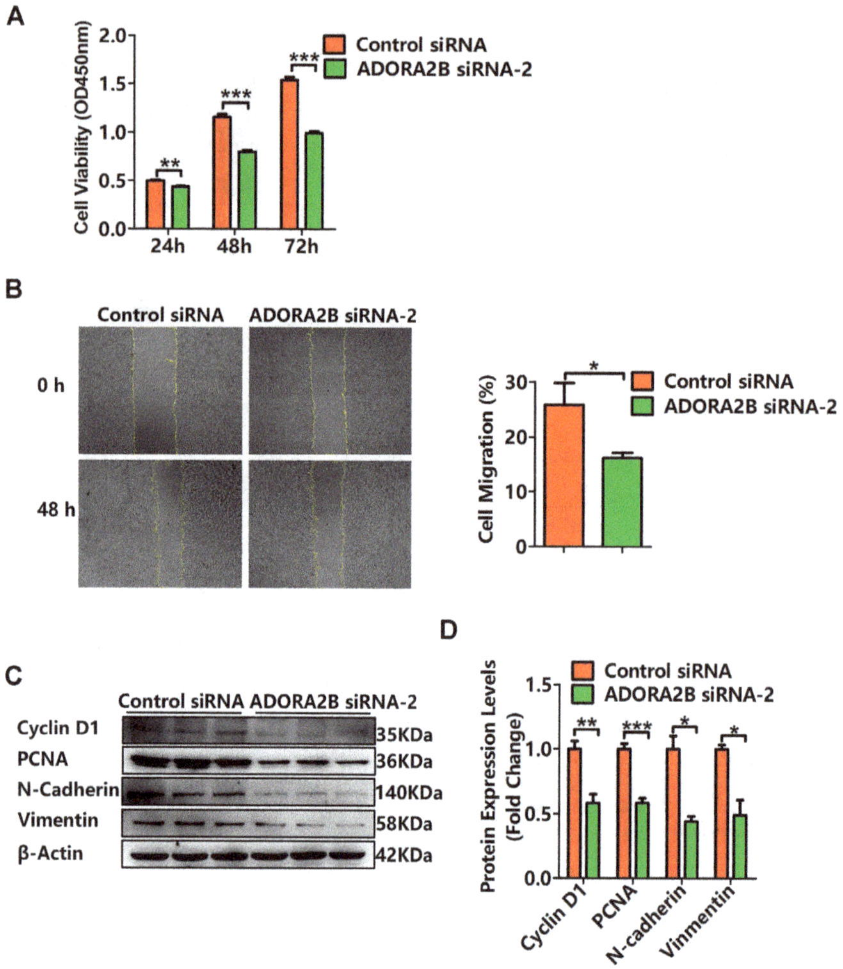

FIGURE 9 | Knockdown of *ADORA2B* inhibited the proliferation and metastasis of LUAD cells. **(A)** The cell viability of LUAD cells transfected with control or *ADORA2B* siRNA was detected by the CCK-8 assay. **(B)** The wound healing assay was used to examine the effect of *ADORA2B* siRNA on A549 cell migration for 48 h (magnification: ×40). **(C)** Relative protein expressions of proliferative (cyclin D1 and PCNA) and metastatic (N-cadherin and vimentin) markers were determined by western blotting. **(D)** Protein quantitative statistics. $^*p < 0.05$, $^{**}p < 0.01$, and $^{***}p < 0.001$ are statistically significant.

to those reported in previous LUAD studies. According to the mRNA expression level, *ADORA2B* ranked among the top 8–33% of all upregulated genes expressed in LUAD, indicating that *ADORA2B* is significantly overexpressed in LUAD (**Figure 1**). Survival analysis showed that the OS time (including the overall, one-year, three-year, and five-year survival rates) in the low *ADORA2B* expression group was significantly longer than that in the high *ADORA2B* expression group. These results indicated that a high *ADORA2B* expression predicted a poor prognosis for LUAD patients (**Figure 4**).

Further analysis using the UALCAN database showed that the mRNA expression levels of *ADORA2B* were significantly higher in LUAD samples than in para-carcinoma tissues. Furthermore, the expression varied depending on the cancer stage, age, smoking habit, nodal metastasis status, and TP53 mutation status. In addition, the copy number of *ADORA2B* was significantly increased in LUAD (**Figure 2**). These associations indicated the impact of *ADORA2B* expression on human health or the types of biological and social factors that contribute to the pathological process of LUAD.

Cancer progression involves a series of histopathological processes (Xie et al., 2017; Chen et al., 2016) and changes in the functions of specific genes that have potential inhibitory or carcinogenic effects on cancer progression (Cui et al., 2018; Klonowska et al., 2016). Therefore, in the present study, we used the web-based tool, cBioPortal, to detect amplification, mutations, and mRNA expression of *ADORA2B* in LUAD. The major types of *ADORA2B* alterations were mRNA low, deep deletion, and amplification. The fraction of genome altered and mutation type, including not mutated, not profiled for mutations, amplification, gain, diploid, shallow deletion, and deep deletion, were analyzed. These mutations may play key roles in cancer progression and prognosis (**Figure 3**). Tumorigenesis is an extremely complex process, and new intricate protein–protein interactions and altered signaling pathways accelerate the pathological process of malignant tumors. *ADORA2B* was reported to be involved in tumor-cell proliferation, tumor-cell metastasis, and tumor microenvironment changes (Desmet et al., 2013; Kasama et al., 2015; Vecchio et al., 2016). To further clarify the role of *ADORA2B* in the progression of LUAD, we performed related functional experiments to verify the function of *ADORA2B*. The results indicated that knockdown of *ADORA2B* inhibited the proliferation and metastasis of LUAD cells and that *ADORA2B* might participate in the proliferation and metastasis of LUAD cells (**Figure 9**).

To identify the functional proteins in LUAD, we used the GeneMANIA web server. Interacting proteins regulate tumor progression. To determine the hierarchy of interacting proteins, we used the LinkedOmics database and drew a heat map of differentially expressed genes correlated with *ADORA2B* expression. In LUAD, *ADORA2B* was predicted to be associated with several *ADORA2B*-associated genes. Among them, *ANXA1* was highly expressed in various malignant tumors (Huang et al., 2015; Okano et al., 2015), and upregulation of ANXA1 levels in the serum was related to the pathological grade and clinical stage of patients with particular forms of LUAD. Knockout of *ANXA1* expression inhibited the proliferation, migration, and invasion of lung carcinoma cells (Fang et al., 2016), while the expression level of *ITGA3* can be used as a diagnostic and prognostic marker for several malignant tumors (Koshizuka et al., 2017; Jiao et al., 2019; Ramovs et al., 2019). *S100A6*, which regulates cytoskeleton protein dynamics, cell proliferation, cell differentiation, calcium metabolism, ubiquitination, and acetylation, was found to promote the proliferation, invasion, migration, and angiogenesis of lung carcinoma cells by inhibiting acetylation of *p53* when overexpressed (Li et al., 2019). KDM2B can reduce the proliferation of carcinoma cells by inhibiting the expression of oncogenes that play important roles in the self-renewal, differentiation, and apoptosis of stem cells (Hong et al., 2016; Goyama and Kitamura, 2017). Therefore, the findings of the present study validated the significance of *ADORA2B* in LUAD (**Figure 5**). *ADORA2B* interacts with these proteins that regulate important cellular processes associated with cancers and diseases.

Enrichment analysis of target gene sets using GSEA can identify important networks involved in protein targeting, mRNA processing, and transcription factors. ADORA2B was revealed to regulate the FAS signaling pathway, EGF receptor signaling pathway, and apoptosis signaling pathway (**Figure 6**). The CD73–adenosine receptor signaling pathway can promote the immunosuppressive effect of the tumor microenvironment, which is closely associated with a poor prognosis of multiple tumors (Chen et al., 2020). Immune cell infiltration analysis results suggested that the expression level of *ADORA2B* was associated with infiltrating immune cells in LUAD, including B cells, macrophages, neutrophils, and dendritic cells (**Figure 7**). These results revealed the indispensable role of *ADORA2B* in the development of LUAD.

The results of our preliminarily bioinformatics analysis suggested that *ADORA2B* can be used as a biomarker for LUAD, and we further confirmed the role of *ADORA2B* in LUAD through *in vitro* experiments. Human LUAD- and bronchial epithelial cell-derived cells lines were cultured *in vitro*, and mRNA and protein levels of *ADORA2B* were analyzed. Our results showed that both the transcription and protein levels of *ADORA2B* were significantly higher in A549 and NCl-H1299 cells than in HBE cells. The expression of genes positively (*ANXA1*, *ITGA3*, and *S100A6*) or negatively (*KDM2B*, *NEB*, and *CBFA2T2*) correlated with *ADORA2B* was consistent with the transcription level of *ADORA2B*. siRNA *ADORA2B* transfection experiments further confirmed these results (**Figure 8**). Our *in vitro* experiments confirmed the predictive and diagnostic role of ADORA2B in LUAD, but there were some limitations of this study. We tried to obtain human LUAD tissues to verify our *in vitro* results; however, it is difficult to acquire human LUAD tissues owing to ethical and technical reasons. If we get an opportunity to acquire LUAD tissues in the future, we will further investigate the role of *ADORA2B* in LUAD.

CONCLUSION

In conclusion, we used several public databases to extract data related to mRNA expression and mutations of *ADORA2B* and to the expression of genes associated with *ADORA2B* in LUAD. Furthermore, we predicted the differentially expressed genes correlated with *ADORA2B* expression in LUAD. Survival analysis showed that the OS time in the low *ADORA2B* expression group was longer than that in the high *ADORA2B* expression group. These results indicated that a high expression of *ADORA2B* predicted a poor prognosis for LUAD patients. Enrichment analysis of target gene sets using GSEA revealed important networks of the *ADORA2B* signaling pathway. Immune infiltration analysis results suggested that the expression level of *ADORA2B* was associated with immune cell infiltration in LUAD. *In vitro* experiments revealed that the relative *ADORA2B* expression levels in LUAD cells were significantly higher than those in normal bronchial epithelial cells. Knockdown of *ADORA2B* inhibited the proliferation and metastasis of LUAD cells, indicating that *ADORA2B* might participate in the proliferation and metastasis of LUAD cells. Taken together, our results revealed the significance of *ADORA2B* expression and its interaction networks in LUAD; the results of our *in vitro* experiments were consistent with those of the bioinformatics analysis. Although A549, NCl-H1299, and HBE cell lines were mainly used in the current experiments, we will verify these results with human and murine LUAD tissues in future studies. Our findings provide valuable insights into *ADORA2B* as a potential diagnostic and prognostic marker for LUAD and thus provide a foundation for further research focusing on LUAD biomarker development.

data were downloaded from the Oncomine database under Series accession number GSE10072 (http://www.ncbi.nlm.nih.gov/geo/query/acc.cgi?acc=GSE10072). Selamat Lung data were downloaded from the Oncomine database under Series accession number GSE32863 (http://www.ncbi.nlm.nih.gov/geo/query/acc.cgi?acc=GSE32863). Stearman Lung data were downloaded from the Oncomine database under Series accession number GSE2514 (http://www.ncbi.nlm.nih.gov/geo/query/acc.cgi?acc=GSE2514). Beer Lung data were downloaded from the Oncomine database under the Array Type: HumanGeneFL Array, Measured 5,338 genes, 7,133 reporters (Beer, D. G., Kardia, S. L., Huang, C. C., Giordano, T. J., Levin, A. M., Misek, D. E., et al., 2002). Gene expression profiles predict survival of patients with lung adenocarcinoma (Nat. Med. 8, 816–824. doi: 10.1038/nm733). Su Lung data were downloaded from the Oncomine database under Series accession number GSE7670 (http://www.ncbi.nlm.nih.gov/geo/query/acc.cgi?acc=GSE7670). Bhattacharjee Lung data were downloaded from the Oncomine database under the Array Type: Human Genome U95A-Av2 Array, Measured 8,603 genes, 12,651 reporters (Bhattacharjee, A., Richards, W. G., Staunton, J., Li, C., Monti, S., Vasa, P., et al., 2001). Classification of human lung carcinomas by mRNA expression profiling reveals distinct adenocarcinoma subclasses (Proc. Natl. Acad. Sci. U S A98, 13790–13795. doi: 10.1073/pnas.191502998). Garber Lung data were downloaded from the Oncomine database under Series accession number GSE3398 (http://www.ncbi.nlm.nih.gov/geo/query/acc.cgi?acc=GSE3398). OncoPrint data were downloaded from the cBioPortal database Shortened URL https://bit.ly/3oTsOd5. Mutation data were downloaded from the cBioPortal database Shortened URL https://bit.ly/2ObTF7t. Clinical attribute data were downloaded from the cBioPortal database Shortened URL https://bit.ly/3rnelHU. LinkedOmics data were downloaded from the LinkedOmics database under ID number ID-62189.

AUTHOR CONTRIBUTIONS

YS and JL designed the study, performed the data analysis, and aided in writing the manuscript. JZ, ZZ, and ZW completed the data download and analysis and *in vitro* experiments. ZJ and ZM evaluated and reviewed the manuscript structure, ideas, and science. All authors read and approved the final manuscript.

FUNDING

This work was supported by the National Natural Science Foundation of China (Grant Number 31800722 to ZM), Tianjin Natural Science Foundation (Grant Number 19JCQNJC11400 to ZM), China Postdoctoral Science Foundation (Grant Number 2019M660030 to YS), Tianjin Health Commission Science and Technology Talent Cultivation Project (Grant Number KJ20040 to ZM), Postdoctoral Fund of the First Affiliated Hospital, Jinan University (Grant Number 809036 to ZJ), and HAI YAN Science Foundation of Harbin Medical University Cancer Hospital (Grant Numbers JJQN 2021-14 and JJMS 2021-30 to JL). We are grateful to the data contributors of Oncomine, UALCAN, cBioPortal, GeneMANIA, LinkedOmics, KM Plotter, and TIMER for providing access to all the data required for this study. We are also grateful to *Editage* for editing the revised manuscript.

REFERENCES

Beer, D. G., Kardia, S. L. R., Huang, C.-C., Giordano, T. J., Levin, A. M., Misek, D. E., et al. (2002). Gene-expression Profiles Predict Survival of Patients with Lung Adenocarcinoma. *Nat. Med.* 8, 816–824. doi:10.1038/nm733

Bhattacharjee, A., Richards, W. G., Staunton, J., Li, C., Monti, S., Vasa, P., et al. (2001). Classification of Human Lung Carcinomas by mRNA Expression Profiling Reveals Distinct Adenocarcinoma Subclasses. *Proc. Natl. Acad. Sci.* 98, 13790–13795. doi:10.1073/pnas.191502998

Borea, P. A., Gessi, S., Merighi, S., and Varani, K. (2016). Adenosine as a Multi-Signalling Guardian Angel in Human Diseases: when, where and How Does it Exert its Protective Effects?. *Trends Pharmacol. Sci.* 37, 419–434. doi:10.1016/j.tips.2016.02.006

Cancer Genome Atlas Research Network (2018). Author Correction: Comprehensive Molecular Profiling of Lung Adenocarcinoma. *Nature* 559, E12. doi:10.1038/s41586-018-0228-6

Chandrashekar, D. S., Bashel, B., Balasubramanya, S. A. H., Creighton, C. J., Ponce-Rodriguez, I., Chakravarthi, B. V. S. K., et al. (2017). UALCAN: a portal for Facilitating Tumor Subgroup Gene Expression and Survival Analyses. *Neoplasia* 19, 649–658. doi:10.1016/j.neo.2017.05.002

Chen, S., Akdemir, I., Fan, J., Linden, J., Zhang, B., and Cekic, C. (2020). The Expression of Adenosine A2B Receptor on Antigen-Presenting Cells Suppresses CD8+ T-Cell Responses and Promotes Tumor Growth. *Cancer Immunol. Res.* 8, 1064–1074. doi:10.1158/2326-6066.CIR-19-0833

Chen, W.-C., Wang, C.-Y., Hung, Y.-H., Weng, T.-Y., Yen, M.-C., and Lai, M.-D. (2016). Systematic Analysis of Gene Expression Alterations and Clinical Outcomes for Long-Chain Acyl-Coenzyme A Synthetase Family in Cancer. *PLoS One* 11, e0155660. doi:10.1371/journal.pone.0155660

Covarrubias, R., Chepurko, E., Reynolds, A., Huttinger, Z. M., Huttinger, R., Stanfill, K., et al. (2016). Role of the CD39/CD73 Purinergic Pathway in Modulating Arterial Thrombosis in Mice. *Arterioscler Thromb. Vasc. Biol.* 36, 1809–1820. doi:10.1161/ATVBAHA.116.307374

Csóka, B., Selmeczy, Z., Koscsó, B., Németh, Z. H., Pacher, P., Murray, P. J., et al. (2012). Adenosine Promotes Alternative Macrophage Activation via A2A and A2B Receptors. *FASEB j.* 26, 376–386. doi:10.1096/fj.11-190934

Cui, X., Jing, X., Yi, Q., Long, C., Tan, B., Li, X., et al. (2018). Systematic Analysis of Gene Expression Alterations and Clinical Outcomes of STAT3 in Cancer. *Oncotarget* 9, 3198–3213. doi:10.18632/oncotarget.23226

Desmet, C. J., Gallenne, T., Prieur, A., Reyal, F., Visser, N. L., Wittner, B. S., et al. (2013). Identification of a Pharmacologically Tractable Fra-1/ADORA2B axis Promoting Breast Cancer Metastasis. *Proc. Natl. Acad. Sci.* 110, 5139–5144. doi:10.1073/pnas.1222085110

Drilon, A., Oxnard, G. R., Tan, D. S. W., Loong, H. H. F., Johnson, M., Gainor, J., et al. (2020). Efficacy of Selpercatinib in *RET* Fusion-Positive Non-small-cell Lung Cancer. *N. Engl. J. Med.* 383, 813–824. doi:10.1056/NEJMoa2005653

Fang, Y., Guan, X., Cai, T., Long, J., Wang, H., Xie, X., et al. (2016). Knockdown of ANXA1 Suppresses the Biological Behavior of Human NSCLC Cells *In Vitro*. *Mol. Med. Rep.* 13, 3858–3866. doi:10.3892/mmr.2016.5022

Fenouillet, E., Mottola, G., Kipson, N., Paganelli, F., Guieu, R., and Ruf, J. (2019). Adenosine Receptor Profiling Reveals an Association between the Presence of Spare Receptors and Cardiovascular Disorders. *Int. J. Mol. Sci.* 20, 5964. doi:10.3390/ijms20235964

Feoktistov, I., and Biaggioni, I. (2011). Role of Adenosine A2B Receptors in Inflammation. *Adv. Pharmacol.* 61, 115–144. doi:10.1016/B978-0-12-385526-8.00005-9

Fishman, P., Bar-Yehuda, S., Liang, B. T., and Jacobson, K. A. (2012). Pharmacological and Therapeutic Effects of A3 Adenosine Receptor Agonists. *Drug Discov. Today* 17, 359–366. doi:10.1016/j.drudis.2011.10.007

Fishman, P., Bar-Yehuda, S., Synowitz, M., Powell, J. D., Klotz, K. N., Gessi, S., et al. (2009). Adenosine Receptors and Cancer. *Handb. Exp. Pharmacol.* 193, 399–441. doi:10.1007/978-3-540-89615-9_14

Garber, M. E., Troyanskaya, O. G., Schluens, K., Petersen, S., Thaesler, Z., Pacyna-Gengelbach, M., et al. (2001). Diversity of Gene Expression in Adenocarcinoma of the Lung. *Proc. Natl. Acad. Sci.* 98, 13784–13789. doi:10.1073/pnas.241500798

Goyama, S., and Kitamura, T. (2017). Epigenetics in normal and Malignant Hematopoiesis: An Overview and Update 2017. *Cancer Sci.* 108, 553–562. doi:10.1111/cas.13168

Hamidzadeh, K., and Mosser, D. M. (2016). Purinergic Signaling to Terminate TLR Responses in Macrophages. *Front. Immunol.* 7, 74. doi:10.3389/fimmu.2016.00074

Hong, X., Xu, Y., Qiu, X., Zhu, Y., Feng, X., Ding, Z., et al. (2016). MiR-448 Promotes Glycolytic Metabolism of Gastric Cancer by Downregulating KDM2B. *Oncotarget* 7, 22092–22102. doi:10.18632/oncotarget.8020

Huang, Y., Zhang, C., Chen, C., Sun, S., Zheng, H., Wan, S., et al. (2015). Investigation of Circulating Antibodies to ANXA1 in Breast Cancer. *Tumor Biol.* 36, 1233–1236. doi:10.1007/s13277-014-2751-x

Jiao, Y., Li, Y., Liu, S., Chen, Q., and Liu, Y. (2019). ITGA3 Serves as a Diagnostic and Prognostic Biomarker for Pancreatic Cancer. *Ott* 12, 4141–4152. doi:10.2147/OTT.S201675

Karmouty-Quintana, H., Weng, T., Garcia-Morales, L. J., Chen, N.-Y., Pedroza, M., Zhong, H., et al. (2013). Adenosine A2B Receptor and Hyaluronan Modulate Pulmonary Hypertension Associated with Chronic Obstructive Pulmonary Disease. *Am. J. Respir. Cel Mol. Biol.* 49, 1038–1047. doi:10.1165/rcmb.2013-0089OC

Kasama, H., Sakamoto, Y., Kasamatsu, A., Okamoto, A., Koyama, T., Minakawa, Y., et al. (2015). Adenosine A2b Receptor Promotes Progression of Human Oral Cancer. *BMC Cancer* 15, 563. doi:10.1186/s12885-015-1577-2

Klonowska, K., Czubak, K., Wojciechowska, M., Handschuh, L., Zmienko, A., Figlerowicz, M., et al. (2016). Oncogenomic Portals for the Visualization and Analysis of Genome-wide Cancer Data. *Oncotarget* 7, 176–192. doi:10.18632/oncotarget.6128

Koeppen, M., Eckle, T., and Eltzschig, H. K. (2011). Interplay of Hypoxia and A2B Adenosine Receptors in Tissue protection. *Adv. Pharmacol.* 61, 145–186. doi:10.1016/B978-0-12-385526-8.00006-0

Koshizuka, K., Hanazawa, T., Kikkawa, N., Arai, T., Okato, A., Kurozumi, A., et al. (2017). Regulation of ITGA 3 by the Anti-tumor miR-199 Family Inhibits Cancer Cell Migration and Invasion in Head and Neck Cancer. *Cancer Sci.* 108, 1681–1692. doi:10.1111/cas.13298

Landi, M. T., Dracheva, T., Rotunno, M., Figueroa, J. D., Liu, H., Dasgupta, A., et al. (2008). Gene Expression Signature of Cigarette Smoking and its Role in Lung Adenocarcinoma Development and Survival. *PLoS One* 3, e1651. doi:10.1371/journal.pone.0001651

Li, P., Lv, X., Zhang, Z., and Xie, S. (2019). S100A6/miR193a Regulates the Proliferation, Invasion, Migration and Angiogenesis of Lung Cancer Cells through the P53 Acetylation. *Am. J. Transl. Res.* 11, 4634–4649.

Mazieres, J., Cropet, C., Montané, L., Barlesi, F., Souquet, P. J., Quantin, X., et al. (2020). Vemurafenib in Non-small-cell Lung Cancer Patients with BRAFV600 and BRAFnonV600 Mutations. *Ann. Oncol.* 31, 289–294. doi:10.1016/j.annonc.2019.10.022

Mertens, T. C. J., Hanmandlu, A., Tu, L., Phan, C., Collum, S. D., Chen, N.-Y., et al. (2018). Switching-off Adora2b in Vascular Smooth Muscle Cells Halts the Development of Pulmonary Hypertension. *Front. Physiol.* 9, 555. doi:10.3389/fphys.2018.00555

Okano, M., Kumamoto, K., Saito, M., Onozawa, H., Saito, K., Abe, N., et al. (2015). Upregulated Annexin A1 Promotes Cellular Invasion in Triple-Negative Breast Cancer. *Oncol. Rep.* 33, 1064–1070. doi:10.3892/or.2015.3720

Okayama, H., Kohno, T., Ishii, Y., Shimada, Y., Shiraishi, K., Iwakawa, R., et al. (2012). Identification of Genes Upregulated in ALK-Positive and EGFR/KRAS/ALK-negative Lung Adenocarcinomas. *Cancer Res.* 72, 100–111. doi:10.1158/0008-5472.CAN-11-1403

Philip, K., Mills, W. T., Davies, J., Chen, N. Y., Karmouty-Quintana, H., Luo, F., et al. (2017). HIF1A Up-regulates the ADORA2B Receptor on Alternatively Activated Macrophages and Contributes to Pulmonary Fibrosis. *FASEB j.* 31, 4745–4758. doi:10.1096/fj.201700219R

Pillai, R. N., Behera, M., Berry, L. D., Rossi, M. R., Kris, M. G., Johnson, B. E., et al. (2017). HER2 Mutations in Lung Adenocarcinomas: a Report from the Lung Cancer Mutation Consortium. *Cancer* 123, 4099–4105. doi:10.1002/cncr.30869

Ramovs, V., Secades, P., Song, J.-Y., Thijssen, B., Kreft, M., and Sonnenberg, A. (2019). Absence of Integrin α3β1 Promotes the Progression of HER2-Driven Breast Cancer *In Vivo*. *Breast Cancer Res.* 21, 63. doi:10.1186/s13058-019-1146-8

Román, M., Baraibar, I., López, I., Nadal, E., Rolfo, C., Vicent, S., et al. (2018). KRAS Oncogene in Non-small Cell Lung Cancer: Clinical Perspectives on the Treatment of an Old Target. *Mol. Cancer* 17, 33. doi:10.1186/s12943-018-0789-x

Russell, P. A., Wainer, Z., Wright, G. M., Daniels, M., Conron, M., and Williams, R. A. (2011). Does Lung Adenocarcinoma Subtype Predict Patient Survival?: a Clinicopathologic Study Based on the New International Association for the Study of Lung Cancer/American Thoracic Society/European Respiratory Society International Multidisciplinary Lung Adenocarcinoma Classification. *J. Thorac. Oncol.* 6, 1496–1504. doi:10.1097/JTO.0b013e318221f701

Selamat, S. A., Chung, B. S., Girard, L., Zhang, W., Zhang, Y., Campan, M., et al. (2012). Genome-scale Analysis of DNA Methylation in Lung Adenocarcinoma and Integration with mRNA Expression. *Genome Res.* 22, 1197–1211. doi:10.1101/gr.132662.111

Shaw, A. T., Felip, E., Bauer, T. M., Besse, B., Navarro, A., Postel-Vinay, S., et al. (2017). Lorlatinib in Non-small-cell Lung Cancer with ALK or ROS1 Rearrangement: an International, Multicentre, Open-Label, Single-Arm First-In-Man Phase 1 Trial. *Lancet Oncol.* 18, 1590–1599. doi:10.1016/S1470-2045(17)30680-0

Stearman, R. S., Dwyer-Nield, L., Zerbe, L., Blaine, S. A., Chan, Z., Bunn, P. A., et al. (2005). Analysis of Orthologous Gene Expression between Human Pulmonary Adenocarcinoma and a Carcinogen-Induced Murine Model. *Am. J. Pathol.* 167, 1763–1775. doi:10.1016/S0002-9440(10)61257-6

Su, L.-J., Chang, C.-W., Wu, Y.-C., Chen, K.-C., Lin, C.-J., Liang, S.-C., et al. (2007). Selection of DDX5 as a Novel Internal Control for Q-RT-PCR from Microarray Data Using a Block Bootstrap Re-sampling Scheme. *BMC Genomics* 8, 140. doi:10.1186/1471-2164-8-140

Tian, Z., Dixon, J., Guo, X., Deal, B., Liao, Q., Zhou, Y., et al. (2021). Co-inhibition of CD73 and ADORA2B Improves Long-Term Cigarette Smoke Induced Lung Injury. *Front. Physiol.* 12, 614330. doi:10.3389/fphys.2021.614330

Vecchio, E. A., Baltos, J. A., Nguyen, A. T. N., Christopoulos, A., White, P. J., and May, L. T. (2018). New Paradigms in Adenosine Receptor Pharmacology: Allostery, Oligomerization and Biased Agonism. *Br. J. Pharmacol.* 175, 4036–4046. doi:10.1111/bph.14337

Vecchio, E. A., Tan, C. Y. R., Gregory, K. J., Christopoulos, A., White, P. J., and May, L. T. (2016). Ligand-independent Adenosine A2B Receptor Constitutive Activity as a Promoter of Prostate Cancer Cell Proliferation. *J. Pharmacol. Exp. Ther.* 357, 36–44. doi:10.1124/jpet.115.230003

Warde-Farley, D., Donaldson, S. L., Comes, O., Zuberi, K., Badrawi, R., Chao, P., et al. (2010). The GeneMANIA Prediction Server: Biological Network Integration for Gene Prioritization and Predicting Gene Function. *Nucleic Acids Res.* 38, W214–W220. doi:10.1093/nar/gkq537

Xie, S., Shen, C., Tan, M., Li, M., Song, X., and Wang, C. (2017). Systematic Analysis of Gene Expression Alterations and Clinical Outcomes of Adenylate Cyclase-Associated Protein in Cancer. *Oncotarget* 8, 27216–27239. doi:10.18632/oncotarget.16111

Yu, H. A., Arcila, M. E., Rekhtman, N., Sima, C. S., Zakowski, M. F., Pao, W., et al. (2013). Analysis of Tumor Specimens at the Time of Acquired Resistance to EGFR-TKI Therapy in 155 Patients with EGFR-Mutant Lung Cancers. *Clin. Cancer Res.* 19, 2240–2247. doi:10.1158/1078-0432.CCR-12-2246

Yu, L., Todd, N. W., Xing, L., Xie, Y., Zhang, H., Liu, Z., et al. (2010). Early Detection of Lung Adenocarcinoma in Sputum by a Panel of microRNA Markers. *Int. J. Cancer* 127, 2870–2878. doi:10.1002/ijc.25289

Zagryazhskaya, A., Gyuraszova, K., and Zhivotovsky, B. (2015). Cell Death in Cancer Therapy of Lung Adenocarcinoma. *Int. J. Dev. Biol.* 59, 119–129. doi:10.1387/ijdb.150044bz

8

Therapeutic Effects of the Bcl-2 Inhibitor on Bleomycin-Induced Pulmonary Fibrosis in Mice

Yicheng He[1], Fei Li[1], Chao Zhang[1], Xinwei Geng[2], Madiha Zahra Syeda[2], Xufei Du[1], Zhehua Shao[1], Wen Hua[1], Wen Li[1], Zhihua Chen[1], Songmin Ying[1,2] and Huahao Shen[1,3]**

[1]Key Laboratory of Respiratory Disease of Zhejiang Province, Department of Respiratory and Critical Care Medicine, Second Affiliated Hospital of Zhejiang University School of Medicine, Hangzhou, China, [2]Department of Pharmacology, Zhejiang University School of Medicine, Hangzhou, China, [3]State Key Lab of Respiratory Disease, Guangzhou, China

***Correspondence:**
Songmin Ying
yings@zju.edu.cn
Huahao Shen
huahaoshen@zju.edu.cn*

Idiopathic pulmonary fibrosis (IPF) is a distressing lung disorder with poor prognosis and high mortality rates. Limited therapeutic options for IPF is a major clinical challenge. Well-known for its anti-apoptotic properties, B-cell lymphoma 2 (Bcl-2) plays a critical role in the pathology of malignancies and inflammatory diseases, including IPF. In this study, we aimed to investigate the therapeutic effect of a Bcl-2 homology domain 3 mimetic inhibitor, ABT-199, on bleomycin (BLM)-induced pulmonary fibrosis in mice, and explore possible underlying mechanism. The lung inflammation and fibrosis model was established by intratracheal instillation of a single dose of BLM. We observed elevated Bcl-2 in the alveolar macrophages and fibroblasts derived from BLM-instilled mice from day 7. Further, we obtained *in vivo* evidence that early therapeutic treatment with Bcl-2 inhibitor ABT-199 from day 3, and late treatment from day 10, both alleviated airway inflammation and lung fibrosis induced by BLM. Our data suggest that ABT-199 might be an effective antifibrotic agent that interferes with profibrogenic cells, which may be a promising therapy in the treatment of clinical IPF patients.

Keywords: idiopathic pulmonary fibrosis, Bcl-2, ABT-199, macrophage, fibroblast

INTRODUCTION

IPF is an interstitial lung disease characterized pathologically by progressive scarring of lung tissue, increased fibroblast proliferation, excessive accumulation of extracellular matrix (ECM), exacerbation of lung inflammation, diffused destruction of alveolar structure and remodeling of the lung architecture (Todd et al., 2012). The clinical symptoms of IPF are progressive dyspnea, wheezing or panting which finally lead to respiratory failure (Chen et al., 2013). This disease is significantly correlated to a dismal outcome with a median survival time of 2–4 yr after diagnosis (Bjoraker et al., 1998). To date, there is no promising medication to effectively cure this disease, which makes it vital to find novel therapeutic targets to treat IPF.

Apoptosis plays a significant role in wound repair and pulmonary epithelial injury leading to fibrosis. Decreased apoptosis of inflammatory cells and fibroblasts results in chronic inflammation

---

Abbreviations: BALF, bronchial alveolar lavage fluid; Bcl-2, B-cell lymphoma 2; BLM, bleomycin; Collagen I, type I collagen; ECM, extracellular matrix; ELISA, enzyme-linked immunosorbent assay; HE, Hematoxylin-Eosin; HYP, hydroxyproline; IL-1β, interleukin-1β; IPF, Idiopathic pulmonary fibrosis; NS, normal saline; α-SMA, α-smooth muscle actin; SPF, Specific Pathogen Free; TGF-β1, transforming growth factor-β1; TNF-α, tumor necrosis factor-α.

which injures the lung and promotes fibrogenesis (Polunovsky et al., 1993). Notably, a marked reduction in the apoptosis of alveolar macrophages plays an integral role in the pathogenesis of pulmonary fibrosis by triggering an immune response (Larson-Casey et al., 2016). There is evidence that the apoptosis rate of alveolar macrophages in bronchial alveolar lavage fluid (BALF) of IPF patients was decreased compared with normal subjects (Drakopanagiotakis et al., 2012). Further, alveolar macrophages could release important profibrotic mediators, such as transforming growth factor-β1 (TGF-β1) (Jain et al., 2013). Overexpression of active TGF-β1 would extend the survival time of lung fibroblasts, which is known to play a crucial role in the pathogenesis of fibrotic processes and ECM protein synthesis (Huang and Natarajan, 2015). Consequently, the persistent existence of lung fibroblasts induces prolonged and severe interstitial lung fibrosis (Sime et al., 1997; Zhou et al., 2013). Therefore, promoting apoptosis of alveolar macrophages and lung fibroblasts may be a potential strategy to decline proinflammatory cytokine production and accelerate the resolution of IPF.

Bcl-2 family proteins exist in the upstream of apoptotic pathways and have a pivotal role in the regulation of apoptosis. More than 20 members with diverse proapoptotic or anti-apoptotic functions are included in Bcl-2 family (Gross et al., 1999). Mounting evidence revealed that during pulmonary fibrosis, deregulation of Bcl-2 family proteins and imbalance between pro- and anti-apoptotic activities may determine the cellular susceptibility to apoptosis, among which Bcl-2 as an anti-apoptotic protein promotes cell survival. The expression of Bcl-2 differs in different cell types, for example, lower expression of Bcl-2 was observed in alveolar epithelial cell after intratracheally instillation of bleomycin (Oltvai et al., 1993). While in fibroblasts and macrophages, the expression of Bcl-2 increased (Kazufumi et al., 1997; Moodley et al., 2003; Nishimura et al., 2007). Thus, using the inhibitors against antiapoptotic Bcl-2 family proteins might prove a promising treatment option for IPF. One such example is the small molecule BH3 domain peptide mimetic ABT-199, a highly potent bioavailable Bcl-2 specific inhibitor (Oltersdorf et al., 2005). It was approved by the US Food and Drug Administration to treat chronic lymphocytic leukemia (Deeks, 2016). Studies have shown that ABT-199 has remarkable therapeutic effects on steroid-insensitive airway inflammation and particulate matter-induced lung inflammation (Tian et al., 2017; Geng et al., 2018). However, the therapeutic potential of ABT-199 against IPF has not been investigated till now. Hence, in the present study, we sought to explore whether Bcl-2 is a promising target for IPF and evaluate the antifibrotic effect of ABT-199 on BLM-induced pulmonary inflammation and lung fibrosis.

MATERIALS AND METHODS

Reagents

ABT-199 was purchased from Selleckchem (TX, United States), and BLM was purchased from Hisun Pfizer Pharmaceuticals Co., Ltd (Zhejiang, China). Hydroxyproline (HYP) assay kit was purchased from Nanjing Jiancheng Biochemical Institute (Nanjing, China). Mouse TGF-β1 and interleukin-6 (IL-6) enzyme-linked immunosorbent assay (ELISA) kits used were from R&D (Minneapolis, MN, United States). Antibody against Bcl-2 (7382) was purchased from Santa Cruz Biotechnology (TX, United States). Antibodies against α-SMA (ab5694) and type I collagen (ab34710) were purchased from Abcam Inc. (Cambridge, MA, United States). BCA Protein Assay kit was purchased from Thermo Fisher Scientific (Waltham, MA, United States).

Animal Model of BLM-induced Pulmonary Fibrosis

8-wk old, male C57BL/6 mice weighing 18–22 g were purchased from the Animal Center of Zhejiang University. The mice were housed in a Specific Pathogen Free (SPF) facility and provided with food and water ad libitum. The pulmonary fibrosis mouse model was established as previously described (Larson-Casey et al., 2016). Briefly, mice were anesthetized *via* intraperitoneal injection of 40 mg/kg pentobarbital sodium solution and then the skin and subcutaneous tissue overlying the proximal portion of the trachea were exposed by a 5 mm transversal incision to allow insertion into the trachea of a needle containing a single dose of BLM 50 μl (2.5 U/kg, BLM group) or the same volume of sterile saline (normal saline, NS group). These two groups were respectively divided into two subgroups, a control group, and ABT-199 treatment group. Mice in the latter group were treated through intratracheal administration of 2 μg/μl ABT-199, suspended in 50 μl PBS, while the mice in control group were treated with an equal volume of PBS. Mice were sacrificed at the indicated times after BLM/saline instillation and their lungs and BALF were collected. The animal study was reviewed and approved by the Institutional Animal Care and Use Committee of Zhejiang University. Experiments with animals were carried out in accordance with the guidelines of the Animal Care and Use Committee of the Zhejiang University School of Medicine.

BALF Collection and Analysis

BALF was collected and centrifuged at 400 g for 10 min at 4°C. Supernatant was stored at −80°C for the analysis of cytokines, while cell pellets were resuspended in 200 μl PBS for total and differential cell counting, numbers of macrophages, lymphocytes and neutrophils in a total of 200 cells were counted and categorized under microscope, according to standard morphological criteria. Total BALF protein was measured using BCA Protein Assay Kit, according to the manufacturer's instructions.

Histological Examination

Lungs were fixed in 4% paraformaldehyde and embedded in paraffin. Sections were stained with Hematoxylin-Eosin (HE) or Masson's trichrome for evaluation of fibrosis under a microscope. The Szapiel score was used to evaluate the degree of parenchymal alveolitis (Szapiel et al., 1979). The area analysis of fibrotic changes was performed according to Ashcroft scale (Ashcroft et al., 1988). Five randomly chosen fields within each lung section were observed at a magnification of ×100 or 200×. Two independent blind observers scored each specimen. A mean score of Szapiel or Ashcroft for each mouse was used for statistical analysis. For detection of fibroblasts and myofibroblasts, the slides were probed with antibodies against type I collagen (collagen I, 1:500) or α-smooth muscle actin (α-SMA, 1:600) as previously described (Rangarajan et al., 2018). Images were acquired on a fluorescence microscope and analyzed using ImageJ software.

Hydroxyproline Assay

The collagen content of lungs was measured by HYP assay kits according to the manufacturer's instructions. Briefly, 0.1 g of lung tissue was weighed and placed into a test tube, 3 ml of 6 mol/L HCl was added, and lungs were then digested for 12 h at 110°C. Later, the samples were neutralized by adjusting pH to 6.0–6.8 with NaOH. Subsequently, ddH_2O was added to make a total volume of 10 ml. Absorbance was measured at 560 nm on a spectrophotometer and amount of HYP was calculated.

Immunofluorescence

BAL cells were collected and fixed in 4% paraformaldehyde for 30 min, permeabilized in 0.2% Triton X-100 (LC262801; Sigma-Aldrich) for 5 min, and then blocked with 5% BSA (Sigma-Aldrich, B2064) for 1 h. Then cells were incubated with the antibody against Bcl-2 (1:1000) at 4°C overnight. Sections were stained with goat anti-mouse IgG secondary antibody (A28180; Invitrogen) (1:5000) for 30 min at room temperature. Slides were then washed and counterstained with DAPI. Finally, slides were observed under a fluorescence microscope (Olympus).

Enzyme-linked Immunosorbent Assay

The levels of TGF-β1 and IL-6 in BALF and lung homogenate were measured by ELISA kits according to the manufacturer's instructions.

Real-time Quantitative PCR

Total RNA was extracted from lungs using Trizol reagent (Takara Biotechnology) according to the manufacturer's instructions. RNA was then reverse transcribed into cDNA using Reverse Transcription Reagents (Takara Biotechnology). Real-time PCR was performed with the SYBR Green Master Mix (Takara Biotechnology) on a StepOne real-time PCR system (Applied Biosystems, Foster City, CA, United States). The relative expression of target genes was normalized against β-actin using the $2^{-\Delta\Delta Ct}$ method. Primer sequences used were as follows: *β-actin* (Forward: 5′-GTCCACCGTGTATGCCTTCT-3′, Reverse: 5′-CTCCTGGTGTCCGAACTGAT-3′); *Il-6* (Forward: 5′-CTGCAAGAGACTTCCATCCAG-3′, Reverse: 5′-AGTGGTATAGACAGGTCTGTTGG-3′); *Tgf-β1* (Forward: 5′-GCGCTCACTGCTCTTGTGACA-3′, Reverse: 5′-GCAATA GTTGGTATCCAGGGCTCT-3′); *Tnf-α* (Forward: 5′-CAC TTGGTGGTTTGCTACGA-3′, Reverse: 5′-GTGGCCCCTGCC ACAAGCAG-3′); *Il-1β* (Forward: 5′-GATCCACACTCTCCA GCTGCA-3′, Reverse: 5′-CAACCAACAAGTGATATTCTC CATG-3′).

Statistical Analysis

Results are expressed as mean ± SD. All data were analyzed using GraphPad Prism Version 7.0 software. Statistical comparisons were performed using Student t-test for two-group comparison and one or two-way ANOVA with a Tukey's *post hoc* test for multiple comparisons. $p < 0.05$ was considered to be statistically significant.

RESULTS

The Expression of Bcl-2 Increased in BALF Cells and Fibroblasts in BLM-induced Pulmonary Fibrosis

To validate the inflammatory response of IPF *in vivo*, we first established a BLM-induced pulmonary inflammation mouse model by intratracheally instilling a single dose of BLM, BALF and lung tissues was collected on day 3, 7 and 14. The findings revealed that BLM induced lung inflammation was dominated by macrophages on day 7 (**Supplementary Figure S1A**). In addition, both the total number of BAL cells and the absolute number of differential cells in the BLM group increased significantly relative to the NS group (**Supplementary Figure S1B**).

We examined the mRNA expression level of Bcl2 in whole lung tissue by qPCR, the results showed no significant statistical difference after BLM administration (**Supplementary Figures S2A–C**). Of note, the percentage of Bcl-2 positive macrophages examined by immunofluorescence increased after BLM instillation on day 7 and 14 (**Figures 1A–C**), suggesting that macrophages accumulate in BALF during inflammatory phase with the expression of Bcl-2 increasing significantly. Moreover, fibroblasts began to grow after the instillation of BLM for 7–14 days, we observed that the expression of Bcl-2 in fibroblasts increased on day 14 (**Figure 1D**).

Early ABT-199 Treatment Attenuated Lung Inflammation and in the Early Inflammation Phase

To test if targeting Bcl-2 could alleviate the inflammatory response after BLM injury, we applied the Bcl-2 inhibitor ABT-199 *in vivo*. ABT-199 (100 μg/mouse) was administrated to mice on day 2 after BLM instillation, and mice were sacrificed on day 3 (**Supplementary Figure S3A**), the results showed no obvious inflammation induced by BLM and no significant effect following ABT-199 administration (**Supplementary Figures S3B–F**). Next, ABT-199 was then administrated to mice every 3 days from day 3 after BLM instillation, and mice were sacrificed on days 7 (**Figure 2A**). Inflammatory cell recruitment and release of cytokines were studied to determine the effects of ABT-199 in BLM-induced lung inflammation. As expected, the number of total cells macrophages in the BALF of ABT-199 treated mice decreased significantly compared to the BLM-only treated group (**Figure 2B**).

In addition, the percentage of Bcl-2 positive macrophages in BALF decreased after 7 days of treatment with ABT-199 (**Figures

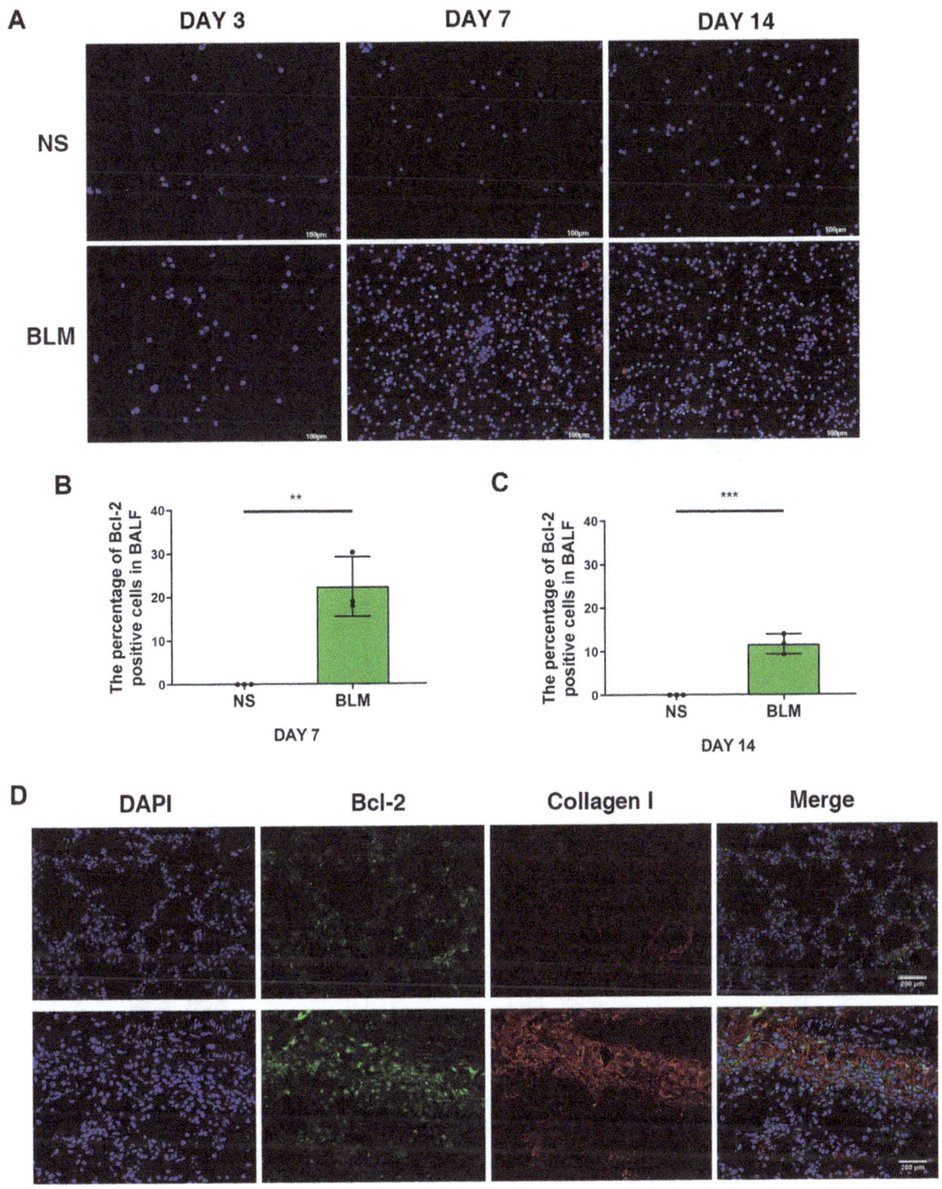

FIGURE 1 | The expression of Bcl-2 was increased in BALF cells and fibroblasts in BLM-induced pulmonary fibrosis. **(A–C)** Intracellular Bcl-2 expression of BAL cells was assessed by immunofluorescence assay, and the percentage of Bcl-2 positive macrophages was determined. **(D)** Representative images of collagen I and Bcl-2 show fluorescent staining in lung tissues of mice induced by BLM at day 14. The data are presented as means ± SD of an experiment performed three times. $^{**}p < 0.01$, $^{***}p < 0.001$. $n = 5$. BLM, bleomycin; BAL, bronchial alveolar lavage; NS, normal saline; Bcl-2, B-cell lymphoma-2.

2C,D). The attenuation of inflammation in ABT-199-treated mice was further supported by histological analysis by H&E staining (**Figures 2E,F**), which demonstrated less inflammation and reduced alveolar wall thickness at indicated time points. Results of Masson's trichrome staining revealed that the ABT-199-treated fibrotic mice had a marked reduction in collagen accumulation and preserved lung architecture as shown by the lower Ashcroft scores (**Figures 2G,H**). To further explore the effect of ABT-199 therapy, we then assessed the level of inflammatory response. Administration of ABT-199 also reduced the BALF protein content in BLM-induced lung injury (**Figure 2I**). Moreover, ABT-199 treatment significantly reduced the concentration of TGF-β1 and IL-6 protein in BALF on day 7 (**Figures 2J,K**).

The continuous attenuation of inflammation in ABT-199-treated mice was further confirmed on day 14 (**Figure 3A**). Less infiltration of inflammatory cells, in which reduced Bcl2 positive macrophage was observed in BALF (**Figures 3B–D**). The inflammation score and Ashcroft score for mice which received ABT-199 was much lower compared to that for BLM-only treated mice (**Figures 3E–H**), accompanied by reduced BALF protein and alleviation of fibrosis factor expression (**Figures 3I–M**). *In*

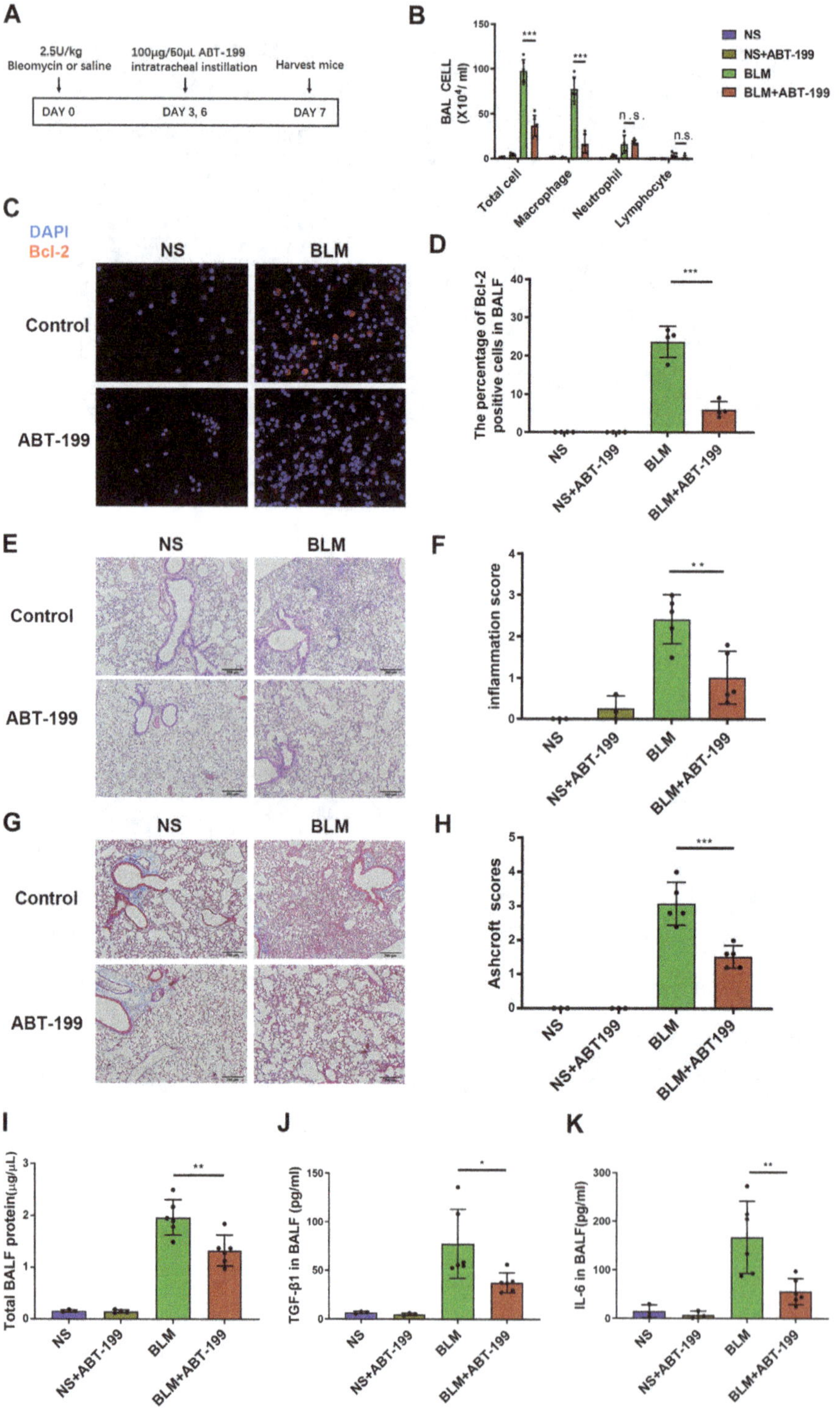

FIGURE 2 | Early ABT-199 treatment attenuated BLM-induced lung inflammation at day 7. **(A)** Treatment scheme. **(B)** After 7 days, the total number of inflammatory cells was quantified and the number of differential cells was calculated. **(C)** Intracellular Bcl-2 expression of BAL cells was assessed by immunofluorescence assay on day 7. **(D)** The percentage of Bcl-2 positive macrophages was determined. **(E)** Representative images of lung sections stained with hematoxylin and eosin (H&E). **(F)** Degree of parenchymal alveolitis was evaluated using Szapiel score. **(G)** Representative images of lung sections stained with Masson's trichrome. **(H)** The area analysis of fibrotic changes according to Ashcroft scale. **(I)** Total BALF protein on day 7 was measured using BCA Protein Assay. **(J,K)** Expressions of TGF-β1 and IL-6 levels in BALF on day 7 were determined using ELISA. The data are presented as means ± SD of an experiment performed three times. n.s., not significant, $^{*}p < 0.05$, $^{**}p < 0.01$, $^{***}p < 0.001$. n = 3–6. BLM, bleomycin; BAL, bronchial alveolar lavage; NS, normal saline; Bcl-2, B-cell lymphoma-2.

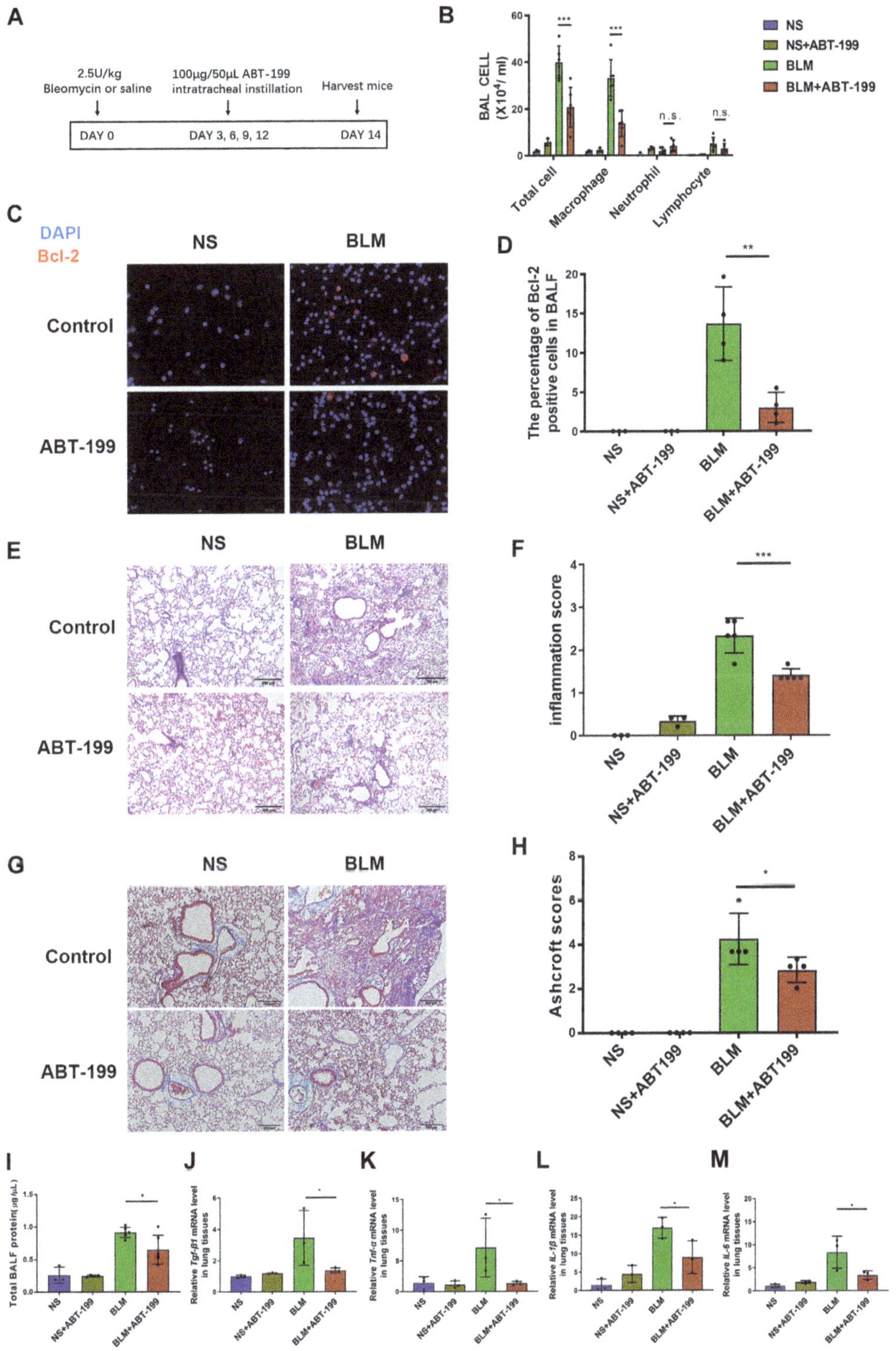

FIGURE 3 | Early ABT-199 treatment attenuated BLM-induced lung inflammation at day 14. **(A)** Treatment scheme. **(B)** After 14 days, the total number of inflammatory cells was quantified and the number of differential cells was calculated. **(C)** Intracellular Bcl-2 expression of BAL cells was assessed by immunofluorescence assay on day 14. **(D)** The percentage of Bcl-2 positive macrophages was determined. **(E)** Representative images of lung sections stained with hematoxylin and eosin (H&E). **(F)** Degree of parenchymal alveolitis was evaluated using Szapiel score. **(G)** Representative images of lung sections stained with Masson's trichrome. **(H)** The area analysis of fibrotic changes according to Ashcroft scale. **(I)** Total BALF protein on day 14 was measured using BCA Protein Assay. **(J–M)** The relative levels of *Tgf-β1, Tnf-α, Il-1β, and Il-6* mRNA transcripts were determined using quantitative PCR. The data are presented as means ± SD of an experiment performed three times. n.s., not significant, *$p < 0.05$, **$p < 0.01$, ***$p < 0.001$. $n = 3$–6. BLM, bleomycin; BAL, bronchial alveolar lavage; NS, normal saline; TGF-β1, transforming growth factor-β1; TNF-α, tumor necrosis factor-α; IL-1β, interleukin-1β; IL-6, interleukin-6.

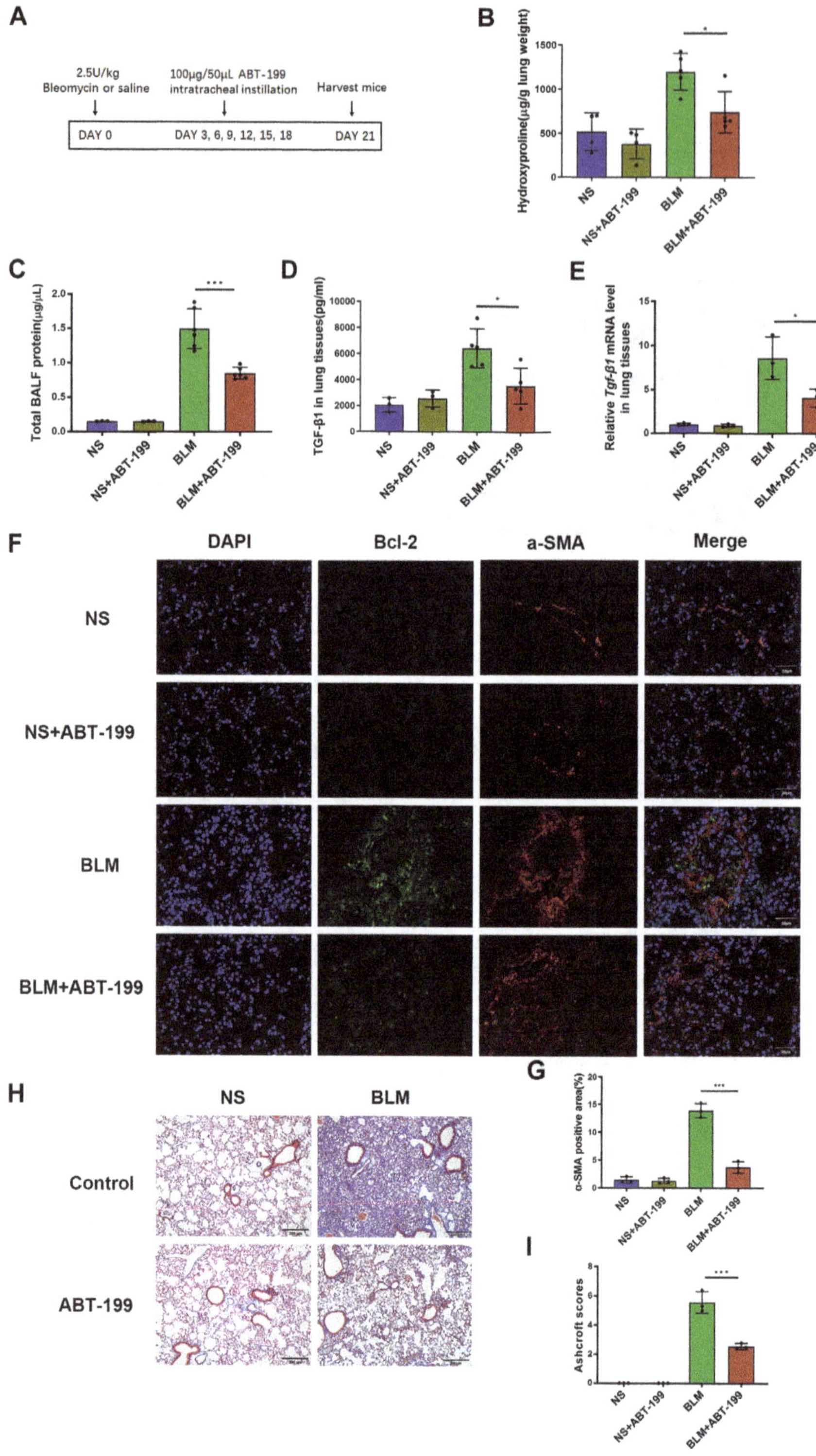

FIGURE 4 | ABT-199 alleviates BLM-induced lung fibrosis. **(A)** Treatment scheme. **(B)** Hydroxyproline contents in lung tissues. **(C)** Total BALF protein on day 21 was measured using BCA Protein Assay. **(D,E)** Expression of TGF-β1 level in the lung tissue were determined using ELISA and real-time PCR. **(F)** Representative images of myofibroblasts in lung tissues by immunofluorescence staining of α-SMA and Bcl-2. **(G)** Quantitative analysis of α-SMA positive areas in lung sections. **(H)** Representative images of lung sections stained with Masson's trichrome. **(I)** The area analysis of fibrotic changes according to Ashcroft scale. The data are presented as means ± SD of an experiment performed three times. *$p < 0.05$, ***$p < 0.001$. $n = 3–6$. BLM, bleomycin; BAL, bronchial alveolar lavage; NS, normal saline; TGF-β1, transforming growth factor-β1; α-SMA, alpha smooth muscle actin.

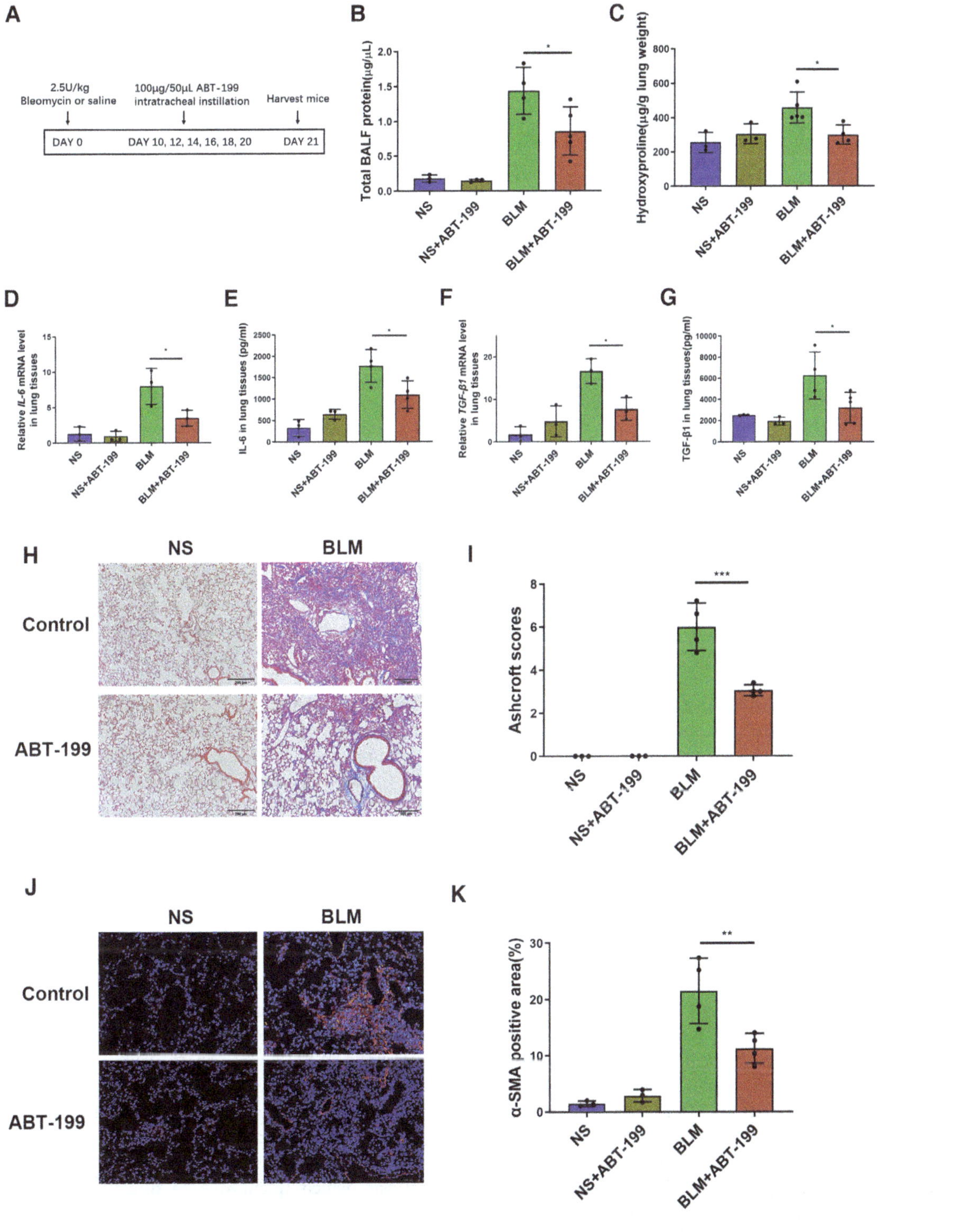

FIGURE 5 | ABT-199 reverses the established lung fibrosis in BLM-injured mice. **(A)** Treatment scheme. **(B)** Total BALF protein was measured using BCA Protein Assay. **(C)** Hydroxyproline contents in lung tissues. **(D,E)** Expression level of IL-6 in the lung tissue was determined using real-time PCR and ELISA. **(F,G)** Expression level of TGF-β1 in the lung tissue was determined using real-time PCR and ELISA. **(H)** Representative images of lung sections stained with Masson's trichrome. **(I)** The area analysis of fibrotic changes according to Ashcroft scale. **(J)** Representative images of myofibroblasts in lung tissues by immunofluorescence staining of α-SMA. **(K)** Quantitative analysis of α-SMA positive areas in lung sections. The data are presented as means ± SD of an experiment performed three times. $^{*}p < 0.05$, $^{**}p < 0.01$, $^{***}p < 0.001$. $n = 3$–6. BLM, bleomycin; Bcl-2, B-cell lymphoma-2; BAL, bronchial alveolar lavage; NS, normal saline; TGF-β1, transforming growth factor-β1; IL-6, interleukin-6.

vitro, we also treated the mouse peritoneal macrophages with ABT-199 and found that 10 μM ABT-199 could induce the apoptosis (**Supplementary Figures S4A,B**). Conclusively, these data indicate that ABT-199 is effective against BLM-induced lung inflammatory response by reducing the number of BAL macrophages.

ABT-199 Significantly Decreased Bcl-2 and Attenuates BLM-induced Lung Fibrosis in Mice

To evaluate the antifibrotic effects of ABT-199 against BLM-induced pulmonary fibrosis in mice, we established a 21 days BLM-induced pulmonary fibrosis mouse model and intratracheally instilled ABT-199 (100 μg/mouse) every 3 days, starting from the third day after BLM administration (**Figure 4A**). The lung hydroxyproline content and BALF protein concentration of fibrotic mice were significantly reduced by ABT-199 treatment (**Figures 4B,C**). Analysis of lung extracts revealed decreased mRNA and protein levels of TGF-β1 in mice following treatment with ABT-199 (**Figures 4D,E**). Furthermore, Bcl2 expression, increased in BLM group and reduced following ABT-199 administration, was shown to be co-localized with α-SMA (**Figure 4F**). Also, quantitative analysis showed that the α-SMA positive areas were smaller in the lungs of ABT-199-treated fibrotic mice than that of fibrotic mice (**Figure 4G**), suggesting a reduction in myofibroblasts. The results of Masson's trichrome staining revealed that the ABT-199-treated fibrotic mice had a marked reduction in collagen accumulation and preserved lung architecture as shown by the lower Ashcroft scores (**Figures 4H,I**), which were consistent with the above findings. Collectively, these results confirmed the therapeutic effect of ABT-199 against BLM-induced pulmonary fibrosis in mice.

ABT-199 Attenuated Established Lung Fibrosis in BLM-injured Mice

To find out whether the inhibition of Bcl-2 protein could attenuate established lung fibrosis during the post-inflammatory phase, we administered ABT-199 every 2 days from day 10 (**Figure 5A**). ABT-199 administration resulted in decreased number of infiltrating macrophages (**Supplementary Figure S5**). Notably, even after collagen has already been deposited, ABT-199 significantly reduced the over-production of total BALF protein the over-accumulation of HYP (**Figures 5B,C**) induced by BLM. Meanwhile, the results of qPCR and ELISA showed that ABT-199 significantly downregulated the expression of pro-fibrotic cytokines (IL-6 and TGF-β1) (**Figures 5D–G**). Histological analysis of lung by Masson's trichrome staining revealed that ABT-199 could effectively attenuate BLM-induced pulmonary fibrosis, mainly by reducing the thickness of alveolar walls and collagen deposition (**Figures 5H,I**). Reduction in myofibroblasts was also shown by the α-SMA positive areas that were smaller in the lungs of ABT-199-treated fibrotic mice than that of fibrotic mice (**Figures 5J,K**). *In vitro*, we also treated mouse embryonic fibroblasts with ABT-199 and found that 100 μM ABT-199 could induce the apoptosis (**Supplementary Figures S6A,B**). In summary, our data confirm the antifibrotic effect of ABT-199 on established lung fibrosis.

DISCUSSION

At present, the medications used clinically to treat IPF are insufficient to prevent or reverse the progression of the disease. Therefore, the development of novel therapeutic approaches against IPF is mandatory. Bcl-2, which is known as an inhibitor of apoptosis promotes cell survival (Llambi and Green, 2011). There is a growing body of evidence that suggests a crucial role for Bcl-2 in the pathogenesis of inflammation, apoptosis and fibrosis induced by various factors in the interstitial lung diseases. In this study, we demonstrated that in a mouse model of BLM-induced pulmonary fibrosis, numerous macrophages were recruited to BALF and fibroblasts proliferated in the lungs. Higher expressions of Bcl-2 was detected in alveolar macrophages and lung fibroblasts, which displays similar expression pattern with α-SMA and the severity of lung fibrosis. Furthermore, we found ABT-199 mediated selective inhibition of Bcl-2 significantly attenuated lung inflammation and fibrosis, even with a late treatment from day 10, when the fibrosis had already been established.

Different experimental models have been developed for understanding the role of Bcl-2 protein in the regulation of apoptosis through fibrosis development, including bleomycin, asbestos, silica, paraquate, chemokine and radiation, among which, the bleomycin model of pulmonary fibrosis is the best characterized murine model. The pathogenesis of IPF is divided into two phases, named the early inflammatory response and the late fibrogenesis. The inflammation phase which is mediated by various inflammatory cells is the initial response after BLM stimulation. In this study, a significant increase in inflammatory cells in BALF from BLM treated mice on day 7 and 14 were detected, especially macrophages, which are known to be the primary source of a variety of pro-inflammatory and fibrogenic cytokines and growth factors (Kendall and Feghali-Bostwick, 2014; Li et al., 2019). Previous studies showed that specific macrophage depletion attenuated lung injury *in vivo* (Redente et al., 2014). Therefore, whether macrophage apoptosis induction be a potential anti-fibrosis therapy remains to be critical and rarely studied.

Our results revealed that the Bcl-2 in alveolar macrophages was increased significantly, suggesting accumulation of macrophages due to their apoptosis resistance in the airway during inflammatory phase. Thus, we wondered if the treatment with Bcl-2 inhibitor ABT-199 would decrease inflammation response in a model of BLM-induced pulmonary fibrosis. Our results confirm that ABT-199 reduced the number of BAL macrophages in the early inflammation phase of lung fibrosis, which might due to direct pro-apoptotic effect on macrophages. In addition, we also observed a decline in the level of various harmful growth factors and cytokines, which is consistent with the fact that macrophages are known to initiate an inflammatory response after injury by secreting these factors, which contribute to the further amplification of inflammatory processes (Bitterman et al., 1982; Lemaire et al., 1986).

Although suppressing inflammatory response has been regarded as an important clinical strategy to treat IPF (Hara et al., 2012). More and more researches proved that anti-inflammatory treatments may not be effective for all IPF patients. The inflammation is significant in early phase of IPF but relieved in late fibrosis phase, which may lead to the failure of traditional anti-inflammatory therapy. Thus, the anti-fibrosis effect of ABT-199 may not be entirely dependent on the inhibition of inflammatory response. Our observation suggested that the lung fibroblasts were established on day 14 and showed increased apoptosis resistance, with high expression of Bcl-2, indicates that fibroblasts were also a target of ABT-199. Therefore, we aimed to evaluate whether ABT-199 could reverse the already existing fibrosis using a late-ABT199 treatment model. As active fibrosis phase is between 7 and 14 days, significantly increased collagen deposition is observed on day 14 (Peng et al., 2013). For this reason, we intratracheally instilled ABT-199 from 10 days after BLM administration, when lung fibrosis was already established. Our data showed that BLM-induced fibrosis was significantly attenuated. Therefore, a direct effect of ABT-199 on fibroblast could have accounted for the antifibrotic effects observed.

Finally, we originally illustrate the potential therapeutic effect of ABT-199 against BLM-induced pulmonary fibrosis in mice, and emphasized that both early and late treatment with ABT-199 attenuated pulmonary fibrosis through its anti-inflammatory, along with anticoagulant effects. Although we propose that ABT-199 could be used as a new medicinal approach against fibrotic diseases such as IPF, further studies are still required to reveal its more comprehensive effects and mechanism of action.

AUTHOR CONTRIBUTIONS

HS and SY proposed this study and designed the paper. YH, XG, and FL completed the manuscript. YH, FL, WH, and ZS completed the experiments. MS, CZ, and XD analyzed the data. SY, HS, WL, and ZC revised the article. All authors read and approved the final manuscript.

REFERENCES

Ashcroft, T., Simpson, J. M., and Timbrell, V. (1988). Simple Method of Estimating Severity of Pulmonary Fibrosis on a Numerical Scale. *J. Clin. Pathol.* 41 (4), 467–470. doi:10.1136/jcp.41.4.467

Bitterman, P. B., Rennard, S. I., Hunninghake, G. W., and Crystal, R. G. (1982). Human Alveolar Macrophage Growth Factor for Fibroblasts. *J. Clin. Invest.* 70 (4), 806–822. doi:10.1172/jci110677

Bjoraker, J. A., Ryu, J. H., Edwin, M. K., Myers, J. L., Tazelaar, H. D., Schroeder, D. R., et al. (1998). Prognostic Significance of Histopathologic Subsets in Idiopathic Pulmonary Fibrosis. *Am. J. Respir. Crit. Care Med.* 157 (1), 199–203. doi:10.1164/ajrccm.157.1.9704130

Chen, X., Zhang, X., Li, X., and Wang, Z. (2013). Who and what Should We Rely on in Early Diagnosis of Idiopathic Pulmonary Fibrosis. *Eur. Respir. J.* 41 (1), 249–250. doi:10.1183/09031936.00142012

Deeks, E. D. (2016). Venetoclax: First Global Approval. *Drugs* 76 (9), 979–987. doi:10.1007/s40265-016-0596-x

Drakopanagiotakis, F., Xifteri, A., Tsiambas, E., Karameris, A., Tsakanika, K., Karagiannidis, N., et al. (2012). Decreased Apoptotic Rate of Alveolar Macrophages of Patients with Idiopathic Pulmonary Fibrosis. *Pulm. Med.* 2012, 1–9. doi:10.1155/2012/981730

Geng, X., Wang, X., Luo, M., Xing, M., Wu, Y., Li, W., et al. (2018). Induction of Neutrophil Apoptosis by a Bcl-2 Inhibitor Reduces Particulate Matter-Induced Lung Inflammation. *Aging* 10 (6), 1415–1423. doi:10.18632/aging.101477

Gross, A., McDonnell, J. M., and Korsmeyer, S. J. (1999). BCL-2 Family Members and the Mitochondria in Apoptosis. *Genes Dev.* 13 (15), 1899–1911. doi:10.1101/gad.13.15.1899

Hara, A., Sakamoto, N., Ishimatsu, Y., Kakugawa, T., Nakashima, S., Hara, S., et al. (2012). S100A9 in BALF Is a Candidate Biomarker of Idiopathic Pulmonary Fibrosis. *Respir. Med.* 106 (4), 571–580. doi:10.1016/j.rmed.2011.12.010

Huang, L. S., and Natarajan, V. (2015). Sphingolipids in Pulmonary Fibrosis. *Adv. Biol. Regul.* 57, 55–63. doi:10.1016/j.jbior.2014.09.008

Jain, M., Rivera, S., Monclus, E. A., Synenki, L., Zirk, A., Eisenbart, J., et al. (2013). Mitochondrial Reactive Oxygen Species Regulate Transforming Growth Factor-β Signaling. *J. Biol. Chem.* 288 (2), 770–777. doi:10.1074/jbc.M112.431973

Kazufumi, M., Sonoko, N., Masanori, K., Takateru, I., and Akira, O. (1997). Expression of Bcl-2 Protein and APO-1 (Fas Antigen) in the Lung Tissue from Patients with Idiopathic Pulmonary Fibrosis. *Microsc. Res. Tech.* 38 (5), 480–487. doi:10.1002/(sici)1097-0029(19970901)38:5<480::Aid-jemt4>3.0.Co;2-m

Kendall, R. T., and Feghali-Bostwick, C. A. (2014). Fibroblasts in Fibrosis: Novel Roles and Mediators. *Front. Pharmacol.* 5, 123. doi:10.3389/fphar.2014.00123

Larson-Casey, J. L., Deshane, J. S., Ryan, A. J., Thannickal, V. J., and Carter, A. B. (2016). Macrophage Akt1 Kinase-Mediated Mitophagy Modulates Apoptosis Resistance and Pulmonary Fibrosis. *Immunity* 44 (3), 582–596. doi:10.1016/j.immuni.2016.01.001

Lemaire, I., Beaudoin, H., Massé, S., and Grondin, C. (1986). Alveolar Macrophage Stimulation of Lung Fibroblast Growth in Asbestos-Induced Pulmonary Fibrosis. *Am. J. Pathol.* 122 (2), 205–211.

Li, G., Jin, F., Du, J., He, Q., Yang, B., and Luo, P. (2019). Macrophage-secreted TSLP and MMP9 Promote Bleomycin-Induced Pulmonary Fibrosis. *Toxicol. Appl. Pharmacol.* 366, 10–16. doi:10.1016/j.taap.2019.01.011

Llambi, F., and Green, D. R. (2011). Apoptosis and Oncogenesis: Give and Take in the BCL-2 Family. *Curr. Opin. Genet. Dev.* 21 (1), 12–20. doi:10.1016/j.gde.2010.12.001

Moodley, Y. P., Misso, N. L. A., Scaffidi, A. K., Fogel-Petrovic, M., McAnulty, R. J., Laurent, G. J., et al. (2003). Inverse Effects of Interleukin-6 on Apoptosis of Fibroblasts from Pulmonary Fibrosis and Normal Lungs. *Am. J. Respir. Cel Mol Biol* 29 (4), 490–498. doi:10.1165/rcmb.2002-0262OC

Nishimura, Y., Nishiike-Wada, T., Wada, Y., Miura, Y., Otsuki, T., and Iguchi, H. (2007). Long-Lasting Production of TGF-B1 by Alveolar Macrophages Exposed to Low Doses of Asbestos without Apoptosis. *Int. J. Immunopathol Pharmacol.* 20 (4), 661–671. doi:10.1177/039463200702000402

Oltersdorf, T., Elmore, S. W., Shoemaker, A. R., Armstrong, R. C., Augeri, D. J., Belli, B. A., et al. (2005). An Inhibitor of Bcl-2 Family Proteins Induces Regression of Solid Tumours. *Nature* 435 (7042), 677–681. doi:10.1038/nature03579

Oltvai, Z. N., Milliman, C. L., and Korsmeyer, S. J. (1993). Bcl-2 Heterodimerizes In Vivo with a Conserved Homolog, Bax, that Accelerates Programmed Cell Death. *Cell* 74 (4), 609–619. doi:10.1016/0092-8674(93)90509-o

Peng, R., Sridhar, S., Tyagi, G., Phillips, J. E., Garrido, R., Harris, P., et al. (2013). Bleomycin Induces Molecular Changes Directly Relevant to Idiopathic Pulmonary Fibrosis: a Model for "active" Disease. *PLoS One* 8 (4), e59348. doi:10.1371/journal.pone.0059348

Polunovsky, V. A., Chen, B., Henke, C., Snover, D., Wendt, C., Ingbar, D. H., et al. (1993). Role of Mesenchymal Cell Death in Lung Remodeling After Injury. *J. Clin. Invest.* 92 (1), 388–397. doi:10.1172/jci116578

Rangarajan, S., Bone, N. B., Zmijewska, A. A., Jiang, S., Park, D. W., Bernard, K., et al. (2018). Metformin Reverses Established Lung Fibrosis in a Bleomycin Model. *Nat. Med.* 24 (8), 1121–1127. doi:10.1038/s41591-018-0087-6

Redente, E. F., Keith, R. C., Janssen, W., Henson, P. M., Ortiz, L. A., Downey, G. P., et al. (2014). Tumor Necrosis Factor-α Accelerates the Resolution of Established Pulmonary Fibrosis in Mice by Targeting Profibrotic Lung Macrophages. *Am. J. Respir. Cel Mol Biol* 50 (4), 825–837. doi:10.1165/rcmb.2013-0386OC

Sime, P. J., Xing, Z., Graham, F. L., Csaky, K. G., and Gauldie, J. (1997). Adenovector-mediated Gene Transfer of Active Transforming Growth Factor-Beta1 Induces Prolonged Severe Fibrosis in Rat Lung. *J. Clin. Invest.* 100 (4), 768–776. doi:10.1172/jci119590

Szapiel, S. V., Elson, N. A., Fulmer, J. D., Hunninghake, G. W., and Crystal, R. G. (1979). Bleomycin-induced Interstitial Pulmonary Disease in the Nude, Athymic Mouse. *Am. Rev. Respir. Dis.* 120 (4), 893–899. doi:10.1164/arrd.1979.120.4.893

Tian, B.-p., Xia, L.-x., Bao, Z.-q., Zhang, H., Xu, Z.-w., Mao, Y.-y., et al. (2017). Bcl-2 Inhibitors Reduce Steroid-Insensitive Airway Inflammation. *J. Allergy Clin. Immunol.* 140 (2), 418–430. doi:10.1016/j.jaci.2016.11.027

Todd, N. W., Luzina, I. G., and Atamas, S. P. (2012). Molecular and Cellular Mechanisms of Pulmonary Fibrosis. *Fibrogenesis Tissue Repair* 5 (1), 11. doi:10.1186/1755-1536-5-11

Zhou, Y., Huang, X., Hecker, L., Kurundkar, D., Kurundkar, A., Liu, H., et al. (2013). Inhibition of Mechanosensitive Signaling in Myofibroblasts Ameliorates Experimental Pulmonary Fibrosis. *J. Clin. Invest.* 123 (3), 1096–1108. doi:10.1172/jci66700

9

Treatment of Sarcoidosis: A Multidisciplinary Approach

*Alicia K. Gerke**

Pulmonary and Critical Care Medicine, Department of Internal Medicine, University of Iowa, Iowa City, IA, United States

Correspondence:
Alicia K. Gerke
alicia-gerke@uiowa.edu

Sarcoidosis is a systemic disease of unknown etiology defined by the presence of noncaseating granulomatous inflammation that can cause organ damage and diminished quality of life. Treatment is indicated to protect organ function and decrease symptomatic burden. Current treatment options focus on interruption of granuloma formation and propagation. Clinical trials guiding evidence for treatment are lacking due to the rarity of disease, heterogeneous clinical course, and lack of prognostic biomarkers, all of which contribute to difficulty in clinical trial design and implementation. In this review, a multidisciplinary treatment approach is summarized, addressing immunuosuppressive drugs, managing complications of chronic granulomatous inflammation, and assessing treatment toxicity. Discovery of new therapies will depend on research into pathogenesis of antigen presentation and granulomatous inflammation. Future treatment approaches may also include personalized decisions based on pharmacogenomics and sarcoidosis phenotype, as well as patient-centered approaches to manage immunosuppression, symptom control, and treatment of comorbid conditions.

Keywords: therapeutics, immunosuppression, sarcoidosis, drug-related side effects and adverse reactions, treatment outcome, granuloma

INTRODUCTION

Sarcoidosis is a systemic disease of unknown etiology that can cause organ dysfunction and diminished quality of life. The disease is diagnosed by a constellation of radiographic, clinical and histopathologic findings; it is most often defined by the presence of noncaseating granulomatous inflammation that occurs in the absence of infection, exposures, malignancy, or alternative immune-related disease. Lung and thoracic lymph nodes are most often involved, but any organ can be affected, with multi-system involvement having a worse prognosis. Treatment is directed at alleviating organ dysfunction, preventing irreversible scarring, and improving quality of life. Herein, we review the indications for treatment, pharmacotherapy, treatment duration, side effects, adjunct non-pharmacologic therapies, and outcomes for patients.

BRIEF PATHOGENESIS

The sarcoidosis granuloma is formed by a distinct conglomeration of multinucleated giant cells and epithelioid macrophages surrounded by a rim of CD4+ T cells (1). Less abundantly, CD8+ T cells and B cells can be found in the surrounding rim. The granulomatous inflammation seen in sarcoidosis is thought to be a dysregulated antigenic response due to an unknown environmental exposure in a genetically susceptible individual. Loci that house antigen presentation genes such as HLA class II and BTNL-2 have been linked to development of sarcoidosis, as well as certain disease phenotypes (2–4). Mycobacterial antigens have been proposed based on studies showing heightened immune responses of both peripheral macrophages and bronchoalveolar (BAL) fluid of patients with sarcoidosis to mycobacterial proteins including mKatG and ESAT-6 (5, 6). Similarly, *Propionibacterium acnes* has also been proposed as an etiologic agent given the higher frequency of genetic material found in sarcoidosis granulomas compared to controls, as well as similar exaggerated immune response to *Priopionibacteria* in sarcoidosis T cells compared to normals (7). It is also likely that dendritic cells play an important role in the presentation of antigen and continued immune response, although the mechanisms are not well-understood (8). More recent data would also suggest that not only is sarcoidosis a disease of heightened Th1 immune response, but also potential dysfunction of regulatory immune cells and immune 'exhaustion' with failure to clear an antigenic agent (9, 10). Therefore, therapeutic targets currently include suppression of inflammation, improvement of the regulatory capacity of the immune system, and modulating the antigen or antigen presenting capacity of the immune system.

The basis of treatment of sarcoidosis is regulation of the heightened immune response and suppression of granulomatous inflammation in order to prevent dangerous interference with organ function (as seen in the eye or the heart) and to prevent eventual scarring and fibrosis as seen in the lungs. Current standard of care focuses on suppressing highly activated macrophages and T cells and their production of cytokines such as TNF-α, IL-1, IFN-γ, and IL-6. More recent study has also suggested a possible role of anti-B cell therapy given the presence of B cells in the granuloma and increased B cell activating factor (BAFF) in sarcoidosis patients (11). Additionally, the increasing evidence of a Th17 response (as seen in autoimmune disease) in addition to a strong Th1 mediated response potentially suggests more therapeutic targets (12). Last, cytokine-specific biologics and treatment of mycobacterial infection have emerged as potential future alternatives. **Figure 1** illustrates current and investigational therapies for sarcoidosis based upon pathogenesis.

TREATMENT APPROACH

To date, treatment of sarcoidosis is largely guided by small, uncontrolled trials and expert consensus (13–19). A few randomized controlled trials (RCTs) have been performed, but trials are limited by the rarity of disease, heterogeneity of disease presentation and progression, and lack of standardized, responsive outcome measures (20, 21). Additionally, even past negative trials may not completely negate the efficacy of certain compounds, as study design is difficult due to the idiosyncrasy of the disease itself (21). A number of suggested treatment algorithms have been published, most of which are based upon initiation of corticosteroids in a symptomatic patient with abnormal function or imaging studies, followed by tapering of steroids over a minimum of 1 year (22, 23). Second and third-line agents can be added based on lack of response to therapy, toxic side effects, or inability to taper corticosteroids (**Table 1**). Importantly, outcomes of symptomatic response and toxicity profile can vary from patient to patient, emphasizing the need for a patient-centered approach. Objective outcomes can include imaging studies (e.g., chest X-rays, computed tomography (CT), positron emission tomography (PET) scans, MRI), pulmonary function tests, walk distance, and laboratory testing (e.g., liver function, blood counts, chemistries, calcium). Subjective assessments can include (but are not limited to) dyspnea, cough, fatigue, cardiac symptoms, neurologic symptoms, and pain. In some patients, the objective and subjective outcomes may not correlate, adding to the complexity of management decisions (24). Therefore, management of patients with sarcoidosis often requires a three-pronged approach: treatment of symptomatic granulomatous inflammation, assessment of comorbid conditions, and tempering of immunosuppressive toxicities (**Figure 2**).

INDICATIONS FOR TREATMENT

Over half of patients with sarcoidosis will incur spontaneous resolution or never have clinical manifestations of the disease, whereas the remaining half will experience a more chronic course, often requiring treatment. Mortality appears to be increasing over time, and burden of disease can be substantial due to complications of the disease or its treatments (25). It is unclear if treatment with corticosteroids alters the natural history of disease; therefore, treatment is recommended only for those with high symptom burden and/or evidence of organ damage (26). For those requiring treatment due to symptoms or suspicion of injury to organs, a stepwise approach to therapy is recommended, although more aggressive therapeutic management can be considered in particularly severe cases of neurologic, ophthalmic, or cardiac involvement (23). In general, there are very few large clinical trials for treatment in sarcoidosis (27). Therefore, in clinical practice, use of corticosteroids and other immunomodulatory agents is often modeled by use on other autoimmune and inflammatory diseases in which suppression of the immune system is desired.

IMMUNOSUPPRESSIVE TREATMENT

Corticosteroids

Corticosteroids are considered first-line treatment by consensus of sarcoidosis providers (28, 29). Multiple uncontrolled studies have shown that corticosteroids suppress production of cytokines that contribute to persistent granuloma formation including TNF-α and

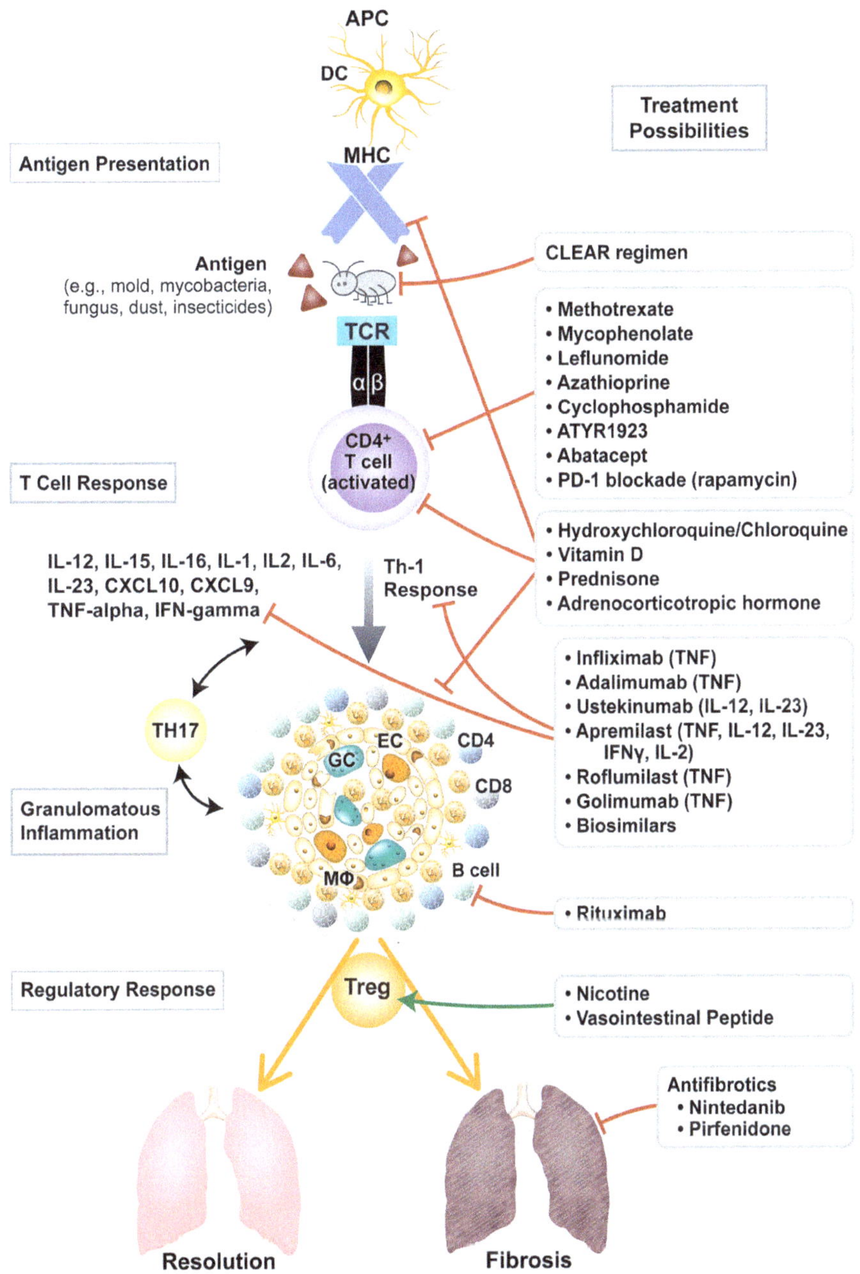

FIGURE 1 | Current and investigational treatments for sarcoidosis based on pathogenesis. Treatments for sarcoidosis target antigen presentation, T cell activation, cytokine/chemokine profiles, propagation of granulomatous inflammation, T-regulatory balance, and the fibrotic response. APC, antigen presenting cell; DC, dendritic cell; MHC, major histocompatibility complex; TCR, T cell receptor; GC, multinucleated giant cell; EC, epitheloid cell; Mφ, macrophage; IL, interleukin; TNF, tumor necrosis factor; IFN, interferon; PD-1, programmed cell death protein-1; CLEAR, Combined Levofloxacin; Ethambutol, Azithromycin and Rifampin.

IFN-γ (30, 31). However, only a small number of RCTs with corticosteroids have been performed (26). Although patients have shown improvement in symptoms and biomarkers in the short-term, current evidence is yet unable to show long-term benefit, alteration of natural history or improved mortality (32). Accordingly, the ideal dosing and length of therapy are unknown. A starting dosage of 20–40 milligrams (mg) per day is generally recommended, although a few select patients with severe disease may be initiated on much higher doses in cases of severe neurosarcoidosis, refractory arrhythmias, ophthalmic disease threatening vision loss, or other severe organ damage (29). Lower induction doses may also be reasonable, particularly in pulmonary sarcoidosis, as one early clinical trial of prednisone established improvement in pulmonary infiltrates with 15 mg per day (33). Similarly, a Finnish study from 2002 in pulmonary sarcoidosis used a protocol of 20 mg of prednisolone per day for eight weeks, 15 mg

TABLE 1 | Common therapeutics for treatment of sarcoidosis*.

	Drug name	Suggested dose range	Special treatment issues/monitoring
First-Line Agents	Corticosteroids (Prednisone)	20–40 mg/day initial Dose, tapered to 7.5–15 mg/day	Bone density Eye exams (glaucoma and cataracts) Body Mass Index
Second-Line Agents	Methotrexate	7.5–25 mg/week orally or subcutaneously	Concurrent need for folic acid. Liver function, kidney function, CBC. Can cause hepatotoxicity, GI distress, pneumonitis, mouth ulcers, bone marrow suppression.
	Hydroxychloroquine	200–400 mg/day	Eye exams for retinopathy. Rarely associated with QT elongation (consider drug interactions).
	Leflunomide	10–20 mg/day	Liver function, kidney function, CBC. Can cause neuropathy, hepatotoxicity, GI distress, pneumonitis, bone marrow suppression. In cases of toxicity, can clear more urgently with cholestyramine.
	Azathioprine	50–200 mg/day	Liver function, kidney function, CBC. Consider TPMT level. Can cause hepatotoxicity, GI distress, hypersensitivity reaction, bone marrow suppression.
	Mycophenolate	500–3,000 mg/day	Liver function, kidney function, CBC. Associated with GI distress, bone marrow suppression. Enteric coated option available (different dose range).
Third-Line Agents	Infliximab	3–5 mg/kg intravenously at weeks 0, 2, and every 4–8 weeks thereafter	Tuberculosis Testing Caution in heart failure. Allergic reactions possible with injections. Associated with demyelination syndrome, malignancy, and sarcoid-like reactions.
	Adalimumab	40 mg subcutaneous every 1–2 weeks	Similar precautions and adverse reactions as infliximab.

Other therapeutic options can be considered in some cases (e.g., cyclophosphamide, rituximab, adrenocorticotropic hormone, pentoxifylline).
CBC, complete blood count; GI, gastrointestinal; mg, milligrams; kg, kilograms; TPMT, thiopurine methyltransferase.

per day for 2 weeks, 10 mg per day for 2 weeks, and then inhaled budesonide for 15 months. The results showed improved pulmonary function over a five-year period in patients with Stage II-III disease (34). Long-term doses above 40 mg per day are not recommended for most cases of sarcoidosis due to high risk of corticosteroid-induced toxicity and little added physiologic benefit. For example, a study in Japan revealed increased morbidity and mortality in patients with cardiac sarcoidosis who were treated with higher doses of corticosteroids (greater than 40 mg per day) compared to lower doses (less than 30 mg per day) (35). Similarly, higher cumulative doses of prednisone in sarcoidosis have been associated with decreased quality of life and increased frequency of emergency department visits (36). Another analysis of differing starting dosages for patients with pulmonary sarcoidosis did not show a strong correlation between outcome and initial dose, indicating that lower doses may be used with similar effect. On the other hand, there was a strong correlation between starting dose and weight gain over a two-year period (37). Taken in total, these studies suggest that toxicity of higher dose corticosteroids is prominent, whereas there appears to be no discernible benefits in disease outcomes on higher doses versus lower doses, particularly for maintenance therapy.

Corticosteroid-Sparing Medications

Although corticosteroids are most often used first-line for sarcoidosis, patients with chronic sarcoidosis requiring prolonged therapy, those with particularly severe disease, and those with significant corticosteroid toxicity may require a corticosteroid-sparing medication. A Delphi consensus of sarcoidosis experts noted that doses of greater than 10 mg of prednisone per day were generally considered too high for long-term therapy and a steroid-sparing agent is often considered in these patients (29). Methotrexate, azathioprine, leflunomide, and mycophenolate are the most common steroid-sparing alternatives applied to treat sarcoidosis. Methotrexate is the most frequently recommended second-line therapy, based on its well-established side effect profile and efficacy in autoimmune disease such as rheumatoid arthritis and psoriasis (29). It is a folic acid antagonist that, through a series of steps, inhibits purine and pyrimidine metabolism, as well as amino acid and polyamine synthesis. The drug may also have other anti-inflammatory effects on T cells, suppressing formation of contributing cytokines by these cells *via* the adenosine a2a receptors (38). Methotrexate has been shown to be an effective steroid-sparing agent in two small clinical intervention studies (one randomized and one non-randomized), where patients showed improvement in vital capacity or symptomatic organ dysfunction while concurrently tapering down on steroids (39, 40). These data are supported by multiple case series and retrospective studies, both in pulmonary and extrapulmonary sarcoidosis (19). A dosage of 7.5 mg to 15 mg per week appears to be effective for most cases, with an overall response rate up to 55%, which may be higher if used in combination with corticosteroids and lower if used as monotherapy (19, 41). However, a significant percentage of patients both in sarcoidosis and rheumatoid arthritis do not respond or have toxicity to methotrexate, which may be reflective of certain pharmacogenomic profiles or genetic predisposition to drug efficacy and/or toxicity (42, 43). The most common adverse events seen with treatment with methotrexate include infections,

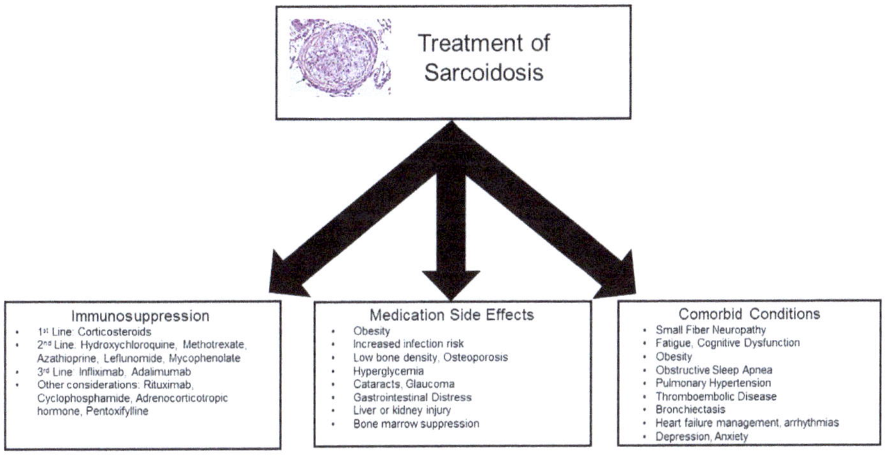

FIGURE 2 | Concepts for treatment of sarcoidosis. Management of patients with sarcoidosis often requires a multidisciplinary approach: treatment of symptomatic granulomatous inflammation, assessment of comorbid conditions, and tempering of immunosuppressive toxicities.

hepatotoxicity, gastrointestinal distress, malaise, and leukopenia. Patients should be started on folic acid concurrently with methotrexate and regular monitoring of liver function, blood counts, and kidney function should be performed.

Similarly, leflunomide, a dihydroorotase inhibitor that inhibits dividing lymphocytes, is often used an alternative (or even additionally, in some cases) to methotrexate in sarcoidosis. Its safety and efficacy are supported by a retrospective study of 76 patients who had progressive sarcoidosis or had failed alternative immunosuppressive medications. A small, but significant improvement was seen in forced vital capacity (FVC) for pulmonary involvement, and a partial or good response was seen in 83% of the patients with extrapulmonary sarcoidosis (44). A steroid-sparing effect was also seen. The side effect and tolerability profiles were similar to studies in other rheumatologic diseases, with diarrhea and liver enzyme elevation being the most common side effects. Respiratory infections and neuropathy were the more serious, but less frequent side effects. A smaller study of 32 patients from 2004 also supported efficacy, with 78% of the patients showing improvement, including in patients who failed to respond to methotrexate (45). Leflunomide has similar lab monitoring requirements to methotrexate. Interestingly, both drugs have been associated with pneumonitis in rheumatoid arthritis, although leflunomide is less common than methotrexate for this confounding reaction (46).

Azathioprine, an inhibitor of purine metabolism, can also be considered as a steroid-sparing agent in patients with sarcoidosis, with similar efficacy compared to methotrexate to improve FVC and diffusing capacity (DLCO), and to taper corticosteroids (47). Azathioprine acts to decrease production circulating T cells and B cells, as well as increase apoptosis of circulating lymphocytes. Toxicity of azathioprine is affected by an individual's thiopurine S-methyltransferase (TPMT) activity which plays a large role in drug metabolism. Genetic deficiency of this enzyme can increase the risk of myelosuppression and hepatotoxicity, although the role for routine testing prior to therapy is unclear given that most people who have myelosuppression do not have deficiency of TPMT (48, 49). The main side effects of azathioprine are gastrointestinal upset, myelosuppression, infections, and potential increased risk of malignancy (47). Side effects are comparable to methotrexate for use in sarcoidosis, although azathioprine did show a higher rate of infections (34.6% vs 18.1%, p=0.01) in one retrospective analysis (47). Doses of 2 mg per kilogram body weight per day were utilized in one study (50), whereas 100–150 mg per day in another (51).

Mycophenolate mofetil (MMF) is another second-line option that acts by inhibiting purine nucleotide synthesis specifically in lymphocytes and decreases production of autoantibodies by B cells; therefore, the drug is used commonly for immunosuppression in a variety of rheumatologic diseases and interstitial lung diseases (52). The largest series reported for use of MMF in sarcoidosis included 37 patients with primarily pulmonary sarcoidosis treated with MMF due to intolerance of an immunosuppressive regimen or treatment failure (53). A trend towards improved DLCO was seen in patients started on MMF, and a steroid-sparing effect was also noted. In a series of patients with neurosarcoidosis, 7 of 8 patients with central nervous system involvement showed remission of disease after 21 months of therapy (54). Three of four patients who had failed alternative immunosuppressive regimens appeared to respond to MMF. However, two patients with sarcoid myopathy did not appear to benefit from MMF. In all patients, no significant side effects were noted, concluding that this drug had a better tolerability profile than other immunosuppressive options and was effective for neurosarcoidosis with central involvement. Another small series of ten patients with chronic pulmonary sarcoidosis treated with MMF found similar steroid-sparing effect and little to no side effects, supporting its utility and tolerability in this patient population (55).

Antimalarials

Chloroquine and hydroxychloroquine have been frequently used in treatment of sarcoidosis based on early randomized trials that showed a long-term benefit with chloroquine (56). However, based on the better safety profile, hydroxychloroquine is most often preferred. The mechanisms of action for hydroxychloroquine are varied; it can interfere with antigen presentation, prevent T cell activation, inhibit toll-like receptor signaling, and reduce inflammatory cytokines by T cells and B cells (57). Hydroxychloroquine has been particularly useful in cutaneous disease, hypercalcemia, and in some cases of neurosarcoidosis (58–60). Although gastrointestinal side effects are commonly reported with use of hydroxychloroquine, they are generally mild and well-tolerated (61).

Inhaled Therapies

Inhaled corticosteroids have not been shown to have clear benefit in patients with sarcoidosis in a RCT (62), but given their low side effect profile and plausible mechanism of decreasing airway inflammation, they may play a role in maintenance, acute airway exacerbations, or cough (63, 64). However, given the lack of data and the likely small effects, consensus of sarcoidosis experts do not recommend inhaled corticosteroids for initial treatment of sarcoidosis (29). Another inhaled therapy, vasoactive intestinal peptide (VIP), has shown some potential effects; a single trial in 20 patients with sarcoidosis revealed that inhaled VIP decreased TNF-α production by alveolar macrophages and increased regulatory T cells in the lung. Reduced cough was seen in 75% of trial subjects, indicating its possible use for symptomatic relief (65). However, subsequent studies are needed to further dictate use of these inhaled therapies in clinical practice.

Tumor Necrosis Factor (TNF) Antagonists and Biosimilars

TNF-α is a predominant cytokine, consistently elevated in active sarcoidosis as a product of macrophage activation, particularly at sites of granuloma formation (31). It is a major contributor to propagation of granulomatous inflammation. TNF-α by is elevated in progressive or steroid-resistant disease (66), and soluble TNF-α receptors are higher in BAL fluid of patients with active disease, signaling a role in pathogenesis (67). For this reason, the use of TNF inhibition has been studied as a therapeutic target. The use of TNF antagonists is supported by numerous compelling case reports and series in refractory sarcoidosis. Both infliximab and adalimumab are monoclonal antibodies targeted against TNF itself, with infliximab being chimeric and adalimumab being a humanized monoclonal antibody. In one double-blind, placebo-controlled Phase II trial of 138 patients with chronic pulmonary sarcoidosis, infliximab significantly increased the percent of predicted FVC compared to baseline by 2.5%, whereas placebo did not (68). The drug was not approved based on the perceived lack of clinical significance. Interestingly, however, post-hoc analysis suggested that patients with more severe disease and those with extrapulmonary disease may have derived the greatest benefit (68, 69). In addition, there were some improvements in reticular opacities on chest x-rays and decreases in inflammatory cytokines. A later examination of the data showed that infliximab had some benefit over placebo as measured by a novel extrapulmonary severity scoring tool, but the effect was not sustained after 24 weeks of therapy (70). However, a more recent long-term retrospective review of patients treated with infliximab for pulmonary and extrapulmonary sarcoidosis disputes this finding, as 58.5% of patients showed improvement of disease on pulmonary imaging up to 85 months of follow-up (71). Currently, infliximab is the most well-studied third-line agent and dosage recommendations are 3–5 mg/kg with maintenance therapy every 4–8 weeks after initial loading. The role of concurrent immunosuppression (e.g., methotrexate) to decrease formation of anti-drug antibodies for TNF inhibitors is unclear in sarcoidosis; its use is based on studies performed in rheumatoid arthritis and Crohn's disease (72–74).

Increasing data for adalumimab would suggest a role for this TNF-α antagonist in sarcoidosis (75, 76). In one double-blind RCT of 16 patients with cutaneous sarcoidosis, adalimumab was associated with improved skin lesions (77). An open-label single-center study of 11 patients with refractory pulmonary sarcoidosis treated with 40 mg weekly of adalimumab showed that four patients had at least a 5% improvement in percent-predicted FVC (seven had stable FVC) and five had an improvement of at least 50 meters in 6-min walk distance (6MWD), with a total of eight who had improvement in one or the other (76). Another prospective observational study of ten patients with sarcoidosis refractory steroids and cytolytics, the PET avid activity seen with active inflammation was reduced in nine patients with the addition of adalumimab to the existing regimen, indicating responsive disease (78). In sarcoidosis patients with refractory posterior uveitis, adalumimab was associated with improvement in 85% of patients and stabilization in the remaining, supporting its use for ophthalmic sarcoidosis (79). Similarly, a recent series of 17 patients with refractory ocular sarcoidosis (predominately chronic relapsing panuveitis) showed efficacy of both adalimumab (40 mg subcutaneously every 2 weeks) and infliximab (5 mg per kg every 4–8 weeks) (80). The drugs were associated with an improvement in cells in the ocular anterior chamber, vitritis, macular thickness, and visual acuity, with a mean follow-up of 34 months. Corticosteroids were able to be tapered off in these cases. Adalimumab may also be effective for a proportion of patients who develop antibodies or resistance to infliximab therapy (81).

On the other hand, etanercept, a fusion protein that antagonizes the TNF receptor, has not shown clear efficacy in treatment of sarcoidosis. Therefore, this drug is not recommended for use in sarcoidosis. An open-label Phase II study in stages 2 and 3 pulmonary sarcoidosis was stopped early due to excessive treatment failures in patients treated with etanercept 25 mg subcutaneously twice weekly (82). Although five of seventeen patients appeared to respond to the drug, there were no clinical predictors of response that could be found, including TNF-α levels in the serum or BAL fluid. Similarly, in a double-blind randomized trial of 18 patients with refractory chronic ocular sarcoidosis, only three of the patients in the etanercept arm were able to decrease corticosteroid use, which was similar to the placebo group (83). This lack of efficacy may imply an inability for the drug to penetrate the vitreous cavity or may reflect the different mechanism of action by targeting the receptor, as compared to inhibition of the cytokine directly or lysing the cells that produce it, as infliximab does (83).

Similarly, ustekinumab and golimumab were tested in a three-arm double-blind RCT in chronic pulmonary sarcoidosis patients with a primary endpoint of FVC change (84). Golimumab is a fully human monoclonal IgG1 antibody specific for TNF-α, administered subcutaneously every month. Ustekinumab is an IL-12 and IL-23 inhibitor. After 16 weeks of therapy, no differences were observed between the intervention groups and placebo for lung function, although trends were seen in improvement of skin sarcoidosis. Interestingly, in this trial, the placebo group had improved lung function also, indicating that perhaps patient selection of spontaneously resolving patients could have biased results toward the null.

The advent of biosimilars has provided another, potentially less expensive, option for clinicians who desire an anti-TNF therapy. The biosimilar to infliximab has been tested in rheumatoid arthritis and found to have equivalent efficacy to its original form (PLANETRA trial) (85). A retrospective cohort study in 29 patients with sarcoidosis patients who received the infliximab biosimilar at a dose of 5 mg/kg/month showed improvement in FVC, health-related quality of life, reduction of standardized uptake value (SUV) on PET scans, and decreased sIL-2R biomarker (86). Another retrospective review of 20 neurosarcoidosis patients showed good efficacy and tolerable adverse events with infliximab biosimilar (87). Although promising, it will be important to follow patients closely who are treated with biosimilars; it is unclear if there are differences in immunogenicity that could complicate treatment dosages or switching of therapies (88).

Anti-B Cell Therapy

Sarcoidosis has been associated with altered B cell homeostasis (89), high BAFF (11, 90), hypergammaglobulinemia, the presence of IgA-producing plasma cells near the granuloma (91), and autoimmune antibodies, suggesting that the humoral immunity may be playing a role. Consequently, it has been suggested that targeting of the B cells may influence the disease process (90). Rituximab, a chimeric monoclonal antibody against CD20+ B cells that reduce the mature circulating population, has been investigated in small studies (92–94). In one prospective phase I/II trial in ten patients with refractory pulmonary disease, five patients had a greater than 5% absolute improvement in FVC and five patients improved their 6MWD by 30 meters, with a total of seven patients having a response of one or the other (94). The results did not correlate with a patient's pre-treatment immunoglobulin levels. Interestingly, two patients died of respiratory failure (thought to be due to progressive sarcoidosis) and there was one hospitalization for infectious pneumonia during the study follow-up. Lower et al. retrospectively assessed patients with ocular sarcoidosis (n=4) who were treated with rituximab and found that the therapy was effective as a steroid-sparing agent for three of the four, and well-tolerated except for neutropenia in two patients which resolved with lower doses and Staphylococcus aureus skin infections in another (95). Two of the sarcoidosis patients also had concurrent lung disease and incurred symptomatic pulmonary improvement. At this time, the role of rituximab as a third or fourth-line agent in sarcoidosis remains unclear, but future elucidation of the B cell actions in sarcoidosis will likely help in clarifying the use of this drug.

Antifibrotics

Antifibrotics, now approved for treatment of idiopathic pulmonary fibrosis and progressive fibrotic interstitial lung diseases (ILDs), are also an enticing possibility for fibrotic sarcoidosis. The INBUILD trial, a positive RCT of nintadenib in various progressive fibrotic interstitial lung diseases included a few patients with fibrotic sarcoidosis (96). In the overall population of all patients, there was less decline in FVC (a difference of 107 ml) over 52 weeks as compared to placebo. The sarcoidosis patients were included in a group termed "other fibrosing ILDs" which included patients with sarcoidosis and exposure-related ILDs. This group made up approximately 12% of the study population, and therefore, the effects on purely sarcoidosis are not entirely clear. A trial of pirfenidone specifically for fibrotic sarcoidosis is also ongoing (NCT03260556). Future studies will be necessary to determine how antifibrotics may be incorporated into the management of sarcoidosis patients.

Other Third-Line Agents

A few other immunosuppressive drugs have been reported as potential options in sarcoidosis, but lack a significant body of evidence in the form of RCTs or larger series. For example, cyclophosphamide has been reported as an effective treatment in corticosteroid-resistant disease in both neurosarcoidosis and cardiac sarcoidosis, and has been associated with a lower relapse rate for patients with neurosarcoidosis (97–99). However, with more responsive disease, the risk profile is less desirable than other steroid-sparing agents, making cyclophosphamide harder to justify for long-term treatment in milder disease. Adrenocorticotropic hormone analogue is also undergoing evaluation based on a multicenter RCT in chronic pulmonary sarcoidosis that showed improvement in lung function, imaging, and quality of life, combined with a steroid sparing effect (100). Although the drug holds historical FDA approval, there are little prior data to support its use in sarcoidosis; therefore, ongoing clinical trials will inform future use of this drug. Although less commonly used due to side effects and pill burden, pentoxifylline is an oral non-selective phosphodiesterase inhibitor that decreases cytokine production by suppression of macrophages. Its use is supported by one small RCT with 27 patients supporting a steroid-sparing effect, and one observational study in newly treated patients showing improvement or stability of disease with use of pentoxifylline (101, 102).

ADDITIONAL THERAPIES UNDER INVESTIGATION

Additional therapies targeting a variety of pathogenic mechanisms are also undergoing further study, but do not have enough evidence yet to be incorporated into treatment recommendations. For example, nicotine acts upon NFκB in macrophages to decrease cytokine production and acts to decrease the Th17/T-reg ratio by its effects on CD4+ lymphocytes, leading to evaluation of this compound as a treatment for sarcoidosis. A small RCT of 13 patients with sarcoidosis treated with transdermal nicotine versus standard treatment alone showed that those treated with nicotine had normalization of their TLR-2 and TLR-9 responsiveness and increased the T-reg response (103). Based on these preliminary data, a clinical trial is ensuing investigating the effect of nicotine on inflammatory biomarkers in patients with sarcoidosis (NCT02265874).

Another trial, entitled the CLEAR trial (Combined Levofloxacin, Ethambutol, Azithromycin and Rifampin), is targeting the hypothesis that mycobacteria are the elusive antigen in some cases of sarcoidosis. A pilot study of thirty patients with cutaneous sarcoidosis showed decrease in size of skin lesions and granulomatous burden with the CLEAR regimen (104). In a similar trial of 15 patients with chronic pulmonary sarcoidosis treated with CLEAR showed an improvement in walk distance, dyspnea (measured by St. George's Respiratory Questionnaire), and FVC, although half of patients had to stop therapy due to intolerance (105). Results from a Phase II RCT in patients with progressive pulmonary sarcoidosis are awaited (NCT02024555).

Other drugs are being repurposed for treatment of sarcoidosis and are actively being investigated. For example, roflumilast, an oral anti-TNF agent approved for asthmatics with frequent exacerbations, is being evaluated for acute exacerbations of fibrotic sarcoidosis (NCT01830959). Apremilast, a phosphodiesterase-4 inhibitor approved for psoriasis that decreases production of TNF-α, interferon γ, IL-2, IL-12, and IL-23 was recently investigated in 15 patients with cutaneous sarcoidosis. In this study, skin lesions improved significantly after 12 weeks of therapy (106). A Phase 2a trial testing abatacept, a CTLA-4–Ig fusion protein that interferes with T-cell activation (currently approved for rheumatoid arthritis), is underway to understand safety and efficacy in chronic sarcoidosis (107). Similarly, a phase I/II trial using ATYR1923 (NCT03824392), a compound that downregulates T cell responses, cytokines and inflammatory fibrosis *via* modulation of neuropilin-2, is also ongoing in pulmonary sarcoidosis (108). Results from these studies may increase options for clinicians treating sarcoidosis.

Additionally, evolving research in granuloma formation and propagation has suggested new potential therapeutic targets. For example, mTORC1 activation of macrophages has been associated with disease progression, and alveolar macrophages from sarcoidosis patients have upregulation of interleukin-1 receptor associated kinases (IRAK1 and IRAK-M) and receptor interacting protein 2 (Rip2) (109, 110). Interference with these pathways may result in decrease of granuloma formation.

The role of vitamin D in prevention or treatment of sarcoidosis has also been debated, based on the potential immunomodulatory role in Th1 inflammation. Vitamin D has been shown *in vitro* to inhibit proliferation of Th1 lymphocytes, as well as suppress antigen presentation and activation of macrophages, all of which could potentially diminish granuloma formation and propagation (111, 112). Vitamin D may also modulate dendritic cell differentiation, decreasing the antigen presenting capabilities of the immune response (113). Clinically, low serum levels of 25-hydroxyvitaminD have been associated with active disease (114). However, treatment of sarcoidosis is complicated by the dysregulated calcium metabolism that occurs with granulomatous inflammation. The macrophage converts vitamin D to its active form, 1,25-dihydroxyvitaminD, *via* 1-alpha-hydroxylase, which is activated in sarcoidosis irregardless of the parathyroid feedback mechanisms which normally control calcium levels. Thereby, up to 10% of patients with sarcoidosis will have hypercalcemia and even a higher percentage will have hypercalciuria, making vitamin D supplementation increasingly risky if not closely monitored. A small clinical trial of 16 sarcoidosis subjects with normal serum ionized calcium levels and vitamin D deficiency showed that treatment with ergocalciferol increased the storage form of vitamin D, whereas decreased the active form (1,25-dihydroxyvitaminD) and angiotensin converting enzyme levels, suggesting an effect on granulomatous inflammation (115). Asymptomatic increases in serum calcium levels were seen in three of the patients in this trial. Larger clinical trials will be necessary for future recommendations regarding vitamin D as a treatment modality regarding both safety and efficacy.

CHOOSING A TREATMENT OPTION

Deciding on the most appropriate treatment regimen for a patient is often a complex interplay of disease characteristics (such as immediate risk of severe organ damage), familiarity of therapies by the clinician, side effect profiles, and patient preferences. The choice can be influenced by a patient's age, alcohol intake, likelihood of pregnancy, concurrent medications, or comorbidities such as diabetes, liver or kidney dysfunction. Given the polypharmacy often involved in the patient regimen, drug interactions should be considered in medication choice. Corticosteroids are most often first line therapy for any type of sarcoidosis, but second or third-line therapies can be considered in cases where corticosteroids are risky (decompensated heart failure, uncontrolled diabetes, severe obesity, uncontrolled hypertension, glaucoma) or these drugs can be added in the more aggressive treatment of life-threatening or severe organ derangement such as can be seen in neurosarcoidosis, ophthalmic injury, or severe infiltrative heart disease. On a more chronic, outpatient regimen, steroid-sparing agents are often used when corticosteroids cannot be reduced to reasonable doses (less than 10–15 mg per day), there is corticosteroid toxicity, or the anticipated course of treatment is lengthy.

Length of Treatment

Duration of therapy, whether with corticosteroids or other immunosuppressive treatment, is generally considered to be approximately 1 year, based on data suggesting an increased risk of relapse with shorter courses (23, 116–118). The British Thoracic Society Sarcoidosis Study found that in patients with asymptomatic, but radiographically evident pulmonary sarcoidosis, who were treated empirically with long-term therapy of 18 months versus "selective" therapy based on development of symptoms or radiographic progression, the patients who received long-term therapy had greater improvements in symptoms, respiratory function, and radiographic appearances than those in the selectively treated group (119). At this point, there are no sensitive or specific biomarkers to predict relapse, leading to blanket generalization of longer duration (120); however, shorter tapers can be considered based on symptoms and overall response to therapy on an individual basis. This is supported by recent data from a prospective study of 21 patients with pulmonary sarcoidosis showing that most of the improvement in pulmonary function (measured by home spirometry), was seen in the first month after initiation of treatment (121). A smaller additional improvement was seen by three months, indicating that steroids may be able to be tapered within the first three months to a tolerable, long-term dose that would lessen the toxicity for patients. Additionally, this study showed that the improvement in fatigue as measured by the Fatigue Assessment Scale (FAS) and dyspnea as measured by the Medical Research Council dyspnea scale also occurred within the first month of treatment (121).

Organ-Specific Therapy

The question of whether there are organ systems which benefit from a particular steroid sparing agent is not wholly clear, and generally, extrapulmonary sarcoidosis is treated with the same algorithms as pulmonary sarcoidosis (28). However, some extrapolations from prior study have suggested preferences for certain therapies depending on sarcoidosis phenotype. For example, hydroxychloroquine has been suggested as quite effective for cutaneous sarcoidosis, but not considered highly effective for pulmonary disease (60). Hydroxychloroquine also impairs 25(OH)D3-1-α-hydroxylase, and therefore, it is often chosen to treat hypercalcemia (59). Similarly, leflunomide seemed to be more effective for lung, skin, eye, and sinus disease, and less so for neurosarcoidosis and musculoskeletal disease in one retrospective study (44). In another series, MMF was quite effective for neurosarcoidosis, resulting in some favoritism of this drug for treatment of neurosarcoidosis (54). However, a more recent review of long-term (median follow-up 8 years) outcomes of a large series of 234 patients from France, found that a lower risk of neurologic relapse was seen in patients treated cyclophosphamide (HR 0.26, 95%CI 0.11–0.59), methotrexate (HR 0.47; 95%CI 0.25–0.87), and hydroxychloroquine (HR 0.37, 95% CI 0.15–0.92) (97). This effect was also seen in risk of overall relapse rate, in addition to neurologic relapse. On the other hand, mycophenolate and azathioprine were not associated with a decreased relapse rate, either overall or specifically in the neurologic system. Infliximab was associated with decreased overall relapse rate (neurologic or other organ), and a trend was seen for decrease in neurologic relapses (HR 0.16, CI 0.021–1.24, p=0.08) Conversely, glucocorticoids alone were associated with a decrease in any organ relapse rate, but not specifically for neurologic relapse, perhaps suggesting a need for dual therapy in these cases. In current management, there are few comparative effectiveness studies that can dictate choice of agent based on organ involvement, and therefore, decisions are often made on tolerability, response, and physician experience.

Predictors of Clinical Course and Treatment Response

Although some demographic and clinical characteristics have been associated with worse outcomes and increased disease severity in the broader sarcoidosis population, there are no patient-specific biomarkers used in clinical practice that can directly predict who will progress and necessitate treatment, nor are there clear biomarkers that will predict relapse in any one individual patient. However, increasing data shows promise for potential biomarkers. Multiple differing HLA haplotypes seem to track with both disease onset and differing presentations, implying that the genetic profile of the immune system can account for some of the varied clinical manifestations (122). For instance, the HLA-A1 and HLA-B8 have been associated with acute onset of sarcoidosis, and HLA-DR14(6) and DR15(2) are associated with chronic disease (123, 124). With further insights into abnormal T-regulatory function, recent data has shown an increased proportion of 'exhausted' T-reg cells is associated with chronic sarcoidosis (125). Conversely, the presence of high levels of functioning T-regs in tissues are associated with more self-limited disease (126). The presence of B cells and aberrant proportions of B cells may also signal poorer outcomes. BAFF has also correlated with multi-system disease, and low NFKβ p65 protein on T cells and B cells has been associated with increased severity of disease (90, 127, 128).

For treatment response, genetic polymorphisms may account for some of the variability in treatment response by therapy. For example, a study of 111 refractory sarcoidosis patients who were started on infliximab or adalimumab showed that patients without the TNF-alpha-308A variant allele (GG genotype) had a three -fold higher response to the TNF antagonists compared to those with the allele (129). Higher soluble TNF-receptor-2 expression levels also seem to correlate with response to infliximab (130). Additionally, a small study of five patients with CD4+ lymphopenia showed both clinical improvement in and an increase in CD4+ T cell counts, suggesting that this phenotype may be particularly responsive to infliximab (131). Increasing research and understanding of the intricate mechanisms of pathophysiology may yield future personalized prognostic markers.

TREATMENT-ASSOCIATED ISSUES

Although immunosuppression dominates the forefront of sarcoidosis therapy, in reality, holistic treatment of patients with sarcoidosis often involves addressing the comorbid conditions associated with the disease and mitigating side effects of immunosuppression. Sarcoidosis can cause a number of "danger situations", including fibrocystic sarcoidosis, sarcoidosis-associated pulmonary hypertension (SAPH), bronchiectasis, and mycetomas (132). Additionally, "parasarcoidosis" syndromes are associated with the disease, including small fiber neuropathy, cognitive dysfunction, chronic pain, and fatigue; each of these issues can cause significant disability and burden upon patients, and often, do not respond desirably to traditional immunosuppressive therapies (25). Last, the immunosuppressive treatments themselves contribute to predictable comorbidities, including infections, fatigue, and malaise. Corticosteroids are highly associated with obesity, malaise, decreased bone density, cataracts, hyperglycemia and edema (133, 134). Additionally, each steroid-sparing agent can be associated with organ toxicities in the liver, kidney, or bone marrow. One cross-sectional study assessing gastrointestinal (GI) side effects in patients from the United States, United Kingdom, and the Netherlands found that the most important GI side effect was weight gain related to corticosteroid use; methotrexate was associated with nausea and diarrhea. Vomiting and weight loss were most associated with azathioprine and mycophenolate (61). Last, paradoxically, some of the drugs used to treat sarcoidosis (e.g., the TNF-antagonists) have been associated with development of a sarcoid-like reaction (135).

Strategies to circumvent detrimental toxicities of both corticosteroids and alternative immunosuppression are important to incorporate into the multidisciplinary management of patients. For example, maintaining routine recommended vaccinations for infections such as influenza or pneumococcus should be considered (136, 137). Additionally, bone health should be addressed upon initiation of corticosteroids and regularly thereafter; clinical risk assessment (yearly) and intermittent bone mineral density testing can be incorporated based on duration of corticosteroid use, age, and risk scores (138). Treatment often includes bisphosphonates or other anti-fracture medications. Bone health management can be somewhat complicated given the need for calcium and vitamin D supplementation, but can be done safely with close monitoring. Similarly, patients should adhere to recommended laboratory monitoring intervals specific to their immunosuppressive medication to avoid irreversible organ injury (139). Regular eye exams can be helpful to evaluate for glaucoma or cataracts that can result from corticosteroid use.

Cavitary Lung Disease and Bronchiectasis

Fibrotic sarcoidosis has been historically difficult to treat given lack of treatment options and resultant complications of fibrosis (140). Pulmonary cavities can occur in patients with sarcoidosis related to progressive fibrosis of the lung (141). Mycetomas, caused by *Aspergillus* within lung cavities, can cause hemoptysis or lead to invasive infection. Similarly, bronchiectasis resultant of fibrotic sarcoidosis can also complicate treatment. In these cases, use of antibiotics and pulmonary therapies including bronchodilators, mucolytics, and chest physiotherapy is often most effective (140). Immunosuppression may be counterproductive in these cases, exacerbating chronic or repeated infection.

Pulmonary Hypertension

Pulmonary arterial hypertension can be a complication of sarcoidosis. It is associated with increased mortality, especially among those individuals awaiting lung transplantation (142, 143). Pulmonary hypertension in sarcoidosis may be due to granulomatous vasculitis, pulmonary artery compression by lymphadenopathy, left heart dysfunction due to myocardial involvement, porto-pulmonary hypertension in those with associated liver disease, parenchymal and vascular destruction due to fibrosis, or hypoxic vasoconstriction related to parenchymal abnormalities. Additionally, the associated risk of thromboembolic disease can lead to pulmonary emboli (and subsequent pulmonary hypertension), requiring a high index of suspicion (144). Pulmonary hypertension should be suspected if there is a drop in functional status or DLCO in cases of stable pulmonary parenchymal disease. Upon CT evaluation, pulmonary artery diameter indexed to body surface area correlates with the presence of sarcoidosis-associated pulmonary hypertension (SAPH) and may raise also suspicion (145).

Because of the varied contributing pathophysiology (some of which may be overlapping), the treatment of pulmonary hypertension in sarcoidosis can be complex. Corticosteroid treatment may result in the improvement of pulmonary pressures in some, but not all cases, reflecting the differing mechanisms of pulmonary hypertension. Case series suggest benefit of prostacyclin analogues in some patients and endothelin receptor antagonists (ERAs) have conflicting data reports (146–148). Retrospective series have shown that ERAs may decrease pulmonary pressures and improve functional and exercise capacity in some individuals (149). However, a RCT of 35 patients randomized to bosentan 125 mg twice daily versus placebo failed to show a functional improvement in walk distance, although this study did show small, but statistically significant, improvement in mean pulmonary artery pressure and pulmonary vascular resistance (PVR) (150). Two of the treated patients had increased need for oxygen, possibly indicating a deleterious effect on the compensatory mechanisms of hypoxic vasoconstriction seen in patients with concomitant parenchymal lung disease. Another study, an open-label proof of concept trial of 21 SAPH patients treated with ambrisentan, showed that, in the patients who completed therapy over 24 weeks, there was a non-statistical improvement in walk distance and dyspnea as measured by the St. Georges Respiratory Questionnaire (146). In this trial, drop-out rate was 52% primarily driven by intolerance of the drug. A more recent retrospective review of the French Pulmonary Hypertension Registry between 2004–2015 showed that patients on pulmonary vasodilator therapy (including phosphodiesterase-5 inhibitors, prostacyclin analogues, and ERAs) appeared to have hemodynamic benefit, but lacked a functional benefit from PAH therapies, similar to results from the bosentan RCT (142). Clinical trials with selexipag (a non-prostanoid prostacyclin receptor agonist) and inhaled treprostinil in patients with SAPH is have recently been initiated (NCT03942211, NCT03814317) with the primary outcome of hemodynamic measurements, including PVR. Given the multiple potential causes of pulmonary hypertension in this population, current optimal management for SAPH is unclear. Vasodilator treatments should be used with caution and careful patient selection is advised.

Lung Transplantation

In case of progressive organ failure, transplantation can be considered in patients with sarcoidosis. Approximately 3% of lung transplants done in the United States are due to sarcoidosis (151). Successful outcomes have been reported for lung, heart, and liver disease, comparable to transplantation for alternative causes (151, 152). Interestingly, despite post-transplant immunosuppression, recurrence of non-necrotizing granulomas in the transplanted organ is common, and thought to be derived from the recipient (153, 154). One analysis of DNA from transbronchial biopsies of lung transplant recipients with recurrent granulomatous inflammation found increased percentage of recipient DNA in the epitheloid clusters suggesting repopulation by host macrophages (154). Granulomas can be found on routine transbronchial biopsies in follow-up and often resolve spontaneously (155). Generally, the presence of granulomatous inflammation does not seem to affect overall survival in most patients (151, 156).

Small Fiber Neuropathy, Cognitive Dysfunction, and Fatigue

Small Fiber Neuropathy in sarcoidosis causes chronic pain, autonomic dysfunction, and altered sensation (157). Treatment for small-fiber neuropathy has been notoriously difficult, with failure to respond to most traditional therapies such as corticosteroids, MTX, AZA, MMF, and therefore, symptomatic treatment for neuropathic pain is usually considered (158). Additionally, the anti-TNF agents, both infliximab and adalumimab, have some suggestion of improving sarcoidosis-related fatigue and cognitive difficulties, as compared to other immunosuppressive agents (159). Intravenous immunoglobulin has also been suggested and has shown efficacy in a proportion of patients (160). ARA 290, a peptide that targets the innate repair receptor to decrease cytokine production and tissue inflammation, is also currently under study given supporting preliminary data in a small RCT of 22 patients showing a reduction in small fiber neuropathy symptoms (including pain) when treated with 28 days of ARA 290 (161).

Fatigue in sarcoidosis is extremely common. Its presence is an interplay of inflammation, musculoskeletal disease, mental health, treatment side effects, and sleep issues (162, 163). Given the association of sarcoidosis and sleep apnea, sleep evaluation is recommended in the workup of fatigue in this population (164). Both armodafinil and dexmethylphenidate have shown some benefit for sarcoid-related fatigue in very small studies of 15 patients or less when added to their immunosuppressive regimen (165, 166). Given the above potential benefits seen with the TNF antagonists, further study with these drugs should include fatigue as an endpoint. Treatment of depression and anxiety, both common confounding ailments, should also be evaluated and considered (167).

Physical Training/Pulmonary Rehabilitation

Physical training studies in sarcoidosis have suggested that a structured physical activity program can improve exercise capacity, muscle strength, and fatigue in sarcoidosis (168, 169). Additionally, physical training regimens appear to improve overall physical and psychological well-being, suggesting a role in the treatment of sarcoidosis. Pulmonary rehabilitation and training have been incorporated into expert consensus recommendations (170).

CONCLUSIONS

Treatment of sarcoidosis is complex and non-standardized for clinicians and patients. Further research is necessary to inform clinical guidelines and provide higher quality evidence for treatment regimens. Drug development is challenging due to the lack of animal model and rudimentary understanding of pathogenesis. Additionally, research should involve clinical trial design and prognostic biomarkers to appropriately select and evaluate those patients who will require therapy. Advancing the knowledge regarding etiology and pathophysiology may one day lead to prevention or cure. Future treatments will likely involve prevention of exposure, treatment of an antigen, mitigation of granulomatous inflammation, and interrupting fibrotic pathways. Management decisions should evolve to include personalized medicine based on pharmacogenomics and sarcoidosis phenotype, as well as patient-centered approaches to incorporate immunosuppression, symptom control, and treatment of comorbid conditions.

AUTHOR CONTRIBUTIONS

The author confirms being the sole contributor of this work and has approved it for publication.

ACKNOWLEDGMENTS

The author would like to acknowledge Dr. Nabeel Hamzeh for his thoughtful edits and suggestions on the final draft.

REFERENCES

Crouser ED, Maier LA, Wilson KC, Bonham CA, Morgenthau AS, Patterson KC, et al. Diagnosis and Detection of Sarcoidosis. An Official American Thoracic Society Clinical Practice Guideline. *Am J Respir Crit Care Med* (2020) 201(8):e26–51. doi: 10.1164/rccm.202002-0251ST

Adrianto I, Lin CP, Hale JJ, Levin AM, Datta I, Parker R, et al. Genome-wide association study of African and European Americans implicates multiple shared and ethnic specific loci in sarcoidosis susceptibility. *PloS One* (2012) 7(8):e43907. doi: 10.1371/journal.pone.0043907

Rossman MD, Thompson B, Frederick M, Maliarik M, Iannuzzi MC, Rybicki BA, et al. HLA-DRB1*1101: a significant risk factor for sarcoidosis in blacks and whites. *Am J Hum Genet* (2003) 73(4):720–35. doi: 10.1086/378097

Grunewald J, Eklund A. Lofgren's syndrome: human leukocyte antigen strongly influences the disease course. *Am J Respir Crit Care Med* (2009) 179 (4):307–12. doi: 10.1164/rccm.200807-1082OC

Richmond BW, Ploetze K, Isom J, Chambers-Harris I, Braun NA, Taylor T, et al. Sarcoidosis Th17 cells are ESAT-6 antigen specific but demonstrate reduced IFN-gamma expression. *J Clin Immunol* (2013) 33(2):446–55. doi: 10.1007/s10875-012-9817-6

Song Z, Marzilli L, Greenlee BM, Chen ES, Silver RF, Askin FB, et al. Mycobacterial catalase-peroxidase is a tissue antigen and target of the adaptive immune response in systemic sarcoidosis. *J Exp Med* (2005) 201 (5):755–67. doi: 10.1084/jem.20040429

Eishi Y. Etiologic link between sarcoidosis and Propionibacterium acnes. *Respir Invest* (2013) 51(2):56–68. doi: 10.1016/j.resinv.2013.01.001

Ten Berge B, Kleinjan A, Muskens F, Hammad H, Hoogsteden HC, Hendriks RW, et al. Evidence for local dendritic cell activation in pulmonary sarcoidosis. *Respir Res* (2012) 13:33. doi: 10.1186/1465-9921- 13-33

Braun NA, Celada LJ, Herazo-Maya JD, Abraham S, Shaginurova G, Sevin CM, et al. Blockade of the programmed death-1 pathway restores sarcoidosis CD4(+) T-cell proliferative capacity. *Am J Respir Crit Care Med* (2014) 190 (5):560–71. doi: 10.1164/rccm.201401-0188OC

Snyder-Cappione JE, Nixon DF, Chi JC, Nguyen ML, Kirby CK, Milush JM, et al. Invariant natural killer T (iNKT) cell exhaustion in sarcoidosis. *Eur J Immunol* (2013) 43(8):2194–205. doi: 10.1002/eji.201243185

Ando M, Goto A, Takeno Y, Yamasue M, Komiya K, Umeki K, et al. Significant elevation of the levels of B-cell activating factor (BAFF) in patients with sarcoidosis. *Clin Rheumatol* (2018) 37(10):2833–8. doi: 10.1007/s10067-018-4183-2

Chen ES. Reassessing Th1 versus Th17.1 in sarcoidosis: new tricks for old dogma. *Eur Respir J* (2018) 51(3). doi: 10.1183/13993003.00010-2018

Drent M, Cremers JP, Jansen TL. Pulmonology meets rheumatology in sarcoidosis: a review on the therapeutic approach. *Curr Opin Rheumatol* (2014) 26(3):276–84. doi: 10.1097/BOR.0000000000000052

Drent M, Cremers JP, Jansen TL, Baughman RP. Practical eminence and experience-based recommendations for use of TNF-alpha inhibitors in sarcoidosis. *Sarcoidosis Vasc Diffuse Lung Dis* (2014) 31(2):91–107.

Baughman RP. Treatment of sarcoidosis. *Panminerva Med* (2013) 55 (2):175–89.

Baughman RP, Nunes H, Sweiss NJ, Lower EE. Established and experimental medical therapy of pulmonary sarcoidosis. *Eur Respir J* (2013) 41(6):1424– 38. doi: 10.1183/09031936.00060612

Cremers JP, Drent M, Bast A, Shigemitsu H, Baughman RP, Valeyre D, et al. Multinational evidence-based World Association of Sarcoidosis and Other Granulomatous Disorders recommendations for the use of methotrexate in sarcoidosis: integrating systematic literature research and expert opinion of sarcoidologists worldwide. *Curr Opin Pulm Med* (2013) 19(5):545–61. doi: 10.1097/MCP.0b013e3283642a7a

Bradley B, Branley HM, Egan JJ, Greaves MS, Hansell DM, Harrison NK, et al. Interstitial lung disease guideline: the British Thoracic Society in collaboration with the Thoracic Society of Australia and New Zealand and the Irish Thoracic Society. *Thorax* (2008) 63(Suppl 5):v1–58. doi: 10.1136/ thx.2008.101691

Brito-Zeron P, Perez-Alvarez R, Pallares L, Retamozo S, Baughman RP, Ramos-Casals M, et al. Sarcoidosis: an update on current pharmacotherapy options and future directions. *Expert Opin Pharmacother* (2016) 17 (18):2431–48. doi: 10.1080/14656566.2016.1258061

Kampstra NA, Grutters JC, van Beek FT, Culver DA, Baughman RP, Renzoni EA, et al. First patient-centred set of outcomes for pulmonary sarcoidosis: a multicentre initiative. *BMJ Open Respir Res* (2019) 6(1): e000394. doi: 10.1136/bmjresp-2018-000394

Moller DR. Negative clinical trials in sarcoidosis: failed therapies or flawed study design? *Eur Respir J* (2014) 44(5):1123–6. doi: 10.1183/09031936.00156314

Llabres M, Brito-Zeron P, Ramos-Casals M, Sellares J. Synthetic pharmacotherapy for pulmonary sarcoidosis. *Expert Opin Pharmacother* (2019) 20(11):1397–404. doi: 10.1080/14656566.2019.1615054

Judson MA. An approach to the treatment of pulmonary sarcoidosis with corticosteroids: the six phases of treatment. *Chest* (1999) 115(4):1158–65. doi: 10.1378/chest.115.4.1158

Cox CE, Donohue JF, Brown CD, Kataria YP, Judson MA. Health-related quality of life of persons with sarcoidosis. *Chest* (2004) 125(3):997–1004. doi: 10.1378/chest.125.3.997

Gerke AK, Judson MA, Cozier YC, Culver DA, Koth LL. Disease Burden and Variability in Sarcoidosis. *Ann Am Thorac Soc* (2017) 14(Supplement_6): S421–S8. doi: 10.1513/AnnalsATS.201707-564OT

Paramothayan NS, Lasserson TJ, Jones PW. Corticosteroids for pulmonary sarcoidosis. *Cochrane Database Syst Rev* (2005) 2:CD001114. doi: 10.1002/14651858.CD001114.pub2

Paramothayan S, Lasserson TJ, Walters EH. Immunosuppressive and cytotoxic therapy for pulmonary sarcoidosis. *Cochrane Database Syst Rev* (2006) 3:CD003536. doi: 10.1002/14651858.CD003536.pub2

Hamzeh NY, Wamboldt FS, Weinberger HD. Management of cardiac sarcoidosis in the United States: a Delphi study. *Chest* (2012) 141(1):154– 62. doi: 10.1378/chest.11-0263

Schutt AC, Bullington WM, Judson MA. Pharmacotherapy for pulmonary sarcoidosis: a Delphi consensus study. *Respir Med* (2010) 104(5):717–23. doi: 10.1016/j.rmed.2009.12.009

Grutters JC, van den Bosch JM. Corticosteroid treatment in sarcoidosis. *Eur Respir J* (2006) 28(3):627–36. doi: 10.1183/09031936.06.00105805

Gerke AK, Hunninghake G. The immunology of sarcoidosis. *Clin Chest Med* (2008) 29(3):379–90, vii. doi: 10.1016/j.ccm.2008.03.014

Paramothayan S, Jones PW. Corticosteroid therapy in pulmonary sarcoidosis: a systematic review. *JAMA* (2002) 287(10):1301–7. doi: 10.1001/jama.287.10.1301

Israel HL, Fouts DW, Beggs RA. A controlled trial of prednisone treatment of sarcoidosis. *Am Rev Respir Dis* (1973) 107(4):609–14. doi: 10.1164/arrd.1973.107.4.609

Pietinalho A, Tukiainen P, Haahtela T, Persson T, Selroos OFinnish Pulmonary Sarcoidosis Study G. Early treatment of stage II sarcoidosis improves 5-year pulmonary function. *Chest* (2002) 121(1):24–31. doi: 10.1378/chest.121.1.24

Yazaki Y, Isobe M, Hiroe M, Morimoto S, Hiramitsu S, Nakano T, et al. Prognostic determinants of long-term survival in Japanese patients with cardiac sarcoidosis treated with prednisone. *Am J Cardiol* (2001) 88 (9):1006–10. doi: 10.1016/S0002-9149(01)01978-6

Judson MA, Chaudhry H, Louis A, Lee K, Yucel R. The effect of corticosteroids on quality of life in a sarcoidosis clinic: the results of a propensity analysis. *Respir Med* (2015) 109(4):526–31. doi: 10.1016/ j.rmed.2015.01.019

Broos CE, Poell LHC, Looman CWN, In 't Veen J, Grootenboers M, Heller R, et al. No evidence found for an association between prednisone dose and FVC change in newly-treated pulmonary sarcoidosis. *Respir Med* (2018) 138S:S31–S7. doi: 10.1016/j.rmed.2017.10.022

Gerards AH, de Lathouder S, de Groot ER, Dijkmans BA, Aarden LA. Inhibition of cytokine production by methotrexate. Studies in healthy volunteers and patients with rheumatoid arthritis. *Rheumatol (Oxford)* (2003) 42(10):1189–96. doi: 10.1093/rheumatology/keg323

Baughman RP, Winget DB, Lower EE. Methotrexate is steroid sparing in acute sarcoidosis: results of a double blind, randomized trial. *Sarcoidosis Vasc Diffuse Lung Dis* (2000) 17(1):60–6.

Lower EE, Baughman RP. Prolonged use of methotrexate for sarcoidosis. *Arch Intern Med* (1995) 155(8):846–51. doi: 10.1001/archinte.155.8.846

Goljan-Geremek A, Bednarek M, Franczuk M, Puscinska E, Nowinski A, Czystowska M, et al. Methotrexate as a single agent for treating pulmonary sarcoidosis: a single centre real-life prospective study. *Pneumonol Alergol Pol* (2014) 82(6):518–33. doi: 10.5603/PiAP.2014.0069

Qiu Q, Huang J, Lin Y, Shu X, Fan H, Tu Z, et al. Polymorphisms and pharmacogenomics for the toxicity of methotrexate monotherapy in patients with rheumatoid arthritis: A systematic review and meta-analysis. *Med (Baltimore)* (2017) 96(11):e6337. doi: 10.1097/MD.0000000000006337

Qiu Q, Huang J, Shu X, Fan H, Zhou Y, Xiao C. Polymorphisms and Pharmacogenomics for the Clinical Efficacy of Methotrexate in Patients with Rheumatoid Arthritis: A Systematic Review and Meta-analysis. *Sci Rep* (2017) 7:44015. doi: 10.1038/srep44015

Sahoo DH, Bandyopadhyay D, Xu M, Pearson K, Parambil JG, Lazar CA, et al. Effectiveness and safety of leflunomide for pulmonary and extrapulmonary sarcoidosis. *Eur Respir J* (2011) 38(5):1145–50. doi: 10.1183/09031936.00195010

Baughman RP, Lower EE. Leflunomide for chronic sarcoidosis. *Sarcoidosis Vasc Diffuse Lung Dis* (2004) 21(1):43–8. doi: 10.1007/s11083-004-5178-y

Conway R, Low C, Coughlan RJ, O'Donnell MJ, Carey JJ. Leflunomide Use and Risk of Lung Disease in Rheumatoid Arthritis: A Systematic Literature Review and Metaanalysis of Randomized Controlled Trials. *J Rheumatol* (2016) 43(5):855–60. doi: 10.3899/jrheum.150674

Vorselaars ADM, Wuyts WA, Vorselaars VMM, Zanen P, Deneer VHM, Veltkamp M, et al. Methotrexate vs azathioprine in second-line therapy of sarcoidosis. *Chest* (2013) 144(3):805–12. doi: 10.1378/chest.12-1728

Booth RA, Ansari MT, Loit E, Tricco AC, Weeks L, Doucette S, et al. Assessment of thiopurine S-methyltransferase activity in patients prescribed thiopurines: a systematic review. *Ann Intern Med* (2011) 154(12):814–23, W-295-8. doi: 10.7326/0003-4819-154-12-201106210-00009

Payne K, Newman W, Fargher E, Tricker K, Bruce IN, Ollier WE. TPMT testing in rheumatology: any better than routine monitoring? *Rheumatol (Oxford)* (2007) 46(5):727–9. doi: 10.1093/rheumatology/kel427

Muller-Quernheim J, Kienast K, Held M, Pfeifer S, Costabel U. Treatment of chronic sarcoidosis with an azathioprine/prednisolone regimen. *Eur Respir J* (1999) 14(5):1117–22. doi: 10.1183/09031936.99.14511179

Lewis SJ, Ainslie GM, Bateman ED. Efficacy of azathioprine as second-line treatment in pulmonary sarcoidosis. *Sarcoidosis Vasc Diffuse Lung Dis* (1999) 16(1):87–92.

Meyer KC. Diagnosis and management of interstitial lung disease. *Transl Respir Med* (2014) 2:4. doi: 10.1186/2213-0802-2-4

Hamzeh N, Voelker A, Forssen A, Gottschall EB, Rose C, Mroz P, et al. Efficacy of mycophenolate mofetil in sarcoidosis. *Respir Med* (2014) 108 (11):1663–9. doi: 10.1016/j.rmed.2014.09.013

Androdias G, Maillet D, Marignier R, Pinede L, Confavreux C, Broussolle C, et al. Mycophenolate mofetil may be effective in CNS sarcoidosis but not in sarcoid myopathy. *Neurology* (2011) 76(13):1168–72. doi: 10.1212/WNL.0b013e318212aafb

Brill AK, Ott SR, Geiser T. Effect and safety of mycophenolate mofetil in chronic pulmonary sarcoidosis: a retrospective study. *Respiration* (2013) 86 (5):376–83. doi: 10.1159/000345596

Morse SI, Cohn ZA, Hirsch JG, Schaeder RW. The treatment of sarcoidosis with chloroquine. *Am J Med* (1961) 30:779–84. doi: 10.1016/0002-9343(61) 90213-3

Schrezenmeier E, Dorner T. Mechanisms of action of hydroxychloroquine and chloroquine: implications for rheumatology. *Nat Rev Rheumatol* (2020) 16(3):155–66. doi: 10.1038/s41584-020-0372-x

Sharma OP. Effectiveness of chloroquine and hydroxychloroquine in treating selected patients with sarcoidosis with neurological involvement. *Arch Neurol* (1998) 55(9):1248–54. doi: 10.1001/archneur.55.9.1248

Baughman RP, Janovcik J, Ray M, Sweiss N, Lower EE. Calcium and vitamin D metabolism in sarcoidosis. *Sarcoidosis Vasc Diffuse Lung Dis* (2013) 30 (2):113–20.

Baughman RP, Lower EE. Evidence-based therapy for cutaneous sarcoidosis. *Clin Dermatol* (2007) 25(3):334–40. doi: 10.1016/j.clindermatol.2007.03.011

Drent M, Proesmans VLJ, Elfferich MDP, Jessurun NT, de Jong SMG, Ebner NM, et al. Ranking Self-reported Gastrointestinal Side Effects of Pharmacotherapy in Sarcoidosis. *Lung* (2020) 198(2):395–403. doi: 10.1007/s00408-020-00323-8

Milman N, Graudal N, Grode G, Munch E. No effect of high-dose inhaled steroids in pulmonary sarcoidosis: a double-blind, placebo-controlled study. *J Intern Med* (1994) 236(3):285–90. doi: 10.1111/j.1365-2796.1994.tb00798.x

Selroos O, Lofroos AB, Pietinalho A, Niemisto M, Riska H. Inhaled budesonide for maintenance treatment of pulmonary sarcoidosis. *Sarcoidosis* (1994) 11(2):126–31.

Baughman RP, Iannuzzi MC, Lower EE, Moller DR, Balkissoon RC, Winget DB, et al. Use of fluticasone in acute symptomatic pulmonary sarcoidosis. *Sarcoidosis Vasc Diffuse Lung Dis* (2002) 19(3):198–204.

Prasse A, Zissel G, Lutzen N, Schupp J, Schmiedlin R, Gonzalez-Rey E, et al. Inhaled vasoactive intestinal peptide exerts immunoregulatory effects in sarcoidosis. *Am J Respir Crit Care Med* (2010) 182(4):540–8. doi: 10.1164/ rccm.200909-1451OC

Loza MJ, Brodmerkel C, Du Bois RM, Judson MA, Costabel U, Drent M, et al. Inflammatory profile and response to anti-tumor necrosis factor therapy in patients with chronic pulmonary sarcoidosis. *Clin Vaccine Immunol* (2011) 18(6):931–9. doi: 10.1128/CVI.00337-10

Dai H, Guzman J, Chen B, Costabel U. Production of soluble tumor necrosis factor receptors and tumor necrosis factor-alpha by alveolar macrophages in sarcoidosis and extrinsic allergic alveolitis. *Chest* (2005) 127(1):251–6. doi: 10.1378/chest.127.1.251

Baughman RP, Drent M, Kavuru M, Judson MA, Costabel U, du Bois R, et al. Infliximab therapy in patients with chronic sarcoidosis and pulmonary involvement. *Am J Respir Crit Care Med* (2006) 174(7):795–802. doi: 10.1164/ rccm.200603-402OC

Baughman RP, Judson MA, Lower EE, Drent M, Costabel U, Flavin S, et al. Infliximab for chronic cutaneous sarcoidosis: a subset analysis from a double-blind randomized clinical trial. *Sarcoidosis Vasc Diffuse Lung Dis* (2016) 32(4):289–95.

Judson MA, Baughman RP, Costabel U, Flavin S, Lo KH, Kavuru MS, et al. Efficacy of infliximab in extrapulmonary sarcoidosis: results from a randomised trial. *Eur Respir J* (2008) 31(6):1189–96. doi: 10.1183/ 09031936.00051907

Russell E, Luk F, Manocha S, Ho T, O'Connor C, Hussain H. Long term follow-up of infliximab efficacy in pulmonary and extra-pulmonary sarcoidosis refractory to conventional therapy. *Semin Arthritis Rheumatol* (2013) 43(1):119–24. doi: 10.1016/j.semarthrit.2012.10.008

Strand V, Balsa A, Al-Saleh J, Barile-Fabris L, Horiuchi T, Takeuchi T, et al. Immunogenicity of Biologics in Chronic Inflammatory Diseases: A Systematic Review. *BioDrugs* (2017) 31(4):299–316. doi: 10.1007/s40259- 017-0231-8

Radstake TR, Svenson M, Eijsbouts AM, van den Hoogen FH, Enevold C, van Riel PL, et al. Formation of antibodies against infliximab and adalimumab strongly correlates with functional drug levels and clinical responses in rheumatoid arthritis. *Ann Rheum Dis* (2009) 68(11):1739–45. doi: 10.1136/ard.2008.092833

Baert F, Noman M, Vermeire S, Van Assche G, DH G, Carbonez A, et al. Influence of immunogenicity on the long-term efficacy of infliximab in Crohn's disease. *N Engl J Med* (2003) 348(7):601–8. doi: 10.1056/ NEJMoa020888

Kamphuis LS, Lam-Tse WK, Dik WA, van Daele PL, van Biezen P, Kwekkeboom DJ, et al. Efficacy of adalimumab in chronically active and symptomatic patients with sarcoidosis. *Am J Respir Crit Care Med* (2011) 184(10):1214–6. doi: 10.1164/ ajrccm.184.10.1214

Sweiss NJ, Noth I, Mirsaeidi M, Zhang W, Naureckas ET, Hogarth DK, et al. Efficacy Results of a 52-week Trial of Adalimumab in the Treatment of Refractory Sarcoidosis. *Sarcoidosis Vasc Diffuse Lung Dis* (2014) 31(1):46–54.

Pariser RJ, Paul J, Hirano S, Torosky C, Smith M. A double-blind, randomized, placebo-controlled trial of adalimumab in the treatment of cutaneous sarcoidosis. *J Am Acad Dermatol* (2013) 68(5):765–73. doi: 10.1016/j.jaad.2012.10.056

Milman N, Graudal N, Loft A, Mortensen J, Larsen J, Baslund B. Effect of the TNF-alpha inhibitor adalimumab in patients with recalcitrant sarcoidosis: a prospective observational study using FDG-PET. *Clin Respir J* (2012) 6 (4):238–47. doi: 10.1111/j.1752-699X.2011.00276.x

Erckens RJ, Mostard RL, Wijnen PA, Schouten JS, Drent M. Adalimumab successful in sarcoidosis patients with refractory chronic non-infectious uveitis. *Graefes Arch Clin Exp Ophthalmol* (2012) 250(5):713–20. doi: 10.1007/s00417-011-1844-0

Riancho-Zarrabeitia L, Calvo-Rio V, Blanco R, Mesquida M, Adan AM, Herreras JM, et al. Anti-TNF-alpha therapy in refractory uveitis associated with sarcoidosis: Multicenter study of 17 patients. *Semin Arthritis Rheum* (2015) 45(3):361–8. doi: 10.1016/j.semarthrit.2015.05.010

Crommelin HA, van der Burg LM, Vorselaars AD, Drent M, van Moorsel CH, Rijkers GT, et al. Efficacy of adalimumab in sarcoidosis patients who developed intolerance to infliximab. *Respir Med* (2016) 115:72–7. doi: 10.1016/j. rmed.2016.04.011

Utz JP, Limper AH, Kalra S, Specks U, Scott JP, Vuk-Pavlovic Z, et al. Etanercept for the treatment of stage II and III progressive pulmonary sarcoidosis. *Chest* (2003) 124(1):177–85. doi: 10.1378/chest.124.1.177

Baughman RP, Lower EE, Bradley DA, Raymond LA, Kaufman A. Etanercept for refractory ocular sarcoidosis: results of a double-blind randomized trial. *Chest* (2005) 128(2):1062–47. doi: 10.1016/S0012-3692 (15)50471-6

Judson MA, Baughman RP, Costabel U, Drent M, Gibson KF, Raghu G, et al. Safety and efficacy of ustekinumab or golimumab in patients with chronic sarcoidosis. *Eur Respir J* (2014) 44(5):1296–307. doi: 10.1183/ 09031936.00000914

Yoo DH, Hrycaj P, Miranda P, Ramiterre E, Piotrowski M, Shevchuk S, et al. A randomised, double-blind, parallel-group study to demonstrate equivalence in efficacy and safety of CT-P13 compared with innovator infliximab when coadministered with methotrexate in patients with active rheumatoid arthritis: the PLANETRA study. *Ann Rheum Dis* (2013) 72 (10):1613–20. doi: 10.1136/ annrheumdis-2012-203090

Schimmelpennink MC, Vorselaars ADM, van Beek FT, Crommelin HA, Deneer VHM, Keijsers RGM, et al. Efficacy and safety of infliximab biosimilar Inflectra((R)) in severe sarcoidosis. *Respir Med* (2018) 138S:S7– S13. doi: 10.1016/j.rmed.2018.02.009

Riller Q, Cotteret C, Junot H, Benameur N, Haroche J, Mathian A, et al. Infliximab biosimilar for treating neurosarcoidosis: tolerance and efficacy in a retrospective study including switch from the originator and initiation of treatment. *J Neurol* (2019) 266(5):1073–8. doi: 10.1007/s00415-019-09234-y

Veltkamp M, Drent M, Baughman RP. Infliximab or biosimilars in sarcoidosis; to switch or not to switch? *Sarcoidosis Vasc Diffuse Lung Dis* (2016) 32(4):280–3.

Lee NS, Barber L, Akula SM, Sigounas G, Kataria YP, Arce S. Disturbed homeostasis and multiple signaling defects in the peripheral blood B-cell compartment of patients with severe chronic sarcoidosis. *Clin Vaccine Immunol* (2011) 18(8):1306–16. doi: 10.1128/CVI.05118-11

Ueda-Hayakawa I, Tanimura H, Osawa M, Iwasaka H, Ohe S, Yamazaki F, et al. Elevated serum BAFF levels in patients with sarcoidosis: association with disease activity. *Rheumatol (Oxford)* (2013) 52(9):1658–66. doi: 10.1093/rheumatology/ket186

Kamphuis LS, van Zelm MC, Lam KH, Rimmelzwaan GF, Baarsma GS, Dik WA, et al. Perigranuloma localization and abnormal maturation of B cells: emerging key players in sarcoidosis? *Am J Respir Crit Care Med* (2013) 187 (4):406–16. doi: 10.1164/rccm.201206-1024OC

Belkhou A, Younsi R, El Bouchti I, El Hassani S. Rituximab as a treatment alternative in sarcoidosis. *Joint Bone Spine* (2008) 75(4):511–2. doi: 10.1016/j.jbspin.2008.01.025

Bomprezzi R, Pati S, Chansakul C, Vollmer T. A case of neurosarcoidosis successfully treated with rituximab. *Neurology* (2010) 75(6):568–70. doi: 10.1212/WNL.0b013e3181ec7ff9

Sweiss NJ, Lower EE, Mirsaeidi M, Dudek S, Garcia JG, Perkins D, et al. Rituximab in the treatment of refractory pulmonary sarcoidosis. *Eur Respir J* (2014) 43(5):1525–8. doi: 10.1183/09031936.00224513

Lower EE, Baughman RP, Kaufman AH. Rituximab for refractory granulomatous eye disease. *Clin Ophthalmol* (2012) 6:1613–8. doi: 10.2147/OPTH.S35521

Flaherty KR, Wells AU, Cottin V, Devaraj A, Walsh SLF, Inoue Y, et al. Nintedanib in Progressive Fibrosing Interstitial Lung Diseases. *N Engl J Med* (2019) 381(18):1718–27. doi: 10.1056/NEJMoa1908681

Joubert B, Chapelon-Abric C, Biard L, Saadoun D, Demeret S, Dormont D, et al. Association of Prognostic Factors and Immunosuppressive Treatment With Long-term Outcomes in Neurosarcoidosis. *JAMA Neurol* (2017) 74 (11):1336–44. doi: 10.1001/jamaneurol.2017.2492

Demeter SL. Myocardial sarcoidosis unresponsive to steroids. Treatment with cyclophosphamide. *Chest* (1988) 94(1):202–3. doi: 10.1378/ chest.94.1.202

Lower EE, Broderick JP, Brott TG, Baughman RP. Diagnosis and management of neurological sarcoidosis. *Arch Intern Med* (1997) 157 (16):1864–8. doi: 10.1001/archinte.157.16.1864

Baughman RP, Sweiss N, Keijsers R, Birring SS, Shipley R, Saketkoo LA, et al. Repository corticotropin for Chronic Pulmonary Sarcoidosis. *Lung* (2017) 195(3):313–22. doi: 10.1007/s00408-017-9994-4

Zabel P, Entzian P, Dalhoff K, Schlaak M. Pentoxifylline in treatment of sarcoidosis. *Am J Respir Crit Care Med* (1997) 155(5):1665–9. doi: 10.1164/ajrccm.155.5.9154873

Park MK, Fontana, Babaali H, Gilbert-McClain LI, Stylianou M, Joo J, et al. Steroid-sparing effects of pentoxifylline in pulmonary sarcoidosis. *Sarcoidosis Vasc Diffuse Lung Dis* (2009) 26(2):121–31.

Julian MW, Shao G, Schlesinger LS, Huang Q, Cosmar DG, Bhatt NY, et al. Nicotine treatment improves Toll-like receptor 2 and Toll-like receptor 9 responsiveness in active pulmonary sarcoidosis. *Chest* (2013) 143(2):461–70. doi: 10.1378/chest.12-0383

Drake WP, Oswald-Richter K, Richmond BW, Isom J, Burke VE, Algood H, et al. Oral antimycobacterial therapy in chronic cutaneous sarcoidosis: a randomized, single-masked, placebo-controlled study. *JAMA Dermatol* (2013) 149(9):1040–9. doi: 10.1001/jamadermatol.2013.4646

Drake WP, Richmond BW, Oswald-Richter K, Yu C, Isom JM, Worrell JA, et al. Effects of broad-spectrum antimycobacterial therapy on chronic pulmonary sarcoidosis. *Sarcoidosis Vasc Diffuse Lung Dis* (2013) 30(3):201–11.

Baughman RP, Judson MA, Ingledue R, Craft NL, Lower EE. Efficacy and safety of apremilast in chronic cutaneous sarcoidosis. *Arch Dermatol* (2012) 148(2):262–4. doi: 10.1001/archdermatol.2011.301

Frye BC, Rump IC, Uhlmann A, Schubach F, Ihorst G, Grimbacher B, et al. Safety and efficacy of abatacept in patients with treatment-resistant SARCoidosis (ABASARC) - protocol for a multi-center, single-arm phase IIa trial. *Contemp Clin Trials Commun* (2020) 19:100575. doi: 10.1016/ j.conctc.2020.100575

Paz S CD, Ferrer M, Crampton S, Burkart C, Ampudia J, Nangle L, et al. Neuropilin-2, the Specific Binding Partner to ATYR1923, Is Expressed in Sarcoid Granulomas and Key Immune Cells. *Am J Respir Crit Care Med* (2020). doi: 10.1164/ajrccm-conference.2020.201.1_MeetingAbstracts.A3099

Talreja J, Talwar H, Ahmad N, Rastogi R, Samavati L. Dual Inhibition of Rip2 and IRAK1/4 Regulates IL-1beta and IL-6 in Sarcoidosis Alveolar Macrophages and Peripheral Blood Mononuclear Cells. *J Immunol* (2016) 197(4):1368–78. doi: 10.4049/jimmunol.1600258

Linke M, Pham HT, Katholnig K, Schnoller T, Miller A, Demel F, et al. Chronic signaling via the metabolic checkpoint kinase mTORC1 induces macrophage granuloma formation and marks sarcoidosis progression. *Nat Immunol* (2017) 18(3):293–302. doi: 10.1038/ni.3655

Boonstra A, Barrat FJ, Crain C, Heath VL, Savelkoul HF, O'Garra A. 1alpha,25-Dihydroxyvitamin d3 has a direct effect on naive CD4(+) T cells to enhance the development of Th2 cells. *J Immunol* (2001) 167(9):4974–80. doi: 10.4049/jimmunol.167.9.4974

Helming L, Bose J, Ehrchen J, Schiebe S, Frahm T, Geffers R, et al. 1alpha,25-Dihydroxyvitamin D3 is a potent suppressor of interferon gamma-mediated macrophage activation. *Blood* (2005) 106(13):4351–8. doi: 10.1182/blood- 2005-03-1029

Piemonti L, Monti P, Sironi M, Fraticelli P, Leone BE, Dal Cin E, et al. Vitamin D3 affects differentiation, maturation, and function of human monocyte-derived dendritic cells. *J Immunol* (2000) 164(9):4443–51. doi: 10.4049/jimmunol.164.9.4443

Kamphuis LS, Bonte-Mineur F, van Laar JA, van Hagen PM, van Daele PL. Calcium and vitamin D in sarcoidosis: is supplementation safe? *J Bone Miner Res* (2014) 29(11):2498–503. doi: 10.1002/jbmr.2262

Capolongo G, Xu LH, Accardo M, Sanduzzi A, Stanziola AA, Colao A, et al. Vitamin-D status and mineral metabolism in two ethnic populations with sarcoidosis. *J Invest Med* (2016) 64(5):1025–34. doi: 10.1136/jim-2016- 000101

Gottlieb JE, Israel HL, Steiner RM, Triolo J, Patrick H. Outcome in sarcoidosis. The relationship of relapse to corticosteroid therapy. *Chest* (1997) 111(3):623–31. doi: 10.1378/chest.111.3.623

Baughman RP, Judson MA. Relapses of sarcoidosis: what are they and can we predict who will get them? *Eur Respir J* (2014) 43(2):337–9. doi: 10.1183/09031936.00138913

Hunninghake GW, Costabel U, Ando M, Baughman R, Cordier JF, du Bois R, et al. ATS/ERS/WASOG statement on sarcoidosis. American Thoracic Society/European Respiratory Society/World Association of Sarcoidosis and other Granulomatous Disorders. *Sarcoidosis Vasc Diffuse Lung Dis* (1999) 16 (2):149–73.

Gibson GJ, Prescott RJ, Muers MF, Middleton WG, Mitchell DN, Connolly CK, et al. British Thoracic Society Sarcoidosis study: effects of long term corticosteroid treatment. *Thorax* (1996) 51(3):238–47. doi: 10.1136/thx.51.3.238

Baughman RP, Judson MA, Teirstein A, Yeager H, Rossman M, Knatterud GL, et al. Presenting characteristics as predictors of duration of treatment in sarcoidosis. *QJM* (2006) 99(5):307–15. doi: 10.1093/qjmed/hcl038

Broos CE, Wapenaar M, Looman CWN, In 't Veen J, van den Toorn LM, Overbeek MJ, et al. Daily home spirometry to detect early steroid treatment effects in newly treated pulmonary sarcoidosis. *Eur Respir J* (2018) 51(1). doi: 10.1183/13993003.02089-2017

Martinetti M, Tinelli C, Kolek V, Cuccia M, Salvaneschi L, Pasturenzi L, et al. The sarcoidosis map": a joint survey of clinical and immunogenetic findings in two European countries. *Am J Respir Crit Care Med* (1995) 152(2):557–64. doi: 10.1164/ajrccm.152.2.7633707

Berlin M, Fogdell-Hahn A, Olerup O, Eklund A, Grunewald J. HLA-DR predicts the prognosis in Scandinavian patients with pulmonary sarcoidosis. *Am J Respir Crit Care Med* (1997) 156(5):1601–5. doi: 10.1164/ ajrccm.156.5.9704069

Judson MA. A sarcoidosis clinician's perspective of MHC functional elements outside the antigen binding site. *Hum Immunol* (2019) 80(1):85– 9. doi: 10.1016/j.humimm.2018.05.007

Taflin C, Miyara M, Nochy D, Valeyre D, Naccache JM, Altare F, et al. FoxP3 + regulatory T cells suppress early stages of granuloma formation but have little impact on sarcoidosis lesions. *Am J Pathol* (2009) 174(2):497–508. doi: 10.2353/ajpath.2009.080580

Miyara M, Amoura Z, Parizot C, Badoual C, Dorgham K, Trad S, et al. The immune paradox of sarcoidosis and regulatory T cells. *J Exp Med* (2006) 203 (2):359–70. doi: 10.1084/jem.20050648

Lee NS, Barber L, Kanchwala A, Childs CJ, Kataria YP, Judson MA, et al. Low levels of NF-kappaB/p65 mark anergic CD4+ T cells and correlate with disease severity in sarcoidosis. *Clin Vaccine Immunol* (2011) 18(2):223–34. doi: 10.1128/CVI.00469-10

Tarasidis A, Arce S. Immune response biomarkers as indicators of sarcoidosis presence, prognosis, and possible treatment: An Immunopathogenic perspective. *Autoimmun Rev* (2020) 19(3):102462. doi: 10.1016/j.autrev.2020.102462

Wijnen PA, Cremers JP, Nelemans PJ, Erckens RJ, Hoitsma E, Jansen TL, et al. Association of the TNF-alpha G-308A polymorphism with TNF-inhibitor response in sarcoidosis. *Eur Respir J* (2014) 43(6):1730–9. doi: 10.1183/09031936.00169413

Verwoerd A, Hijdra D, Vorselaars AD, Crommelin HA, van Moorsel CH, Grutters JC, et al. Infliximab therapy balances regulatory T cells, tumour necrosis factor receptor 2 (TNFR2) expression and soluble TNFR2 in sarcoidosis. *Clin Exp Immunol* (2016) 185(2):263–70. doi: 10.1111/cei.12808

Crouser ED, Lozanski G, Fox CC, Hauswirth DW, Raveendran R, Julian MW. The CD4+ lymphopenic sarcoidosis phenotype is highly responsive to anti-tumor necrosis factor-{alpha} therapy. *Chest* (2010) 137(6):1432–5. doi: 10.1378/chest.09-2576

Judson MA. Developing better drugs for pulmonary sarcoidosis: determining indications for treatment and endpoints to assess therapy based on patient and clinician concerns. *F1000Res* (2019) 8:2149. doi: 10.12688/f1000research.20696.1

Sweiss NJ, Lower EE, Korsten P, Niewold TB, Favus MJ, Baughman RP. Bone health issues in sarcoidosis. *Curr Rheumatol Rep* (2011) 13(3):265–72. doi: 10.1007/s11926-011-0170-1

Khan NA, Donatelli CV, Tonelli AR, Wiesen J, Ribeiro Neto ML, Sahoo D, et al. Toxicity risk from glucocorticoids in sarcoidosis patients. *Respir Med* (2017) 132:9–14. doi: 10.1016/j.rmed.2017.09.003

Chopra A, Nautiyal A, Kalkanis A, Judson MA. Drug-Induced Sarcoidosis- Like Reactions. *Chest* (2018) 154(3):664–77. doi: 10.1016/j.chest.2018.03.056

Tavana S, Argani H, Gholamin S, Razavi SM, Keshtkar-Jahromi M, Talebian AS, et al. Influenza vaccination in patients with pulmonary sarcoidosis: efficacy and safety. *Influenza Other Respir Viruses* (2012) 6(2):136–41. doi: 10.1111/j.1750-2659.2011.00290.x

Mirsaeidi M, Ebrahimi G, Allen MB, Aliberti S. Pneumococcal vaccine and patients with pulmonary diseases. *Am J Med* (2014) 127(9):886 e1–8. doi: 10.1016/j.amjmed.2014.05.010

Buckley L, Guyatt G, Fink HA, Cannon M, Grossman J, Hansen KE, et al. 2017 American College of Rheumatology Guideline for the Prevention and Treatment of Glucocorticoid-Induced Osteoporosis. *Arthritis Rheumatol* (2017) 69(8):1521–37. doi: 10.1002/art.40137

Singh JA, Saag KG, Bridges SLJr., Akl EA, Bannuru RR, Sullivan MC, et al. 2015 American College of Rheumatology Guideline for the Treatment of Rheumatoid Arthritis. *Arthritis Care Res (Hoboken)* (2016) 68(1):1–25. doi: 10.1002/acr.22783

Bonham CA, Strek ME, Patterson KC. From granuloma to fibrosis: sarcoidosis associated pulmonary fibrosis. *Curr Opin Pulm Med* (2016) 22 (5):484–91. doi: 10.1097/MCP.0000000000000301

Hours S, Nunes H, Kambouchner M, Uzunhan Y, Brauner MW, Valeyre D, et al. Pulmonary cavitary sarcoidosis: clinico-radiologic characteristics and natural history of a rare form of sarcoidosis. *Med (Baltimore)* (2008) 87 (3):142–51. doi: 10.1097/MD.0b013e3181775a73

Boucly A, Cottin V, Nunes H, Jais X, Tazi A, Prevot G, et al. Management and long-term outcomes of sarcoidosis-associated pulmonary hypertension. *Eur Respir J* (2017) 50(4). doi: 10.1183/13993003.00465-2017

Shlobin OA, Nathan SD. Management of end-stage sarcoidosis: pulmonary hypertension and lung transplantation. *Eur Respir J* (2012) 39(6):1520–33. doi: 10.1183/09031936.00175511

Ungprasert P, Crowson CS, Matteson EL. Association of Sarcoidosis With Increased Risk of VTE: A Population-Based Study, 1976 to 2013. *Chest* (2017) 151(2):425–30. doi: 10.1016/j.chest.2016.09.009

Huitema MP, Spee M, Vorselaars VM, Boerman S, Snijder RJ, van Es HW, et al. Pulmonary artery diameter to predict pulmonary hypertension in pulmonary sarcoidosis. *Eur Respir J* (2016) 47(2):673–6. doi: 10.1183/ 13993003.01319-2015

Judson MA, Highland KB, Kwon S, Donohue JF, Aris R, Craft N, et al. Ambrisentan for sarcoidosis associated pulmonary hypertension. *Sarcoidosis Vasc Diffuse Lung Dis* (2011) 28(2):139–45.

Fisher KA, Serlin DM, Wilson KC, Walter RE, Berman JS, Farber HW. Sarcoidosis-associated pulmonary hypertension: outcome with long-term epoprostenol treatment. *Chest* (2006) 130(5):1481–8. doi: 10.1378/ chest.130.5.1481

Foley RJ, Metersky ML. Successful treatment of sarcoidosis-associated pulmonary hypertension with bosentan. *Respiration* (2008) 75(2):211–4. doi: 10.1159/000089815

Barnett CF, Bonura EJ, Nathan SD, Ahmad S, Shlobin OA, Osei K, et al. Treatment of sarcoidosis-associated pulmonary hypertension. A two-center experience. *Chest* (2009) 135(6):1455–61. doi: 10.1378/chest.08-1881

Baughman RP, Culver DA, Cordova FC, Padilla M, Gibson KF, Lower EE, et al. Bosentan for sarcoidosis-associated pulmonary hypertension: a double- blind placebo controlled randomized trial. *Chest* (2014) 145(4):810–7. doi: 10.1378/chest.13-1766

Taimeh Z, Hertz MI, Shumway S, Pritzker M. Lung transplantation for pulmonary sarcoidosis. Twenty-five years of experience in the USA. *Thorax* (2016) 71(4):378–9. doi: 10.1136/thoraxjnl-2015-207497

Zaidi AR, Zaidi A, Vaitkus PT. Outcome of heart transplantation in patients with sarcoid cardiomyopathy. *J Heart Lung Transplant* (2007) 26(7):714–7. doi: 10.1016/j.healun.2007.05.006

Collins J, Hartman MJ, Warner TF, Muller NL, Kazerooni EA, McAdams HP, et al. Frequency and CT findings of recurrent disease after lung transplantation. *Radiology* (2001) 219(2):503–9. doi: 10.1148/ radiology.219.2.r01ma12503

Ionescu DN, Hunt JL, Lomago D, Yousem SA. Recurrent sarcoidosis in lung transplant allografts: granulomas are of recipient origin. *Diagn Mol Pathol* (2005) 14(3):140–5. doi: 10.1097/01.pas.0000176765.26047.6f

Meyer KC. Lung Transplantation for Sarcoidosis. *Sarcoidosis Vasc Diffuse Lung Dis* (2019) 36(2):92–107. doi: 10.36141/svdld.v36i2.7163

Schultz HH, Andersen CB, Steinbruuchel D, Perch M, Carlsen J, Iversen M. Recurrence of sarcoid granulomas in lung transplant recipients is common and does not affect overall survival. *Sarcoidosis Vasc Diffuse Lung Dis* (2014) 31(2):149–53.

Hoitsma E, Marziniak M, Faber CG, Reulen JP, Sommer C, De Baets M, et al. Small fibre neuropathy in sarcoidosis. *Lancet* (2002) 359(9323):2085–6. doi: 10.1016/S0140-6736(02)08912-2

Heij L, Dahan A, Hoitsma E. Sarcoidosis and pain caused by small-fiber neuropathy. *Pain Res Treat* (2012) 2012:256024. doi: 10.1155/2012/256024

Elfferich MD, Nelemans PJ, Ponds RW, De Vries J, Wijnen PA, Drent M. Everyday cognitive failure in sarcoidosis: the prevalence and the effect of anti-TNF-alpha treatment. *Respiration* (2010) 80(3):212–9. doi: 10.1159/ 000314225

Parambil JG, Tavee JO, Zhou L, Pearson KS, Culver DA. Efficacy of intravenous immunoglobulin for small fiber neuropathy associated with sarcoidosis. *Respir Med* (2011) 105(1):101–5. doi: 10.1016/j.rmed.2010.09.015

Dahan A, Dunne A, Swartjes M, Proto PL, Heij L, Vogels O, et al. ARA 290 improves symptoms in patients with sarcoidosis-associated small nerve fiber loss and increases corneal nerve fiber density. *Mol Med* (2013) 19:334–45. doi: 10.2119/molmed.2013.00122

Eklund A, du Bois RM. Approaches to the treatment of some of the troublesome manifestations of sarcoidosis. *J Intern Med* (2014) 275 (4):335–49. doi: 10.1111/joim.12198

de Kleijn WP, De Vries J, Lower EE, Elfferich MD, Baughman RP, Drent M. Fatigue in sarcoidosis: a systematic review. *Curr Opin Pulm Med* (2009) 15 (5):499–506. doi: 10.1097/MCP.0b013e32832d0403

Turner GA, Lower EE, Corser BC, Gunther KL, Baughman RP. Sleep apnea in sarcoidosis. *Sarcoidosis Vasc Diffuse Lung Dis* (1997) 14(1):61–4.

Lower EE, Malhotra A, Surdulescu V, Baughman RP. Armodafinil for sarcoidosis-associated fatigue: a double-blind, placebo-controlled, crossover trial. *J Pain Symptom Manage* (2013) 45(2):159–69. doi: 10.1016/j.jpainsymman.2012.02.016

Lower EE, Harman S, Baughman RP. Double-blind, randomized trial of dexmethylphenidate hydrochloride for the treatment of sarcoidosis- associated fatigue. *Chest* (2008) 133(5):1189–95. doi: 10.1378/chest.07-2952

Bosse-Henck A, Koch R, Wirtz H, Hinz A. Fatigue and Excessive Daytime Sleepiness in Sarcoidosis: Prevalence, Predictors, and Relationships between the Two Symptoms. *Respiration* (2017) 94(2):186–97. doi: 10.1159/ 000477352

Marcellis R, Van der Veeke M, Mesters I, Drent M, De Bie R, De Vries G, et al. Does physical training reduce fatigue in sarcoidosis? *Sarcoidosis Vasc Diffuse Lung Dis* (2015) 32(1):53–62.

Strookappe B, Swigris J, De Vries J, Elfferich M, Knevel T, Drent M. Benefits of Physical Training in Sarcoidosis. *Lung* (2015) 193(5):701–8. doi: 10.1007/ s00408-015-9784-9

Strookappe B, Saketkoo LA, Elfferich M, Holland A, De Vries J, Knevel T, et al. Physical activity and training in sarcoidosis: review and experience- based recommendations. *Expert Rev Respir Med* (2016) 10(10):1057–68. doi: 10.1080/17476348.2016.1227244

10

The Application of Transbronchial Lung Cryobiopsy and Uniportal and Tubeless Video-Assisted Thoracic Surgery in the Multidisciplinary Diagnosis of Interstitial Lung Disease

Qian Han[1,2†], Xiaobo Chen[1,2†], Xin Xu[2,3†], Weiping Qian[1,2], Gui Zhao[1,2], Mengmeng Mao[1,2], Bingpeng Guo[1,2], Shu Xia[1,2], Guilin Peng[2,3], Jianxing He[2,3], Yingying Gu[2,4], Shiyue Li[1,2] and Qun Luo[1,2]**

[1]Department of Respiratory Medicine, The First Affiliated Hospital of Guangzhou Medical University, Guangzhou, China, [2]National Clinical Research Center for Respiratory Disease, Guangzhou Institute of Respiratory Health, Guangzhou, China, [3]Department of Cardio-thoracic Surgery, The First Affiliated Hospital of Guangzhou Medical University, Guangzhou, China, [4]Department of Pathology, Guangzhou Institute of Respiratory Health, Guangzhou, China

***Correspondence:**
Qun Luo
luoqunx@163.com
Shiyue Li
lishiyuo@188.com

†These authors have contributed equally to this work

The application of transbronchial lung cryobiopsy (TBLC) and uniportal and tubeless video-assisted thoracic surgery (UT-VATS) in the multidisciplinary diagnosis of interstitial lung disease (ILD) has not been demonstrated in real-world clinical practice. This prospective study included 137 patients with no definitive diagnosis who were the subject of two multidisciplinary discussion (MDD) sessions. As indicated in the first MDD, 67 patients underwent UT-VATS and 70 underwent TBLC. The specificity of biopsy information and its contribution to final MDD diagnosis were evaluated in the second MDD. The post-operative complications and hospitalization costs associated with the two biopsy methods were compared. UT-VATS was favored for patients initially diagnosed with idiopathic pulmonary fibrosis (IPF), bronchiolitis-associated interstitial lung disease (RB-ILD)/desquamative interstitial pneumonia (DIP) and undefined idiopathic interstitial pneumonia (UIIP), while TBLC was preferred for pulmonary lymphangioleiomyomatosis (PLAM) and pulmonary alveolar proteinosis (PAP). The spirometry parameters were better in patients who underwent UT-VATS than those who underwent TBLC. UT-VATS provided more specific pathological results than TBLC (85.7 vs 73.7%, p = 0.06). In patients initially diagnosed with UIIP, pathological information from UT-VATS was more clinically useful than that obtained from TBLC, although both tests contributed similarly to cases initially diagnosed as interstitial pneumonia with auto-immune features (IPAF)/connective tissue disease-related ILD (CTD-ILD). The safety of UT-VATS was comparable with TBLC although TBLC was cheaper during hospitalization (US$4,855.7 vs US$3,590.9, p < 0.001). multidisciplinary discussion decisions about biopsies were driven by current knowledge of sampling and diagnosis capacity as well as potential risks of different biopsy methods. The current MDD considered UT-VATS more informative than TBLC in cases initially diagnosed as UIIP although they were equally valuable in patients initially diagnosed with IPAF/CTD-ILD.

Keywords: multidisciplinary diagnosis, interstitial lung disease, cryobiopsy, uniportal and tubeless video-assisted thoracic surgery, pathological diagnosis

INTRODUCTION

Interstitial lung diseases (ILDs) represent a heterogeneous group of non-neoplastic pulmonary disorders that manifest with varying patterns of parenchymal inflammation and fibrosis of the lungs (Demedts and Costabel, 2002). A specific diagnosis is essential to determine appropriate therapeutic interventions and prognosis. Diagnosis following multidisciplinary discussion (MDD) is considered the gold standard in ILD diagnosis (Flaherty et al., 2004; Chaudhuri et al., 2016; De Sadeleer et al., 2018). Nonetheless MDD pathways are largely heterogeneous due to the absence of specific guidelines. The American Thoracic Society (Raghu et al.)/ European Respiratory Society (ERS) joint statement recommends a two-round MDD process and emphasizes the necessity for lung biopsy and utilization of histopathologic information in reaching a final diagnosis (Raghu et al., 2018).

Current guidelines emphasize the significant role of surgical lung biopsy (SLB) in the diagnosis of undefined ILDs, with video-assisted thoracic surgery (VATS) preferred to open thoracotomy (Raghu et al., 2011; Raghu et al., 2018; Travis et al., 2013). Nonetheless traditional VATS is burdened by relatively high morbidity and mortality (Han et al., 2015; Luo et al., 2013; Fibla et al., 2012a; Fibla et al., 2012b; Sigurdsson et al., 2009). The development of uniportal and tubeless VATS (UT-VATS) under spontaneous ventilation anesthesia offers a safe and feasible option in the diagnosis of ILDs (Peng et al., 2017). Recent studies suggest that transbronchial lung cryobiopsy (TBLC) may be an alternative method for obtaining large and well-preserved samples of lung parenchyma. It is less invasive and associated with fewer complications and a lower mortality rate than SLB (Colella et al., 2018; Tomassetti et al., 2016; Johannson et al., 2016).

Little is known about how this two-round MDD model is implemented in real-world practice. It is unclear what proportion of cases require biopsy; and how much pathological information, with different biopsies performed, contributes to the final MDD diagnosis and patient management. In this prospective study, we aimed to evaluate the application of UT-VATS and TBLC, under the current MDD schema, in the diagnostic algorithm of undefined ILDs. The option by the MDD on biopsy methods was described, and the contribution of different biopsy methods in a spectrum of certain ILD subtypes was evaluated by MDD.

METHODS

Patient Selection and Data Archiving

This was a single center, non-randomized, prospective study that involved consecutive patients referred to the ILD Center, First Affiliated Hospital of Guangzhou Medical University, between June 1st and Dec 1st, 2019. According to the patient triage algorithm at our Center, all referred patients were reviewed at MDD sessions (see below) and the initial diagnosis of ILD was based on clinical-radiological information. Prior to this, complete data (clinical and imaging findings) of each patient were collated.

To ensure integrity and consistency of clinical data, case report forms (CRFs) were used to record patient information, including general information (age, sex, smoking status), exposure history (environmental, occupational, medications), history of physician-diagnosed connective tissue disease (CTD), CTD-related symptoms, signs and serological results, and spirometry. The CRFs were a modified form of the American College of Chest Physicians (ACCP) ILD questionnaire (with CHEST copyright permission) and an ILD questionnaire adopted by the Firestone Institute for Respiratory Health in Canada (by courtesy of MK).

Study Protocol

The MDD session was held online via a regional research network, and hosted by an expert panel that comprised one pulmonologist (LQ), one respiratory radiologist (ZQS), one thoracic pathologist (GYY) and one rheumatologist (YSH) from our institute, each with recognized expertise in the management of ILDs for at least 10 years.

As per our practice, two MDD sessions were usually needed to agree a final diagnosis of ILD. The first MDD session produced an initial diagnosis but where histological data were required for accurate diagnosis, a multidisciplinary decision would be made to perform a biopsy with careful scrutiny of the indications for VATS or TBLC based on dominant distribution of lesions on high-resolution CT (HRCT) and spirometry data (**Figure 1**). All patients gave informed consent. The eligibility and exclusion criteria are described in the supplemental materials (**Supplementary Table S1**).

Following biopsy, a second MDD session was conducted to review complete clinical, radiological and pathological data and agree a final diagnosis. The evaluation of the pathological diagnosis by the MDD produced one of four grades: Grade 1, histological information was specific to indicate a definitive ILD subtype and sufficient to alter the initial clinical-radiological diagnosis; grade 2, histological information was specific and sufficient to support the initial clinical-radiological diagnosis; grade 3, albeit non-specific, the histological information provided supplementary information for ILD subtype and thereby aided treatment decision, i.e., germinal center formation, lymphoid aggregates, vasculitis; grade 4, the histological information failed to provide diagnostic or therapeutic clues for a given case. The detailed "Pathological evaluation form" is shown in the supplemental materials (**Supplementary Table S2**).

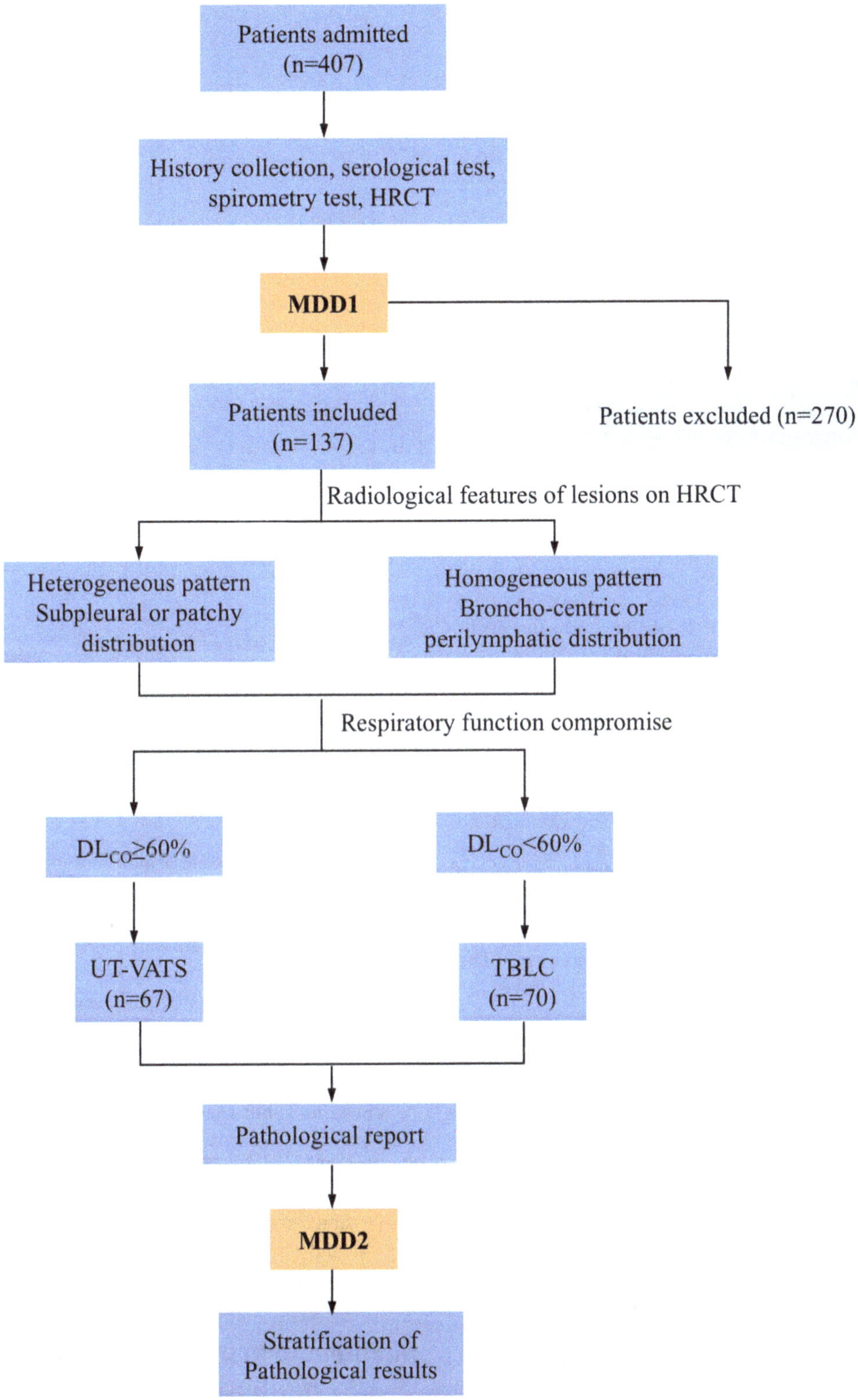

FIGURE 1 | Flowchart of the study. Patients admitted to the institute underwent MDD1 after history collection, serological testing, spirometry and HRCT. A decision was made whether to perform a biopsy and which method (UT-VATS or TBLC) to utilize, the latter based on radiological features of lesions as well as respiratory compromise of patients. MDD2 was held with pathological reports available. Stratification of pathological results was performed based on specificity as well as their contribution to the final MDD diagnosis. MDD: multidisciplinary discussion, HRCT: high resolution computed tomography. UT-VATS: uniportal and tubeless-video-assisted thoracic surgery, TBLC: transbronchial lung cryobiopsy, FVC: forced vital capacity, DL_{CO}: carbon-monoxide diffusion coefficient.

Uniportal and Tubeless Video-Assisted Thoracic Surgery and Transbronchial Lung Cryobiopsy

The biopsy location for both procedures was confirmed by the pulmonologist and radiologist on the MDD panel following review of a pre-operative HRCT. Two specimens from different lobes were routinely harvested for UT-VATS; in TBLC, several samples from different segments of the selected lobe were collected. Sample characteristics were evaluated by individual sample size as well as sample number.

The UT-VATS was performed as previously described (Peng et al., 2017) by an experienced cardiothoracic team in our institute (XX and PGL). Briefly, under intravenous anesthesia with a laryngeal mask airway, a 30°/5 mm thoracoscope (Stryker, United States) was inserted into the pleural cavity to exclude any dense or extensive lung-pleura adhesions. Ring-forceps were used to hold the targeted pulmonary segment and the parenchyma gently pulled out of the chest wall. Wedge resection was performed for biopsy and the residual lung tissue sutured. A chest tube was placed into the chest cavity followed by subcutaneous tissue closure. After expansion of the lung through the chest tube and laryngeal mask, the "tubeless" state was realized by rapid removal of the chest tube and subsequent suture of the skin incision.

TBLC was performed by two experienced bronchoscopists (LSY and CXB) under general sedation using an endotracheal tube airway. Samples were obtained using a flexible cryoprobe with a diameter of 1.9 mm (Erbokryo CA, Erbe, Germany) under fluoroscopic guidance. The gas source of the cryosurgical system was CO_2 with a working pressure of 55–60 bar. The freezing time was 3–6 s, adjusted according to the sample size. Samples were harvested from different bronchopulmonary segments of selected lobes.

The study was registered at clinicaltrials.gov (NCT03958162) and approved by the local independent ethics committee (The First Affiliated Hospital of Guangzhou Medical University; reference number: 2018-85).

Statistical Analysis

Statistical analyses were performed using IBM SPSS Statistics 20.0 (IBM Corporation, Armonk, NY, United States). Qualitative values are presented as numbers with percentages and compared by Chi-Square test or Fisher's exact test. Quantitative values are expressed as mean with standard error of mean (SEM) or median with interquartile range and compared by independent t-test or Mann-Whitney test. Kappa coefficient (κ) was used to determine the agreement between pathological results or initial clinical-radiological diagnoses and final diagnoses. A p value < 0.05 was considered statistically significant.

RESULTS

General Conditions of the Study Population

Between June and Dec 2019, 407 consecutive patients who visited our institute for the first time were initially determined to have ILD.

TABLE 1 | Characteristics of patients undergoing UT-VATS or TBLC.

	UT-VATS (n = 67)	TBLC (n = 70)	p value
Age[b]	54.0 (20–70)	50.0 (21–72)	0.27
Male/female, n	39/28	28/42	0.04
Smoking history, no/yes, n	28/39	16/54	0.03
FVC%[a]	81.3 (2.7)	71.8 (2.8)	0.01
FEV1%[a]	80.7 (2.6)	73.0 (2.8)	0.05
DL_{CO}%[a]	68.7 (2.4)	47.2 (2.5)	<0.001
Biopsy location, n	–	–	–
LUL	10	NA	–
LL(lingular)L	42	NA	–
LL(lower)L	53	44	–
RUL	1	4	–
RML	9	NA	–
RLL	8	295	–
Sample number, n	–	–	–
1	14 (20.9)	1 (1.4)	–
2	50 (74.6)	1 (1.4)	–
3	3 (4.5)	8 (11.4)	–
4	–	9 (12.9)	–
5	–	31 (44.3)	–
>5	–	20 (28.6)	–
Sample number[b]	2 (1–3)	5 (1–8)	–
Sample size[b], cm²/mm²	5.3 (1–32.0)[c]	9.0 (1–40.0)d	–

Values are presented as
[a]mean (SEM)
[b]median (interquartile range) where appropriate.
[c]: cm²
[d]: mm²
UT-VATS: uniportal and tubeless-video-assisted thoracic surgery, TBLC: transbronchial lung cryobiopsy, FVC: forced vital capacity, FEV1: forced expiratory volume in 1 s, DL_{CO}: carbon-monoxide diffusion coefficient. LUL: left upper lobe, RUL: right upper lobe, RML: right middle lobe, RLL: right lower lobe.

Of these, 137 (33.7%) were eligible and included in this study. As indicated by the first MDD session, 67 patients underwent UT-VATS and 70 underwent TBLC. The two cohorts did not differ significantly in age but there were more female and never-smoking patients in the TBLC compared with the UT-VATS cohort, and spirometry parameters (FVC, FEV1 and DL_{CO}%) in the UT-VATS were better than those in the TBLC cohort (**Table 1**).

Biopsy Specimens

As shown in **Table 1**, a total of 123 samples (median: 2, range: 1–3) were obtained by UT-VATS and 343 (median: 5, range:1–8) by TBLC. The mean individual sample size was 5.3 (range: 1–32) cm² for UT-VATS and 9.0 (range: 1–40.0) mm² for TBLC. The VATS samples were mainly from the left lobe, especially the left lingular and lower lobes; TBLC samples were mainly from the lower lobes, especially the right lower lobe.

Multidisciplinary Discussion Choice of Biopsy Methods

The choice of biopsy method and altered MDD diagnosis following the addition of pathological information are listed in **Table 2**. The multidisciplinary team was inclined to select UT-VATS as the biopsy method where the initial diagnosis was idiopathic pulmonary fibrosis (IPF) (76.9%, 10/13), respiratory bronchiolitis-associated interstitial lung disease (RB-ILD)/

TABLE 2 | The alteration of MDD diagnosis after the addition of pathological information.

Pre-biopsy dx	Post-biopsy dx		p value
	UT-VATS (n = 67)	TBLC (n = 70)	
IPF (n = 13)	IPF 8	IPF 3	0.40
	RBILD/DIP 2	–	
COP (n = 1)	NA	COP 1	–
RBILD/DIP (n = 7)	RBILD/DIP 2	RBILD/DIP 2	0.15
	IPF 2	–	
	HP 1	–	
LIP (n = 2)	NSIP 1	LIP 1	–
UIIP (n = 37)	UIIP 9	UIIP 8	0.46
	HP 4	IPF 3	
	IPF 3	NSIP 1	
	RBILD/DIP 2	Pneumoconiosis 1	
	IPAF 1	HP 1	
	LIP 1	ACIF 1	
	Vasculitis 1	–	
	ACIF 1	–	
IPAF (n = 34)	IPAF 12	IPAF 20	0.10
	Sarcoidosis 1	–	
–	HP 1	–	
CTD-ILD (n = 22)	CTD-ILD 9	CTD-ILD 12	0.43
	–	IPF 1	
HP (n = 3)	IPAF 1	HP 1	–
	–	Infection 1	
Sarcoidosis (n = 1)	Sarcoidosis 1	NA	–
PAP (n = 5)	PAP 1	PAP 4	–
PLAM (n = 4)	NA	PLAM 4	–
Vasculitis (n = 1)	Vasculitis 1	NA	–
Pneumoconiosis (n = 1)	Lipid pneumonia 1	–	–
PLCH (n = 2)	UIIP 1	PLCH 1	–
IPH (n = 1)	NA	IPH 1	–
PAM (n = 1)	NA	PAM 1	–
Infection (n = 1)	NA	Infection 1	–

UT-VATS: uniportal and tubeless-video-assisted thoracic surgery, TBLC: transbronchial lung cryobiopsy, IPF: idiopathic pulmonary fibrosis, NSIP: non-specific interstitial pneumonia, COP: cryptogenic organizing pneumonia, RB-ILD: respiratory bronchiolitis interstitial lung disease, DIP: desquamative interstitial pneumonia, LIP: lymphocyte interstitial pneumonia, ACIF: airway-lefted interstitial fibrosis, UIIP: undefined interstitial pneumonia, IPAF: interstitial pneumonia with autoimmune features, CTD-ILD: connective tissue disease-related ILD, HP: hypersensitivity pneumonitis, PAP: pulmonary alveolar proteinosis, PLAM: pulmonary lymphangioleiomyomatosis, PLCH: pulmonary Langerhans cell histiocytosis, IPH: idiopathic pulmonary hemosiderosis, PAM: pulmonary alveolar microlithiasis.

desquamative interstitial pneumonia (DIP) (71.4%, 5/7) or unclassifiable idiopathic interstitial pneumonia (UIIP) (59.5%, 22/37); TBLC was more likely to be selected when the initial diagnosis was pulmonary lymphangioleiomyomatosis (PLAM) (100%, 4/4), pulmonary alveolar proteinosis (PAP) (80%, 4/5), connective tissue disease-related ILD (CTD-ILD) (59.1%, 13/22) or interstitial pneumonia with auto-immune features (IPAF) (58.8%, 20/34).

Pathological Diagnoses

There was a borderline significant increase in specific pathological diagnosis for the UT-VATS compared with TBLC cohort (85.7 vs 73.7%, p = 0.06). For UT-VATS, the most common pathological diagnosis was usual interstitial pneumonia (UIP), followed by non-specific interstitial pneumonia (NSIP) and RB-ILD/DIP; for TBLC, UIIP was most commonly encountered, followed by NSIP and UIP (**Figure 2**). The kappa coefficient between pathological result and final diagnosis was 0.8 (95% CI: 0.7–0.9) for UT-VATS and 0.7 (95% CI: 0.6–0.8) for TBLC.

A total of 42.5% (65 out of 153) of pathological diagnoses were derived from patients diagnosed with IPAF/CTD-ILD, with NSIP as the dominant pattern (38.5%, 25/65), followed by UIP (33.8%, 22/65) (**Supplementary Figure S1**). The spectrum of connective tissue diseases in this study encompassed idiopathic inflammatory myopathy (IIM), rheumatoid arthritis (RA) and systemic sclerosis (SSc). The distribution of pathological patterns was not significantly different between the two cohorts (p = 0.26) (**Table 3**).

Stratification of the Pathological Information

As mentioned above, the pathological information was stratified based on its specificity as well as its contribution to the final MDD diagnosis. The grade distribution of pathological results was significantly different for UT-VATS and TBLC (p = 0.02): compared with TBLC, UT-VATS was more likely to alter the initial clinical-radiological diagnosis (grade1: 34.3 vs 12.9%, p = 0.003) and provide more informative results (grade 4: 9.0 vs 20.0%, p = 0.06) to the second MDD session. As shown in **Figure 2**, among cases with specific pathological diagnoses, those initially diagnosed as UIIP accounted for a majority of diagnosis-altered cases (62.5%, 20/32), followed by RB-ILD/DIP (9.4%, 3/32). Those initially diagnosed as IPAF accounted for a great proportion of diagnosis-unchanged cases (35.1%, 26/74), followed by CTD-ILD (24.3%, 18/74) and IPF (13.5%, 10/74). A subgroup analysis based on ILD subtype and focused on cases initially diagnosed as UIIP and IPAF/CTD-ILD showed that histological information from UT-VATS appeared more informative than that obtained from TBLC for cases initially diagnosed as UIIP (grade 4: 13.6 vs 40.0%, p = 0.06). Nonetheless UT-VATS and TBLC contributed similarly to the final diagnosis for cases initially diagnosed as IPAF/CTD-ILD (total p = 0.14, grade 4: 8.7 vs 15.2%, p = 0.47) (**Table 4**).

Safety and Cost

Pneumothorax occurred in 5.7% (4/70) of patients who underwent TBLC. There were no significant differences in severe bleeding, acute exacerbation or 90-days mortality between UT-VATS and TBLC cohorts. The total and post-operative length of hospital stay were comparable for both methods although the hospitalization cost of UT-VATS was much higher (US$4,855.7 vs US$3,590.9, p < 0.001) (**Table 5**).

DISCUSSION

This prospective study illustrated the two-round MDD decision-making process in the diagnostic algorithm of ILD. The first MDD reflected the choice of experts on candidates and methods of biopsies, and the second revealed the performance of different biopsy methods in patients with distinct ILD subtypes: pathological information via UT-VATS was more clinically useful than that from TBLC for cases initially diagnosed as UIIP, although both methods contributed similarly to cases

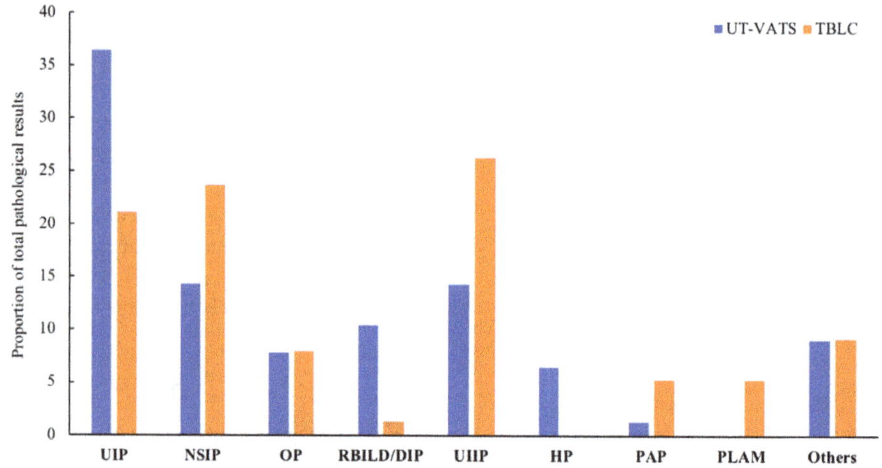

FIGURE 2 | The distribution of pathological diagnoses by different biopsy methods. UT-VATS: uniportal and tubeless-video-assisted thoracic surgery, TBLC: transbronchial lung cryobiopsy, UIP: usual interstitial pneumonia, NSIP: non-specific interstitial pneumonia, OP: organizing pneumonia, RB-ILD: respiratory bronchiolitis interstitial lung disease, DIP: desquamative interstitial pneumonia, UIIP: undefined interstitial pneumonia, HP: hypersensitivity pneumonitis, PAP: pulmonary alveolar proteinosis, PLAM: pulmonary lymphangioleiomyomatosis, Others: including LIP (lymphocyte interstitial pneumonia), sarcoidosis, PLCH (pulmonary Langerhans cell histiocytosis), IPH (idiopathic pulmonary hemosiderosis) and PAM (pulmonary alveolar microlithiasis).

TABLE 3 | The distribution of pathological diagnosis in IPAF/CTD-ILD patients.

	UT-VATS (*n* = 29)				–	TBLC (*n* = 36)			
–	UIP	NSIP	OP	DIP	UIIP	UIP	NSIP	OP	UIIP
IPAF	8	4	1	1	1	6	11	2	4
IIM-ILD	1	4	2	0	1	1	4	2	1
RA-ILD	3	2	0	0	0	1	0	0	1
SSc-ILD	1	0	0	0	0	1	0	1	1
Total	13	10	3	1	2	9	15	5	7

UT-VATS: uniportal and tubeless-video-assisted thoracic surgery, TBLC: transbronchial lung cryobiopsy. UIP: usual interstitial pneumonia, NSIP: non-specific interstitial pneumonia, OP: organizing pneumonia, DIP: desquamative interstitial pneumonia, UIIP: undefined idiopathic interstitial pneumonia, IPAF: interstitial pneumonia with autoimmune features, IIM-ILD: idiopathic inflammatory myositis-related interstitial lung disease, RA-ILD: rheumatoid arthritis-related interstitial lung disease, SSc-ILD: systemic sclerosis -related interstitial lung disease.

TABLE 4 | The stratification of pathological information with different biopsy methods

	UT-VATS	TBLC	*p* value
Total, n	67	70	0.02
Grade 1	23 (34.3)	9 (12.9)	0.003
Grade 2	33 (49.3)	41 (58.6)	0.27
Grade 3	5 (7.5)	6 (8.6)	0.81
Grade 4	6 (9.0)	14 (20.0)	0.06
Initial dx UIIP, n	22	15	0.27
Grade 1	13 (59.1)	7 (46.7)	0.46
Grade 2	1 (4.5)	0 (0)	0.40
Grade 3	5 (22.7)	2 (13.3)	0.47
Grade 4	3 (13.6)	6 (40.0)	0.06
Initial dx IPAF/CTD-ILD, n	23	33	0.14
Grade 1	2 (8.7)	0 (0)	0.08
Grade 2	19 (82.6)	25 (75.8)	0.54
Grade 3	0 (0)	3 (9.1)	0.14
Grade 4	2 (8.7)	5 (15.2)	0.47

Values are presented as number (%) unless specified. UT-VATS: uniportal and tubeless-video-assisted thoracic surgery, TBLC: transbronchial lung cryobiopsy, UIIP: undefined interstitial pneumonia, IPAF: interstitial pneumonia with autoimmune features, CTD-ILD: connective tissue disease-related interstitial lung disease. Grade 1: specific diagnosis with final diagnosis altered; grade 2: specific diagnosis without final diagnosis altered; grade 3: non-specific diagnosis with supplementary information provided; grade 4: non-informative diagnosis.

initially diagnosed as IPAF/CTD-ILD. The safety of UT-VATS was comparable with that of TBLC although the latter appeared to cost less during the hospitalization.

MDD is considered the gold standard in the diagnosis of ILD given its improvement of diagnostic confidence. Although different pathways that follow a multidisciplinary approach to ILD are largely heterogeneous and need further validation, the two-round MDD method is recommended in the ATS/ERS joint statement (Raghu et al., 2018). We implemented this mode in real-world practice and included a pulmonologist, radiologist, pathologist and rheumatologist in the MDD team. The first round MDD aimed to confirm which patients required a biopsy along with the appropriate biopsy method. SLB is regarded as the most reliable tool to provide diagnostic and prognostic information but is associated with substantial morbidity and mortality. In recent years, TBLC has been proposed as an alternative to SLB in the diagnosis of ILD, with a comparable diagnostic yield and less invasive nature (Tomassetti et al., 2016; Johannson et al., 2016; Ravaglia et al., 2016; Kronborg-White et al., 2017), although results are conflicting (Troy et al., 2020; Romagnoli et al., 2019). In the present study, the counterpart of TBLC was uniportal and tubeless VATS (UT-VATS), characterized by spontaneous ventilation anesthesia and absence of postoperative chest tube drainage, thereby mitigating the peri-procedure risk and postoperative discomfort (Peng et al., 2017). Based on current knowledge of the utility and safety of biopsy procedures, our MDD team was inclined to select UT-VATS in cases initially diagnosed as IPF and RB-ILD/DIP; TBLC appeared to be favored more in cases initially

TABLE 5 | Complications and hospitalization costs for different biopsy methods.

	UT-VATS (n = 67)	TBLC (n = 70)	p value
Pneumothorax, n	NA	4 (5.7)	NA
Severe bleeding, n	0 (0)	0 (0)	NA
Acute exacerbation, n	2 (3.0)	3 (4.3)	0.68
90-days mortality, n	0 (0)	0 (0)	NA
Hospitalization days[a]	13.0 (4.0)	13.0 (5.5)	0.57
Post-operative hospitalization days[a]	6.0 (3.0)	5.0 (3.0)	0.2
Total expense[a], US$	4885.7 (1586.0)	3590.9 (2927.0)	0.001

Values are presented as number (%) or
[a]median (interquartile range).
UT-VATS: uniportal and tubeless-video-assisted thoracic surgery, TBLC: transbronchial lung cryobiopsy.

diagnosed as PLAM and PAP. This choice may be related to the radiological features of lesions: SLB is preferred in the presence of a heterogeneous pattern with subpleural or patchy distribution, while TBLC is preferred in the presence of a homogeneous pattern with broncho-centric or perilymphatic distribution (Colby et al., 2017).

The major concern raised for TBLC is that a smaller sample from a single locus may not provide the representative data that are obtained from multiple biopsies from multiple lobes via SLB, especially for UIP pattern (Raparia et al., 2016; Patel et al., 2016). Tomassetti et al. reported the comparable change of initial clinical-radiological diagnosis with the addition of histological information from TBLC or SLB (26 vs 36%), and more cases were finally diagnosed as IPF on TBLC (50 vs 39%), albeit with lower inter-pathologist agreement (Tomassetti et al., 2016); similarly, Troy et al. showed a higher proportion of probable UIP relative to UIP pattern in TBLC, while the converse was observed with SLB samples (Troy et al., 2020), indicating that the heterogeneous pattern of IPF may be more reliable on SLB samples. A smoking history combined with typical radiological changes, i.e. bronchial thickening followed by centrilobular nodules and ground-glass opacity (GGO) in RB-ILD and extensive bilateral GGO with a peripheral and basal predominance in DIP, is usually sufficient to diagnose these ILD subtypes causally associated with smoking (Kumar et al., 2018). Nonetheless it should be noted that there is a high chance of overlap of various smoking-related ILDs, such as RB-ILD/DIP and IPF, in which cases confirmation of the dominant lesion is essential for diagnosis orientation and patient management (Bak and Lee, 2017). We identified an altered diagnosis of RB-ILD/DIP and IPF in four cases with UT-VATS samples, raising the possibility that a representative area of the disease or a coexistent fibrotic process could be presented in a higher proportion of SLB samples.

Another concern in decision-making relates to safety. Since low pulmonary function has been suggested to be associated with a higher rate of complications (Ravaglia et al., 2016), the MDD team adopted DL_{CO}<45% predicted to exclude biopsy candidates and DL_{CO}<60% to refuse UT-VATS. These cut-off values may partly explain the comparable incidence of procedure-related complications between UT-VATS and TBLC groups. The improved surgical technique with less injury and fast track compared with conventional VATS procedure would increase safety for these selected patients (Peng et al., 2017). Among the adverse events related to TBLC, pneumothorax was the most common (5.7%) but the lower incidence compared with many previous studies (Tomassetti et al., 2016; Ravaglia et al., 2016) seems to correlate with the distribution of dominant lesions in the TBLC group, i.e., broncho-centric or perilymphatic distribution. No severe bleeding occurred in our cohort, partly due to intubation with the rigid bronchoscope and prophylactic placement of a Fogarty balloon.

The second round MDD evaluated the pathological information in terms of its specificity as well as its contribution to the final MDD diagnosis. In line with previous data (Colby et al., 2017), the majority of UT-VATS samples were obtained from two lobes and TBLC samples were from different segments of one lobe (mostly lower lobes). There were one to three biopsies with average size of 5.3cm^2 and one to eight samples with average size of 9.0 mm^2 in UT-VATS and TBLC groups, respectively. The specific pathological yield in the UT-VATS cohort was borderline higher than that in the TBLC group (85.7 vs 73.7%, p = 0.06). The final diagnosis agreed more with UT-VATS than with TBLC (κ = 0.8 vs κ = 0.7), indicating a considerably higher diagnostic confidence for UT-VATS over TBLC.

Apart from histological specificity, biopsy information, albeit non-specific, is valuable if it provides diagnostic clues or suggests a management strategy: the observation of lymphoid aggregates, germinal centers, lymphoplasmacytic inflammation, vasculitis or pleuritis may indicate the underlying "CTD color" (Fischer and Richeldi, 2014), while multiple foci of peribronchiolar metaplasia may favor HP to a great extent (Churg et al., 2017). We therefore stratified the pathological information into four grades based on non-diagnostic supplementary information provided as well as histological specificity, and grades 1–3 were deemed clinically helpful. We found that UT-VATS samples appeared more informative than TBLC samples across the whole ILD spectrum (91.0 vs 80.0%, p = 0.06) as well as in cases initially diagnosed as UIIP (86.4 vs 60.0%, p = 0.06). These data indicated that following the first round MDD options, pathological information derived from UT-VATS contributed more to the final MDD diagnosis than information obtained from TBLC.

The proportion of patients who underwent biopsy at our institute was relatively higher than previously reported (33.7 vs 7.5–40.3%) (Singh et al., 2017). This may have been attributable to the great number of patients diagnosed with CTD-ILD or IPAF (23/67, 34.3% in UT-VATS and 33/70, 47.1% in TBLC groups, respectively). The necessity for lung biopsy in ILD patients with autoimmune features remains controversial: although the UIP pattern may offer SSc-ILD patients a comparable prognosis to those with a NSIP pattern (Bouros et al., 2002), it may indicate a worse outcome in patients with RA-ILD, IIM-ILD and IPAF (Antoniou et al., 2009) (Kim et al., 2015; Oldham et al., 2016). Recently, it was revealed in the INBUILD trial that nintedanib could slow the decline in FVC in patients with progressive fibrosing ILD other than IPF, and benefits were observed only when those with a UIP-like pattern were grouped together (Flaherty et al., 2019). These results led pulmonologists and rheumatologists to propose a combination therapy of anti-inflammatory and anti-fibrotic agents in patients with autoimmune diseases characterized by a UIP-pattern. In the current study, we found that most histopathological data for IPAF/CTD-ILD patients, albeit specific, did not alter the diagnosis. Although patients with UIP pattern were prescribed the combination therapy mentioned before and closely monitored, the response to therapy and disease behavior are the subject of another study. Regarding biopsy methods, UT-VATS and TBLC contributed similarly to the final MDD diagnosis in providing clinically useful pathological information, and the distribution of histological pattern was similar between UT-VATS and TBLC groups ($p = 0.26$). This may be partly explained by the distribution of lung injury pattern for this subtype: usually symmetrical, basilar and non-subpleural predominant, thus allowing good sampling with TBLC.

There was no significant difference between UT-VATS and TBLC groups in post-operative hospitalization days, although this may be relatively longer compared with previous data because we usually advise our patients to wait for 3–4 days after the procedure for pathological results and a final MDD decision. The hospitalization expense was higher in the UT-VATS group, mainly attributable to the cost of the procedure, so a patient's ability to pay may also affect choice of biopsy method.

Our study has several limitations. Although it was recommended that the MDD team should decide candidates for biopsy and the biopsy method, there remains no consensus or guideline on how to make the decision. The non-randomized nature of this study may have led to a selection bias. Direct comparison of the techniques is also difficult since they were performed in different patients. Nonetheless our objective was to evaluate TBLC and UT-VATS, each with well-known advantages and disadvantages for sampling and safety, in the real-world clinical practice within the context of MDD. The organizational scheme of this study may provide additional information for the application of biopsy methods in different ILD subtypes, rather than just emphasizing priority or alteration. Second, this study included a limited number of patients so subgroup analysis was difficult to perform in most ILD subtypes. Future studies that focus on a certain subgroup may better inform the application of different biopsy methods under different circumstances. Finally, this study involved patients and MDD experts from only one center, and the counterpart of TBLC in our study was a highly sophisticated surgical technique that has not been widely implemented in other institutes. Results may differ for other institutes. It should be remembered though that improving conventional procedures is just as important, possibly more so, than developing new ones.

CONCLUSION

In conclusion, this prospective study demonstrated the option and evaluation of different biopsy methods in the ILD diagnostic algorithm within the two-round MDD context. MDD decisions about biopsies are driven by the current knowledge of risk-benefit of different biopsy methods as well as the working diagnosis of a given patient. Our study provides a robust rationale for future studies investigating the MDD implementation regarding the selection of biopsy methods in ILD diagnostic schema.

ETHICS STATEMENT

The studies involving human participants were reviewed and approved by The First Affiliated Hospital of Guangzhou Medical University. The patients/participants provided their written informed consent to participate in this study.

AUTHOR CONTRIBUTIONS

QH, XC, XX, SL, JH, and QL designed the study. QH, XC, XX, SL, and QL coordinated the study. QH, WQ, GZ, and QL included patients. XC and SL performed transbronchial lung cryobiopsy. XX, GP, and JH performed tubeless video-assisted thoracic surgery. QH, XC, SL, XX, YG, and QL participated in multidisciplinary discussion. YG performed blinded tissue pathology. WQ, GZ, BG, and SX participated in data collection. QH, XC, XX, and MM performed statistical analyses. QH, XC, XX, SL, and QL wrote the first draft of the manuscript. All authors critically revised the manuscript for intellectually important content. All authors gave final approval for the publication of the work, and all accepted responsibility for the integrity of the work.

REFERENCES

Antoniou, K. M., Margaritopoulos, G., Economidou, F., and Siafakas, N. M. (2009). Pivotal Clinical Dilemmas in Collagen Vascular Diseases Associated with Interstitial Lung Involvement. *Eur. Respir. J.* 33 (4), 882–896. doi:10.1183/09031936.00152607

Bak, S. H., and Lee, H. Y. (2017). Overlaps and Uncertainties of Smoking-Related Idiopathic Interstitial Pneumonias. *Copd* 12, 3221–3229. doi:10.2147/COPD.S146899

Bouros, D., Wells, A. U., Nicholson, A. G., Colby, T. V., Polychronopoulos, V., Pantelidis, P., et al. (2002). Histopathologic Subsets of Fibrosing Alveolitis in Patients with Systemic Sclerosis and Their Relationship to Outcome. *Am. J. Respir. Crit. Care Med.* 165 (12), 1581–1586. doi:10.1164/rccm.2106012

Chaudhuri, N., Spencer, L., Greaves, M., Bishop, P., Chaturvedi, A., and Leonard, C. (2016). A Review of the Multidisciplinary Diagnosis of Interstitial Lung Diseases: A Retrospective Analysis in a Single UK Specialist Centre. *Jcm* 5 (8), 66. doi:10.3390/jcm5080066

Churg, A., Wright, J. L., and Ryerson, C. J. (2017). Pathologic Separation of Chronic Hypersensitivity Pneumonitis from Fibrotic Connective Tissue Disease-Associated Interstitial Lung Disease. *Am. J. Surg. Pathol.* 41 (10), 1403–1409. doi:10.1097/PAS.0000000000000885

Colby, T. V., Tomassetti, S., Cavazza, A., Dubini, A., and Poletti, V. (2017). Transbronchial Cryobiopsy in Diffuse Lung Disease: Update for the Pathologist. *Arch. Pathol. Lab. Med.* 141 (7), 891–900. doi:10.5858/arpa.2016-0233-RA

Colella, S., Haentschel, M., Shah, P., Poletti, V., and Hetzel, J. (2018). Transbronchial Lung Cryobiopsy in Interstitial Lung Diseases: Best Practice. *Respiration* 95 (6), 383–391. doi:10.1159/000488910

De Sadeleer, L. J., Meert, C., Yserbyt, J., Slabbynck, H., Verschakelen, J. A., Verbeken, E. K., et al. (2018). Diagnostic Ability of a Dynamic Multidisciplinary Discussion in Interstitial Lung Diseases. *Chest* 153 (6), 1416–1423. doi:10.1016/j.chest.2018.03.026

Demedts, M., and Costabel, U. (2002). ATS/ERS International Multidisciplinary Consensus Classification of the Idiopathic Interstitial Pneumonias. *Eur. Respir. J.* 19 (5), 794–796. doi:10.1183/09031936.02.00492002

Fibla, J. J., Brunelli, A., Cassivi, S. D., and Deschamps, C. (2012a). Aggregate Risk Score for Predicting Mortality after Surgical Biopsy for Interstitial Lung Disease. *Interactive CardioVascular Thorac. Surg.* 15 (2), 276–279. doi:10.1093/icvts/ivs174

Fibla, J. J., Molins, L., Blanco, A., Royo, Í., Martínez Vallina, P., Martínez, N., et al. (2012b). Video-assisted Thoracoscopic Lung Biopsy in the Diagnosis of Interstitial Lung Disease: a Prospective, Multi-center Study in 224 Patients. *Arch. Bronconeumol. (English Edition)* 48 (3), 81–85. doi:10.1016/j.arbres.2011.11.002

Fischer, A., and Richeldi, L. (2014). Cross-disciplinary Collaboration in Connective Tissue Disease-Related Lung Disease. *Semin. Respir. Crit. Care Med.* 35 (2), 159–165. doi:10.1055/s-0034-1371530

Flaherty, K. R., King, T. E., Jr., Raghu, G., Lynch, J. P., 3rd, Colby, T. V., Travis, W. D., et al. (2004). Idiopathic Interstitial Pneumonia. *Am. J. Respir. Crit. Care Med.* 170 (8), 904–910. doi:10.1164/rccm.200402-147OC

Flaherty, K. R., Wells, A. U., Cottin, V., Devaraj, A., Walsh, S. L. F., Inoue, Y., et al. (2019). Nintedanib in Progressive Fibrosing Interstitial Lung Diseases. *N. Engl. J. Med.* 381 (18), 1718–1727. doi:10.1056/NEJMoa1908681

Han, Q., Luo, Q., Xie, J.-X., Wu, L.-L., Liao, L.-Y., Zhang, X.-X., et al. (2015). Diagnostic Yield and Postoperative Mortality Associated with Surgical Lung Biopsy for Evaluation of Interstitial Lung Diseases: A Systematic Review and Meta-Analysis. *J. Thorac. Cardiovasc. Surg.* 149 (5), 1394–1401.e1. doi:10.1016/j.jtcvs.2014.12.057

Johannson, K. A., Marcoux, V. S., Ronksley, P. E., and Ryerson, C. J. (2016). Diagnostic Yield and Complications of Transbronchial Lung Cryobiopsy for Interstitial Lung Disease: A Systematic Review and Meta-Analysis. *Ann. ATS* 13 (10), 1828–1838. doi:10.1513/AnnalsATS.201606-461SR

Kim, H.-C., Ji, W., Kim, M. Y., Colby, T. V., Jang, S. J., Lee, C.-K., et al. (2015). Interstitial Pneumonia Related to Undifferentiated Connective Tissue Disease. *Chest* 147 (1), 165–172. doi:10.1378/chest.14-0272

Kronborg-White, S., Folkersen, B., Rasmussen, T. R., Voldby, N., Madsen, L. B., Rasmussen, F., et al. (2017). Introduction of Cryobiopsies in the Diagnostics of Interstitial Lung Diseases - Experiences in a Referral center. *Eur. Clin. Respir. J.* 4 (1), 1274099. doi:10.1080/20018525.2016.1274099

Kumar, A., Cherian, S. V., Vassallo, R., Yi, E. S., and Ryu, J. H. (2018). Current Concepts in Pathogenesis, Diagnosis, and Management of Smoking-Related Interstitial Lung Diseases. *Chest* 154 (2), 394–408. doi:10.1016/j.chest.2017.11.023

Luo, Q., Han, Q., Chen, X., Xie, J., Wu, L., and Chen, R. (2013). The Diagnosis Efficacy and Safety of Video-Assisted Thoracoscopy Surgery (VATS) in Undefined Interstitial Lung Diseases: a Retrospective Study. *J. Thorac. Dis.* 5 (3), 283–288. doi:10.3978/j.issn.2072-1439.2013.04.12

Oldham, J. M., Adegunsoye, A., Valenzi, E., Lee, C., Witt, L., Chen, L., et al. (2016). Characterisation of Patients with Interstitial Pneumonia with Autoimmune Features. *Eur. Respir. J.* 47 (6), 1767–1775. doi:10.1183/13993003.01565-2015

Patel, N. M., Borczuk, A. C., and Lederer, D. J. (2016). Cryobiopsy in the Diagnosis of Interstitial Lung Disease. A Step Forward or Back? *Am. J. Respir. Crit. Care Med.* 193 (7), 707–709. doi:10.1164/rccm.201511-2313ED

Peng, G., Liu, M., Luo, Q., Chen, H., Yin, W., Wang, W., et al. (2017). Spontaneous Ventilation Anesthesia Combined with Uniportal and Tubeless Thoracoscopic Lung Biopsy in Selected Patients with Interstitial Lung Diseases. *J. Thorac. Dis.* 9 (11), 4494 4501. doi:10.21037/jtd.2017.10.76

Raghu, G., Collard, H. R., Egan, J. J., Martinez, F. J., Behr, J., Brown, K. K., et al. (2011). An Official ATS/ERS/JRS/ALAT Statement: Idiopathic Pulmonary Fibrosis: Evidence-Based Guidelines for Diagnosis and Management. *Am. J. Respir. Crit. Care Med.* 183 (6), 788–824. doi:10.1164/rccm.2009-040GL

Raghu, G., Remy-Jardin, M., Myers, J. L., Richeldi, L., Ryerson, C. J., Lederer, D. J., et al. (2018). Diagnosis of Idiopathic Pulmonary Fibrosis. An Official ATS/ERS/JRS/ALAT Clinical Practice Guideline. *Am. J. Respir. Crit. Care Med.* 198 (5), e44–e68. doi:10.1164/rccm.201807-1255ST

Raparia, K., Aisner, D. L., Allen, T. C., Beasley, M. B., Borczuk, A., Cagle, P. T., et al. (2016). Transbronchial Lung Cryobiopsy for Interstitial Lung Disease Diagnosis: A Perspective from Members of the Pulmonary Pathology Society. *Arch. Pathol. Lab. Med.* 140 (11), 1281–1284. doi:10.5858/arpa.2016-0258-SA

Ravaglia, C., Bonifazi, M., Wells, A. U., Tomassetti, S., Gurioli, C., Piciucchi, S., et al. (2016). Safety and Diagnostic Yield of Transbronchial Lung Cryobiopsy in Diffuse Parenchymal Lung Diseases: A Comparative Study versus Video-Assisted Thoracoscopic Lung Biopsy and a Systematic Review of the Literature. *Respiration* 91 (3), 215–227. doi:10.1159/000444089

Romagnoli, M., Colby, T. V., Berthet, J.-P., Gamez, A. S., Mallet, J.-P., Serre, I., et al. (2019). Poor Concordance between Sequential Transbronchial Lung Cryobiopsy and Surgical Lung Biopsy in the Diagnosis of Diffuse Interstitial Lung Diseases. *Am. J. Respir. Crit. Care Med.* 199 (10), 1249–1256. doi:10.1164/rccm.201810-1947OC

Sigurdsson, M. I., Isaksson, H. J., Gudmundsson, G., and Gudbjartsson, T. (2009). Diagnostic Surgical Lung Biopsies for Suspected Interstitial Lung Diseases: a Retrospective Study. *Ann. Thorac. Surg.* 88 (1), 227–232. doi:10.1016/j.athoracsur.2009.04.002

Singh, S., Collins, B. F., Sharma, B. B., Joshi, J. M., Talwar, D., Katiyar, S., et al. (2017). Interstitial Lung Disease in India. Results of a Prospective Registry. *Am. J. Respir. Crit. Care Med.* 195 (6), 801–813. doi:10.1164/rccm.201607-1484OC

Tomassetti, S., Wells, A. U., Costabel, U., Cavazza, A., Colby, T. V., Rossi, G., et al. (2016). Bronchoscopic Lung Cryobiopsy Increases Diagnostic Confidence in the Multidisciplinary Diagnosis of Idiopathic Pulmonary Fibrosis. *Am. J. Respir. Crit. Care Med.* 193 (7), 745–752. doi:10.1164/rccm.201504-0711OC

Travis, W. D., Costabel, U., Hansell, D. M., King, T. E., Jr., Lynch, D. A., Nicholson, A. G., et al. (2013). An Official American Thoracic Society/European Respiratory Society Statement: Update of the International Multidisciplinary Classification of the Idiopathic Interstitial Pneumonias. *Am. J. Respir. Crit. Care Med.* 188 (6), 733–748. doi:10.1164/rccm.201308-1483ST

Troy, L. K., Grainge, C., Corte, T. J., Williamson, J. P., Vallely, M. P., Cooper, W. A., et al. (2020). Diagnostic Accuracy of Transbronchial Lung Cryobiopsy for Interstitial Lung Disease Diagnosis (COLDICE): a Prospective, Comparative Study. *Lancet Respir. Med.* 8 (2), 171–181. doi:10.1016/S2213-2600(19)30342-X

11

ΔCT Value of Amplified Refractory Mutation System Predicts Efficacy of EGFR-TKIs in Advanced Non–Small-Cell Lung Cancer

Min Chen[1,2†], Wenqi Huang[3†], Dongyong Yang[4†], Jincheng Huang[4], Gong Li[5], Xiaoqing Wang[1], Nanjie Xiao[1], Weijian Zhang[6], Jian Guan[1], Shuang Wang[7,8*] and Laiyu Liu[3*]*

[1]Department of Radiation Oncology, Nanfang Hospital, Southern Medical University, Guangzhou, China, [2]Department of Radiation Oncology, Peking University Shenzhen Hospital, Shenzhen, China, [3]Chronic Airways Diseases Laboratory, Department of Respiratory and Critical Care Medicine, Nanfang Hospital, Southern Medical University, Guangzhou, China, [4]Department of Respiratory and Critical Care Medicine, Second Affiliated Hospital of Fujian Medical University, Quanzhou, China, [5]Guangdong Provincial Hospital of Traditional Chinese Medicine, Guangzhou, China, [6]Department of Radiation Oncology, The First Affiliation Hospital of Fujian Medical University, Fuzhou, China, [7]Department of Pathology, Nanfang Hospital, Southern Medical University, Guangzhou, China, [8]Department of Pathology, School of Basic Medical Sciences, Southern Medical University, Guangzhou, China

***Correspondence:**
Jian Guan
guanjian5461@163.com
Shuang Wang
shuangw@126.com
Laiyu Liu
liuly5461@163.com

[†]These authors have contributed equally to this work and share first authorship.

Purpose: This multi-center retrospective study determines whether the ΔCT value of the Amplified Refractory Mutation System (ARMS) predicts the efficacy of epidermal growth factor receptor (EGFR) tyrosine kinase inhibitors (TKIs) in EGFR-mutant advanced non–small-cell lung cancer (NSCLC).

Patients and methods: Patients who harbored an exon 19 deletion (19Del) or L858R mutation detected by the ARMS and previously received treatment of EGFR-TKIs as a monotherapy were enrolled. A total of 108 NSCLC patients in four hospitals were enrolled. We divided the patients into a high ΔCT group (Group H) and a low ΔCT group (Group L) by the Martingale residuals analysis and log-rank test. The primary outcome was progression-free survival (PFS). Univariate analysis and multivariable regression were applied to compare the PFS between the groups.

Result: The Martingale residuals analysis and log-rank test were applied to find the cutoff ΔCT value (0.8). In the 108 patients we enrolled, 59 were in group L and 49 were in group H. Patients' demographics and clinical characteristics, including age, sex, smoking history, pathology, mutation sites, TNM stage, and line of TKIs therapy, were not significantly different between group L and group H. The median PFS was 11.1 months in group L and 6.9 months in group H, and the difference showed statistical significance ($p < 0.001$). Moreover, the objective response rates (ORRs) in group L was significantly higher than in group H (61.0 vs 34.7%, $p = 0.002$). The median OS was 25.0 months in group L and 20.0 months in group H ($p = 0.046$).

Conclusion: The ΔCT value of ARMS could be an efficacy predictor for EGFR-TKI treatment in advanced EGFR-mutant NSCLC.

Keywords: ΔCT, ARMS, efficacy, EGFR-TKIs, NSCLC

INTRODUCTION

Lung cancer is the most common cancer leading to cancer-related deaths worldwide. More than 70% of patients with lung cancer are diagnosed with advanced non–small-cell lung cancer (NSCLC) (Siegel et al., 2017). Many clinical trials have demonstrated the superiority of epidermal growth factor receptor (EGFR) tyrosine kinase inhibitors (TKIs) over chemotherapy in the treatment of patients with advanced NSCLC harboring EGFR mutations (Maemondo et al., 2010; Mitsudomi et al., 2010; Rosell et al., 2012; Yang et al., 2013; Wu et al., 2014). Therefore, EGFR-TKIs have been recommended as the standard of care for first-line treatment for EGFR-mutant NSCLC, especially for those who harbored a drug sensitivity-associated mutation including exon 19 deletion (19Del) and exon 21 L858R. However, these clinical trials also showed that the efficacy of EGFR-TKIs was not so satisfactory in a nonnegligible proportion of NSCLCs harboring sensitive EGFR mutations. In the studies we have mentioned above (Maemondo et al., 2010; Mitsudomi et al., 2010; Rosell et al., 2012; Yang et al., 2013; Wu et al., 2014), 20–44% patients who harbored EGFR mutation had a best response of stable disease (SD) or progressive disease (PD) and 8–15% patients had a best response of PD. Still a significant minority of patients had a primary resistance or poor progression of disease (PFS) to EGFR-TKIs when harbored sensitive EGFR mutations.

Distinguishing patients who are most likely to experience an expected response to EGFR-TKIs from those who are not likely to show a response has emerged as a crucial issue. Although previous studies had reported several resistance mechanisms of EGFR TKIs for EGFR-mutant NSCLC patients, in many cases, the mechanisms remain unclear (Costa et al., 2014; Beau-Faller et al., 2014; Ogino et al., 2007; Engelman et al., 2007). Efforts are still needed to explore the reasons for the various rates of resistance to EGFR-TKIs for EGFR-mutant NSCLC.

The correlation of intratumor heterogeneity of tumor and drug resistance has been widely studied in recent years (Turner and Reis-Filho, 2012; Jamal-Hanjani et al., 2015; Mangano et al., 2015). For the EGFR heterogeneity in lung cancer, recent reports have indicated that tumors are composed of mixed populations of mutant EGFR and wild-type EGFR cells, suggesting that the intratumor heterogeneity does indeed exist (Jiang et al., 2008; Taniguchi et al., 2008; Wei et al., 2014; Cai et al., 2015). Furthermore, several groups have demonstrated that the intratumor heterogeneity of EGFR-mutant NSCLC associated with the efficacy of EGFR-TKIs. They demonstrated that patients with higher relative abundance of EGFR mutation showed longer PFS (Jiang et al., 2008; Taniguchi et al., 2008; Zhou et al., 2011; Zhao et al., 2014a; Zhao et al., 2014b). These reports gave a great inspiration to the development of the therapeutic strategy of EGFR-TKIs. Researchers advised that for patients who harbored a high ratio of EGFR mutation in tumor, EGFR-TKI was effective to control the progression of tumor, but for the low, monotherapy of EGFR-TKIs may be not enough. However, until now, there was not any effective and convenient ways for clinicians to distinguish whether a patient is harboring a high ratio of EGFR mutation in tumor or not. Therefore, there is an urgent need to develop a method to assess the abundance of *EGFR* mutations in NSCLC in clinical practice. The Amplified Refractory Mutation System (ARMS) had widely been applied in the detection of EGFR mutation in recent years (Shaozhang et al., 2014). Mutant allele assays were run with a gene reference assay, which was designed to a mutation-free region of the gene. The mutational status of a sample was determined by calculating the ΔCT value between amplification reactions for a mutant allele assay and gene reference assay, as follows: ΔCT = Ct (mutant allele assay) – Ct (gene reference assay). Mutation or not is determined by the Ct value and ΔCT value. The reference gene was a relatively conserved region of the EGFR gene. Thus, Ct (gene reference assay) could effectively reflect the DNA level of the EGFR gene. For the tumor samples with EGFR mutation, the ΔCT value could reflect the relative level of EGFR mutation in the tumor sample. Therefore, we assume that patients with a lower ΔCT value may harbor a high ratio of EGFR mutation and may associate with better response to EGFR-TKIs. Furthermore, we divided the EGFR-mutant NSCLC into a low ΔCT value and a high ΔCT value to explore whether the ΔCT value of the tumor sample could be a predictor for the efficacy of EGFR-TKIs in EGFR-mutant NSCLC patients.

Patients and Methods

Patients

A total of 108 Chinese patients were enrolled in this study from four medical centers in China including Nanfang Hospital of Southern Medical University, the first affiliated hospital of Fujian Medical University, the second affiliated hospital of Fujian Medical University, and Guangdong Province Traditional Medical Hospital between March 2013 and Jan 2015. The criteria for the patients enrolled in this retrospective study were as follows: 1. Diagnosed with advanced NSCLC and harbored a drug sensitivity-associated mutation site (19Del and L858R). 2. EGFR mutations were tested by ARMS (Shanghai Yuanqi Bio-Pharmaceutical Company Limited, Shanghai, China) and previously received treatment of EGFR-TKIs including gefitinib, erlotinib and icotinib as a monotherapy. The data we collected of all patients were from the electronic medical record system in the four medical centers.

Epidermal Growth Factor Receptor Mutation Analysis

EGFR mutation testing was performed on formalin-fixed paraffin-embedded (FFPE) specimens from primary tumor obtained from bronchoscopic biopsy or CT-guided core biopsy before any tumor-related treatment. The HE-stained section of FFPE was assessed again to establish the pathological diagnosis. Some of the FFPE samples were trimmed according to the HE-stained section to make sure that the samples we would test were all tumors. The genomic DNA was isolated and purified from tumor specimens using the DNeasy Blood & Tissue Kit (Qiagen,

Valencia, CA, United States) according to the manufacturer's instructions. EGFR mutation detection was performed according to the principles of the ARMS, using the Human EGFR Gene Mutation Detection Kit (PCR Fluorescence Probe) (Shanghai Yuanqi Bio-Pharmaceutical Company Limited, Shanghai, China) on the MX3005P QPCR system (Agilent, Santa Clara, CA, United States), according to manufacturers' recommendations. It covered 23 EGFR mutation hotspots within exons 18, 19, 20 and 21. The results were analyzed according to the criteria defined by the manufacturer's instructions. Positive results were defined as Ct (mutant allele assay) - Ct (gene reference assay) < ΔCT (cutoff). We divided the patients into two groups by the media ΔCT value.

Statistical Analyses

The primary end point was progression-free survival (PFS), and the second end points were the objective response rate (ORR) and primary resistance. In patients with measurable disease, the tumor burden was assessed by the Response Evaluation Criteria in Solid Tumor (RECIST) and categorized as a complete response (CR), partial response (PR), stable disease (SD), or progressive disease (PD) (Eisenhauer et al., 2009). PFS was calculated from the time from commencement of EGFR-TKIs treatment to PD according to the RECIST criteria or death resulting from any cause. OS was calculated from the time from commencement of EGFR-TKI treatment to death. The definition of primary resistance to EGFR-TKIs was not uniform among researchers, and in this study, we defined it as patients who had progressive disease to EGFR TKI without initial objective response (Cortot and Janne, 2014). The Kaplan–Meier method was applied to analyze the PFS or OS, and the Cox proportional hazard model was applied to explore the statistical difference in PFS between different groups. A comparison of ORRs and rates of primary resistance in different groups was made using $\chi 2$ tests. A two-sided p value of less than 0.05 was considered statistically significant.

RESULT

Patient Characteristics

A total of 108 patients who fully met the enrollment criteria were enrolled in the present study. In all the patients, the median age was 61 (ranged from 40 to 83 years); 52 were males and 56 were females; 63 were never smokers and 45 were current or former smokers; three were non-adenocarcinoma and 105 were adenocarcinoma; 57 patients harbored a 19Del mutation and 51 harbored a L858R mutation; and 87 patients received EGFR-TKI as the first-line therapy, 20 patients received EGFR-TKI as the second line therapy, and 1 received EGFR-TKI as the third-line therapy.

Epidermal Growth Factor Receptor Mutation Groups

Martingale residuals analysis was applied, and a non-linear relationship was noted between the ΔCT value and PFS of the patients (**Figures 1A,B**). The risk of event went down with an increasing ΔCT value when ΔCT < −1, remained steadily when −1 > ΔCT <1, and increased when ΔCT >1. Thus, we applied log-ranking analysis to find the cutoff ΔCT value. The ΔCT value corresponding to the maximum log-rank value was defined as the cutoff ΔCT value and was 0.8, which agreed with the tendency in the Martingale residuals analysis (**Figure 1C**).

59 patients had a ΔCT value less than 0.8 (group L), and 49 patients had a ΔCT value greater than 0.8 (group H). The median of age was similar between group L and group H (60 vs 61, p = 0.499). 49.2% of group L and 55.1% of group H were female (p = 0.538). The proportions of never smokers in group L and group H were similar (71.2 vs 71.4%, p = 0.978), and 19Del was more frequent in group L than L858R mutation (61.0 vs 42.9%, p = 0.060). The TNM stage and line of TKI therapy were all well balanced between the two groups (p = 0.356, p = 0.818). Treatment with different EGFR-TKIs was balanced between the two groups (p = 0.422) (**Table 1**).

Efficacy of Different ΔCT Value Groups

All the patients were received TKIs from Jan 2013 to Dec 2015 in the four hospitals. The last follow-up date was Aug 9, 2021.100 (92.6%) patients experienced a disease progression, and 36 (33.3%) of the patients were still alive or concord.

The median PFS was 11.1 months (95% CI, 9.8–12.3) in group L and 6.9 months (95% CI, 5.1–8.6) in group H, and the difference showed statistical significance (p < 0.001) (**Figure 2A**). Multivariate analysis shows that the ΔCT value was the variable that mostly influences the PFS (**Table 2**).

The rate of primary resistance in group H was significantly higher than in group L (26.5% *vs* 5.1%, p = 0.002). ORRs in group L were significantly higher than in group H (61.0% *vs* 34.7%, p = 0.002). The median OS was 24.0 months (95% CI, 19.8–28.2) in group L and 19.0 months in group H (95% CI, 15.4–22.6), which was statistically significant (p = 0.046). (**Table 3; Figure 2B**).

In addition, for patients who either harbored 19Del or L858R mutation, patients in group L had better PFS than those in group H. For patients who harbored 19Del mutation, the median PFS was 10.8 months (95% CI, 10.2–11.4) in group L and 6.8 months (95% CI, 5.3–8.4) in group H, and the difference was statistically significant (p = 0.001) (**Figure 2C**). For patients who harbored L858R mutation, the median PFS was 12.8 months (95% CI, 8.8–16.7) in group L and 6.1 months (95% CI, 3.3–9.1) in group H, and the difference showed statistical significance (p < 0.001) (**Figure 2D**).

Efficacy of EGFR 19Del and EGFR 21 L858R Mutation

The PFS of patients who harbored 19Del mutation was 9.1 months (95% CI, 7.9–10.2), and in patients who harbored L858R mutation, PFS was 10.6 months (95% CI, 8.5–12.7). The difference between the two group was not significant (p = 0.634) (**Figure 2A**). ORRs in patients who harbored 19Del were higher than in those who harbored L858R mutation, while the difference showed no significance (59.7 vs 39.2%, p = 0.034). However, the rate of

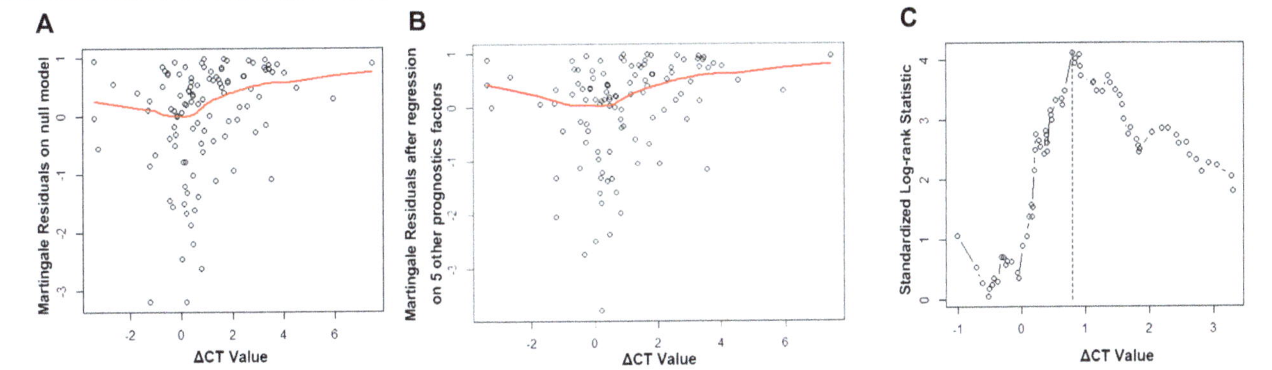

FIGURE 1 | Martingale residuals analysis and standard log-rank analysis. **(A)** Martingale residuals analysis of the association between the ΔCT value and progression-free survival (PFS). **(B)** Martingale residuals analysis of the association between the ΔCT value and PFS by age, gender, smoking status, mutation sites, and therapy line (first-line or second-line therapy). **(C)** Standard log-rank statistic to determine the cutoff value.

TABLE 1 | Patient demographics and clinical characteristics.

		ΔCT value				
		Group L (n = 59)		Group H (n = 49)		
Variable	**Total**	**No. of patients**	**%**	**No. of patients**	**%**	**P**
Age, years						0.499
Median (range)	61 (40–83)	60 (40–83)		61 (41–79)		
Sex						0.538
Male	52	30	50.8	22	44.9	
Female	56	29	49.2	27	55.1	
Smoking history						0.978
Never-smoker	77	42	71.2	35	71.4	
Current or former-smoker	31	17	28.8	14	28.6	
Pathology						0.412
Non-adeno	3	2	3.4	1	1.9	
Adeno	105	57	96.6	48	98.1	
Mutation site						0.060
19Del	57	36	61.0	21	42.9	
L858R	51	23	39.0	28	57.1	
TNM stage						0.356
IIIB	7	5	8.5	2	4.1	
IV	101	54	91.5	47	95.9	
Line of therapy						0.818
First	87	48	81.4	39	79.6	
Second	21	11	18.6	10	20.4	
EGFR-TKIs						0.422
Gefitinib	50	26	44.1	24	49.0	
Erlotinib	44	27	45.8	17	34.7	
Icotinib	14	6	10.2	8	16.3	

Group L: patients with a lower ΔCT value; group H: patients with a higher ΔCT value; adeno: adenocarcinoma.

primary resistance was significantly higher in patients with L858R mutation than those with 19Del (23.5 vs 6.3%, $p = 0.018$) (**Table 4**).

In addition, for patients in group L, the PFS of the patients who harbored 19Del was 10.8 months (95% CI, 10.2–11.4) and the PFS of the patients who harbored L858R was 12.8 months (95% CI, 8.8–16.7) (p = 0.222) (**Figure 3B**). For patients in group H, the PFS of the patients who harbored 19Del mutation was 6.8 months (95% CI, 5.3–8.4) and the PFS of the patients who harbored L858R was 6.2 months (95% CI, 3.3–9.1) (p = 0.551) (**Figure 3C**).

DISCUSSION

Our study put forward a new possible predictor for efficacy of EGFR-TKIs. We first put forward that the ΔCT value from the ARMS-PCR in EGFR mutation testing could be a predictor for efficacy of EGFR-TKI treatment for advanced EGFR-mutant NSCLC. Patients with a lower ΔCT value of EGFR mutations may benefit more than those with a higher ΔCT value of EGFR mutations according to the statistically different PFS between the groups, and PFS of the two groups had no overlaps. This might

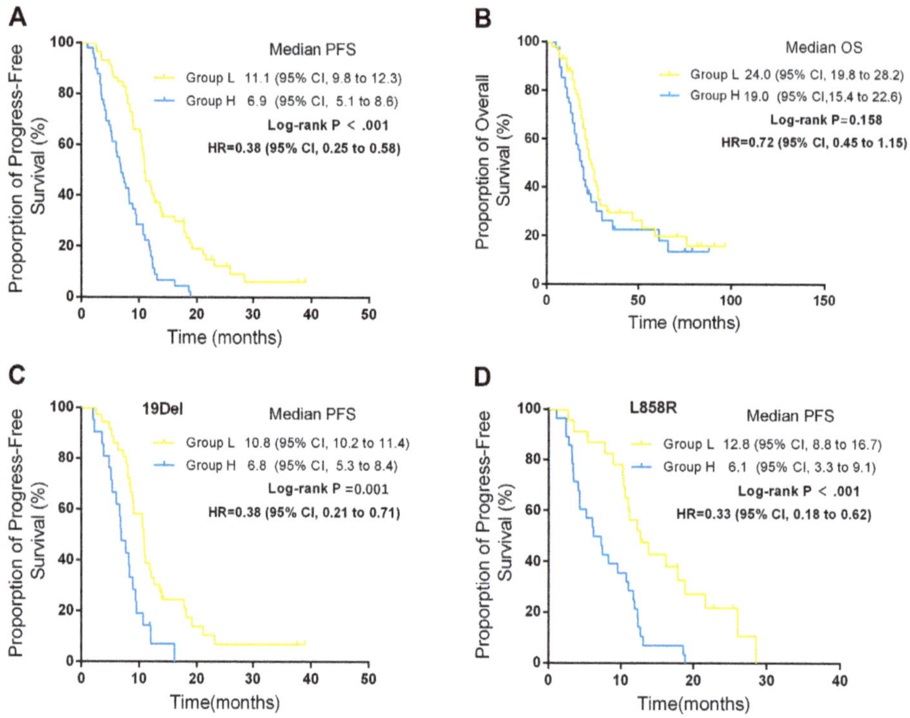

FIGURE 2 | Progression-free survival (PFS) and overall survival (OS) between different ΔCT value groups. **(A)** PFS between different ΔCT value groups. **(B)** OS between different ΔCT value groups. **(C)** PFS between different ΔCT value groups in patients harboring *EGFR* 19Del. **(D)** PFS between different ΔCT value groups in patients harboring *EGFR* L858R.

TABLE 2 | Multivariate analyses of PFS by Cox regression analysis.

Variable	HR	95% CI	*p* Value
ΔCT value groups			
Group L	0.358	0.231–0.555	<0.001
Group H		Reference	
Mutation site			
19Del	1.299	0.848–1.989	0.229
L858R		Reference	
Gender			
Male	1.055	0.612–1.820	0.847
Female		Reference	
Age	0.980	0.956	1.004
Smoking or not			
Never-smoker	1.311	0.727–2.363	0.368
Current or former-smoker		Reference	
Line of therapy			
First	1.311	0.727–2.363	0.096
Second		Reference	

PFS, progression free survival; HR, hazard ratio; CI, confidence interval.

partly explain why some patients who harbored sensitive EGFR mutation did not experience an expected duration of response to EGFR-TKIs. Just like the previous studies, the data of the present study made us not only to focus on whether the patients harbored an EGFR mutation but also to consider the relative abundance of EGFR mutations when making therapeutic strategies for NSCLC (Jiang et al., 2008; Taniguchi et al., 2008; Zhou et al., 2011; Zhao et al., 2014a; Zhao et al., 2014b). What is further than the previous research was that we put forward a predictor that could be conveniently applied in clinical practice. By relatively quantifying the EGFR mutations in tumor tissue according to ΔCT value, patients with a low ΔCT value of EGFR mutations could receive EGFR-TKI treatment because they would benefit the most. However, for patients with a high ΔCT value of EGFR mutations, monotherapy of EGFR-TKIs may not be enough to control the tumor progression. Owing to the fact that 45.4% of the patients were still alive or concord, overall survival was required further to follow up.

Sheng et al. (2015) conducted a meta-analysis including 26 studies and showed that patients with NSCLC and EGFR exon 19 deletion had a longer PFS, OS, and higher ORR compared with exon 21 L858R mutation after EGFR-TKI therapy. Zhang et al. (2017) thought they may be two distinct diseases. However, it remains unclear why the difference in the outcome exists between the two mutation sites. In our study, ignoring the absence of statistical significance, exon 19Del was more frequent in the group of the low ΔCT value and showed higher rate of ORR and lower rate of primary resistance to EGFR-TKIs than exon 21 L858R. Although the PFS showed similarity in the two groups, it may be a clue for researchers to find out the reason why exon 19Del has a better response to EGFR-TKIs. For us, studies with large samples will be conducted to further our findings.

There were some advantages and disadvantages in the present study. The first advantage is that this was a multi-center retrospective study and all the data we recorded were from the electronic medical record system, which made our result more reliable. The second advantage is that the

TABLE 3 | Efficacy of different ΔCT value groups.

Variable	Total	ΔCT value				P
		Group L (*n* = 59)		Group H (*n* = 49)		
		No. of patients	%	No. of patients	%	
PFS, days						<0.001
Median		11.1		6.9		
95% CI		9.8 to 12.3		5.1 to 8.6		
OS, days						0.158
Median		24.0		19.0		
95% CI		19.8–28.2		15.4–22.6		
Primary resistance						0.002
Yes	16	3	5.6	13	24.1	
No	92	56	94.9	36	73.5	
Tumor response						0.002
CR	0	0	0	0	0	
PR	53	36	61.0	17	34.7	
SD	39	20	33.9	19	38.8	
PD	16	3	5.1	13	26.5	

PFS, progression free survival; OS, overall survival; CR, complete response; PR, partial response; SD, stable disease; PD, progressive disease; CI, confidence interval.

TABLE 4 | Efficacy of EGFR 19Del and EGFR 21 L858R mutation.

Variable	Total	Mutation sites				P
		E19Del (n = 57)		L858R (n = 51)		
		No. of patients	%	No. of patients	%	
PFS, months						0.643
Median		9.1		10.6		
95% CI		7.9–10.2		8.5–12.7		
OS, months						
Median		25.3		21.6		0.241
95% CI		21.0–29.7		18.0–25.2		
Primary resistance						0.018
Yes	16	4	6.3	12	23.5	
No	92	53	93.7	39	76.5	
Tumor response						0.026
CR	0	0	0	0	0	
PR	54	34	59.7	20	39.2	
SD	38	19	33.3	19	37.3	
PD	16	4	7.0	12	23.5	

PFS, progress free survival; OS, overall survival; CR, complete response; PR, partial response; SD, stable disease; PD, progressive disease; CI, confidence interval.

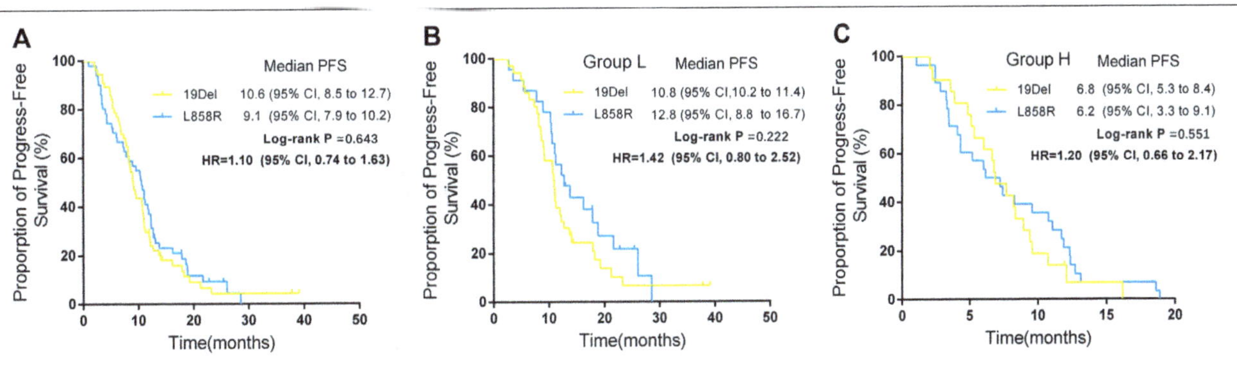

FIGURE 3 | Progression free survival (PFS) between different mutation sites and groups. **(A)** PFS between different mutation sites. **(B)** PFS between different mutation sites in group L. **(C)** PFS between different mutation sites in group H.

predictor we found in this study was much more applicable in clinical practice than in other previous studies.

The first limitation of this study is that the patients in our study had a tumor response evaluation per 8–12 weeks after EGFR-TKIs were taken. However, the proportion of patients had an evaluation per 8–10 weeks and per 11–12 weeks, which were not significantly different. The second limitation is that the follow-up of OS was not regular in our study and might lead to a large bias. However, our aim of this study was to explore whether the ΔCT value affects the efficacy of EGFR-TKIs. The third one was that only one site of the tumor sample was obtained from each patient. Nonetheless, we trimmed some of the tumor sample to ensure that every sample content is a cancerous cell to make our results more reliable. Wei et al. (2014) have demonstrated that the EGFR mutation ratio showed a high level of concordance in primary tumors and when the tumor content is more than 50% in a tumor sample, a randomly chosen sample would reliably represent the type and ratio of mutations of EGFR in primary tumors.

CONCLUSION

In summary, our study suggests that the ΔCT value of EGFR mutations could predict the efficacy of EGFR-TKI treatment in EGFR mutant NSCLC. We hope this indicator would contribute to more accurate technologies to evaluate the ratio of EGFR mutation in tumors.

AUTHOR CONTRIBUTIONS

LL, SW, GJ, and MC contributed to the conception and design of the study. MC, WH and DY performed the statistical analysis and wrote the first draft of the manuscript. JH, GL, XW, NX, and WZ organized the database. All authors contributed to manuscript revision and read and approved the submitted version.

REFERENCES

Beau-Faller, M., Prim, N., Ruppert, A.-M., Nanni-Metéllus, I., Lacave, R., Lacroix, L., et al. (2014). Rare EGFR Exon 18 and Exon 20 Mutations in Non-small-cell Lung Cancer on 10 117 Patients: a Multicentre Observational Study by the French ERMETIC-IFCT Network. *Ann. Oncol.* 25, 126–131. doi:10.1093/annonc/mdt418

Cai, W., Lin, D., Wu, C., Li, X., Zhao, C., Zheng, L., et al. (2015). Intratumoral Heterogeneity of ALK-Rearranged and ALK/EGFR Coaltered Lung Adenocarcinoma. *J. Clin. Oncol.* 33, 3701–3709. doi:10.1200/jco.2014.58.8293

Cortot, A. B., and Janne, P. A. (2014). Molecular Mechanisms of Resistance in Epidermal Growth Factor Receptor-Mutant Lung Adenocarcinomas. *Eur. Respir. Rev.* 23, 356–366. doi:10.1183/09059180.00004614

Costa, C., Molina, M. A., Drozdowskyj, A., Giménez-Capitán, A., Bertran-Alamillo, J., Karachaliou, N., et al. (2014). The Impact of EGFR T790M Mutations and BIM mRNA Expression on Outcome in Patients with EGFR-Mutant NSCLC Treated with Erlotinib or Chemotherapy in the Randomized Phase III EURTAC Trial. *Clin. Cancer Res.* 20, 2001–2010. doi:10.1158/1078-0432.CCR-13-2233

Eisenhauer, E. A., Therasse, P., Bogaerts, J., Schwartz, L. H., Sargent, D., Ford, R., et al. (2009). New Response Evaluation Criteria in Solid Tumours: Revised RECIST Guideline (Version 1.1). *Eur. J. Cancer* 45, 228–247. doi:10.1016/j.ejca.2008.10.026

Engelman, J. A., Zejnullahu, K., Mitsudomi, T., Song, Y., Hyland, C., Park, J. O., et al. (2007). MET Amplification Leads to Gefitinib Resistance in Lung Cancer by Activating ERBB3 Signaling. *Science* 316, 1039–1043. doi:10.1126/science.1141478

Jamal-Hanjani, M., Quezada, S. A., Larkin, J., and Swanton, C. (2015). Translational Implications of Tumor Heterogeneity. *Clin. Cancer Res.* 21, 1258–1266. doi:10.1158/1078-0432.CCR-14-1429

Jiang, S. X., Yamashita, K., Yamamoto, M., Piao, C. J., Umezawa, A., Saegusa, M., et al. (2008). EGFR Genetic Heterogeneity of Nonsmall Cell Lung Cancers Contributing to Acquired Gefitinib Resistance. *Int. J. Cancer* 123, 2480–2486. doi:10.1002/ijc.23868

Maemondo, M., Inoue, A., Kobayashi, K., Sugawara, S., Oizumi, S., Isobe, H., et al. (2010). Gefitinib or Chemotherapy for Non-small-cell Lung Cancer with Mutated EGFR. *N. Engl. J. Med.* 362, 2380–2388. doi:10.1056/NEJMoa0909530

Mangano, A., Lianos, G. D., Mangano, A., Boni, L., and Dionigi, G., (2015). Intratumor Heterogeneity: Origins, Clinical Significance and Optimal Strategies for Cancer Treatment. *Future Oncol.* 11, 561–564. doi:10.2217/fon.14.296

Mitsudomi, T., Morita, S., Yatabe, Y., Negoro, S., Okamoto, I., Tsurutani, J., et al. (2010). Gefitinib versus Cisplatin Plus Docetaxel in Patients with Non-small-cell Lung Cancer Harbouring Mutations of the Epidermal Growth Factor Receptor (WJTOG3405): an Open Label, Randomised Phase 3 Trial. *Lancet Oncol.* 11, 121–128. doi:10.1016/S1470-2045(09)70364-X

Ogino, A., Kitao, H., Hirano, S., Uchida, A., Ishiai, M., Kozuki, T., et al. (2007). Emergence of Epidermal Growth Factor Receptor T790M Mutation during Chronic Exposure to Gefitinib in a Non Small Cell Lung Cancer Cell Line. *Cancer Res.* 67, 7807–7814. doi:10.1158/0008-5472.CAN-07-0681

Rosell, R., Carcereny, E., Gervais, R., Vergnenegre, A., Massuti, B., Felip, E., et al. (2012). Erlotinib versus Standard Chemotherapy as First-Line Treatment for European Patients with Advanced EGFR Mutation-Positive Non-small-cell Lung Cancer (EURTAC): a Multicentre, Open-Label, Randomised Phase 3 Trial. *Lancet Oncol.* 13, 239–246. doi:10.1016/S1470-2045(11)70393-X

Shaozhang, Z., Ming, Z., Haiyan, P., Aiping, Z., Qitao, Y., Xiangqun, S., et al. (2014). Comparison of ARMS and Direct Sequencing for Detection of EGFR Mutation and Prediction of EGFR-TKI Efficacy between Surgery and Biopsy Tumor Tissues in NSCLC Patients. *Med. Oncol.* 31, 926. doi:10.1007/s12032-014-0926-3

Sheng, M., Wang, F., Zhao, Y., Li, S., Wang, X., Tao, S., et al. (2015). Comparison of Clinical Outcomes of Patients with Non-small-cell Lung Cancer Harbouring Epidermal Growth Factor Receptor Exon 19 or Exon 21 Mutations after Tyrosine Kinase Inhibitors Treatment: a Meta-Analysis. *Eur. J. Clin. Pharmacol.* 72, 1. doi:10.1007/s00228-015-1966-0

Siegel, R. L., Miller, K. D., and Ahmedin, J. (2017). Cancer Statistics, 2017. *CA Cancer J. Clin.* 67, 7–30. doi:10.3322/caac.21387

Taniguchi, K., Okami, J., Kodama, K., Higashiyama, M., and Kato, K., (2008). Intratumor Heterogeneity of Epidermal Growth Factor Receptor Mutations in Lung Cancer and its Correlation to the Response to Gefitinib. *Cancer Sci.* 99, 929–935. doi:10.1111/j.1349-7006.2008.00782.x

Turner, N. C., and Reis-Filho, J. S. (2012). Genetic Heterogeneity and Cancer Drug Resistance. *Lancet Oncol.* 13, e178–e185. doi:10.1016/s1470-2045(11)70335-7

Wei, B., Yang, K., Zhao, J., Chang, Y., Ma, Z., Dong, B., et al. (2014). Quantification of EGFR Mutations in Primary and Metastatic Tumors in Non-small Cell Lung Cancer. *J. Exp. Clin. Cancer Res.* 33 (5), 5. doi:10.1186/1756-9966-33-5

Wu, Y.-L., Zhou, C., Hu, C.-P., Feng, J., Lu, S., Huang, Y., et al. (2014). Afatinib versus Cisplatin Plus Gemcitabine for First-Line Treatment of Asian Patients with Advanced Non-small-cell Lung Cancer Harbouring EGFR Mutations (LUX-Lung 6): an Open-Label, Randomised Phase 3 Trial. *Lancet Oncol.* 15, 213 222. doi:10.1016/s1470-2045(13)70604-1

Yang, J. C., Hirsh, V., Schuler, M., Yamamoto, N., O'Byrne, K. J., Mok, T. S., et al. (2013). Symptom Control and Quality of Life in LUX-Lung 3: a Phase III Study of Afatinib or Cisplatin/pemetrexed in Patients with Advanced Lung Adenocarcinoma with EGFR Mutations. *J. Clin. Oncol.* 31, 3342–3350. doi:10.1200/JCO.2012.46.1764

Zhang, Y., Chen, G., Chen, X., Fang, W., Gao, F., Yang, Y., et al. (2017). The Comparison of EGFR-TKI Failure Modes and Subsequent Management between Exon 19 Deletion and Exon 21 L858R Mutation in Advanced Non-small-cell Lung Cancer. *J. Cancer* 8, 1865–1871. doi:10.7150/jca.19867

Zhao, J., Wang, X., Xue, L., Xu, N., Ye, X., Zeng, H., et al. (2014). The Use of Mutation-specific Antibodies in Predicting the Effect of EGFR-TKIs in Patients with Non-small-cell Lung Cancer. *J. Cancer Res. Clin. Oncol.* 140, 849–857. doi:10.1007/s00432-014-1618-2

Zhao, Z.-R., Wang, J.-F., Lin, Y.-B., Wang, F., Fu, S., Zhang, S.-L., et al. (2014). Mutation Abundance Affects the Efficacy of EGFR Tyrosine Kinase Inhibitor Readministration in Non-small-cell Lung Cancer with Acquired Resistance. *Med. Oncol.* 31, 810. doi:10.1007/s12032-013-0810-6

Zhou, Q., Zhang, X.-C., Chen, Z.-H., Yin, X.-L., Yang, J.-J., Xu, C.-R., et al. (2011). Relative Abundance of EGFR Mutations Predicts Benefit from Gefitinib Treatment for Advanced Non-small-cell Lung Cancer. *J. Clin. Oncol.* 29, 3316–3321. doi:10.1200/jco.2010.33.3757

12

Enhancing Extracellular Adenosine Levels Restores Barrier Function in Acute Lung Injury through Expression of Focal Adhesion Proteins

Wei Wang[1], Ning-yuan Chen[2], Dewei Ren[3], Jonathan Davies[4], Kemly Philip[2], Holger K. Eltzschig[5], Michael R. Blackburn[2,6], Bindu Akkanti[7], Harry Karmouty-Quintana[2,6,7] and Tingting Weng[2,6]**

[1]Department of Thoracic Surgery, Renmin Hospital of Wuhan University, Wuhan, China, [2]Department of Biochemistry and Molecular Biology, McGovern Medical School, The University of Texas Health Science Center at Houston, Houston, TX, United States, [3]Houston Methodist J.C. Walter Jr. Transplant Center, Houston Methodist Hospital, Houston, TX, United States, [4]Division of Neonatal-Perinatal Medicine, Department of Pediatrics, Baylor College of Medicine, Houston, TX, United States, [5]Department of Anesthesiology, McGovern Medical School, The University of Texas Health Science Center at Houston, Houston, TX, United States, [6]UTHealth Pulmonary Center of Excellence, Houston, TX, United States, [7]Divisions of Critical Care, Pulmonary and Sleep Medicine, Department of Internal Medicine, McGovern Medical School, The University of Texas Health Science Center at Houston, Houston, TX, United States

***Correspondence:**
Harry Karmouty-Quintana
harry.karmouty@uth.tmc.edu
Tingting Weng
tingting.weng@uth.tmc.edu

Background: Acute respiratory distress syndrome (ARDS) is a clinical presentation of acute lung injury (ALI) with often fatal lung complication. Adenosine, a nucleoside generated following cellular stress provides protective effects in acute injury. The levels of extracellular adenosine can be depleted by equilibrative nucleoside transporters (ENTs). ENT inhibition by pharmaceutical agent dipyridamole promotes extracellular adenosine accumulation and is protective in ARDS. However, the therapeutic potential of dipyridamole in acute lung injury has not yet been evaluated.

Methods: Adenosine acts on three adenosine receptors, the adenosine A1 (Adora1), A2a (Adora2a), the A2b (Adora2b) or the adenosine A3 (Adora 3) receptor. Accumulation of adenosine is usually required to stimulate the low-affinity Adora2b receptor. In order to investigate the effect of adenosine accumulation and the contribution of epithelial-specific ENT2 or adora2b expression in experimental ALI, dipyridamole, and epithelial specific ENT2 or Adora2b deficient mice were utilized. MLE12 cells were used to probe downstream Adora2b signaling. Adenosine receptors, transporters, and targets were determined in ARDS lungs.

Results: ENT2 is mainly expressed in alveolar epithelial cells and is negatively regulated by hypoxia following tissue injury. Enhancing adenosine levels with ENT1/ENT2 inhibitor dipyridamole at a time when bleomycin-induced ALI was present, reduced further injury. Mice pretreated with the ADORA2B agonist BAY 60-6583 were protected from bleomycin-induced ALI by reducing vascular leakage (558.6 ± 50.4 vs. 379.9 ± 70.4, $p < 0.05$), total bronchoalveolar lavage fluid cell numbers (17.9 ± 1.8 to 13.4 ± 1.4 e4, $p < 0.05$), and neutrophil infiltration (6.42 ± 0.25 vs. 3.94 ± 0.29, $p < 0.05$). While mice lacking *Adora2b* in AECs were no longer protected by dipyridamole. We also identified occludin and focal adhesion kinase as downstream targets of ADORA2B, thus providing a novel mechanism for adenosine-mediated barrier protection. Similarly, we also observed similar enhanced ADORA2B (3.33 ± 0.67 to 16.12 ± 5.89, $p < 0.05$) and decreased occludin (81.2 ± 0.3 to 13.3 ± 0.4, $p < 0.05$) levels in human Acute respiratory distress syndrome lungs.

Conclusion: We have highlighted a role of dipyridamole and adenosine signaling in preventing or treating ALI and identified Ent2 and Adora2b as key mediators in important for the resolution of ALI.

Keywords: barrier function, pulmonary edema, ARDS, focal adhesion, equilibrative nucleoside transporters (ENTs), alveolar type 2 cell

INTRODUCTION

Acute respiratory distress syndrome (ARDS) is a clinical presentation of acute lung injury (ALI) characterized by progressive arterial hypoxemia, and dyspnea (Nuckton et al., 2002) caused primarily by pulmonary edema (Ware and Matthay, 2000; Matthay et al., 2012). According to the Berlin definition, ARDS is the presence of bilateral opacities from chest imaging, pulmonary edema not due to cardiac failure or fluid overload, and arterial oxygenation calculated by the PaO_2/FiO_2 ratio. A ratio less than 300 mmHg is termed mild, less than 200 is termed moderate, and less than 100 is severe (Ranieri et al., 2012). The etiology of ARDS is complex and multifactorial: sepsis, pneumonia, major trauma, blood transfusion, smoke inhalation, and aspiration of salt water, fresh water or gastric contents can all promote ALI (Ware and Matthay, 2000). ARDS affects approximately 200,000 Americans and has a mortality of approximately 45% (Flori et al., 2005;). Currently there are no effective treatment options for ARDS (Matthay and Zemans, 2011). This has been painfully apparent in the current COVID-19 pandemic where the vast majority of patients that succumb present with an atypical form of ARDS (Gong et al., 2020; Li and Ma, 2020; Liang et al., 2020), this underscores our need to develop new treatment options for this devastating disease.

Disruption of epithelial and endothelial barrier function is a hallmark of ALI (Ware, 2006). The lung epithelium usually maintains an impermeable network through interactions of numerous structural proteins, including tight junction and focal adhesion proteins. Disruption of tight junction and focal adhesion proteins, including occludins, claudins and focal adhesion kinase (FAK), in epithelial cells promotes the permeability of alveolar epithelium and facilitates the progression of ARDS (Ma et al., 2013; Suzuki, 2013). Preserved epithelial barrier function is inversely associated with mortality of patients with ARDS (Matthay and Zemans, 2011; Fanelli and Ranieri, 2015), suggesting signaling pathways regulating the expression and/or functions of the tight junction and focal adhesion proteins may be a valid therapeutic target for ARDS.

Recently, several studies suggest extracellular adenosine as a potential therapeutic agent for the prevention of lung damage (Kong et al., 2006; Eckle et al., 2009; Eltzschig, 2009; Eltzschig et al., 2013; Karmouty-Quintana et al., 2013). Extracellular adenosine is enhanced in areas with injury and is generated by the breakdown of precursor nucleotides including ATP, ADP and AMP by nucleotidases CD39 and CD73 (Eltzschig et al., 2013; Karmouty-Quintana et al., 2013; Idzko et al., 2014). Adenosine functions through activation of G-protein-coupled receptors (Adora1, Adora2a, Adora2b, and Adora3), and increased extracellular adenosine is normally associated with enhanced barrier functions and decreased ALI (Blackburn et al., 2009; Eckle et al., 2009).Blocking equilibrative nucleoside transporters (ENTs) with dipyridamole or by genetically deleting *Ent2* significantly enhanced extracellular adenosine in the alveoli, and as a result suppressed pulmonary inflammation and vascular leakage in ventilator-induced lung injury (Eckle et al., 2013; Morote-Garcia et al., 2013). In contrast, genetic depletion of CD73, a nucleotidase that is essential for adenosine generation, increased inflammation as well as pulmonary vascular leakage (Eltzschig et al., 2005; Reutershan et al., 2009; Hasko et al., 2011; Thompson et al., 2011). However, the therapeutic potential of enhancing extracellular adenosine levels at a time when acute injury is already established has not yet been evaluated. In addition, the mechanisms of how extracellular adenosine regulates the integrity of pulmonary epithelium and endothelium are not well understood.

Several mouse models of ALI has been developed, including mechanical ventilation, sepsis, acid aspiration, and ischemia-reperfusion induced ALI (Rosenthal et al., 1998; Matute-Bello et al., 2008). However, none of them truly recapitulate features of human ARDS. Intratracheal (i.t.) bleomycin is one of the most commonly used models of ALI in mice. Bleomycin is a chemotherapeutic agent derived from *Streptomyces* verticillus, and it is clinically used to treat a variety of human cancers. However, one of the adverse effect of bleomycin therapy is lung injury and pulmonary fibrosis (Froudarakis et al., 2013; Martin W. G. et al., 2005). Intratracheal bleomycin induced ALI reproduces many features of ARDS, including neutrophil infiltration and increased levels of pro-inflammatory cytokines such as interleukin (IL)-1β, IL-6, IL-1R1, keratinocyte chemoattractant (KC), tumor necrosis factor (TNF)-A at the early inflammatory stage (Matute-Bello et al., 2008; Williamson et al., 2015). Furthermore, profibrotic cytokines such as Granulocyte colony-stimulating factor (G-CSF),

Granulocyte-macrophage colony-stimulating factor (GM-CSF), interferon (IFN)-γ, and IL-4 and the subsequent development of fibrosis at the late stage (Matute-Bello et al., 2008; Williamson et al., 2015). This acute and chronic phases of i.t.- bleomycin instillation reflect the acute and chronic phases of ARDS in human that is characterized by and acute inflammatory onset, hypoxemia and subsequent fibrotic tissue deposition (Matthay and Zemans, 2011).

Accordingly, in the present study, using the intratracheal bleomycin-induced ALI model, we demonstrate that elevating adenosine levels acutely is protective against ALI, both prophylactically and therapeutically. We also demonstrate that activation of Adora2b is important to restore barrier function by modulating the expression of focal adhesion proteins.

MATERIALS AND METHODS

Generation and Genotyping of Mouse Lines

All of the animal experiments were reviewed and approved by the Animal Welfare Committee at the University of Texas Health Science Center at Houston. *Ent2*$^{f/f}$ C57BL6 mice were gifts from Dr Eltzschig's lab at the University of Colorado Denver (Eckle et al., 2013; Grenz et al., 2012a). Conditional SPC-CreER-*Ent2*$^{f/f}$ and SPC-CreER-*Adora2b*$^{f/f}$ mice were obtained by crossing *Ent2*$^{f/f}$ and *Adora2b*$^{f/f}$ with SPC-CreER mice. Age and gender matched littermate SPC-CreER mice used as controls for SPC-CreER-*Ent2*$^{f/f}$ and SPC-Cre-*Adora2b*$^{f/f}$. All of the mice were housed in a pathogen-free environment with adequate food and water. No evidence of fungal, parasitic, or bacterial infection was observed.

Mouse Treatment

The SPC-CreER-*Ent2*$^{f/f}$, SPC-CreER-*Adora2b*$^{f/f}$ and control SPC-CreER were injected intraperitoneally (i.p.) with ~75 mg/kg tamoxifen once every 24 h for a total of five consecutive days to induced the cre recombination. A week after the last tamoxifen injection, mice were injected intratracheally with bleomyicn as previously described (Zhou et al., 2009). Briefly, 10–12 week old female C57BL/6 mice were anesthetized with freshly made avertin (250 mg/kg) and instilled intratracheally with saline or 2.5 U/kg bleomycin (Teva Parenteral Medicine, Irvine, CA). The lungs and bronchoalveolar lavage fluid (BAL) were collected for analysis on day 3 or day 7 after bleomycin injection.

Dipyridamole (Sigma-Aldrich, St. Louis, MO) was diluted in 400 ul DMSO, then 2 ml 100% ethanol and then 18 ml sterile corn oil to a final concentration of 1 mg/ml. For the therapeutic model, two days after bleomycin injection, mice were injected i.p. with 5 mg/kg dipyridamole (Sigma-Aldrich, St. Louis, MO) twice daily or with 500 μg/kg BAY 60-6583 (Tocris, Minneapolis, MN) daily (Wang et al., 2013; Zimmerman et al., 2013). Control mice were injected with same volume of vehicle. The lungs and bronchoalveolar lavage fluid (BAL) were collected for analysis on day 7. To avoid animal death, only female mice were used in this study because male mice are more vulnerable to i.t. bleomycin-induced fibrosis.

Evans Blue Measurement of Vascular Permeability

Mice were i.p. injected with 0.2 ml Evans blue dye (0.5% in PBS) (17). Four hours after dye administration, mice were anesthetized with freshly made avertin (250 mg/kg) and lungs were exposed and perfused with PBS. Lungs were then isolated, weighted and incubated in 1 ml formamide overnight at 55°C to extract dye. Dye concentrations were measured spectrophotometrically at 610 nm. The content of Evans blue dye was determined by generating a standard curve from dye dilutions.

Quantitative Real-Time PCR

Cells or lung tissues were lyzed using TRIZOL Reagent (Thermo Fisher Scientific, Fair Lawn, NJ, United States), and total RNA were extracted using RNeasy mini Kit (Qiagen). Then RNA were treated with Heat&Run gDNA remover kit (ArcticZymes) and reverse transcripted into cDNA using Transcriptor First strand cDNA synthesis (Roche). Real-time PCR was carried out using LightCycler 96 using the following primers: Mouse *Ent1* forward: 5′- CTTGGGATTCAGGGTCAGAA-3′, Mouse *Ent1* reverse: 5′- ATCAGGTCACACGACACCAA -3′; Mouse *Ent2* forward: 5′- CATGGAAACTGAGGGGAAGA -3′, Mouse *Ent2* reverse: 5′- GTTCCAAAGGCCTCACAGAG-3′; Mouse β-Actin forward: 5′- GGCTGTATTCCCCTCCATCG-3′; Mouse β-Actin forward: 5′- CCAGTTGGTAACAATGCCATGT -3′. Data was quantified using the comparative Ct method and presented as mean ratio to β-actin.

BAL Collection and Differential Cell Count

Mice were anesthetized with avertin, the trachea was exposed and lavaged four times with 0.3 ml PBS containing 10 μM dipyridamole, 10 μM αβ-methylene ADP, and 10 μM 5′-deoxycoformycin (Sigma-Aldrich), which will pool about 1 ml bronchoalveolar lavage (BAL) fluid. Total number of BAL cells was counted using a hemocytometer. Cellular differentials were determined by cytospinning BAL aliquots onto microscope slides and staining with Diff-Quick (Dade Behring, Deerfield, IL).

Adenosine Measurement

Adenosine concentration in BAL fluid was measured as described previously (45). Briefly, BAL fluid was centrifuged at highest speed to clear cells and debris. 200 μl BAL supernatant was analyzed by reverse-phase high-performance liquid chromatography (HPLC) as described previously (45). Representative peaks were identified and quantified using external standard curves.

Albumin Measurement

The albumin level in BAL was determined using the mouse albumin ELISA kit (Immunology Consultants Laboratory, Inc., Portland, OR, United States). Briefly, BAL samples and standards were added to predesignated wells coated with anti-albumin antibody for 30 min. After the unbound proteins were rinsed, appropriately diluted Enzyme antibody was added and incubated for an additional 30 min. Then the wells were rinsed again and incubated with TMB Substrate Solution for 10 min. Finally, the reactions were stopped by adding Stop Solution to each well. The absorbance (450 nm) of the contents of each well was measured by plate reader and albumin concentration was calculated based on the standard curve.

Cell Culture and Hypoxia Exposure

MLE12 cells (ATCC) were cultured in RPMI Media 1,640 (Life Technologies, Grand Island, NY, United States) containing 10% fetal bovine serum and 100 U/ml penicillin G, and 100 µg/ml. RLE-6 TN was purchased from ATCC and grown in Dulbecco's Modified Eagle's medium, nutrient mixture F-12 Ham (1:1) supplemented with 10% fetal bovine serum, 40 mmol/L HEPES, 100 U/ml penicillin G, and 100 µg/ml. To study the role of Adora2b on junction proteins and transepithelial electric resistance, cells were serum-starved overnight, treated with 10 µg/ml ADA (Roche) for 30 min, followed by incubation in 500 nM BAY 60-6583, and/or 1 µM MRS 1754, and/or 10 µM H89, then the cells were placed in a sealed hypoxia chamber and exposed to 2% oxygen supplied with 95% N_2 and 5% CO_2 for 1–6 h.

To measure calpain activity, cells were serum-starved, treated with different compounds and exposed to normal air or 2% oxygen for 1 h. Calpain activities were determined using the Calpain-Glo™ protease Assay Kit (Promega, Madison, WI, United States). Experiments were repeated 3 times and triplicated.

Transepithelial Electric Resistance (TEER) Measurement

RLE-6TN cells were seeded on Transwell inserts (0.4-µm pore size, 12-mm inside diameter; Corning Incorporated, Corning, NY) at a density of 1 × 10^5 cells/cm^2. TEER was measured by EVOM2 (World Precision Instruments, Sarasota, FL, United States). When the electrical resistance between the apical and basolateral surfaces of the monolayers was >400 Ω/cm^2, cells were serum-starved overnight, treated with 10 µg/ml ADA for 30 min, followed by incubation in 1 nM BAY 60-6583, and/or 100 nM MRS 1754, and/or 10 µM H89, then the cells were placed in a sealed hypoxia chamber and exposed to 2% oxygen supplied with 95% N_2 and 5% CO_2. TEER was measured 0, 0.5, 1, 2, 4 and 6 h after hypoxia exposure.

Western Blot

Cells or lung samples were collected and lysed in RIPA lysis buffer (50 mM Tris-HCl PH 7.4, 150 mM NaCl, 1% NP-40) containing both protease and phosphatase inhibitor cocktail (Thermo Fisher Scientific, Fair Lawn, NJ, United States). Western blots were carried out as previously described using primary rabbit anti-ENT1 (Abgent, San Diego, CA, United States), rabbit anti-ENT2 (Abcam), rabbit anti-occludin, rabbit anti-phosphorylated FAK, rabbit anti FAK, rabbit anti ZO-1, rabbit anti claudin-1 (Cell signaling, Boston, MA, United States), mouse anti-CD73 antibodies (ThermoFisher Scientific), mouse anti-Hif-1α antibodies (Novus Biological, Littleton, CO, United States), or mouse anti-β-Actin antibodies (Sigma) and corresponding secondary antibodies conjugated to horseradish peroxidase (Jackson ImmunoResearch, West Grove, PA, United States). Finally, the membranes were developed with Pierce ECL Western Blotting Substrate (Thermo Fisher scientific, Fair Lawn, NJ, United States).

H&E Staining and Immunohistochemistry

Mouse lungs were fixed in 10% formaldehyde for at least 24 h. Lungs were then dehydrated, paraffin embedded and sectioned at a thickness of 5 µm. For Hematoxylin and Eosin (H&E), staining sections were rehydrated, incubated with Hematoxylin Solution, Gill No. 3 (Sigma) and then incubated with aqueous 1% Eosin Y solution (Sigma). Finally, slides were dehydrated and mounted in Cytoseal™ XYL (ThemoFisher scientific, Waltham, MA, United States).

For ENT1, ENT2 and neutrophil staining, sections were rehydrated, quenched with 3% hydrogen peroxide, incubated in citric buffer (VectorLabs, Burlingame, CA, United States) for antigen retrieval, and blocked with Avidin/Biotin Blocking System (VectorLabs) and then 5% normal goat serum. After that, the sections were incubated with anti-ENT1, ENT2 (1:200, Abcam), and Anti-Neutrophil antibody NIMP-R14 (1:500, rabbit polyclonal, Abcam, Cambridge, MA, United States) overnight at 4°C. Slides were then incubated with appropriate secondary antibodies (1:1,000, VectorLabs) for 1 h and ABC Elite streptavidin reagents for 30 min at room temperature. Finally, slides were developed with Vector blue (VectorLabs) or 3,3-diaminobenzidine (Sigma-Aldrich, St. Louis, MO, United States) and counter-stained with methyl green. Stained slides were blindly counted for the numbers of positive stained neutrophils at ×20 objective. Ten random areas per lung were analyzed to get the final average number of infiltrated neutrophil.

Human Lung Collection

Normal and ARDS lungs were purchased from the International Institute for the Advancement of Medicine (IIAM) Usage of these tissues was performed under IRB: HSC-MS-08-0354. Discarded lungs for transplantation were considered normal if they did not have a history of chronic lung injury, presented with a partial pressure of oxygen (PaO_2) fraction of inspired oxygen (FIO_2) ratio PaO_2/FIO_2 over 300 mmHg and the absence of bilateral opacities by chest imaging. Discarded lungs for transplantation that met the Berlin definition of ARDS: presence of bilateral opacities from chest imaging, pulmonary edema not due to cardiac failure or fluid overload and arterial oxygenation calculated by the PaO_2/FiO_2 ratio less than 300 mmHg (Ranieri et al., 2012), were used for our study. Samples from four normal and three ARDS lungs were analyzed.

CD73 Activity Assay

Pulverized normal and ARDS lungs were lysed in NP-40 lysis buffer (1% NP-40, 150 mM NaCl, 50 mM Tris-Cl, PH 8.0) containing protease inhibitor cocktail (ThermoFisher). Protein concentration were determined using the Pierce™ BCA protein assay kit (ThermoFisher). For each assay, five ug lung lysate was mixed with assay buffer (10 mM HEPES, 10 mM $MgCl_2$, 10 µM DCF and 200 mM AMP), and immediately incubated at 37°C for 30 min. At the end of the incubation, reaction was inactivated by

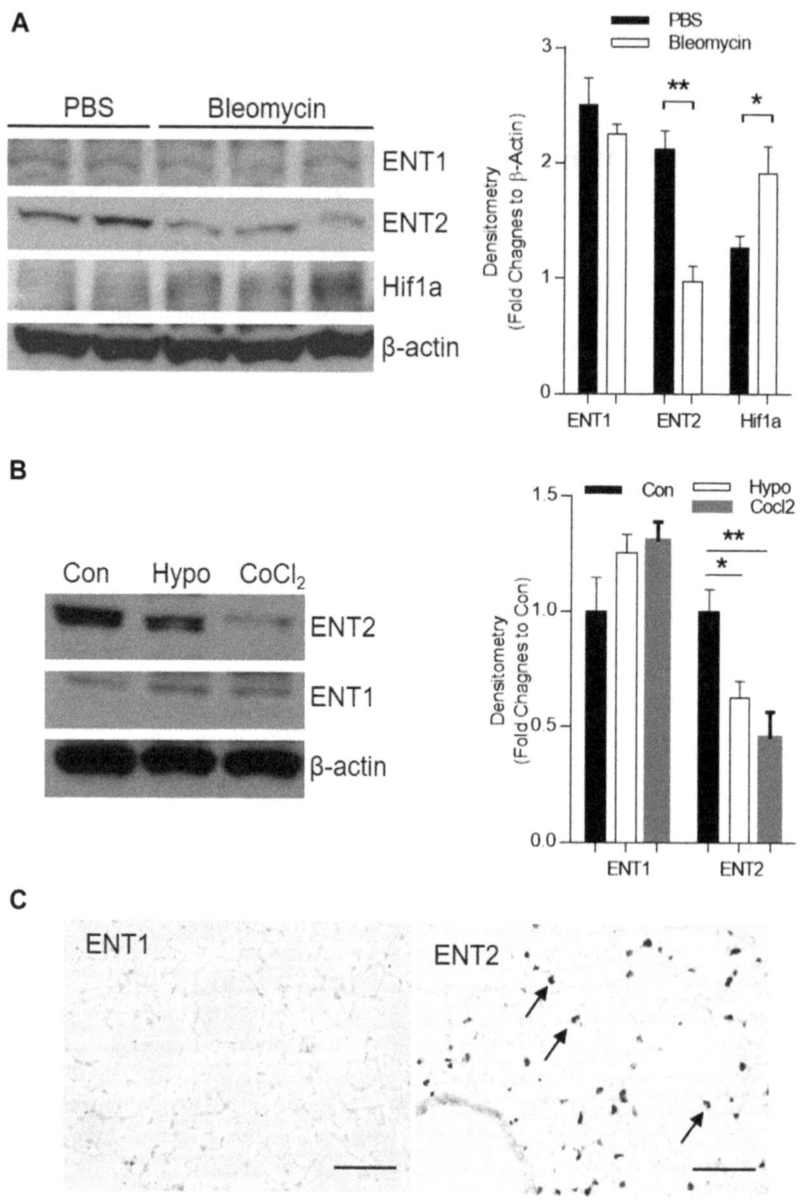

FIGURE 1 | ENT2 expression is decreased in bleomycin-induced ALI. C57BL6 mice were i.t. injected with 2.5 U/kg bleomycin and lungs were collected for analysis on day 3. **(A)** Left Panel: The protein expression of ENT1, ENT2, and Hif1a were determined using western blot. β-Actin was used as an internal control. Right Panel: Densitometry of the Western Blot image were analyzed and data were presented as fold changes to β-Actin ± MSE. $^{*}p < 0.05$, $^{**}p < 0.01$. **(B)** Primary alveolar epithelial type II (AECII) were isolated from normal mouse lungs and exposed to 2% oxygen, or 100 mM $CoCl_2$ for 24 h. Right Panel: Densitometry of the Western Blot image were analyzed and data were presented as fold changes to Control (Con) ± MSE. $^{*}p < 0.05$, $^{**}p < 0.01$. **(C)** Cellular localization of ENT1 and ENT2 (brown, arrow) was visualized using immunohistochemistry in a normal healthy mouse lung. The protein levels of ENT1, ENT2, and β-Actin were determined using western blot. n = 3, $^{*}p < 0.05$ vs. control. Scale bar = 100 μm.

incubating the mixture at 95°C for 5 min. Adenosine levels were measured using HPLC as described above. The activites of CD73 were integrated as the amount of adenosine synthesized per minutes per Gram of total protein.

Statistical Analysis

For scientific rigor, all *in vitro* cell culture experiments were repeated at least three times and each treatment was at least duplicated. For experiments having no more than two treatment groups, two-tailed student t-tests were used to assess whether the means of two groups were statistically different from each other. Otherwise, one-way or two-way ANOVA were used to determine whether there were significant differences among treatments. If so, Tukey's multiple comparison test were carried out to determine whether there were significant differences between any of the two treatments. The data were considered significant with $p < 0.05$. All results were presented as Mean ± SEM to indicate variability.

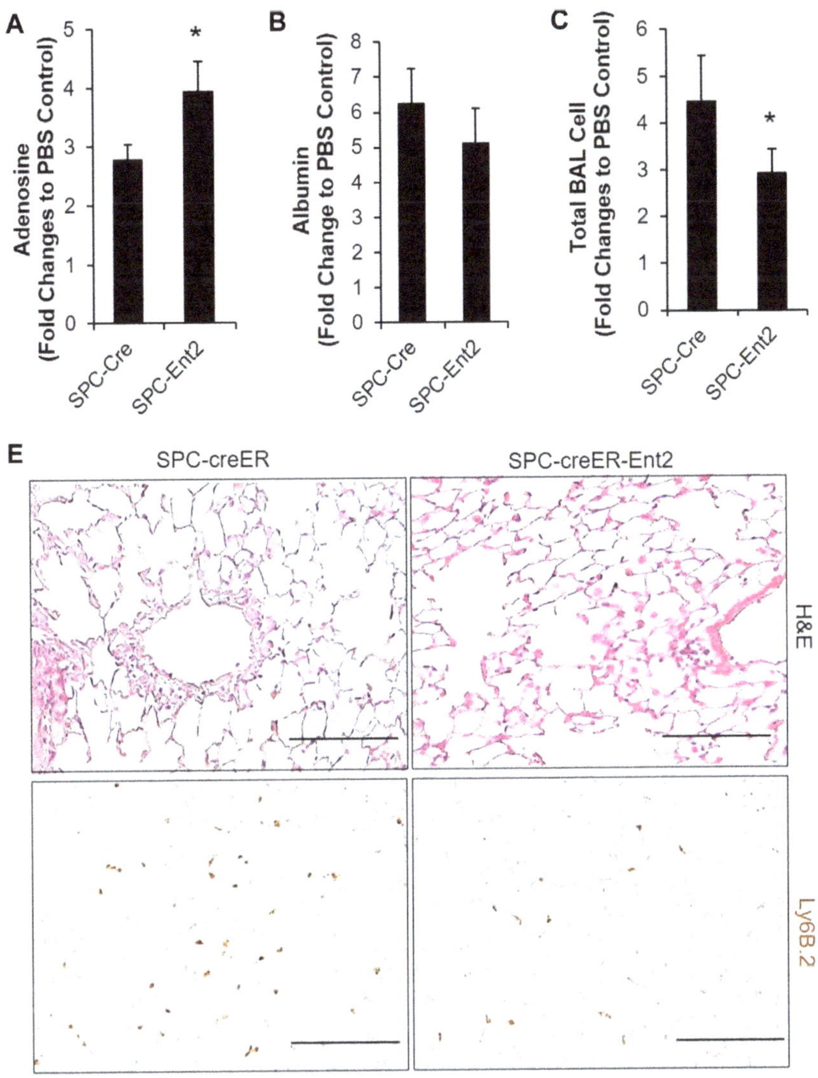

FIGURE 2 | Bleomycin-induced ALI is attenuated in mice with epithelial specific deletion of Ent2. SPC-CreER- Ent2−/− mice or littermate SPC-CreER controls were i.p. injected with 75 mg/ml tamoxifen daily for 5 days. One week after the first tamoxifen injection, mice were I.t. injected with 2.5 U/kg bleomycin. On day 3, BAL adenosine **(A)** and albumin levels **(B)**, and total BAL cell number **(C)** were analyzed. **(D)** Neutrophil infiltration was determined by staining with anti-Ly6B.2, and cell number per high powered filed were counted. **(E)** Representative H&E and Ly6b staining showing pulmonary inflammation and neutrophil infiltration in different groups of lungs. n ≥ 4, $^{*}p < 0.05$, $^{**}p < 0.01$ vs. Control. $\#p < 0.05$ vs. wild type bleomycin. Scale bar = 100 μm.

RESULTS

The Expression of ENT2, but not ENT1, is Negatively Regulated by Hypoxia Following Tissue Injury

Extracellular adenosine is generated following injury and can be transported by ENTs into the cells and then depleted in the extracellular space (Karmouty-Quintana et al., 2013). To understand whether ENT expression is suppressed following bleomycin-induced acute lung injury and partially contributes to the increase of extracellular adenosine levels, we examined the transcript and protein expression of ENTs in the lungs of mice instilled with bleomycin (i.t.) after 3 days. ENT2 protein levels were decreased in the lungs of mice treated with bleomycin (**Figure 1A**), suggesting that ENT2 might be the transporter which is more actively regulated following lung injury. Previous studies have demonstrated that hypoxia is one of the important regulators of ENTs (Eckle et al., 2013). Indeed, we observed an increased expression of hypoxia-inducible factor 1 alpha (Hif-1a) following bleomycin treatment (**Figure 1A**), suggesting that hypoxia is present in the injured lungs and might be the mechanism that leads to decreased ENT expression. To further understand whether hypoxia directly regulates ENT expression, we isolated primary alveolar epithelial type II cells (AECII) from mice and exposed them to 2% oxygen or $CoCl_2$, a chemical

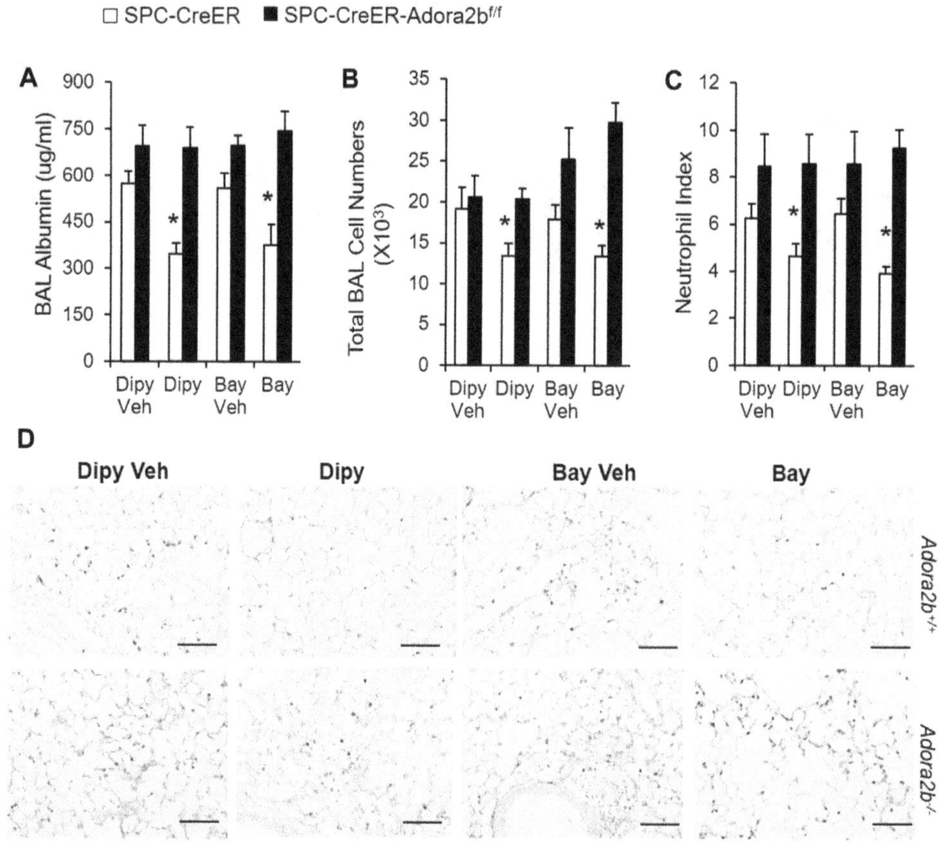

FIGURE 3 | Bleomycin-induced ALI in mice with Adora2b deletion specially in alveolar epithelial cells. SPC-Cre-Adora2b−/− mice and littermate controls were I.p. injected with 75 mg/ml tamoxifen daily for 5 days to induce Cre recombination. One week after the first tamoxifen injection, mice were pretreated with vehicle control, 5 mg/kg dipyridamole or 500 ug/kg BAY 60-6583 1 h before I.t. injected with 2.5 U/kg bleomycin and then continuously injected with dipyridamole twice daily or BAY 60-6583 once daily until day 3 for analysis. **(A)** BAL albumin levels were measured to show vascular leakage. **(B)** Total BAL cell numbers were counted to determine pulmonary inflammation. **(C)** Neutrophil index was calculated by counting the number of neutrophil per high power field from slides stained with anti-Ly6B.2 antibody. n = 5, $^*p < 0.05$ vs. corresponding Veh control using student t-test. **(D)** Representative lung sections stained with Ly6B.2 to show neutrophil infiltration. n ≥ 4, $^*p < 0.05$ vs. vehicle using one way ANOVA followed by Bonferroni's multiple comparisons test. Scale bar = 100 μm.

inducer of Hif-1a. Consistent with the results we observed using whole lung lysates, ENT2 but not ENT1 expression was dramatically down-regulated by both hypoxia and $CoCl_2$ (**Figure 1B**), suggesting that hypoxia following acute lung injury can suppress ENT2 expression in a Hif-1a dependent manner. Immunohistochemistry demonstrated that ENT2 is mainly located in alveolar epithelial cells (arrow) in normal mouse lungs (**Figure 1C**). Taken together, our findings demonstrate that ENT2, but not Ent1, is repressed by hypoxia during ALI induced by bleomycin.

ENT2 Is the Major Transporter to Regulate BAL Adenosine Levels

Our immunostaining mainly located ENT2 in alveolar epithelial cells, suggesting that alveolar epithelial cells might be the key cells to mediate the ENT2 regulation of extracellular adenosine levels. To define this, we crossed SPC-CreER mice with mice carrying a floxed allele of *Ent2* to generate transgenic mice with *Ent2* deficient specifically in alveolar epithelial cells. Seven days after inducing the cre recombinase with tamoxifen, SPC-CreER-*Ent2* mice were administrated with bleomycin and compared with SPC-CreER controls. SPC-CreER-*Ent2* mice had significantly enhanced extracellular adenosine levels (**Figure 2A**) in association with attenuated vascular leakage (**Figure 2B**) and inflammatory cell infiltration (**Figure 2C**) compared to controls. Further differential cell counts revealed that SPC-CreER-*Ent2* mice presented with reduced neutrophil cell infiltration (**Figure 2D,E**). In summary, these findings demonstrate a selective protective role for epithelial ENT2 in bleomycin-induced lung injury.

Adenosine Through Adora2b Is Important to Protect Lungs From Acute Injury

We have demonstrated that elevation of extracellular adenosine is limited by epithelial ENT2 and is associated with increased

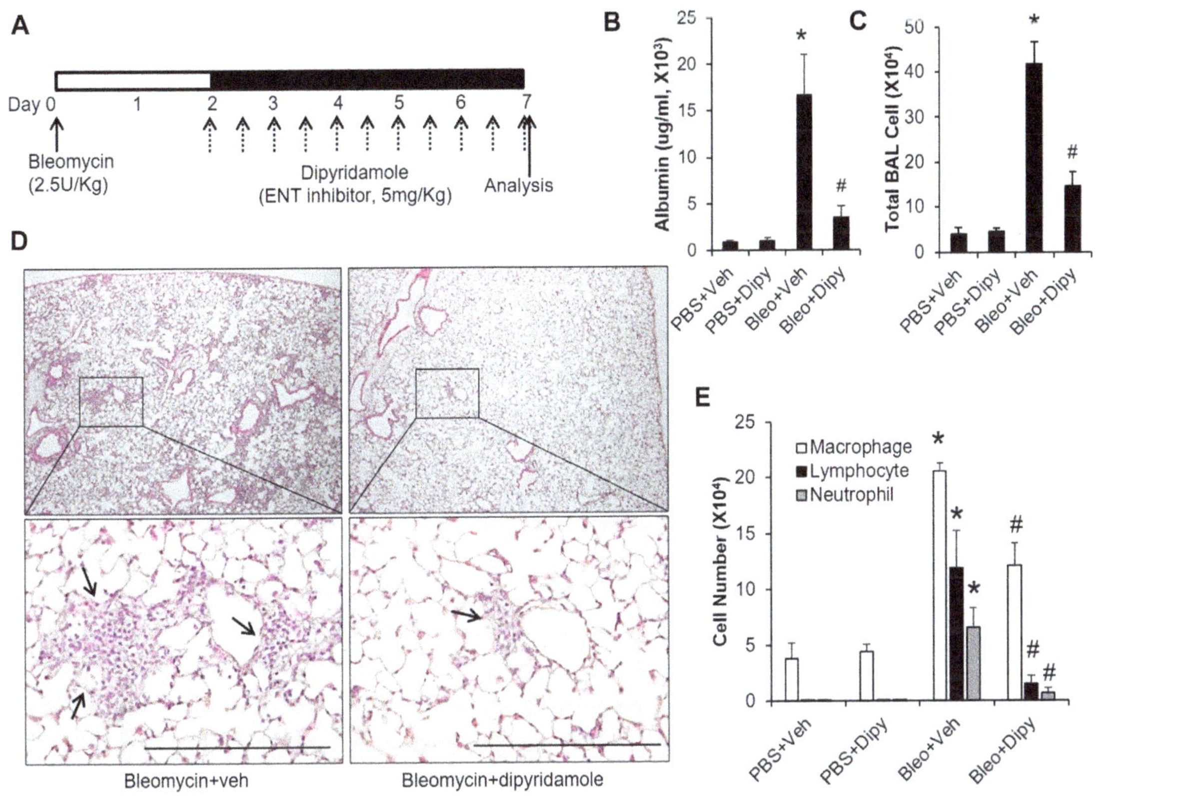

FIGURE 4 | Therapeutic effect of dipyridamole on established ALI. **(A)** A diagram showing how mice were treated with dipyridamole and bleomycin. Mice injected with same volume of Vehicle were used as control. **(B)** BAL albumin levels were measured from different treatment groups. **(C)** BAL total cell numbers were counted. **(D)** Lungs from bleomycin and/or dipyridamole treated mice were sectioned and stained with H&E. Representative pictures were shown. Scale bar = 500 μM. **(E)** Differential assay was performed to determine the degree of macrophage, lymphocyte and neutrophil trafficking into the lungs. $n \geq 5$, $^*p < 0.05$ vs. PBS. $\#p < 0.05$ vs. bleomycin using one way ANOVA followed by Bonferroni's multiple comparisons test. Scale bar = 200 μm.

protection from lung injury. Next, we want to investigate which adenosine receptor is involved in this protection. Previous studies in a mouse model of VILI indicate that adenosine, through the Adora2b receptor, is the major pathway that promotes barrier protection (Eckle et al., 2013). Based on these notions, we hypothesize that Adora2b is the major adenosine receptor that mediates this protection.

Previous studies shown that Adora2b is mainly expressed in alveolar epithelial cells, and Adora2b in epithelial cells is essential to mediate the protective role of adenosine in ventilation induced acute lung injury (Cagnina et al., 2009; Eckle et al., 2013). To determine whether epithelial Adora2b is also important for the protection of barrier function in our model of acute lung injury, we generated mice with Adora2b deleted specially in alveolar epithelial type II cells by crossing SPC-creER mice with mice carrying a floxed allele of Adora2b, and induced ALI in these mice with bleomycin. Compared to SPC-Cre mice, in SPC-cre-*Adora2b*$^{f/f}$ mice, dipyridamole or BAY 60-6583 (an Adora2B agonist) treatment can no longer alleviate vascular leakage (**Figure 3A**), inflammation (**Figure 3B,D**), neutrophil infiltration (**Figure 3C,D**) after bleomycin exposure. Taken together, our study suggests that epithelial Adora2b is important to mediate the protective role of extracellular adenosine in bleomycin-induced acute lung injury.

Inhibiting ENTs at a Time Point When Acute Lung Injury is Already Established Protects Lungs From Bleomycin-Induced Injury

Based on the above findings that extracellular adenosine plays a role in preventing bleomycin-induced injury, we next established another model to see whether adenosine is also beneficial in treating already established ALI. In this model, mice were intratracheally instilled with bleomycin; after 2 days, mice were i.p injected with dipyridamole twice daily until day 7 for analysis (**Figure 4A**). Dipyridamole significantly reduced vascular leakage (**Figure 4B**) as indicated by the amount of albumin leaking into the BAL. Pulmonary inflammation was also dramatically suppressed as shown by both total BAL cell count (**Figure 4C**) and H&E staining (**Figure 4D**). Next, we performed differential assays to understand which inflammatory cells were trafficking into the lungs. We observed that both lymphocytes and neutrophils, which are significantly induced by bleomycin, were repressed by dipyridamole treatment (**Figure 4E**). These findings indicate that inhibiting ENTs at a time point when acute

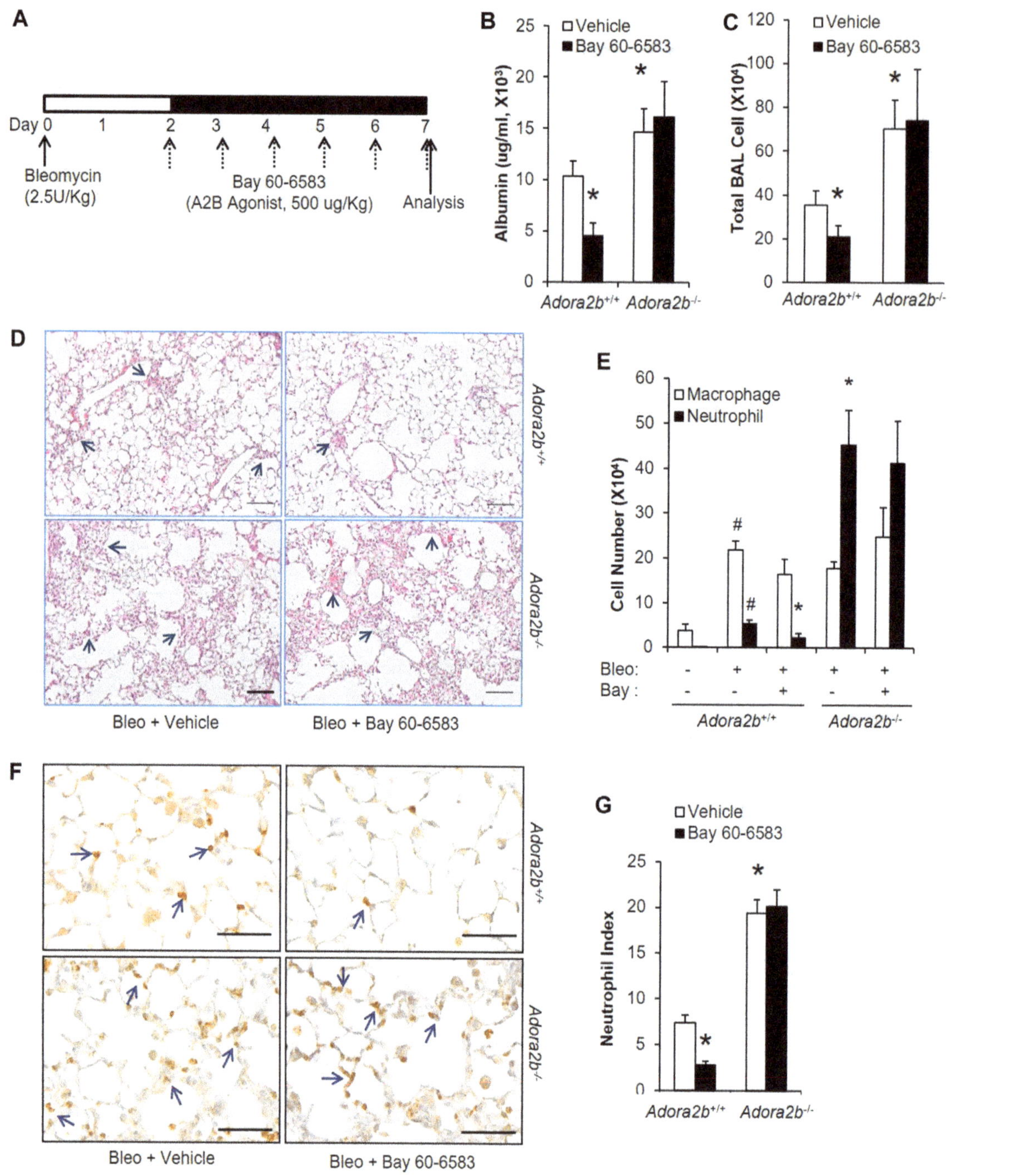

FIGURE 5 | Therapeutic effect of BAY 60-6583 on established ALI in *Adora2b+/+* and *Adora2b−/−* mice. **(A)** A diagram showing how *Adora2b+/+* and *Adora2b−/−* mice were treated with BAY 60-6583 and bleomycin. **(B)** BAL albumin levels were measured to show the levels of vascular leakage. **(C)** BAL total cell number was counted. **(D)** Representative H&E stainings of lungs from bleomycin and/or dipyridamole treated mice. Arrows pointing areas with inflammation. Scale bar = 500 μM. **(E)** Differential assay was performed to determine the number of macrophage and neutrophil in the lungs. **(F)** Mouse lung sections from different treatment group were stained with anti-Ly6B.2 to visualize neutrophil expression and localization. Arrow: positive stained neutrophils. Scale bar = 100 μM. **(G)** The number of neutrophil for each treatment group was quantitated. N = 5, **p* < 0.05 vs. wildtype bleomycin vehicle. #*p* < 0.05 vs. wild type PBS using one way ANOVA followed by Bonferroni's multiple comparisons test.

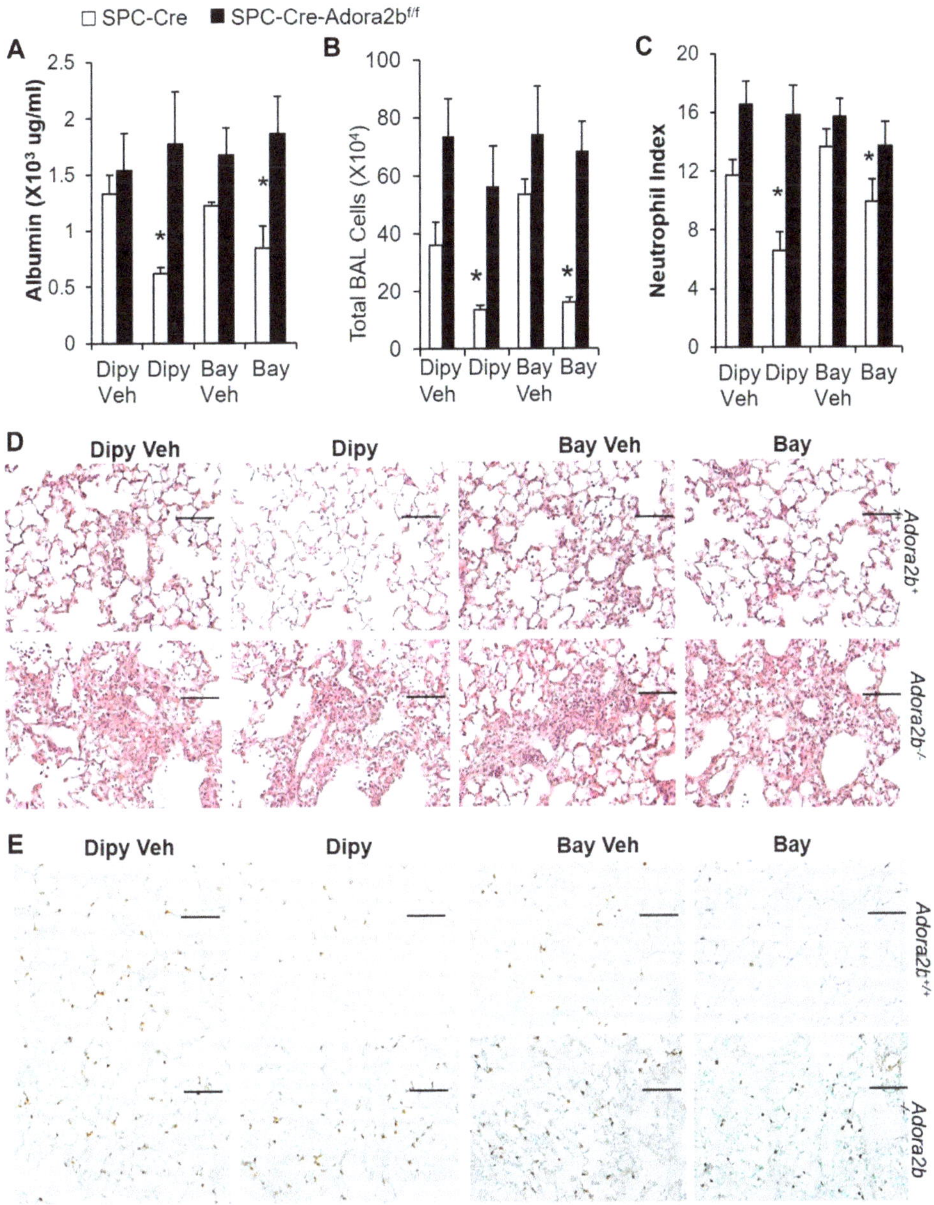

FIGURE 6 | Effect of Dipyridamole and BAY 60-6583 on established ALI in mice with Adora2b knockout specifically in alveolar epithelial cells (SPC-Cre-Adora2blox/lox). *SPC-Cre* and *SPC-Cre-Adora2blox/lox* mice were treated with 2.5 U/kg bleomycin through i.t. Two days later, mice were treated with 5 mg/kg dipyridmole twice daily or 500 ug/kg BAY 60-6583 daily until day 7. BAL albumin **(A)** and total BAL cells **(B)** were measured. **(C)** Lung sections were stained with anti-Ly6B.2 for neutrophil index. **(D)** Representative H&E staining showed pulmonary inflammation and injury in various groups. **(E)** Representative lung sections stained with Ly6B.2 to show neutrophil infiltration. n = 5, $^{*}p < 0.05$ vs. vehicle using one way ANOVA followed by Bonferroni's multiple comparisons test. Scale bar = 100 μm.

lung injury is already established can also protect lungs from bleomycin-induced injury.

Adenosine Through Adora2b is Important for Lungs to Recover From Acute Injury

After having shown that adenosine through Adora2b is important to prevent bleomycin-induced acute injury, we wanted to understand whether Adora2b is also the major adenosine receptor mediating the therapeutic effect of adenosine on established acute lung injury. To study the role of Adora2b in treating acute lung injury, wildtype (*Adora2b*$^{+/+}$) or *Adora2b*$^{-/-}$ mice were subjected to bleomycin injury, followed by i.p injection of BAY 60-6583 starting on day 2 and continuing daily for 5 days (**Figure 5A**). BAY 60-6583 dramatically attenuated bleomycin-induced lung injury by reducing vascular leakage (**Figure 5A**) and

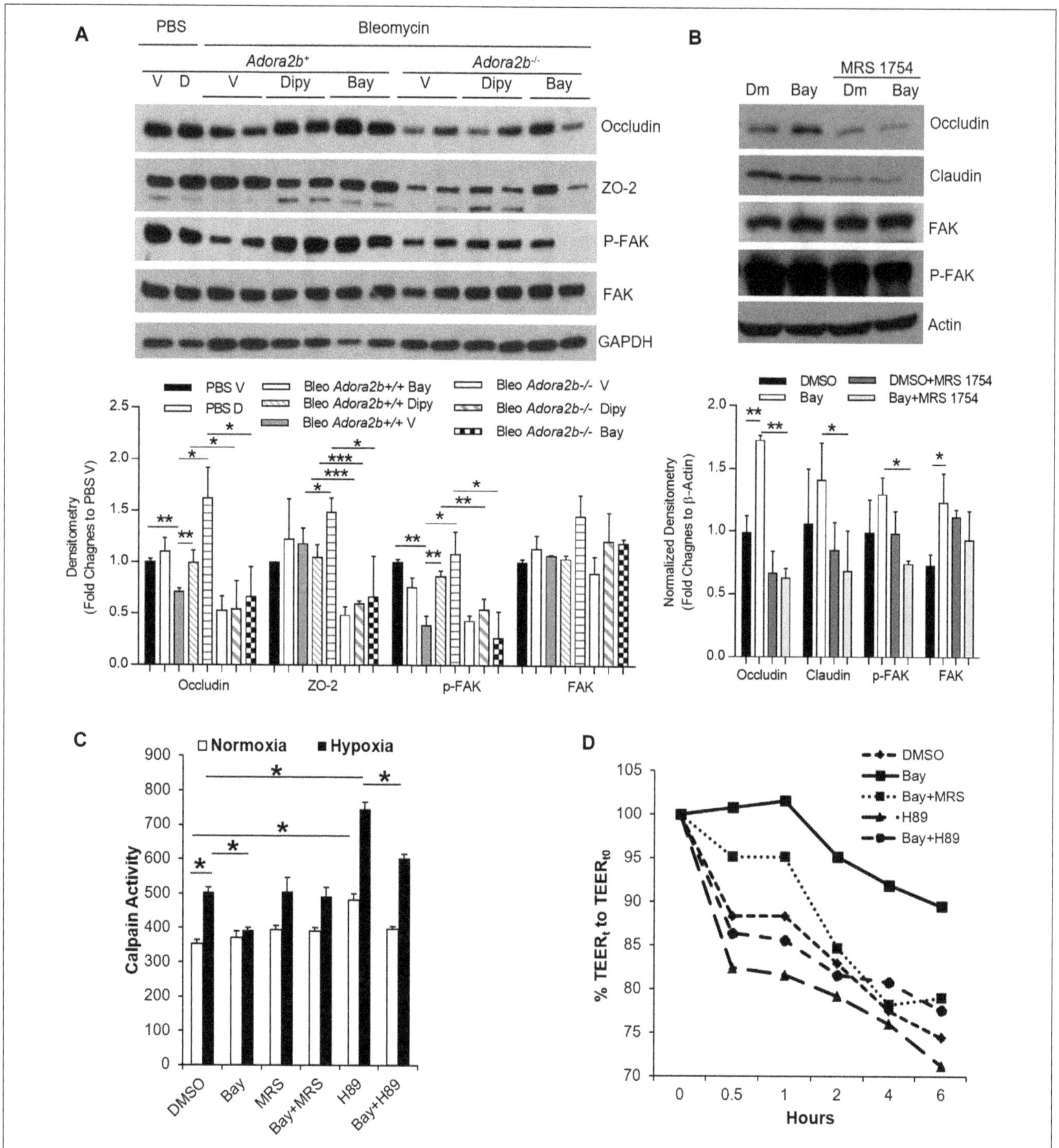

FIGURE 7 | The regulation of Adora2b on junction proteins. *Adora2b*$^{+/+}$ or *Adora2b*$^{-/-}$ mice were I.t injected with 2.5 U/kg bleomycin. Two days later, mice were treated with 5 mg/kg dipyridmole twice daily or 500 ug/kg BAY 60-6583 daily until day 7 for analysis. **(A)** Upper panel: whole lung samples were collected from different treatment group for western blot analysis of Occludin and ZO-2 or phosphorylated FAK (*p*-FAK) and FAK. Lower panel: The Densitometry of the Western Blot image were analyzed. Data were presented as Fold Change to PBS Vehicle± SD. n ≥ 4, *$p < 0.05$, **$p < 0.01$. ***$p < 0.001$. **(B, D,E)** MLE12 cells were serum starved overnight, pretreated with ADA for 30 min, treated with 500 nM BAY 60-6583 or 1 μM MRS 1754 or 10 μM H89, and then exposed to 2% oxygen for 6 h for western blot and 1 h for Calpain activity. **(B)** Upper panel: Expression of Occludin and Claudin-1, and *p*-FAK and FAK were examined using western blot. Lower Panel: Densitometry of the Western Blot image were analyzed. Data were presented as Normalized fold changes to β-Actin ± SD. *$p < 0.05$, **$p < 0.01$. **(C)** Calpain activities were measured and quantitated. *$p < 0.05$ one way ANOVA followed by Bonferroni's multiple comparisons test vs. DMSO control. **(D)** RLE-6TN cells were serum starved overnight, pretreated with ADA for 30 min, treated with 500 nM BAY 60-6583 or 1 μM MRS 1754 or 10 μM H89, and then exposed to 2% oxygen for 0–6 h, transepithelial electrical resistance (TEER) were measured and normalized to 0 h n = 3 independent experiments.

inflammation (**Figure 5B,C**) in wildtype mice. However, the protection of BAY 60-6583 was completely abolished in the absence of Adora2b (**Figure 5A–C**). Moreover, *Adora2b*$^{-/-}$ mice exhibited increased vascular leakage and inflammation compared to *Adora2b*$^{+/+}$ mice (**Figure 5A–C**). Differential assay indicated a significant increase in neutrophil trafficking into the lungs in *Adora2b*$^{-/-}$ mice compared to wildtype controls, and the inhibition of BAY 60-6583 on neutrophil infiltration that we observed in wildtype mice was completely eliminated in *Adora2b*$^{-/-}$ mice (**Figure 5D**). To visualize neutrophil trafficking into the lungs, we stained the lung sections with anti-Neutrophil antibody NIMP-R14. We found the number of neutrophils was significantly increased when Adora2b was deficient (**Figure 5E,F**), and BAY 60-6583 dramatically inhibited neutrophil infiltration in *Adora2b*$^{+/+}$ mice but not in *Adora2b*$^{-/-}$ mice (**Figure 5E,F**).

We have shown that epithelial Adora2b is important to prevent bleomycin-induce lung injury. Next, we wanted to determine whether epithelial Adora2b is also important for the treatment of established ALI. SPC-Cre or SPC-cre-*Adora2b*$^{f/f}$ mice were i.t. administrated with bleomycin. After 2 days, mice were i.p injected with BAY 60-6583 or dipyridamole for five consecutive days. SPC-Cre mice treated with either BAY 60-6583 or dipyridamole had better lung recovery with ameliorated vascular leakage (**Figure 6A**), inflammation (**Figure 6B,D**) and neutrophil infiltration (**Figure 6C,E**). However, neither BAY 60-6583 nor dipyridamole attenuated bleomycin-induced lung injury in mice lacking Adora2b in alveolar epithelial cells (**Figure 6A–C**). Taken together, our findings suggest that epithelial Adora2b is important for lungs to recover from bleomycin-induced acute injury.

Adenosine Through Adora2b Maintains Epithelial Integrity by Preventing the Degradation of Junction Proteins

Based on the above findings, we know that adenosine through Adora2b is important not only to prevent but also to treat acute lung injury. However, the underlying mechanisms are not known. The lung epithelial monolayer is assembled through the interactions of numerous structural proteins, including occludins, claudins and focal adhesion kinase (FAK). Evidence has suggested that deteriorated expression of these proteins in epithelial cells promotes the permeability of the alveolar epithelium and facilitates the progression of ALI. To understand whether adenosine signaling affects the structural proteins, we first characterized the expression of these structural proteins in bleomycin-induced lung injury in different treatment groups. As shown in **Figure 7A**, the levels of occludin and phosphorylated FAK (*p*-FAK) were decreased in wildtype mice exposed to bleomycin for 7 days. Interestingly, both dipyridamole and BAY 60-6583 recovered the levels of occludin and pFAK to about the same levels as uninjured controls. Moreover, if Adora2b was absent (*Adora2b*$^{-/-}$ mice), the expression of *p*-FAK was more significantly decreased by bleomycin, and dipyridamole and BAY 60-6583 could no longer recover occludin and *p*-FAK levels (**Figure 7A**). In addition, the tight junction protein ZO-2 is highly dysregulated in Adora2b$^{-/-}$ mice, representing massive loss of epithelial integrity in *Adora2b*$^{-/-}$ mice. However, dipyridamole failed and BAY 60-6583 only slightly recover the ZO-2 levels in wildtype mice, indicating that ZO-2 might not directly regulated by the Adenosine through Adora2b receptors (**Figure 7A**). Taking together, these results suggest that adenosine through Adora2b may directly regulate the levels of occludin-1 and *p*-FAK.

To determine whether adenosine through Adora2b directly regulates the levels of occludin and *p*-FAK in epithelial cells, we pretreated MLE12 cells, an immortalized alveolar epithelial type II cell line, with BAY 60-6583 and incubated in 2% oxygen for 6 h. BAY 60-6583 significantly increased the levels of occludin and the effect of BAY 60-6583 on occludin could be fully blocked by MRS 1754, an Adora2b antagonist (**Figure 7B**). Although levels of *p*-FAK and claudin-1 was unaffected by BAY 60-6583, they are largely suppressed in cells treated with MRS 1754 (**Figure 7B**), suggesting a role of adenosine through Adora2b in protecting the protein levels of FAK and claudin-1 under hypoxia exposure. Overall, these findings suggest that a role of Adora2b in regulation of occludin, FAK and *p*-FAK.

Since both occludin and FAK could be degraded by calpain, a protease which can be activated in acute lung injury and under stress conditions such as hypoxia (Liu et al., 2012), we hypothesized that adenosine through adora2b may maintain occludin and FAK levels in hypoxia and ALI by inhibiting calpain activity. To test this, we measured calpain activity in MLE12 cells pre-treated with BAY 60-6583 and then exposed them to hypoxia for 1 h. Calpain activity was significantly increased after hypoxia exposure and was dramatically inhibited by BAY 60-6583 (**Figure 7C**). The inhibition of BAY 60-6583 could be neutralized by MRS 1754 (**Figure 7C**). Calpain activity has been shown to be repressed by protein kinase A (PKA), a kinase that can be activated by adenosine through Adora2b. To determine whether BAY 60-6583 can suppress calpain activity through PKA activation, we treated MLE12 cells with H89, a PKA inhibitor. H89 significantly increased calpain activity, even in the presence of BAY 60-6583 (**Figure 7C**). Moreover, to examine whether calpain activity is directly correlated with epithelial leakage, we measured transepithelial resistance (TEER) in cells treated with different compounds and exposed to 2% oxygen for 6 h. Since MLE-12 cells can not form monolayer, we chose RLE-6TN for the TEER measurement. As shown in **Figure 7D**, the TEER is negatively correlated with the calpain activity shown in **Figure 7C** (BAY 60-6583 slowed down hypoxia-induced TEER loss, while H89 dramatically accelerated the decrease in TEER compared to control). Moreover, the protection of BAY 60-6583 was attenuated by both MRS 1754 and H89. Taken together, our data provide a novel mechanism for Adora2b-mediated protection in epithelial leakage and demonstrate that adenosine through Adora2b may attenuate occludin and FAK degradation in ALI by inhibiting calpain activity through PKA activation.

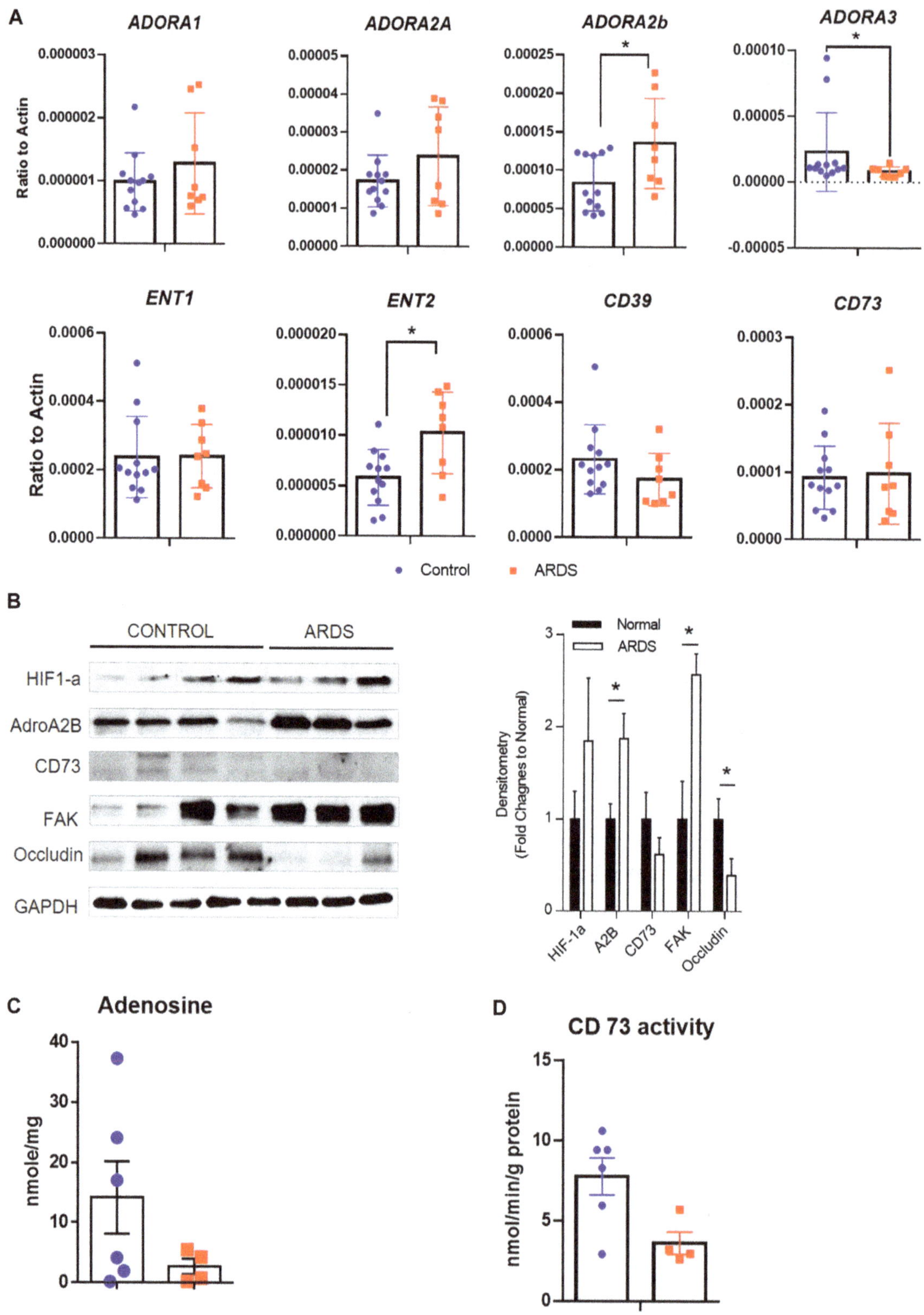

FIGURE 8 | Expression of adenosine receptors, transporters and enzymes in human ARDS lungs. **(A)** The transcript expression of adenosine receptors (ADORA1, ADORA2A, ADORA2B and ADORA3), transporters (ENT1 and ENT2) as well as enzymes (CD39 and CD73) were determined in human normal and ARDS lungs using realtime PCR. **(B)** Left Panel: The protein expression of HIF-1a, ADORA2B, CD73 as well as tight junction proteins were determined in normal and ARDS lungs using western blot. Right Panel: Densitometry of the Western Blot image were analyzed and data were presented as fold changes to Normal control ± MSE. *$p < 0.05$. **(C)** The levels of adenosine were measured using HPLC. **(D)** The activities of CD73 were determined in control and ARDS lungs. *$p < 0.05$ using student t-test.

Levels of Adenosine Signaling Proteins and Structural Proteins are Differently Expressed in Human ARDS Lungs

Lastly, to understand whether similar adenosine signaling is activated in human ARDS lungs, we examined the levels of adenosine receptors and transporters, as well as enzymes for adenosine synthesis in human normal and ARDS lungs. Consistent with the important roles of Adora2b in acute lung injury in mice, *ADORA2B was* the only adenosine receptor having elevated transcript and protein levels in ARDS lungs, interestingly ADORA3 levels were attenuated in ARDS lungs (**Figure 8A,B**). Surprisingly, *ENT2* levels were also increased in ARDS lungs (**Figure 8A**) in association with reduced adenosine levels (**Figure 8C**) and decreased CD73 activities (**Figure 8D**). Moreover, the levels of tight junction protein occludin was decreased in ARDS lungs compared to normal lungs (**Figure 8B**), suggesting that lost epithelial barrier function is also present in human ARDS lungs. Taken together, our data suggest failed adenosine accumulation in response to injury in ARDS lungs may be the potential reason for dampened barrier functions and severe pulmonary damage in ALI. .

DISCUSSION

ARDS is an inflammatory lung disease that is characterized with noncardiogenic pulmonary edema, massive lung inflammation and severe hypoxemia (Bakowitz et al., 2012). Due to the limited clinical management of this disorder, ALI is among the leading causes of death in intensive care units (Bakowitz et al., 2012). This has been overemphasized in the recent COVID-19 pandemic where patients present with rapid-onset ARDS accompanied by a cytokine release storm, severe hypoxemia (Goh et al., 2020) accounting for mortality rates of up to 88.1% (Richardson et al., 2020) Therefore, novel therapeutic approaches targeted to dampen lung inflammation and pulmonary edema during ALI are urgently needed. The release of adenosine from injury tissue has been highlighted as an endogenous mechanism for tissue protection in several murine models of ALI, including ALI induced by high-pressure mechanical ventilation, lipopolysaccharide (LPS) and bleomycin (Eckle et al., 2009; Karmouty-Quintana et al., 2013). Our study implicates the role of adenosine transport inhibitor dipyridamole, which prevents adenosine re-uptake and enhances extracellular adenosine levels, in tissue protection from bleomycin-induced ALI. We observed that dipyridamole play a therapeutic role in bleomycin-induced ALI. Subsequent studies using epithelial specific Ent2 knockout mice, we demonstrated that epithelial Ent2 is important to regulate extracellular adenosine levels. Moreover, we identified epithelial Adora2b as the major adenosine receptor contributing to the protective effects of dipyridamole, and occludin and focal adhesion kinase (FAK) as potential targets of adenosine through Adora2b, thus providing a novel mechanism for adenosine-mediated barrier protection (**Figure 9**). Taken together, we have highlighted a role of adenosine signaling in preventing or treating ALI and identified Ent2 and Adora2b as key mediators in establishing pulmonary protection from bleomycin-induced ALI.

Previous studies identified adenosine as an endogenous protective molecule during lung injury (Eckle et al., 2009; Karmouty-Quintana et al., 2013). In response to tissue injury, ATP and ADP are released from injured cells and quickly metabolized to adenosine monophosphate (AMP) in the extracellular space. Amp is then converted to adenosine by ecto-5′-nucleotidase (CD73). Equilibrative nucleoside transporters can re-uptake extracellular adenosine which allows adenosine to freely cross the extracellular cell membrane according to its concentration gradient (Grenz et al., 2011; Eltzschig et al., 2012; Eckle et al., 2013). Dampened ALI was observed using strategies aiming to inhibit extracellular adenosine levels, including genetic deletion of CD73 or CD39 (Grenz et al., 2007; Hart et al., 2011; Hasko et al., 2011) or treating mice with adenosine deaminase (ADA) which rapidly converts adenosine to inosine. On the other hand, enhancing extracellular adenosine signaling by preventing adenosine re-uptake through ENTs attenuates ALI (Eckle et al., 2013; Morote-Garcia et al., 2013). Our findings are consistent with these studies by targeting ENT as a therapeutic method for the treatment of bleomycin-induced ALI. Inhibiting ENTs with the pharmacological agent dipyridamole ameliorates established lung injury in association with enhanced extracellular adenosine concentrations. Similar protection was also observed in mice with selective deletion of *Ent2* specifically in alveolar epithelial type II cells. Dipyridamole is a FDA-approved medication used as a vasodilator for the treatment of blood clot formation and stroke (De Schryver et al., 2007; Sacco et al., 2008). Compared to mice ENTs, dipyridamole has a more potent inhibition effect on human ENTs (Yao et al., 1997), suggesting that dipyridamole could be an even more beneficial drug in the treatment of patients by lowering the off-target effects.

In this study, we identified Adora2b as the major adenosine receptor involved in the protective effect of dipyridamole mediated lung protection. Adenosine signals through four G-protein coupled receptors (Adora1, Adora2a, Adora2b and Adora3) (Hasko et al., 2008; Blackburn et al., 2009; Eltzschig, 2009; Karmouty-Quintana et al., 2013). Adora2b plays a beneficial role in tissue protection during acute injuries (Csoka et al., 2010; Eltzschig et al., 2009b; Grenz et al., 2012b). The expression levels of Adora2b is elevated as an adaption to hypoxia and inflammation, and it in turn activates a cascade of genes which are implicated in promoting barrier function, attenuating vascular leakage, and preventing inflammation and neutrophil infiltration (Eckle et al., 2009; Koeppen et al., 2011). A study by Eckle and colleagues also suggested that Adora2b promotes fluid clearance from the alveolus and attenuates pulmonary edema (Eckle et al., 2008). Consistent with previous findings, we observed attenuated ALI in mice administrated with Adora2b agonist BAY 60-6583 and enhanced ALI in mice with global deletion of Adora2b. Since Adora2b expression is mainly observed in alveolar epithelial type II cells (Cagnina et al., 2009; Eckle et al., 2013), we also generated mice with Adora2b specifically knocked out in alveolar epithelial cells and detected a similar level of lung injury comparable to global Adora2b

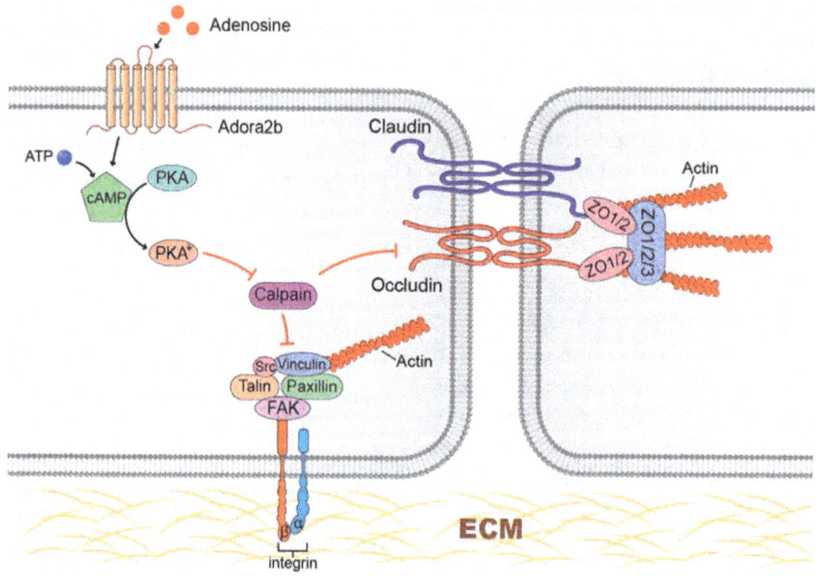

FIGURE 9 | Working model of Adora2b activation in regulating tight junction and focal adhesion junction proteins. Adora2b activation increases cAMP levels by activation of adenylyl cyclase, thus activated protein kinase A (PKA). Activated PKA then inhibits hypoxia-induced calpain activity, protects occludin and FAK degradation, and maintains the epithelial integrity.

knockout mice and loss of protection from dipyridamole and BAY 60-6583. Our studies provide important proof for BAY 60-6583 as a therapeutic medicine for the treatment of ALI.

Previous studies provide proof of concept for adenosine signaling in adaption to hypoxia and inflammation in a wide range of injury models (Eltzschig and Carmeliet, 2011; Eltzschig et al., 2014). In response to hypoxia, transcription factor hypoxia-inducible factor (HIF) is stabilized, which subsequently activates several components of the adenosine signaling pathway, including CD39 and CD73 which elevate extracellular adenosine generation (Eltzschig et al., 2009a; Synnestvedt et al., 2002; Thompson et al., 2004) and Adora2b which enhances the protective adenosine signal (Kong et al., 2006; Eltzschig and Carmeliet, 2011; Eckle et al., 2014; Eltzschig et al., 2014). Moreover, hypoxia also suppresses ENT1 and ENT2 expression by promoting the binding of HIF to their promoters, thus inhibiting adenosine re-uptake and enhancing adenosine downstream signaling events (Eltzschig et al., 2005; Eckle et al., 2013; Morote-Garcia et al., 2013). Consistent with these studies, we observed HIF-1a stabilization following bleomycin exposure in association with a decreased ENT2 expression in the lung. Dampened ENT2 expression is also observed in primary alveolar epithelial cells exposed to hypoxia or HIF-1a stabilizer $CoCl_2$, suggesting the observed down-regulation of ENT2 in ALI could be directly regulated by hypoxia. Taken together, our data provide evidence that the hypoxia-adenosine response is an important mechanism mediating the endogenous protection of ALI. Surprisingly, contrary to the enhanced adenosine levels in response to ALI in mice, we detected decreased adenosine levels in the lungs of ARDS patients. The decreased adenosine levels could be resulted from decreased CD73 activities and elevated adenosine transportation and elimination by ENT2 in ARDS lungs. It is important to mention that the ARDS lungs were collected from patients that succumbed to ARDS, thus it is conceivable that in these patients, insufficient accumulation of adenosine may have been a factor leading to their demise.

Although the role of extracellular adenosine signaling in inflammation has been explored to some extent (Eltzschig, 2011; Eltzschig and Carmeliet, 2011; Eltzschig et al., 2013; Idzko et al., 2014), the downstream mechanisms that mediate the role of adenosine in preventing epithelial permeability is not well studied. The integrity of the epithelial monolayer is critical for the protection of barrier-function (Kirchner et al., 2005; Lucas et al., 2009). Compared to endothelial damage, epithelial damage has more adverse effects on lung injury due to the destruction of the lung architecture that leads to prolonged changes in gas exchange and disordered repair (Martin T. R. et al., 2005). Studies show that preserved epithelial barrier function is inversely associated with mortality of patients with ALI (Martin T. R. et al., 2005; Matthay and Wiener-Kronish, 1990). These conclusions are consistent with our findings that Adora2b in epithelial cells, but not endothelial cells, prevents vascular leakage. Several tight junction and focal adhesion proteins are involved to maintain the integrity of epithelium, including occludins, claudins and focal adhesion kinase (FAK) (Ma et al., 2013; Suzuki, 2013). Deregulation of these proteins in epithelial cells promotes the permeability of the epithelium and facilitates the progression of injury (Jiang et al., 1998; Koval, 2009; Ma et al., 2013). Under stress conditions, cellular permeability can be accelerated by the activation of calpain protease which promotes the degradation of FAK and tight junction proteins and disrupts the cell-cell connection (Chun and Prince, 2009; Heijink et al., 2012; Pereira et al., 2014; Wang et al., 2012). In our study, we found the levels of tight junction protein occludin was decreased in both human ARDS lungs and mouse lungs treated with bleomycin, suggesting a loss of epithelial barrier function in both human and mouse ALI. However, the expression of FAK is elevated in ARDS lungs possibly due to increased infiltration of inflammatory cells such as T lymphocyte and macrophages that also have high FAK expression (Chapman and Houtman, 2014; Hart et al., 2011). We also discovered that adenosine-through Adora2b inhibits hypoxia-induced calpain activation through the activation of cyclic AMP (cAMP) and protein kinase A (PKA), and as a result prevents occludin-1 degradation and epithelial permeability (**Figure 9**). Indeed, under hypoxia condition, our data showed that BAY 60-6583 significantly increased the levels of occludin in MLE12 cells, and the effect of BAY 60-6583 on occludin could be fully blocked by Adora2b antagonist MRS 1754. Although levels of *p*-FAK and claudin-1 was unaffected by BAY 60-6583, they were largely suppressed in cells treated with MRS 1754 (**Figure 7B**), suggesting a role of adenosine through Adora2b in protecting the hypoxia-induced protein degradation of FAK and Claudin-1. FAK protein may be relatively more stable under hypoxia condition, that is probably why it can be slightly upregulated in Bay 606583 treated cells but not obviously affected by MRS 1754. Our results are consistent with previous findings showing improved ALI in mouse treated with a calpain inhibitor (Cuzzocrea et al., 2000; Liu et al., 2012). Although further studies are needed to understand how calpain is activated by hypoxia, and which calpain is directed targeted by adora2b/PKA, our findings identified calpain as a novel downstream target of Adora2b and provide evidence for the development of drugs aimed at targeting adenosine signaling and calpain as a therapeutic treatment of ALI.

In addition to providing evidence for the role of adenosine signaling in preventing ALI, our studies also identified dipyridamole and BAY 60-6583 as therapeutic agents in the treatment of established ALI. Previous studies showed a beneficial role of adenosine in a wide range of acute injury models, including sepsis (Csoka et al., 2010), and lung (Zhou et al., 2011; Eckle et al., 2013), kidney (Bauerle et al., 2011; Grenz et al., 2012b) and gastrointestinal injuries (Eltzschig et al., 2009b). However, all of these studies initiate adenosine treatment before inducing tissue injury and implicate only the prophylactic role of adenosine signaling in ALI. Here we demonstrate that treating mice with dipyridamole or BAY 60-6583 two days after bleomycin exposure, a time point when ALI is already established, still improve the barrier function by decreasing inflammation and neutrophil infiltration. Our findings are of particular importance for the treatment of ARDS patients who have already developed symptoms of ALI in the intensive care unit, and provide important preclinical proof for enhancing adenosine signaling as a therapeutic method for the treatment of ARDS patients.

Taken together, our findings identified adenosine signaling as an important endogenous pathway to not only prevent but also treat ALI. Inhibiting adenosine re-uptake by pharmaceutical agent dipyridamole could be a therapeutic strategy to enhance adenosine signaling through Adora2b that in turn prevents calpain activity and preserves epithelial integrity. Our results provide important pre-clinical data for the use of dipyridamole and adenosine receptor agonists in the treatment of ALI.

AUTHOR CONTRIBUTIONS

TW, HKQ, and MRB, designed the study and drafted the manuscript. WW, TW, NC, JD, and KP performed the experiments, collected the data and contributed to the statistical analysis. HKE, DR, and BA interpreted the data, and reviewed the manuscript.

ACKNOWLEDGMENTS

We thank Kelly A Volcik from the Department of Biochemistry and Molecular Biology, McGovern Medical School, the University of Texas Health Science Center at Houston for proof-reading the manuscript.

REFERENCES

Bakowitz, M., Bruns, B., and McCunn, M. (2012). Acute lung injury and the acute respiratory distress syndrome in the injured patient. *Scand. J. Trauma Resusc. Emerg. Med.* 20, 54. doi:10.1186/1757-7241-20-54

Bauerle, J. D., Grenz, A., Kim, J.-H., Lee, H. T., and Eltzschig, H. K. (2011). Adenosine generation and signaling during acute kidney injury. *J. Am. Soc. Nephrol.* 22 (1), 14–20. doi:10.1681/ASN.2009121217

Blackburn, M. R., Vance, C. O., Morschl, E., and Wilson, C. N. (2009). Adenosine receptors and inflammation. *Handb. Exp. Pharmacol.* 193, 215–269. doi:10.1007/978-3-540-89615-9_8

Cagnina, R. E., Ramos, S. I., Marshall, M. A., Wang, G., Frazier, C. R., and Linden, J. (2009). Adenosine A2B receptors are highly expressed on murine type II alveolar epithelial cells. *Am. J. Physiol. Lung Cell. Mol. Physiol.* 297 (3), L467 L474. doi:10.1152/ajplung.90553.2008

Chapman, N. M., and Houtman, J. C. D. (2014). Functions of the FAK family kinases in T cells: beyond actin cytoskeletal rearrangement. *Immunol. Res.* 59 (1–3), 23–34. doi:10.1007/s12026-014-8527-y

Chun, J., and Prince, A. (2009). TLR2-induced calpain cleavage of epithelial junctional proteins facilitates leukocyte transmigration. *Cell Host and Microbe* 5 (1), 47–58. doi:10.1016/j.chom.2008.11.009

Csóka, B., Németh, Z. H., Rosenberger, P., Eltzschig, H. K., Spolarics, Z., Pacher, P., et al. (2010). A2B adenosine receptors protect against sepsis-induced mortality by dampening excessive inflammation. *J. Immunol.* 185 (1), 542–550. doi:10.4049/jimmunol.0901295

Cuzzocrea, S., McDonald, M. C., Mazzon, E., Siriwardena, D., Serraino, I., Dugo, L., et al. (2000). Calpain inhibitor I reduces the development of acute and chronic inflammation. *Am. J. Pathol.* 157 (6), 2065–2079. doi:10.1016/S0002-9440(10)64845-6

De Schryver, E. L., Algra, A., and van Gijn, J. (2007). Dipyridamole for preventing stroke and other vascular events in patients with vascular disease. *Cochrane Database Syst. Rev.* 3, CD001820. doi:10.1002/14651858.CD001820.pub3

Eckle, T., Grenz, A., Laucher, S., and Eltzschig, H. K. (2008). A2B adenosine receptor signaling attenuates acute lung injury by enhancing alveolar fluid clearance in mice. *J. Clin. Invest.* 118 (10), 3301–3315. doi:10.1172/JCI34203

Eckle, T., Hughes, K., Ehrentraut, H., Brodsky, K. S., Rosenberger, P., Choi, D. S., et al. (2013). Crosstalk between the equilibrative nucleoside transporter ENT2 and alveolar Adora2b adenosine receptors dampens acute lung injury. *FASEB J.* 27 (8), 3078–3089. doi:10.1096/fj.13-228551

Eckle, T., Kewley, E. M., Brodsky, K. S., Tak, E., Bonney, S., Gobel, M., et al. (2014). Identification of hypoxia-inducible factor HIF-1A as transcriptional regulator of the A2B adenosine receptor during acute lung injury. *J. Immunol.* 192 (3), 1249–1256. doi:10.4049/jimmunol.1100593

Eckle, T., Koeppen, M., and Eltzschig, H. K. (2009). Role of extracellular adenosine in acute lung injury. *Physiology* 24, 298–306. doi:10.1152/physiol.00022.2009

Eltzschig, H. K. (2011). Targeting hypoxia-induced inflammation. *Anesthesiology* 114 (2), 239–242. doi:10.1097/ALN.0b013e3182070c66

Eltzschig, H. K., Abdulla, P., Hoffman, E., Hamilton, K. E., Daniels, D., Schönfeld, C., et al. (2005). HIF-1-dependent repression of equilibrative nucleoside transporter (ENT) in hypoxia. *J. Exp. Med.* 202 (11), 1493–1505. doi:10.1084/jem.20050177

Eltzschig, H. K., Bratton, D. L., and Colgan, S. P. (2014). Targeting hypoxia signalling for the treatment of ischaemic and inflammatory diseases. *Nat. Rev. Drug Discov.* 13 (11), 852–869. doi:10.1038/nrd4422

Eltzschig, H. K., and Carmeliet, P. (2011). Hypoxia and inflammation. *N. Engl. J. Med.* 364 (7), 656–665. doi:10.1056/NEJMra0910283

Eltzschig, H. K., Köhler, D., Eckle, T., Kong, T., Robson, S. C., and Colgan, S. P. (2009a). Central role of Sp1-regulated CD39 in hypoxia/ischemia protection. *Blood* 113 (1), 224–232. doi:10.1182/blood-2008-06-165746

Eltzschig, H. K., Rivera-Nieves, J., and Colgan, S. P. (2009b). Targeting the A2B adenosine receptor during gastrointestinal ischemia and inflammation. *Expert Opin. Ther. Targets* 13 (11), 1267–1277. doi:10.1517/14728220903241666

Eltzschig, H. K., Sitkovsky, M. V., and Robson, S. C. (2013). Purinergic signaling during inflammation. *N. Engl. J. Med.* 368 (13), 1260. doi:10.1056/NEJMc1300259

Eltzschig, H. K., Sitkovsky, M. V., and Robson, S. C. (2012). Purinergic signaling during inflammation. *N. Engl. J. Med.* 367 (24), 2322–2333. doi:10.1056/NEJMra1205750

Eltzschig, H. K. (2009). Adenosine: an old drug newly discovered. *Anesthesiology* 111 (4), 904–915. doi:10.1097/ALN.0b013e3181b060f2

Fanelli, V., and Ranieri, V. M. (2015). Mechanisms and clinical consequences of acute lung injury. *Ann. ATS* 12 (Suppl. 1), S3–S8. doi:10.1513/AnnalsATS.201407-340MG

Flori, H. R., Glidden, D. V., Rutherford, G. W., and Matthay, M. A. (2005). Pediatric acute lung injury prospective evaluation of risk factors associated with mortality. *Am. J. Respir. Crit. Care Med.* 171 (9), 995–1001. doi:10.1164/rccm.200404-544OC

Froudarakis, M., Hatzimichael, E., Kyriazopoulou, L., Lagos, K., Pappas, P., Tzakos, A. G., et al. (2013). Revisiting bleomycin from pathophysiology to safe clinical use. *Crit. Rev. Oncol. Hematol.* 87 (1), 90–100. doi:10.1016/j.critrevonc.2012.12.003

Goh, K. J., Choong, M. C., Cheong, E. H., Kalimuddin, S., Duu Wen, S., Phua, G. C., et al. (2020). Rapid progression to acute respiratory distress syndrome: review of current understanding of critical illness from COVID-19 infection. *Ann. Acad. Med. Singapore* 49 (1), 1–9. doi:10.47102/annals-acadmedsg.202057

Gong, Y., Ma, T.-C., Xu, Y.-Y., Yang, R., Gao, L.-J., Wu, S.-H., et al. (2020). Early research on COVID-19: a bibliometric analysis. *Innovation* 1 (2), 100027. doi:10.1016/j.xinn.2020.100027

Grenz, A., Bauerle, J. D., Dalton, J. H., Ridyard, D., Badulak, A., Tak, E., et al. (2012a). Equilibrative nucleoside transporter 1 (ENT1) regulates postischemic blood flow during acute kidney injury in mice. *J. Clin. Invest.* 122 (2), 693–710. doi:10.1172/JCI60214

Grenz, A., Kim, J.-H., Bauerle, J. D., Tak, E., Eltzschig, H. K., and Clambey, E. T. (2012b). Adora2b adenosine receptor signaling protects during acute kidney injury via inhibition of neutrophil-dependent TNF-α release. *J. Immunol.* 189 (9), 4566–4573. doi:10.4049/jimmunol.1201651

Grenz, A., Homann, D., and Eltzschig, H. K. (2011). Extracellular adenosine: a safety signal that dampens hypoxia-induced inflammation during ischemia. *Antioxid. Redox Signaling* 15 (8), 2221–2234. doi:10.1089/ars.2010.3665

Grenz, A., Zhang, H., Hermes, M., Eckle, T., Klingel, K., Huang, D. Y., et al. (2007). Contribution of E-NTPDasel (CD39) to renal protection from ischemia-reperfusion injury. *FASEB J.* 21 (11), 2863–2873. doi:10.1096/fj.06-7947com

Hart, M. L., Grenz, A., Gorzolla, I. C., Schittenhelm, J., Dalton, J. H., and Eltzschig, H. K. (2011). Hypoxia-inducible factor-1α-dependent protection from intestinal ischemia/reperfusion injury involves ecto-5′-nucleotidase (CD73) and the A2B adenosine receptor. *J. Immunol.* 186 (7), 4367–4374. doi:10.4049/jimmunol.0903617

Haskó, G., Csóka, B., Koscsó, B., Chandra, R., Pacher, P., Thompson, L. F., et al. (2011). Ecto-5′-Nucleotidase (CD73) decreases mortality and organ injury in sepsis. *J. Immunol.* 187 (8), 4256–4267. doi:10.4049/jimmunol.1003379

Haskó, G., Linden, J., Cronstein, B., and Pacher, P. (2008). Adenosine receptors: therapeutic aspects for inflammatory and immune diseases. *Nat. Rev. Drug Discov.* 7 (9), 759–770. doi:10.1038/nrd2638

Heijink, I. H., Brandenburg, S. M., Postma, D. S., and van Oosterhout, A. J. M. (2012). Cigarette smoke impairs airway epithelial barrier function and cell-cell contact recovery. *Eur. Respir. J.* 39 (2), 419–428. doi:10.1183/09031936.00193810

Idzko, M., Ferrari, D., and Eltzschig, H. K. (2014). Nucleotide signalling during inflammation. *Nature* 509 (7500), 310–317. doi:10.1038/nature13085

Jiang, W. G., Bryce, R. P., Horrobin, D. F., and Mansel, R. E. (1998). Regulation of tight junction permeability and occludin expression by polyunsaturated fatty acids. *Biochem. Biophys. Res. Commun.* 244 (2), 414–420. doi:10.1006/bbrc.1998.8288

Karmouty-Quintana, H., Xia, Y., and Blackburn, M. R. (2013). Adenosine signaling during acute and chronic disease states. *J. Mol. Med.* 91 (2), 173–181. doi:10.1007/s00109-013-0997-1

Kirchner, E. A., Mols, G., Hermle, G., Muehlschlegel, J. D., Geiger, K. K., Guttmann, J., et al. (2005). Reduced activation of immunomodulatory transcription factors during positive end-expiratory pressure adjustment based on volume-dependent compliance in isolated perfused rabbit lungs. *Br. J. Anaesth.* 94 (4), 530–535. doi:10.1093/bja/aei078

Koeppen, M., Eckle, T., and Eltzschig, H. K. (2011). Interplay of hypoxia and A2B adenosine receptors in tissue protection. *Adv. Pharmacol.* 61, 145–186. doi:10.1016/B978-0-12-385526-8.00006-0

Kong, T., Westerman, K. A., Faigle, M., Eltzschig, H. K., and Colgan, S. P. (2006). HIF-dependent induction of adenosine A2B receptor in hypoxia. *FASEB J.* 20 (13), 2242–2250. doi:10.1096/fj.06-6419com

Koval, M. (2009). Tight junctions, but not too tight: fine control of lung permeability by claudins. *Am. J. Physiol. Lung Cell. Mol. Physiol.* 297 (2), L217–L218. doi:10.1152/ajplung.00196.2009

Li, X., and Ma, X. (2020). Acute respiratory failure in COVID-19: is it "typical" ARDS?. *Crit. Care* 24 (1), 198. doi:10.1186/s13054-020-02911-9

Liang, D., Shi, L., Zhao, J., Liu, P., Sarnat, J. A., Gao, S., et al. (2020). Urban air pollution may enhance COVID-19 case-fatality and mortality rates in the United States. *Innovation* 1 (3), 100047. doi:10.1016/j.xinn.2020.100047

Liu, D., Yan, Z., Minshall, R. D., Schwartz, D. E., Chen, Y., and Hu, G. (2012). Activation of calpains mediates early lung neutrophilic inflammation in ventilator-induced lung injury. *Am. J. Physiol. Lung Cell. Mol. Physiol.* 302 (4), L370–L379. doi:10.1152/ajplung.00349.2011

Lucas, R., Verin, A. D., Black, S. M., and Catravas, J. D. (2009). Regulators of endothelial and epithelial barrier integrity and function in acute lung injury. *Biochem. Pharmacol.* 77 (12), 1763–1772. doi:10.1016/j.bcp.2009.01.014

Ma, Y., Semba, S., Khan, M. R. I., Bochimoto, H., Watanabe, T., Fujiya, M., et al. (2013). Focal adhesion kinase regulates intestinal epithelial barrier function via redistribution of tight junction. *Biochim. Biophys. Acta* 1832 (1), 151–159. doi:10.1016/j.bbadis.2012.10.006

Martin, T. R., Hagimoto, N., Nakamura, M., and Matute-Bello, G. (2005). Apoptosis and epithelial injury in the lungs. *Proc. Am. Thorac. Soc.* 2 (3), 214–220. doi:10.1513/pats.200504-031AC

Martin, W. G., Ristow, K. M., Habermann, T. M., Colgan, J. P., Witzig, T. E., and Ansell, S. M. (2005). Bleomycin pulmonary toxicity has a negative impact on the outcome of patients with Hodgkin's lymphoma. *J. Clin. Oncol.* 23 (30), 7614 7620. doi:10.1200/JCO.2005.02.7243

Matthay, M. A., Ware, L. B., and Zimmerman, G. A. (2012). The acute respiratory distress syndrome. *J. Clin. Invest.* 122 (8), 2731–2740. doi:10.1172/jci60331

Matthay, M. A., and Wiener-Kronish, J. P. (1990). Intact epithelial barrier function is critical for the resolution of alveolar edema in humans. *Am. Rev. Respir. Dis.* 142 (6 Pt. 1), 1250–1257. doi:10.1164/ajrccm/142.6_Pt_1.1250

Matthay, M. A., and Zemans, R. L. (2011). The acute respiratory distress syndrome: pathogenesis and treatment. *Annu. Rev. Pathol. Mech. Dis.* 6, 147–163. doi:10.1146/annurev-pathol-011110-130158

Matute-Bello, G., Frevert, C. W., and Martin, T. R. (2008). Animal models of acute lung injury. *Am. J. Physiol. Lung Cell. Mol. Physiol.* 295 (3), L379–L399. doi:10.1152/ajplung.00010.2008

Morote-Garcia, J. C., Köhler, D., Roth, J. M., Mirakaj, V., Eldh, T., Eltzschig, H. K., et al. (2013). Repression of the equilibrative nucleoside transporters dampens inflammatory lung injury. *Am. J. Respir. Cell. Mol. Biol.* 49 (2), 296–305. doi:10.1165/rcmb.2012-0457OC

Nuckton, T. J., Alonso, J. A., Kallet, R. H., Daniel, B. M., Pittet, J.-F., Eisner, M. D., et al. (2002). Pulmonary dead-space fraction as a risk factor for death in the acute respiratory distress syndrome. *N. Engl. J. Med.* 346 (17), 1281–1286. doi:10.1056/NEJMoa012835

Pereira, M. B. M., Santos, A. M., Gonçalves, D. C., Cardoso, A. C., Consonni, S. R., Gozzo, F. C., et al. (2014). αB-crystallin interacts with and prevents stress-activated proteolysis of focal adhesion kinase by calpain in cardiomyocytes. *Nat. Commun.* 5, 5159. doi:10.1038/ncomms6159

Ranieri, V. M., Ranieri, V. M., Rubenfeld, G. D., Thompson, B. T., Ferguson, N. D., Caldwell, E., et al. (2012). Acute respiratory distress syndrome: the Berlin Definition. *JAMA* 307 (23), 2526–2533. doi:10.1001/jama.2012.5669

Reutershan, J., Vollmer, I., Stark, S., Wagner, R., Ngamsri, K. C., and Eltzschig, H. K. (2009). Adenosine and inflammation: CD39 and CD73 are critical mediators in LPS-induced PMN trafficking into the lungs. *FASEB J.* 23 (2), 473–482. doi:10.1096/fj.08-119701

Richardson, S., Hirsch, J. S., Narasimhan, M., Crawford, J. M., McGinn, T., Davidson, K. W., et al. (2020). Presenting characteristics, comorbidities, and outcomes among 5700 patients hospitalized with COVID-19 in the New York city area. *JAMA*, 323, 2052–2059. doi:10.1001/jama.2020.6775

Rosenthal, C., Caronia, C., Quinn, C., Lugo, N., and Sagy, M. (1998). A comparison among animal models of acute lung injury. *Crit. Care Med.* 26 (5), 912–916. doi:10.1097/00003246-199805000-00027

Sacco, R. L., Diener, H.-C., Yusuf, S., Cotton, D., Ôunpuu, S., Lawton, W. A., et al. 2008). Aspirin and extended-release dipyridamole versus clopidogrel for recurrent stroke. *N. Engl. J. Med.* 359 (12), 1238–1251. doi:10.1056/NEJMoa0805002

Suzuki, T. (2013). Regulation of intestinal epithelial permeability by tight junctions. *Cell. Mol. Life Sci.* 70 (4), 631–659. doi:10.1007/s00018-012-1070-x

Synnestvedt, K., Furuta, G. T., Comerford, K. M., Louis, N., Karhausen, J., Eltzschig, H. K., et al. (2002). Ecto-5′-nucleotidase (CD73) regulation by hypoxia-inducible factor-1 mediates permeability changes in intestinal epithelia. *J. Clin. Invest.* 110 (7), 993–1002. doi:10.1172/jci0215337

Thompson, L. F., Eltzschig, H. K., Ibla, J. C., Van De Wiele, C. J., Resta, R., Morote-Garcia, J. C., et al. (2004). Crucial role for ecto-5′-nucleotidase (CD73) in vascular leakage during hypoxia. *J. Exp. Med.* 200 (11), 1395–1405. doi:10.1084/jem.20040915

Thompson, L. F., Picher, M., and Blackburn, M. R. (2011). Animal models of airway diseases. *Subcell Biochem.* 55, 195–234. doi:10.1007/978-94-007-1217-1_8

Wang, C., Schwab, L. P., Fan, M., Seagroves, T. N., and Buolamwini, J. K. (2013). Chemoprevention activity of dipyridamole in the MMTV-PyMT transgenic mouse model of breast cancer. *Cancer Prev. Res.* 6 (5), 437–447. doi:10.1158/1940-6207.CAPR-12-0345

Wang, T., Wang, L., Moreno-Vinasco, L., Lang, G. D., Siegler, J. H., Mathew, B., et al. (2012). Particulate matter air pollution disrupts endothelial cell barrier via calpain-mediated tight junction protein degradation. *Part. Fibre Toxicol.* 9, 35. doi:10.1186/1743-8977-9-35

Ware, L. (2006). Pathophysiology of acute lung injury and the acute respiratory distress syndrome. *Semin. Respir. Crit. Care Med.* 27 (4), 337–349. doi:10.1055/s-2006-948288

Ware, L. B., and Matthay, M. A. (2000). The acute respiratory distress syndrome. *N. Engl. J. Med.* 342 (18), 1334–1349. doi:10.1056/nejm200005043421806

Williamson, J. D., Sadofsky, L. R., and Hart, S. P. (2015). The pathogenesis of bleomycin-induced lung injury in animals and its applicability to human idiopathic pulmonary fibrosis. *Exp. Lung Res.* 41 (2), 57–73. doi:10.3109/01902148.2014.979516

Yao, S. Y. M., Ng, A. M. L., Muzyka, W. R., Griffiths, M., Cass, C. E., Baldwin, S. A., et al. (1997). Molecular cloning and functional characterization of nitrobenzylthioinosine (NBMPR)-sensitive (es) and NBMPR-insensitive (ei) equilibrative nucleoside transporter proteins (rENT1 and rENT2) from rat tissues. *J. Biol. Chem.* 272 (45), 28423–28430. doi:10.1074/jbc.272.45.28423

Zhou, Y., Schneider, D. J., and Blackburn, M. R. (2009). Adenosine signaling and the regulation of chronic lung disease. *Pharmacol. Ther.* 123 (1), 105–116. doi:10.1016/j.pharmthera.2009.04.003

Zhou, Y., Schneider, D. J., Morschl, E., Song, L., Pedroza, M., Karmouty-Quintana, H., et al. (2011). Distinct roles for the A2B adenosine receptor in acute and chronic stages of bleomycin-induced lung injury. *J. Immunol.* 186 (2), 1097–1106. doi:10.4049/jimmunol.1002907

Zimmerman, M. A., Tak, E., Ehrentraut, S. F., Kaplan, M., Giebler, A., Weng, T., et al. (2013). Retracted: equilibrative nucleoside transporter (ENT)-1-dependent elevation of extracellular adenosine protects the liver during ischemia and reperfusion. *Hepatology* 58 (5), 1766–1778. doi:10.1002/hep.26505

13

Identification of Proteomic Signatures in Chronic Obstructive Pulmonary Disease Emphysematous Phenotype

Shuang Bai[1], Rui Ye[1], Cuihong Wang[1], Pengbo Sun[1], Di Wang[1], Yong Yue[2], Huiying Wang[2], Si Wu[3], Miao Yu[3], Shuhua Xi[4*†] and Li Zhao[1*†]

[1]Department of Pulmonary and Critical Care Medicine, Shengjing Hospital of China Medical University, Shenyang, China, [2]Department of Radiology, Shengjing Hospital of China Medical University, Shenyang, China, [3]Department of Biobank, Shengjing Hospital of China Medical University, Shenyang, China, [4]Department of Environmental and Occupational Health, School of Public Health, China Medical University, Shenyang, China

***Correspondence:**
Shuhua Xi
shxi@cmu.edu.cn
Li Zhao
lzhaoli@163.com

[†]These authors have contributed equally to this work

Chronic obstructive pulmonary disease (COPD) is a highly heterogeneous disease. Emphysematous phenotype is the most common and critical phenotype, which is characterized by progressive lung destruction and poor prognosis. However, the underlying mechanism of this structural damage has not been completely elucidated. A total of 12 patients with COPD emphysematous phenotype (COPD-E) and nine patients with COPD non-emphysematous phenotype (COPD-NE) were enrolled to determine differences in differential abundant protein (DAP) expression between both groups. Quantitative tandem mass tag–based proteomics was performed on lung tissue samples of all patients. A total of 29 and 15 lung tissue samples from patients in COPD-E and COPD-NE groups, respectively, were used as the validation cohort to verify the proteomic analysis results using western blotting. Gene ontology (GO) and Kyoto Encyclopedia of Genes and Genomes (KEGG) enrichment analyses were conducted for DAPs. A total of 4,343 proteins were identified, of which 25 were upregulated and 11 were downregulated in the COPD-E group. GO and KEGG analyses showed that wound repair and retinol metabolism–related pathways play an essential role in the molecular mechanism of COPD emphysematous phenotype. Three proteins, namely, KRT17, DHRS9, and FMO3, were selected for validation. While KRT17 and DHRS9 were highly expressed in the lung tissue samples of the COPD-E group, FMO3 expression was not significantly different between both groups. In conclusion, KRT17 and DHRS9 are highly expressed in the lung tissue of patients with COPD emphysematous phenotype. Therefore, these proteins might involve in wound healing and retinol metabolism in patients with emphysematous phenotype and can be used as phenotype-specific markers.

Keywords: chronic obstructive pulmonary disease, emphysematous phenotype, proteomics, KRT17, DHRS9

INTRODUCTION

Chronic obstructive pulmonary disease (COPD) emphysematous phenotype is characterized by lung tissue destruction and distal airspace over inflation (Alford et al., 2010; Camp et al., 2014; Wang et al., 2018). In contrast to patients with other COPD phenotypes, those with emphysematous phenotype typically manifest symptoms such as severe dyspnea, decreased exercise tolerance, and physiological complications. Moreover, patients with emphysematous phenotype have a higher mortality than those with non-emphysematous phenotype (Fan et al., 2014; Criner et al., 2018; Bai et al., 2020). Some emphysematous smokers do not exhibit airflow limitation (Oelsner et al., 2014), despite showing similar pathophysiological features to those with COPD (Bai et al., 2020). Unfortunately, there are few biomarkers that could be useful to predict the emphysema phenotype in COPD patients. And pharmaceutical intervention to reverse lung destruction or inhibit pulmonary damage is not available for these patients (Vogelmeier et al., 2017; Janssen et al., 2019).

Low blood eosinophils, elevated plasmin-mediated degradation of cross-linked fibrin, and hypermethylation of microRNA-7 are regarded as the features of emphysematous phenotype (Papaioannou et al., 2017; Manon-Jensen et al., 2019; Rosas-Alonso et al., 2020), but their potential to serve as prognostic biomarkers needs further validation. Moreover, the underlying molecular mechanism of COPD emphysematous phenotype remains unclear. Besides, imbalances between proteases/antiproteases and oxidants/antioxidants, enhanced inflammatory response (Lan et al., 2019; Zeng et al., 2020), and dysfunctional tissue repair in the lung parenchyma and interstitium play an important role in the pathogenetic mechanisms of emphysema (Jiang et al., 2017; Belgacemi et al., 2020; Hu et al., 2020). However, the underlying mechanisms remain poorly understood.

Proteomics reflects proteins expression changes, which are occurring in organisms. It is an important tool to understand pathogenesis and identify disease biomarkers. Tandem mass tag (TMT) quantitative proteomics is a reliable approach to measure protein content, and it has been increasingly used to identify pathogenetic mechanisms and human disease biomarkers (Mertins et al., 2018; Dziekan et al., 2020; Wang et al., 2020). While most proteomic studies in patients with COPD have used bronchoalveolar lavage fluid (Tu et al., 2014), sputum (Titz et al., 2015), and blood (Sridhar et al., 2019), only a few have used lung tissue samples. Furthermore, as per our understanding, the studies that specifically addressed COPD emphysematous phenotype are not available. Since COPD is a highly heterogeneous disease, the proteomic analysis focused on its emphysematous phenotype has remarkable significance.

In this study, we conducted proteomic analysis of lung tissue samples using TMT quantitative proteomic techniques to identify key molecules and their underlying mechanisms in patients with COPD emphysematous phenotype.

MATERIALS AND METHODS

Patients

Patients with COPD were recruited based on the criteria previously described (Bai et al., 2020). In brief, the inclusion criteria were as follows: 40- to 80-year-old patients diagnosed with COPD, more than 10 pack-years of smoking history, preparing for chest surgery, and read and signed informed consent. Patients with other respiratory diseases, autoimmune diseases, or infections that occurred within 4 weeks before surgery were excluded. All enrolled patients were assigned to two groups: the COPD emphysematous phenotype (COPD-E) group and the COPD non-emphysematous phenotype (COPD-NE) group, according to the diagnosis of investigators and results of image analysis. Chest computed tomography (CT) scans revealed obvious emphysema in COPD-E patients and almost no emphysema in COPD-NE patients. The patients in both groups were matched for sex, age, and smoking history. The study protocol was approved by the Ethics Committee of Shengjing Hospital of China Medical University (Shenyang, China; Ethical no. 2016PS342K). For each patient included, written informed consent was obtained.

CT Scanning

Chest CT scans were obtained for all patients using Philips Brilliance iCT 256 (Philips, Surrey, United Kingdom), TOSHIBA Aquilion ONE (Toshiba, Tokyo, Japan), Siemens SOMATOM Definition Flash (Siemens, Forchheim, Germany), or GE Optima CT660 (GE, Milwaukee, WI, United States). All scans were obtained at a deep inspiratory breath hold. The following parameters were applied in the examination: tube voltage, 120 kV; tube current, 180 mA; and reconstruction matrix, 512 × 512. Two radiologists performed radiological measurements. The detailed CT acquisition parameters are shown in**Supplementary Table S1**.

Emphysema Screening

Chest CT scans of the patients were acquired from the CT workstation (Neusoft, Shenyang, China), and the image analyses were performed using Pulmonary Toolkit in Matlab (R2016a) (The MathWorks, Inc., Natick, MA, United States). The degree of emphysema was determined quantitatively according to our previous study (Bai et al., 2020). In brief, voxels with a CT value less than −950 HU were identified as the emphysematous area. The emphysema index was defined as the lung volume fraction of voxels with a CT value below −950 HU at a full inspiration (Camp et al., 2009; Coxson et al., 2014). The emphysema percentile density was defined as the 15th percentile lung density derived from the distribution histogram of whole lung CT voxel (Dirksen et al., 2009). The raw data of all CT images were entered into the analysis software, following which the results were obtained.

Sample Preparation

Samples were prepared as described previously (Sun et al., 2019; Bai et al., 2020). In brief, lung tissue samples were obtained as far as possible from the tumor (at least 5 cm from the boundary). Lung parenchyma, pulmonary vessels, and small airways were equal approximately in each sample. Each specimen was cleaned with normal saline and dried. The collected lung tissue samples were frozen with liquid nitrogen immediately and stored at −80°C until use.

The lung tissue samples were lysed using the SDT (4% SDS (w/v); 0.1 M DTT; 100 mM Tris-HCl, pH 7.6) lysis method. The BCA method was used to determine protein concentration. Every three tissue samples of COPD-NE patients were pooled together to form the three biological replicates in the COPD-NE group, and every four tissue samples of COPD-E patients were pooled together to form the three biological replicates in the COPD-E group. The filter-aided proteome preparation method was used to perform protein collection (Wiśniewski et al., 2009). In brief, lysates were mixed with 8 M urea in the filter unit of Microcon devices (Millipore, Bedford, MA, United States) and centrifuged to remove the low-molecular-weight material. Subsequently, 0.05 M iodoacetamide in 8 M urea was added to the concentrate followed by centrifugation. The resulting concentrate was diluted with 8 M urea and concentrated again. Finally, endoproteinase was added to digest proteins, and the digests were centrifuged to collect peptides. The concentration of peptide was measured at OD280. An equal amount of peptide was used from each sample, and all peptides were labeled using the TMT10 labeling kit (Thermo Fisher Scientific, Waltham, MA, United States) as described in the manufacturer's instructions. Then, the labeled peptides were mixed, and the high-pH reversed-phase peptide fractionation kit was used to perform grading subsequently. Briefly, the fractionation column was equilibrated with acetonitrile and 0.1% trifluoroacetic acid, and the labeled peptides were loaded into the column. After adding pure water, the samples were centrifuged at a low speed for desalination treatment. Finally, the column-bound peptides were gradient-eluted with increasing concentrations of high-pH acetonitrile solutions. Each eluted peptide sample was dried in vacuum and reconstituted in 0.1% formic acid. The peptide concentration of each sample was measured at OD280.

Liquid Chromatography-Tandem Mass Spectrometry Analysis

A high-performance liquid chromatography liquid-phase system (Thermo Fisher Scientific, Waltham, MA, United States) was used to separate the graded samples passed consecutively through the loading and analytical columns at 300 nl/min. Subsequently, a Q Exactive mass spectrometer (Thermo Fisher Scientific, Waltham, MA, United States) was used to perform LC-MS/MS analysis. The following parameters were applied for detection: positive ion mode; the precursor ion scanning range was 300–1800 m/z; the first-order mass spectrum resolution was 70,000 at 200 m/z; the automatic gain control target was 1e6; maximum IT at 50 ms; and dynamic exclusion at 60 s. The collection method of peptide fragments' mass-to-mass ratio was as follows: 20 fragment spectra (MS2 scans) were collected after each full scan; the MS2 activation type was high-energy collision dissociation; and the isolation window was 2 m/z. In addition, the secondary MS resolution was 35,000 at 200 m/z, with a normalized collision energy of 30 eV and 0.1% underfill.

Protein Identification and Quantification

Proteins were identified in the UniProt database using Mascot 2.2 and Proteome Discoverer 1.4 software. The selection criteria for the trusted peptides were as follows: FDR < 0.01; peptide mass of ±20 ppm; and fragment mass tolerance of 0.1 Da. Protein quantification was performed in accordance with only the unique peptides' median of the protein. By calculating the relative expression ratio of the target protein to the reference protein for all samples in each group, the protein abundant differences between the two groups were compared. Finally, all peptide ratios were normalized using the median protein ratio.

Bioinformatics Analysis

Gene ontology (GO) and Kyoto Encyclopedia of Genes and Genomes (KEGG) pathways were analyzed using Blast2GO and KEGG automatic annotation server software, respectively. Fisher's exact test was used to compare the distribution of target proteins in the GO and KEGG pathways and perform enrichment analysis. Protein cluster analysis was conducted using the ComplexHeatmap R package (R version 3.4). The expression matrix of target proteins was normalized prior to the generation of the hierarchical cluster heat map. Protein interaction network analysis of target proteins was based on the STRING database and visualized with Cytoscape software (version 3.6.0). The overall scheme of TMT quantitative proteomics is shown in **Figure 1**.

Western Blot Analysis

Western blotting was performed according to our previous protocols (Bai et al., 2020). In brief, total protein extracts were prepared using RIPA lysis buffer, and the concentration of protein was estimated using the BCA method. In sodium dodecyl sulfate–polyacrylamide gel electrophoresis, equal amounts of denatured proteins were loaded. Each sample protein was transferred from gel to a polyvinylidene fluoride membrane, blocked with 5% non-fat milk, and incubated overnight with the primary antibody at 4°C. On the following day, secondary antibodies were added to incubate the membrane for 1 h. For chemiluminescence detection, protein bands were revealed using enhanced chemiluminescence reagent. The following primary antibodies were used: anti-KRT17 (ab51056) and anti-FMO3 (ab126711) from Abcam (Cambridge, Cambridgeshire, United Kingdom) and anti-DHRS9 and anti-GAPDH from Proteintech (Chicago, IL, United States).

Statistical Analysis

All statistical analyses were performed using GraphPad Prism 7 (GraphPad, La Jolla, CA, United States), except for bioinformatics analysis. Bioinformatics-related statistical software and methods are described in *Bioinformatics Analysis*. Student's *t*-test was used to compare means between two groups of normally distributed data. For data with non-normal distribution, the Mann–Whitney U test was used. The comparison of two groups of categorical variable data was analyzed by Fisher's exact probability. Continuous variables are expressed as the mean ± standard error of mean. Linear regression analysis was conducted for regression and correlation analyses. $p < 0.05$ was regarded as statistically significant.

RESULTS

Demographic and Radiological Features

In total, 16 patients in the COPD-NE group and 29 patients in the COPD-E group were recruited between September 2016 and June 2019. Lung tissue samples of 9 patients in the COPD-NE group and 12 patients in the COPD-E group were used for proteomic

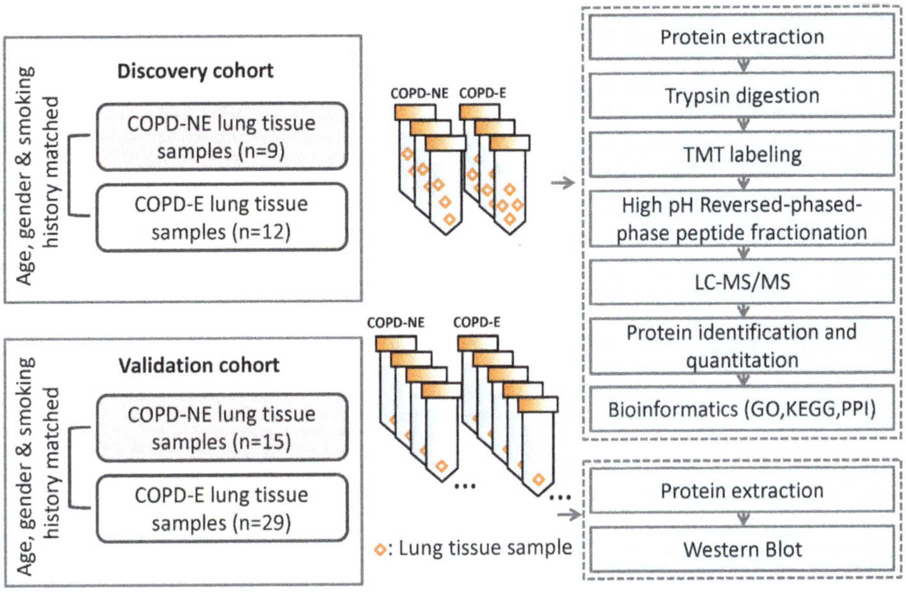

FIGURE 1 | Schematic diagram of tandem mass tag–based quantitative proteomic analysis. For the discovery cohort, every three tissue samples of COPD-NE patients were pooled together to form the three biological replicates in the COPD-NE group, and every four tissue samples of COPD-E patients were pooled together to form the three biological replicates in the COPD-E group. Liquid chromatography-tandem mass spectrometry analysis was performed for the discovery cohort. For the validation cohort, every lung tissue sample was used as an independent one. Western blot was performed to validate the results of liquid chromatography-tandem mass spectrometry analysis.

TABLE 1 | Demographic and spirometric features of the discovery cohort.

	COPD-NE	COPD-E	*p* value
Patients, *n*	9	12	–
Age, years	62.11 ± 2.80	65 ± 1.94	0.39
Gender	–	–	1.00
Male, *n* (%)	9 (100.0)	12 (100.0)	
Female, *n* (%)	0	0	–
Smokers	–	–	0.12
Current, *n* (%)	5 (55.6)	11 (91.7)	–
Ex-smoker, *n* (%)	4 (44.4)	1 (8.3)	–
Years of smoking	37.78 ± 4.26	42.75 ± 2.45	0.30
Pack-years	36.11 ± 9.64	46.71 ± 5.59	0.33
Post-bronchodilator (COPD-NE, *n* = 8; COPD-E, *n* = 12)			
FEV1 (%)	67.91 ± 7.10	68.29 ± 5.55	0.97
FEV1/FVC	60.89 ± 3.20	57.22 ± 2.58	0.38

Data represent the mean ± SEM of demographic and spirometric features of all patients in each group; COPD, chronic obstructive pulmonary disease; FEV1, forced expiratory volume in 1 s; FVC, forced vital capacity.

TABLE 2 | Demographic and spirometric features of the validation cohort.

	COPD-NE	COPD-E	*p* value
Patients, *n*	15	29	–
Age, years	62.33 ± 1.90	64.41 ± 1.27	0.36
Gender	–	–	0.60
Male, *n* (%)	13 (86.67)	27 (93.10)	–
Female, *n* (%)	2 (13.33)	2 (6.90)	–
Smokers	–	–	0.41
Current, *n* (%)	11 (73.33)	25 (86.21)	–
Ex-smoker, *n* (%)	4 (26.67)	4 (13.79)	–
Years of smoking	33.67 ± 3.10	40.28 ± 1.76	0.05
Pack-years	41.00 ± 6.51	43.29 ± 3.50	0.74
Post-bronchodilator (COPD-NE, *n* = 13; COPD-E, *n* = 27)			
FEV1 (%)	69.75 ± 4.84	72.25 ± 3.25	0.64
FEV1/FVC	62.17 ± 2.06	60.12 ± 1.57	0.41

Data represent the mean ± SEM of demographic and spirometric features of all patients in each group; COPD, chronic obstructive pulmonary disease; FEV1, forced expiratory volume in 1 s; FVC, forced vital capacity.

analysis. These 21 lung tissues were collected between September 2016 and March 2018 and defined as the discovery cohort. Until June 2019, all samples had been collected and defined as the validation cohort. The validation cohort consisted of 15 COPD-NE lung tissues and 29 COPD-E lung tissues, of which 8 COPD-NE specimens and 12 COPD-E specimens were involved in the discovery cohort. For general features and pulmonary function parameters, there were no significant differences between both groups in the discovery and validation cohorts. However, both cohorts predominantly consisted of male patients, and the discovery cohort consisted of only male patients. In the validation cohort, patients of the COPD-E group had a longer smoking history than those in the COPD-NE group. However, there were no significant differences in pack-years between the two groups. One patient in the discovery cohort and four in the validation cohort did not have pulmonary function test results after bronchodilator administration (**Table 1**, **Table 2**).

In the discovery cohort, patients in the COPD-E group showed a higher emphysema index (2.94 ± 1.12 vs. 11.56 ± 2.78, p = 0.02) and lower emphysema percentile density

TABLE 3 | Radiological parameters of the discovery and validation cohorts.

	COPD-NE	COPD-E	*p* value
Discovery cohort			
Patients, *n*	9	12	–
% of air	82.72 ± 1.57	84.46 ± 0.79	0.30
Volume of air (cm^3)	2,2419 ± 274.50	2,2635 ± 175.30	0.57
% of tissue	17.28 ± 1.57	15.54 ± 0.79	0.30
Volume of tissue (cm^3)	467.10 ± 27.20	465.50 ± 22.61	0.96
Emphysema index (%)	2.94 ± 1.12	11.56 ± 2.78	0.02*
Emphysema percentile density (HU)	-911.80 ± 8.30	-944.60 ± 8.40	0.01*
Mean airway lumen radius (mm)	7.02 ± 0.27	6.50 ± 0.28	0.21
Mean airway wall thickness (mm)	3.11 ± 0.21	3.65 ± 0.28	0.16
Ratio of mean airway wall thickness to mean radius	0.44 ± 0.037	0.57 ± 0.06	0.10
Validation cohort			
Patients, *n*	15	28[a]	–
% of air	80.59 ± 1.38	83.00 ± 0.78	0.11
Volume of air (cm^3)	2090 ± 229.70	2,2372 ± 145.30	0.28
% of tissue	19.41 ± 1.38	11.04 ± 0.78	0.11
Volume of tissue (cm^3)	448.10 ± 21.68	454.70 ± 17.71	0.82
Emphysema index (%)	4.80 ± 1.31	10.93 ± 1.66	0.02*
Emphysema percentile density (HU)	-912.50 ± 7.55	-936.60 ± 5.25	0.01*
Mean airway lumen radius (mm)	6.68 ± 0.27	6.55 ± 0.21	0.70
Mean airway wall thickness (mm)	3.47 ± 0.22	3.69 ± 0.22	0.53
Ratio of mean airway wall thickness to mean radius	0.53 ± 0.06	0.56 ± 0.03	0.62

Data represent the mean ± SEM of radiological parameters for all patients in each group.
[a]Raw radiological data were not available for one patient in the COPD-E group of the validation cohort. COPD, chronic obstructive pulmonary disease.
**p < 0.05.*

(−911.80 ± 8.30 vs. −944.60 ± 8.40, $p = 0.01$) than those in the COPD-NE group. This result suggested that COPD-E patients had more severe emphysema lesions than COPD-NE patients (**Table 3**). Other airway-related parameters, including proportion of air and tissue, were not significantly different between both groups. The CT scan results did not show large differences between the validation and discovery cohorts. Raw radiological data were not available for one patient in the validation cohort; this patient was not included in this analysis.

Protein Identification and Differential Abundant Protein Screening

A total of 31,479 peptides, including 27,157 unique peptides, were identified by mass spectrometry, and 4,343 proteins were finally identified. All identified proteins and related information are shown in**Supplementary Table S2**. The mass spectrometry proteomics data have been deposited to the ProteomeXchange Consortium (http://proteomecentral.proteomexchange.org) *via* the iProX partner repository with the dataset identifier PXD023900 (Ma et al., 2019). DAPs were identified using the following screening criteria: COPD-E/COPD-NE ratio greater than 1.2-fold (upregulation greater than 1.2-fold or downregulation less than 0.83-fold) and $p < 0.05$. A total of 36 DAPs were identified, of which 25 were upregulated and 11 were downregulated. The type I cytoskeletal 17 (KRT17) protein expression in the COPD-E group was 1.54-fold higher than that in the COPD-NE group, as the protein with the most obvious differences between the two groups. All DAPs are listed in **Table 4**, and a volcano plot showing the distribution of DAPs is illustrated in **Figure 2A**. Hierarchical cluster analysis showed that the samples were clustered into two categories, which were the same groups as the original groups. The clustering results are shown in **Figure 2B**.

Functional Enrichment and Protein–Protein Interaction Network of DAPs

GO functional annotation and enrichment analysis was performed for all DAPs, the results of which are shown in **Supplementary Table S3**. The GO terms were ordered according to the *p* value, and the top 20 enriched GO terms included eight terms in the biological pathway, six terms in the molecular function, and six terms in the cellular component. The biological pathway was mainly related to tissue refactoring and wound healing, including regulation of response to wound, regulation of wound healing, pathways that downregulate wound-related response and healing, response to external stimuli, and defense response. The molecular function was predominantly related to protein binding; protein–lipid complex binding and lipoprotein particle binding had the highest enrichment factor (0.23). For the cellular component, most DAPs were found in the extracellular matrix and some in organelles. Enrichment analysis results of the top 20 enriched GO terms with smallest *p* values are displayed in **Figure 3A**. GO terms at level 2 are on higher positions in the hierarchy of GO terms. Level 2 GO terms describe the properties of proteins more comprehensively, and all of the level 2 GO terms involved in GO enrichment are shown in **Figure 3B**. The metabolic process may occupy an important position in emphysematous phenotype–related biological pathways; besides, growth, cell proliferation, and developmental

TABLE 4 | Differential abundant proteins in the COPD-E and COPD-NE groups.

Accession	Description	Gene name	COPD-E/COPD-NE ratio	*p* value
Q04695	Keratin, type I cytoskeletal 17	KRT17	1.54	0.037*
P02745	Complement C1q subcomponent subunit A	C1QA	1.48	<0.001***
Q9BXD5	N-acetylneuraminate lyase	NPL	1.45	0.040*
P02794	Ferritin heavy chain	FTH1	1.38	0.019*
P48061	Stromal cell–derived factor 1	CXCL12	1.38	0.015*
P39900	Macrophage metalloelastase	MMP12	1.35	0.024*
P02747	Complement C1q subcomponent subunit C	C1QC	1.34	0.031*
P0DOX8	Immunoglobulin lambda-1 light chain	—	1.33	0.039*
P02679	Fibrinogen gamma chain	FGG	1.32	<0.001***
P02746	Complement C1q subcomponent subunit B	C1QB	1.31	0.012*
Q9NP78	ATP-binding cassette sub-family B member 9	ABCB9	1.30	0.024*
Q8TED4	Glucose-6-phosphate exchanger SLC37A2	SLC37A2	1.28	0.021*
P0C0L4	Complement C4-A	C4A	1.28	0.020*
P02671	Fibrinogen alpha chain	FGA	1.27	0.003**
M0R2J8	Doublecortin domain–containing protein 1	DCDC1	1.26	<0.001***
P02675	Fibrinogen beta chain	FGB	1.26	0.001**
Q9BPW9	Dehydrogenase/reductase SDR family member 9	DHRS9	1.25	0.005**
P02649	Apolipoprotein E	APOE	1.24	0.041*
P31513	Dimethylaniline monooxygenase [N-oxide–forming] 3	FMO3	1.23	0.022*
P18428	Lipopolysaccharide-binding protein	LBP	1.23	0.028*
Q9BXN1	Asporin	ASPN	1.23	0.038*
P02743	Serum amyloid P-component	APCS	1.22	0.023*
Q5T6F0	DDB1- and CUL4-associated factor 12	DCAF12	1.21	0.004**
P04003	C4b-binding protein alpha chain	C4BPA	1.21	0.036*
P35542	Serum amyloid A-4 protein	SAA4	1.20	0.025*
Q96D46	60S ribosomal export protein NMD3	NMD3	0.83	0.011*
P33764	Protein S100-A3	S100A3	0.83	0.049*
P31415	Calsequestrin-1	CASQ1	0.82	0.007**
P28906	Hematopoietic progenitor cell antigen CD34	CD34	0.81	0.016*
P15090	Fatty acid–binding protein, adipocyte	FABP4	0.81	0.033*
P43155	Carnitine O-acetyltransferase	CRAT	0.80	0.032*
P16671	Platelet glycoprotein 4	CD36	0.79	0.008**
Q96B54	Zinc finger protein 428	ZNF428	0.78	0.017*
P22748	Carbonic anhydrase 4	CA4	0.78	0.014*
P17152	Transmembrane protein 11, mitochondrial	TMEM11	0.76	0.018*
P30486	HLA class I histocompatibility antigen, B-48 alpha chain	HLA-B	0.76	0.014*

*$p < 0.05$, **$p < 0.01$, ***$p < 0.001$.

process were also involved. Binding was the most predominant molecular function of DAPs. In addition to the extracellular matrix, organelles may be the portion that DAPs were mainly distributed in.

To understand the mechanisms and signaling pathways that DAPs may participate in the pathogenesis of COPD emphysematous phenotype, we performed KEGG pathway annotation and enrichment analysis of all DAPs; the specific results are shown in**Supplementary Table S4**. KEGG enrichment analysis showed that most DAPs were involved in metabolic and inflammatory pathways, including nitrogen metabolism, PPAR signaling, NF-κB signaling, and cholesterol metabolism. All KEGG terms with *p* values less than 0.05 are shown in **Figure 4A** and ordered according to the *p* value. The top 20 KEGG terms with largest enriched protein numbers are shown in **Figure 4B**.

PPI network analysis was used to analyze the interaction between DAPs. As shown in **Figure 5**, 16 out of 36 DAPs had interaction nodes. Apolipoprotein E is the DAP that has most interactions with other DAPs, which indicates it may serve as a key molecule in the mechanism of emphysema. Besides, serum amyloid P-component, various chains of fibrinogen, and different subcomponent subunits of the complement interact with each other. These DAPs were related to the pathways in the results of GO and KEGG enrichment analyses. Therefore, these interactions may play roles in the pathogenesis of emphysematous phenotype, as well.

Validation and Functional Annotation of DAPs

The expression of KRT17, dehydrogenase/reductase short-chain alcohol dehydrogenase/reductase (SDR) family member 9 (DHRS9), and dimethylaniline monooxygenase 3 (FMO3) was determined. Each lung tissue sample obtained from a subject was used as an independent sample in western blot. Western blotting results showing the expression of these proteins in the lung tissue samples of the validation cohort are shown in **Figure 6**. The protein expression of KRT17 (COPD-NE, n = 13, COPD-E, n =

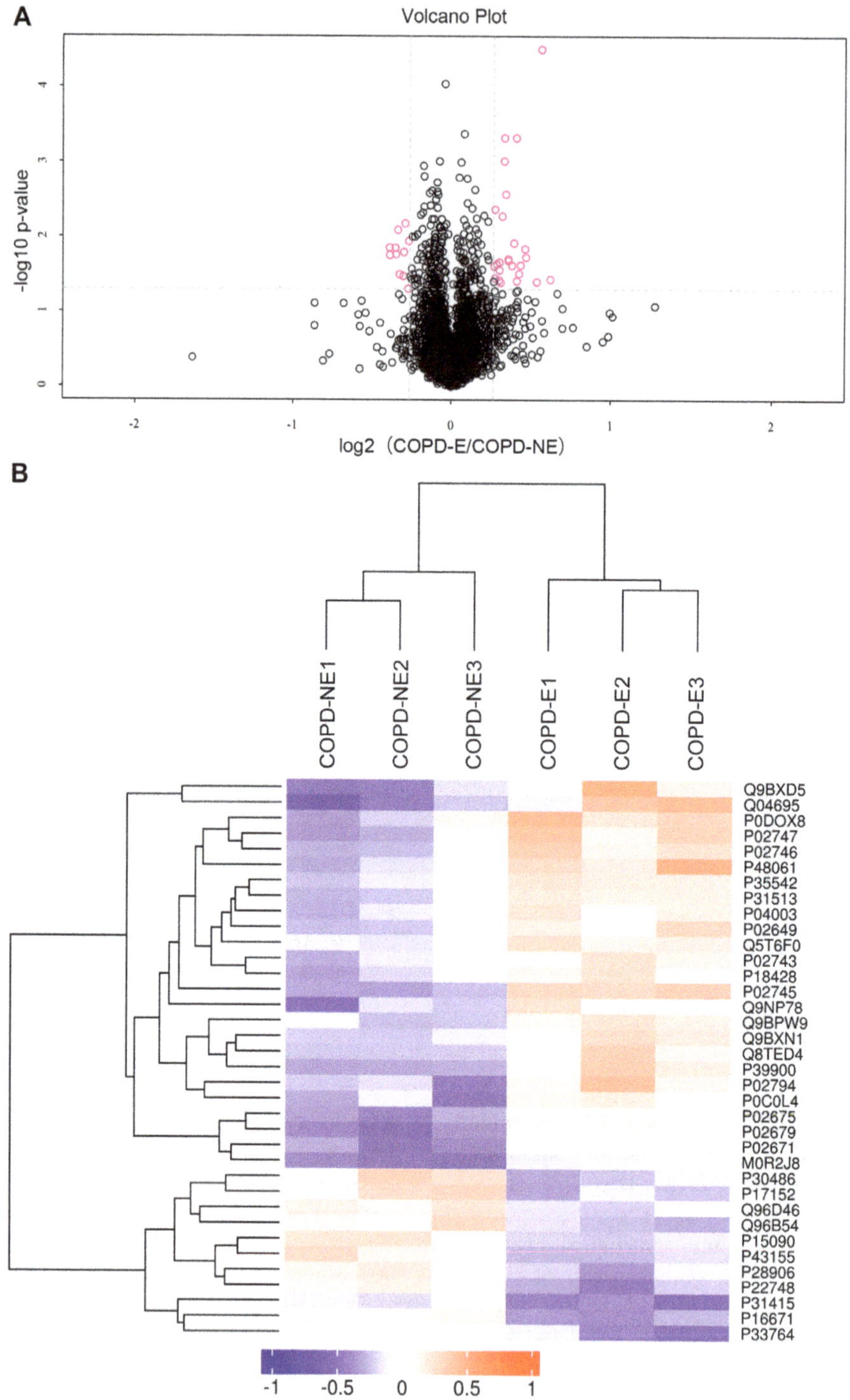

FIGURE 2 | Quantification and hierarchical clustering of differential abundant proteins (DAPs) in COPD emphysmetous phenotype. **(A)** Volcano plot of DAPs. **(B)** Hierarchical clustering heat map of DAPs.

24; $p < 0.01$) and DHRS9 (COPD-NE, $n = 13$, COPD-E, $n = 24$; $p < 0.01$) in the COPD-E group was higher than that in the COPD-NE group. However, the FMO3 expression was not significantly different between both groups. Western blotting results of all lung tissue samples are shown in **Supplementary Figure S1**.

The annotation results showed that KRT17 acts as a cytoskeletal protein and takes part in the process of cell growth and development, while DHRS9 participates in multiple metabolic pathways, such as retinol and steroid hormone biosynthesis (**Table 5**).

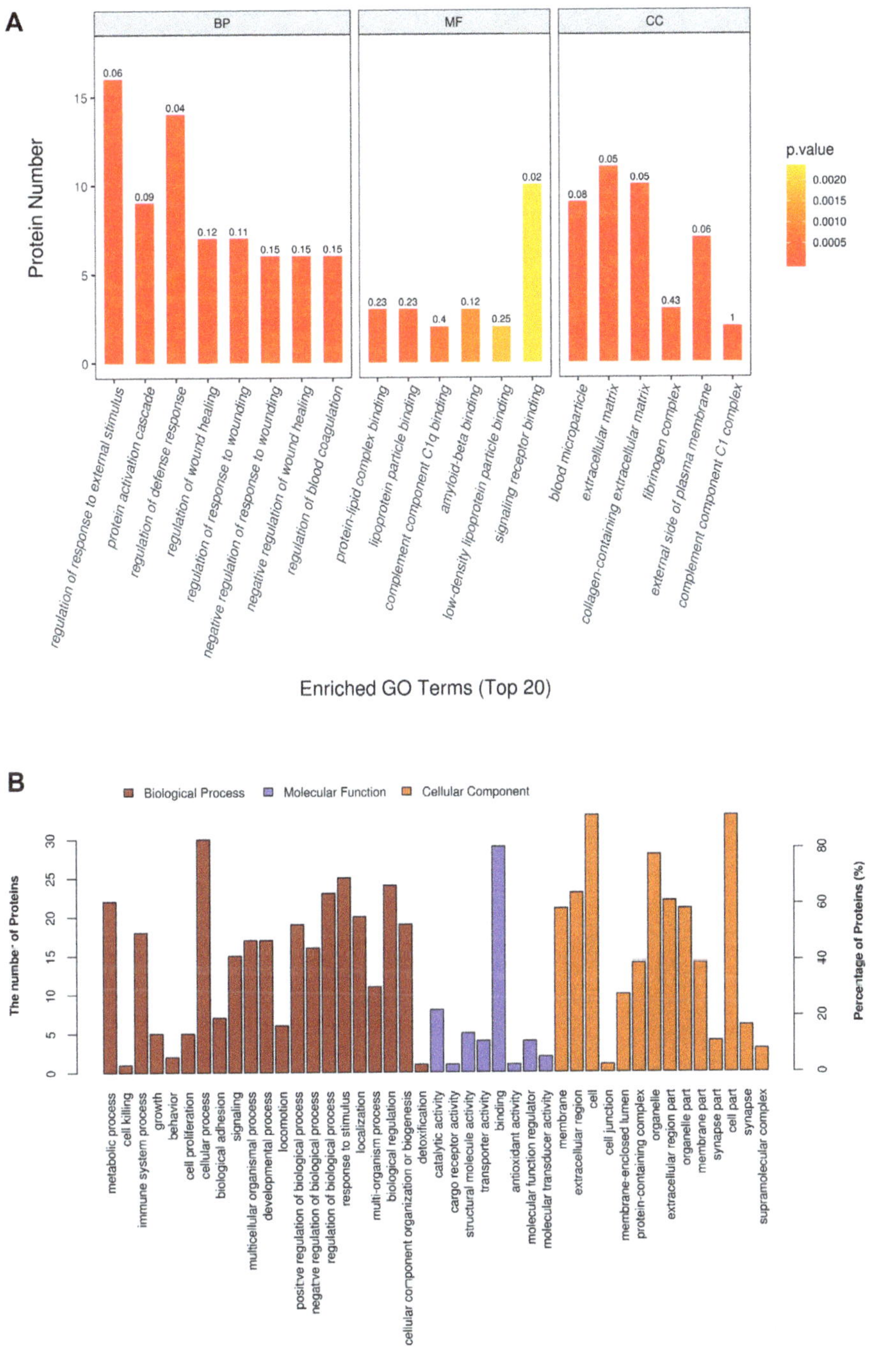

FIGURE 3 | Gene ontology (GO) enrichment analysis of differential abundant proteins. **(A)** Top 20 enriched terms with smallest *p* values in GO enrichment analysis. **(B)** All level 2 GO terms involved in GO enrichment analysis.

DISCUSSION

Patients with COPD emphysematous phenotype account for a considerable portion in clinics. Patients with this phenotype manifest progressive destruction of lung tissue and poor response to current pharmaceutical interventions of COPD (Janssen et al., 2019). With an aim of exploring the specific mechanism underlying the development of this phenotype, the proteome of lung tissues from patients with COPD emphysematous phenotype was studied using TMT quantitative proteomics. A total of 4,343 proteins were identified, out of which 36 were DAPs. Of these, 25 DAPs were upregulated and 11 DAPs were downregulated. This result was comparable with that of other proteomic analyses on lung tissue (Sun et al., 2019; Wu et al., 2020). Functional enrichment analysis of DAPs showed that tissue repair and cell

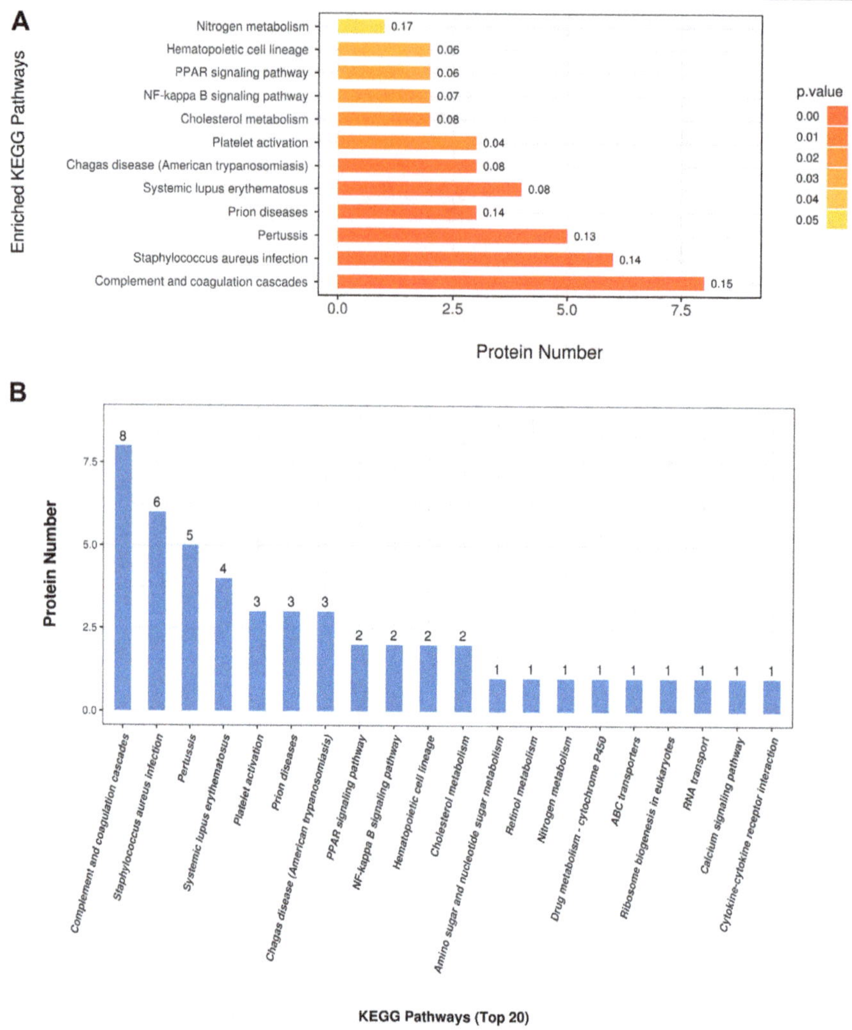

FIGURE 4 | Kyoto Encyclopedia of Genes and Genomes (KEGG) enrichment analysis of differential abundant proteins. **(A)** Enriched terms in KEGG enrichment analysis with *p* values less than 0.05. **(B)** Top 20 KEGG terms with largest enriched protein numbers in KEGG enrichment results.

proliferation and development were primarily related to the pathogenesis of emphysematous phenotype, in addition to inflammatory response, collagen disruption, and other well-recognized mechanisms in emphysema (Lan et al., 2019). Moreover, cholesterol-related, retinol-related, and other lipid-related metabolic pathways were enriched in KEGG pathway analysis. These results suggested that the impaired ability to repair injured tissue and lipid metabolism disorder might play an essential role in the development of prominent lung tissue destruction in COPD emphysematous phenotype. The differential expression of KRT17 and DHRS9 was validated in the lung tissue samples of patients with COPD emphysematous phenotype. Therefore, KRT17 and DHRS9 might affect the pathogenesis of COPD emphysematous phenotype by regulating tissue repair and lipid metabolism and act as phenotype-specific proteomic signatures.

Tissue repair is an essential process for all organisms to protect and maintain the normal structure and function. As structural destruction and collagen fibril disorder are prominently observed in patients with COPD emphysematous phenotype, the impaired ability to repair lung parenchymal and interstitial cells might play a significant role in its pathogenesis (Hu et al., 2020). The WNT/β-catenin pathway is a classical pathway involved in lung growth and development, and cell proliferation and differentiation (Königshoff and Eickelberg, 2010). Downregulation of this pathway will result in the retardation of tissue repair (Kneidinger et al., 2011; Uhl et al., 2015). Under normal conditions, WNT activates the JNK pathway by forming a complex with small G-proteins to promote cytoskeletal rearrangement during embryonic development (Wiggan and Hamel, 2002; Zhang et al., 2018). Moreover, the canonical WNT signaling pathway promotes the proliferation of type II alveolar epithelial cells (AECIIs) and *trans*-differentiation of AECIIs to type I alveolar epithelial cells (AECIs) that replenish injured ones in the damaged process of emphysema. In contrast, the non-canonical WNT signaling pathway inhibits proliferation

TABLE 5 | Annotation of KRT17 and DHRS9.

Accession	Gene name	ID	Annotation term
Q04695	*KRT17*	GO:0070268	BP: cornification
		GO:0008544	BP: epidermis development
		GO:0031069	BP: hair follicle morphogenesis
		GO:0045109	BP: intermediate filament organization
		GO:0031424	BP: keratinization
		GO:0030307	BP: positive regulation of cell growth
		GO:0051798	BP: positive regulation of hair follicle development
		GO:0045727	BP: positive regulation of translation
		GO:0007165	BP: signal transduction
		GO:0071944	CC: cell periphery
		GO:0005829	CC: cytosol
		GO:0070062	CC: extracellular exosome
		GO:0005882	CC: intermediate filament
		GO:0045111	CC: intermediate filament cytoskeleton
		GO:0042289	MF: MHC class II protein binding
		GO:0032395	MF: MHC class II receptor activity
		GO:0005200	MF: structural constituent of cytoskeleton
		hsa05150	*Staphylococcus aureus* infection
		hsa04915	Estrogen signaling pathway
Q9BPW9	*DHRS9*	GO:0042904	BP: 9-cis-retinoic acid biosynthetic process
		GO:0008209	BP: androgen metabolic process
		GO:0030855	BP: epithelial cell differentiation
		GO:0042448	BP: progesterone metabolic process
		GO:0042572	BP: retinol metabolic process
		GO:0005789	CC: endoplasmic reticulum membrane
		GO:0030176	CC: integral component of endoplasmic reticulum membrane
		GO:0004022	MF: alcohol dehydrogenase (NAD) activity
		GO:0047044	MF: androstan-3-alpha,17-beta-diol dehydrogenase activity
		GO:0047023	MF: androsterone dehydrogenase activity
		GO:0016854	MF: racemase and epimerase activity
		GO:0004745	MF: retinol dehydrogenase activity
		GO:0047035	MF: testosterone dehydrogenase (NAD+) activity
		hsa00830	retinol metabolism

BP: biological pathway; CC: cellular component; MF: molecular function.

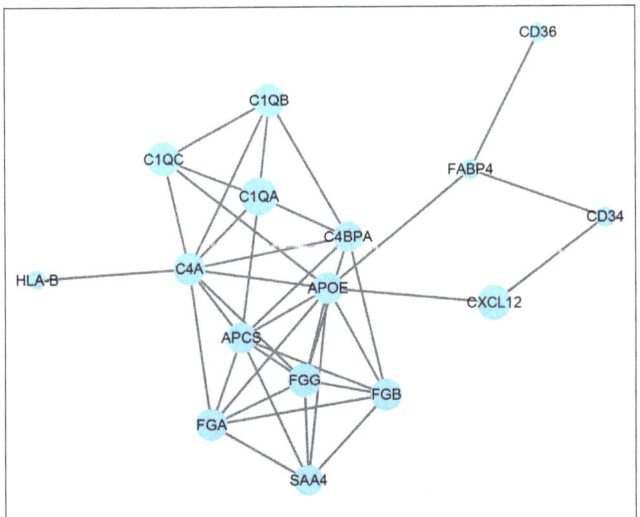

FIGURE 5 | Protein–protein interaction (PPI) network of differential abundant proteins.

and *trans*-differentiation processes (Skronska-Wasek et al., 2017). KRT17 is an important component of cytoskeleton. Functional annotation of DAPs showed that KRT17 participates in cell growth and development and cytoskeletal composition. Therefore, KRT17 has a potential to serve as an important target of the WNT/β-catenin signaling pathway. Both canonical and non-canonical WNT signaling pathways may rearrange or affect the abundance of cytoskeletal component—KRT17, resulting in the severe tissue destruction in patients with COPD emphysematous phenotype. Some studies have confirmed that the expression of cyclin D1, MMP7, c-Myc, and other vital targets of the WNT/β-catenin pathway is increased in KRT17-overexpressing cells (Wang et al., 2019). However, the mechanism through which canonical and non-canonical WNT signaling pathways interact with KRT17 warrants further studies, and the specific roles of KRT17 in the development of COPD and emphysema are still to be explored.

Retinoic acid is synthesized from retinol, and it regulates lung development and alveolar formation in the human body. Some studies have shown that retinoic acid can inhibit the activation of YAP signaling and epithelial-mesenchymal FGF signaling pathways, which promotes the proliferation and inhibits the differentiation of alveolar epithelial cells (Ng-Blichfeldt et al., 2018). In addition, retinoic acid can downregulate pro-apoptotic

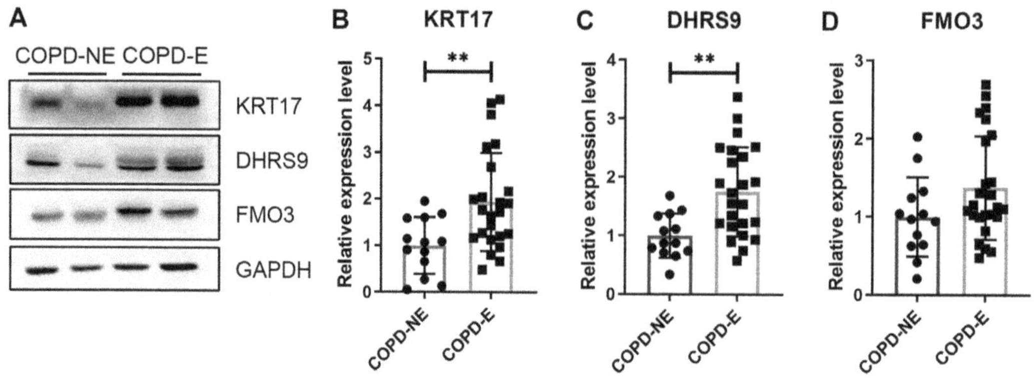

FIGURE 6 | Type I cytoskeletal 17 (KRT17) and dehydrogenase/reductase SDR family member 9 (DHRS9) expressions are increased in the lung tissue samples of patients with chronic obstructive pulmonary disease emphysematous phenotype (COPD-E). **(A)** Western blotting results of KRT17, DHRS9, and FMO3 expressions in the lung tissue samples of COPD non-emphysematous phenotype (COPD-NE) and COPD-E groups. **(B-D)** Quantification of KRT17 (COPD-NE, n = 13; COPD-E, n = 24), DHRS9 (COPD-NE, n = 13; COPD-E, n = 24), and FMO3 (COPD-NE, n = 13; COPD-E, n = 25) protein expressions. $^{**}p < 0.01$.

genes and inhibit the apoptosis of alveolar epithelial cells (Chatterjee and Chatterji, 2017). Therefore, the functional enrichment of DAPs in cholesterol and retinol metabolism in this study suggests aberrant proliferation and differentiation caused by impaired lipid metabolism. DHRS9 is a member of the SDR family. Crosstalk between DHRS9 and retinaldehyde dehydrogenase 1 (Raldh1) exerts important regulatory functions in the synthesis of retinoic acid. Unlike other members of the SDR family (e.g., Rdh10 and Rdh2), DHRS9 knockdown increased retinoic acid synthesis in RALDH1-overexpressing cells (Wang et al., 2011). Combined with the results of functional annotation and enrichment, DHRS9 can modulate the synthesis of retinoic acid, which in turn regulates the proliferation and differentiation of alveolar epithelial cells (Ng-Blichfeldt et al., 2018). Furthermore, clinical studies have confirmed that DHRS9 can regulate inflammation (Morichika et al., 2019) as well as the balance between MMP9 and TIMP1 (Mao et al., 2003) in cells. These results suggest that DHRS9 is predominantly involved in the pathogenic mechanism of emphysema in patients with COPD emphysematous phenotype, but specific molecular mechanisms are still unclear and remain to be explored.

Serum (Sridhar et al., 2019), expectorated sputum (Titz et al., 2015), and bronchoalveolar lavage fluid (Tu et al. 2014) samples have been used in previous proteomic studies to analyze the COPD-related proteome. However, the number of detected DAPs was relatively small and easily influenced by a systemic disease. Lung tissue is the direct affected site of COPD emphysematous phenotype. Therefore, lung tissue samples are the most suitable to identify key molecules involved in the mechanism underlying emphysema pathogenesis. To the best of our knowledge, this is the first proteomic analysis that focuses on emphysematous phenotype, to detect the specific DAPs in this phenotype.

There are some limitations to our study. Due to the fact that only few COPD patients were able to meet the inclusion criteria of our study, there are certain difficulties to collect lung tissue samples and the number of lung tissue samples in the validation cohort was relatively small. Moreover, there was an overlap between lung tissues from the discovery and validation cohorts. Furthermore, though wound repair and retinol metabolism may be the processes that KRT17 and DHRS9 participated in, they have not yet been demonstrated and explored in this study. In the future, more lung tissue samples from COPD patients should be involved and in-depth research studies should be conducted to explore the mechanism of COPD emphysematous phenotype development, including experiments *in vivo* and *in vitro*.

CONCLUSION

A total of 36 DAPs were identified in lung tissue samples from patients in the COPD emphysematous phenotype group. Of these, 25 DAPs were upregulated and 11 DAPs were downregulated. KRT17 and DHRS9 were found to take part in the pathogenesis of emphysema. Moreover, wound repair and retinol metabolism may be the processes they participated. Therefore, KRT17 and DHRS9 can be used as phenotype-specific proteomic signatures in patients with COPD emphysematous phenotype.

AUTHOR CONTRIBUTIONS

SB, SX and LZ substantially contributed to the conception and design of the manuscript. SB, RY, CW, PS, DW, YY, HW, SW, MY, SX and LZ contributed to the acquisition, analysis, and interpretation of data. SB, SX and LZ drafted the article, and SB, RY, CW, PS, DW, YY, HW, SW, MY, SX, and LZ revised it critically and substantially. SB, RY, CW, PS, DW, YY, HW, SW, MY, SX, and LZ approved the final version and accepted accountability for all aspects of the study. Corresponding authors SX and LZ contributed equally to this study.

ACKNOWLEGEMENT

The authors would like to thank the Biological Sample Library of Shengjing Hospital for help of getting tissue samples.

REFERENCES

Alford, S. K., van Beek, E. J. R., McLennan, G., and Hoffman, E. A. (2010). Heterogeneity of Pulmonary Perfusion as a Mechanistic Image-Based Phenotype in Emphysema Susceptible Smokers. *Proc. Natl. Acad. Sci.* 107 (16), 7485–7490. doi:10.1073/pnas.0913880107

Bai, S., Ye, R., Wang, C., Sun, P., and Zhao, L. (2020). Comparative Analysis of Pathophysiological Parameters between Emphysematous Smokers and Emphysematous Patients with COPD. *Sci. Rep.* 10 (1), 420. doi:10.1038/s41598-019-57354-2

Belgacemi, R., Luczka, E., Ancel, J., Diabasana, Z., Perotin, J.-M., Germain, A., et al. (2020). Airway Epithelial Cell Differentiation Relies on Deficient Hedgehog Signalling in COPD. *EBioMedicine* 51, 102572. doi:10.1016/j.ebiom.2019.11.033

Camp, P. G., Coxson, H. O., Levy, R. D., Pillai, S. G., Anderson, W., Vestbo, J., et al. (2009). Sex Differences in Emphysema and Airway Disease in Smokers. *Chest* 136 (6), 1480–1488. doi:10.1378/chest.09-0676

Camp, P. G., Ramirez-Venegas, A., Sansores, R. H., Alva, L. F., McDougall, J. E., Sin, D. D., et al. (2014). COPD Phenotypes in Biomass Smoke- versus Tobacco Smoke-Exposed Mexican Women. *Eur. Respir. J.* 43 (3), 725–734. doi:10.1183/09031936.00206112

Chatterjee, A., and Chatterji, U. (2017). All -Trans Retinoic Acid Ameliorates Arsenic-Induced Oxidative Stress and Apoptosis in the Rat Uterus by Modulating MAPK Signaling Proteins. *J. Cel. Biochem.* 118 (11), 3796–3809. doi:10.1002/jcb.26029

Coxson, H. O., Leipsic, J., Parraga, G., and Sin, D. D. (2014). Using Pulmonary Imaging to Move Chronic Obstructive Pulmonary Disease beyond FEV1. *Am. J. Respir. Crit. Care Med.* 190 (2), 135–144. doi:10.1164/rccm.201402-0256PP

Criner, G. J., Sue, R., Wright, S., Dransfield, M., Rivas-Perez, H., and Wiese, T. (2018). A Multicenter Randomized Controlled Trial of Zephyr Endobronchial Valve Treatment in Heterogeneous Emphysema (LIBERATE). *Am. J. Respir. Crit. Care Med.* 198 (9), 1151–1164. doi:10.1164/rccm.201803-0590OC10.1164/rccm.201808-1477le

Dirksen, A., Piitulainen, E., Parr, D. G., Deng, C., Wencker, M., Shaker, S. B., et al. (2009). Exploring the Role of CT Densitometry: a Randomised Study of Augmentation Therapy in 1-antitrypsin Deficiency. *Eur. Respir. J.* 33 (6), 1345–1353. doi:10.1183/09031936.00159408

Dziekan, J. M., Wirjanata, G., Dai, L., Go, K. D., Yu, H., Lim, Y. T., et al. (2020). Cellular thermal Shift Assay for the Identification of Drug-Target Interactions in the Plasmodium Falciparum Proteome. *Nat. Protoc.* 15 (6), 1881–1921. doi:10.1038/s41596-020-0310-z

Fan, L., Xia, Y., Guan, Y., Zhang, T.-f., and Liu, S.-y. (2014). Characteristic Features of Pulmonary Function Test, CT Volume Analysis and MR Perfusion Imaging in COPD Patients with Different HRCT Phenotypes. *Clin. Respir. J.* 8 (1), 45–54. doi:10.1111/crj.12033

Hu, Y., Ng-Blichfeldt, J.-P., Ota, C., Ciminieri, C., Ren, W., Hiemstra, P. S., et al. (2020). Wnt/β-catenin Signaling Is Critical for Regenerative Potential of Distal Lung Epithelial Progenitor Cells in Homeostasis and Emphysema. *Stem Cells* 38 (11), 1467–1478. doi:10.1002/stem.3241

Janssen, R., Piscaer, I., Franssen, F. M. E., and Wouters, E. F. M. (2019). Emphysema: Looking beyond Alpha-1 Antitrypsin Deficiency. *Expert Rev. Respir. Med.* 13 (4), 381–397. doi:10.1080/17476348.2019.1580575

Jiang, J., Xiao, K., and Chen, P. (2017). NOTCH Signaling in Lung Diseases. *Exp. Lung Res.* 43 (4-5), 217–228. doi:10.1080/01902148.2017.1306599

Kneidinger, N., Yildirim, A. Ö., Callegari, J., Takenaka, S., Stein, M. M., Dumitrascu, R., et al. (2011). Activation of the WNT/β-Catenin Pathway Attenuates Experimental Emphysema. *Am. J. Respir. Crit. Care Med.* 183 (6), 723–733. doi:10.1164/rccm.200910-1560OC

Königshoff, M., and Eickelberg, O. (2010). WNT Signaling in Lung Disease. *Am. J. Respir. Cel Mol Biol.* 42 (1), 21–31. doi:10.1165/rcmb.2008-0485TR

Lan, Y.-W., Yang, J.-C., Yen, C.-C., Huang, T.-T., Chen, Y.-C., Chen, H.-L., et al. (2019). Predifferentiated Amniotic Fluid Mesenchymal Stem Cells Enhance Lung Alveolar Epithelium Regeneration and Reverse Elastase-Induced Pulmonary Emphysema. *Stem Cel Res Ther.* 10 (1), 163. doi:10.1186/s13287-019-1282-1

Ma, J., Chen, T., Wu, S., Yang, C., Bai, M., Shu, K., et al. (2019). iProX: an Integrated Proteome Resource. *Nucleic Acids Res.* 47 (D1), D1211–d1217. doi:10.1093/nar/gky869

Manon-Jensen, T., Langholm, L. L., Rønnow, S. R., Karsdal, M. A., Tal-Singer, R., Vestbo, J., et al. (2019). End-product of Fibrinogen Is Elevated in Emphysematous Chronic Obstructive Pulmonary Disease and Is Predictive of Mortality in the ECLIPSE Cohort. *Respir. Med.* 160, 105814. doi:10.1016/j.rmed.2019.105814

Mao, J. T., Tashkin, D. P., Belloni, P. N., Baileyhealy, I., Baratelli, F., and Roth, M. D. (2003). All- Trans Retinoic Acid Modulates the Balance of Matrix Metalloproteinase-9 and Tissue Inhibitor of Metalloproteinase-1 in Patients with Emphysema *. *Chest* 124 (5), 1724–1732. doi:10.1378/chest.124.5.1724

Mertins, P., Tang, L. C., Krug, K., Clark, D. J., Gritsenko, M. A., Chen, L., et al. (2018). Reproducible Workflow for Multiplexed Deep-Scale Proteome and Phosphoproteome Analysis of Tumor Tissues by Liquid Chromatography-Mass Spectrometry. *Nat. Protoc.* 13 (7), 1632–1661. doi:10.1038/s41596-018-0006-9

Morichika, D., Miyahara, N., Fujii, U., Taniguchi, A., Oda, N., Senoo, S., et al. (2019). A Retinoid X Receptor Partial Agonist Attenuates Pulmonary Emphysema and Airway Inflammation. *Respir. Res.* 20 (1), 2. doi:10.1186/s12931-018-0963-0

Ng-Blichfeldt, J.-P., Schrik, A., Kortekaas, R. K., Noordhoek, J. A., Heijink, I. H., Hiemstra, P. S., et al. (2018). Retinoic Acid Signaling Balances Adult Distal Lung Epithelial Progenitor Cell Growth and Differentiation. *EBioMedicine* 36, 461–474. doi:10.1016/j.ebiom.2018.09.002

Oelsner, E. C., Hoffman, E. A., Folsom, A. R., Carr, J. J., Enright, P. L., Kawut, S. M., et al. (2014). Association between Emphysema-like Lung on Cardiac Computed Tomography and Mortality in Persons without Airflow Obstruction. *Ann. Intern. Med.* 161 (12), 863–873. doi:10.7326/m13-2570

Papaioannou, A. I., Kostikas, K., Papaporfyriou, A., Angelakis, L., Papathanasiou, E., Hillas, G., et al. (2017). Emphysematous Phenotype Is Characterized by Low Blood Eosinophils: A Cross-Sectional Study. *COPD: J. Chronic Obstructive Pulm. Dis.* 14 (6), 635–640. doi:10.1080/15412555.2017.1386644

Rosas-Alonso, R., Galera, R., Sánchez-Pascuala, J. J., Casitas, R., Burdiel, M., Martínez-Cerón, E., et al. (2020). Hypermethylation of Anti-oncogenic MicroRNA 7 Is Increased in Emphysema Patients. *Archivos de Bronconeumología (English Edition)* 56 (8), 506–513. doi:10.1016/j.arbres.2019.10.01710.1016/j.arbr.2019.10.019

Skronska-Wasek, W., Mutze, K., Baarsma, H. A., Bracke, K. R., Alsafadi, H. N., Lehmann, M., et al. (2017). Reduced Frizzled Receptor 4 Expression Prevents WNT/β-Catenin-driven Alveolar Lung Repair in Chronic Obstructive Pulmonary Disease. *Am. J. Respir. Crit. Care Med.* 196 (2), 172–185. doi:10.1164/rccm.201605-0904OC

Sridhar, S., Liu, H., Pham, T.-H., Damera, G., and Newbold, P. (2019). Modulation of Blood Inflammatory Markers by Benralizumab in Patients with Eosinophilic Airway Diseases. *Respir. Res.* 20 (1), 14. doi:10.1186/s12931-018-0968-8

Sun, P., Ye, R., Wang, C., Bai, S., and Zhao, L. (2019). Identification of Proteomic Signatures Associated with COPD Frequent Exacerbators. *Life Sci.* 230, 1–9. doi:10.1016/j.lfs.2019.05.047

Titz, B., Sewer, A., Schneider, T., Elamin, A., Martin, F., Dijon, S., et al. (2015). Alterations in the Sputum Proteome and Transcriptome in Smokers and Early-Stage COPD Subjects. *J. Proteomics* 128, 306–320. doi:10.1016/j.jprot.2015.08.009

Tu, C., Mammen, M. J., Li, J., Shen, X., Jiang, X., Hu, Q., et al. (2014). Large-scale, Ion-Current-Based Proteomics Investigation of Bronchoalveolar Lavage Fluid in Chronic Obstructive Pulmonary Disease Patients. *J. Proteome Res.* 13 (2), 627–639. doi:10.1021/pr4007602

Uhl, F. E., Vierkotten, S., Wagner, D. E., Burgstaller, G., Costa, R., Koch, I., et al. (2015). Preclinical Validation and Imaging of Wnt-Induced Repair in Human 3D Lung Tissue Cultures. *Eur. Respir. J.* 46 (4), 1150–1166. doi:10.1183/09031936.00183214

Vogelmeier, C. F., Criner, G. J., Martinez, F. J., Anzueto, A., Barnes, P. J., Bourbeau, J., et al. (2017). Global Strategy for the Diagnosis, Management, and Prevention of Chronic Obstructive Lung Disease 2017 Report. GOLD Executive Summary. *Am. J. Respir. Crit. Care Med.* 195 (5), 557–582. doi:10.1164/rccm.201701-0218PP

Wang, C., de Mochel, N. S. R., Christenson, S. A., Cassandras, M., Moon, R., Brumwell, A. N., et al. (2018). Expansion of Hedgehog Disrupts Mesenchymal Identity and Induces Emphysema Phenotype. *J. Clin. Invest.* 128 (10), 4343–4358. doi:10.1172/jci99435

Wang, C., Kane, M. A., and Napoli, J. L. (2011). Multiple Retinol and Retinal Dehydrogenases Catalyze All-Trans-Retinoic Acid Biosynthesis in Astrocytes. *J. Biol. Chem.* 286 (8), 6542–6553. doi:10.1074/jbc.M110.198382

Wang, T., Shen, H., Deng, H., Pan, H., He, Q., Ni, H., et al. (2020). Quantitative Proteomic Analysis of Human Plasma Using Tandem Mass Tags to Identify Novel Biomarkers for Herpes Zoster. *J. Proteomics* 225, 103879. doi:10.1016/j.jprot.2020.103879

Wang, Z., Yang, M.-Q., Lei, L., Fei, L.-R., Zheng, Y.-W., Huang, W.-J., et al. (2019). Overexpression of KRT17 Promotes Proliferation and Invasion of Non-small Cell Lung Cancer and Indicates Poor Prognosis. *Cmar* 11, 7485–7497. doi:10.2147/cmar.s218926

Wiggan, O., and Hamel, P. A. (2002). Pax3 Regulates Morphogenetic Cell Behavior *In Vitro* Coincident with Activation of a PCP/non-canonical Wnt-Signaling cascade. *J. Cel Sci.* 115 (Pt 3), 531–541. doi:10.1242/jcs.115.3.531

Wiśniewski, J. R., Zougman, A., Nagaraj, N., and Mann, M. (2009). Universal Sample Preparation Method for Proteome Analysis. *Nat. Methods* 6 (5), 359–362. doi:10.1038/nmeth.1322

Wu, M., Wu, Y., Huang, J., Wu, Y., Wu, H., Jiang, B., et al. (2020). Protein Expression Profile Changes of Lung Tissue in Patients with Pulmonary Hypertension. *Peer. J* 8, e8153. doi:10.7717/peerj.8153

Zeng, H., Li, T., He, X., Cai, S., Luo, H., Chen, P., et al. (2020). Oxidative Stress Mediates the Apoptosis and Epigenetic Modification of the Bcl-2 Promoter via DNMT1 in a Cigarette Smoke-Induced Emphysema Model. *Respir. Res.* 21 (1), 229. doi:10.1186/s12931-020-01495-w

Zhang, P., Hu, C., Li, Y., Wang, Y., Gao, L., Lu, K., et al. (2018). Vangl2 Is Essential for Myocardial Remodeling Activated by Wnt/JNK Signaling. *Exp. Cel Res.* 365 (1), 33–45. doi:10.1016/j.yexcr.2018.02.012

14

Multi-Pharmaceutical Activities of Chinese Herbal Polysaccharides in the Treatment of Pulmonary Fibrosis: Concept and Future Prospects

Xianbo Wu[1†], Jianli Huang[2†], Jie Wang[2], Yihua Xu[3], Xinwei Yang[1], Minghan Sun[4] and Jianyou Shi[5*]*

[1]School of Sports Medicine and Health, Chegdu Sport University, Chengdu, China, [2]Guizhou University of Traditional Chinese Medicine, Guiyang, China, [3]Chengdu University of Traditional Chinese Medicine, Chengdu, China, [4]Central of Reproductive Medicine, Department of Obstetrics and Gynecology, School of Medicine, Sichuan Academy of Medical Sciences and Sichuan Provincial People's Hospital, University of Electronic Science and Technology of China, Chengdu, China, [5]Personalized Drug Therapy Key Laboratory of Sichuan Province, Sichuan Academy of Medical Science and Sichuan Provincial People's Hospital, School of Medicine of University of Electronic Science and Technology of China, Chengdu, China

***Correspondence:**
Jianyou Shi
shijianyoude@126.com
Minghan Sun
sunminghan26@gmail.com

[†]These authors have contributed equally to this work and share first authorship

Pulmonary fibrosis is a fatal chronic progressive respiratory disease, characterized by continuous scarring of the lung parenchyma, leading to respiratory failure and death. The incidence of PF has increased over time. There are drugs, yet, there are some limitations. Hence, it is of importance to find new therapies and new drugs to replace the treatment of pulmonary fibrosis. In recent years, there have been a great number of research reports on the treatment of traditional Chinese medicine polysaccharides in various system fields. Among them, the treatment of PF has also gained extensive attention. This review summarized the source of polysaccharides, the drug activity of traditional Chinese medicine, and the protective effects on targets of Pulmonary fibrosis. We hope it can inspire researchers to design and develop polysaccharides, serving as a reference for potential clinical therapeutic drugs.

Keywords: pulmonary fibrosis, traditional Chinese medicine, polysaccharide, transforming growth factor-β, extracellular matrix, collagen-1, biological activity

INTRODUCTION

Pulmonary fibrosis (PF) is a large category of pulmonary diseases refers to the proliferation of fibroblasts and the accumulation of a large amount of extracellular matrix (ECM), accompanied by inflammatory damage, and tissue structure destruction, which can cause breathing difficulties, cough, hypoxemia, and hinder gas exchange, eventually leading to respiratory failure (Phan et al., 2021). PF's pathogenesis has undergone fibroblast activation, migration, proliferation and differentiation into myofibroblasts, inducing ECM aggregation, destroying the pulmonary parenchyma, changing the expansion of the pulmonary and the diffusion of O2/CO2, resulting in respiratory abnormalities caused by insufficient gas exchange (limitation reduced pulmonary volume and diffusing capacity) (Ruigrok et al., 2021). The triggering factors for fibrosis include genetic susceptibility and other risk factors, such as persistent viruses, bacterial infections, cigarettes, drug damage, and other medical diseases. Hereditary factors account for the largest proportion among them, one that the cause is unknown and the most common type of the disease is called idiopathic PF. (Richeldi et al., 2017; Majewski and Piotrowski, 2020). Radiology of chest

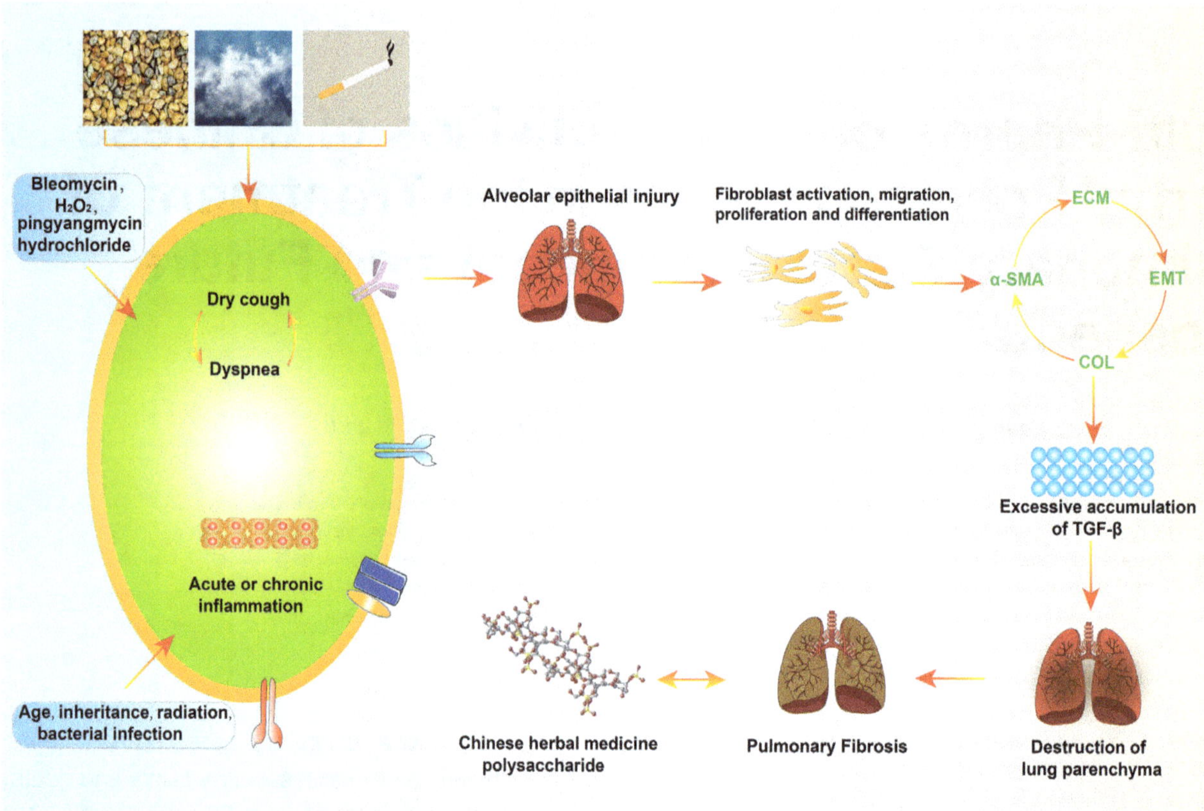

FIGURE 1 | Pathogenic factors and development process of pulmonary fibrosis.

high-resolution CT showed that about 90% of patients had interstitial changes, the histology of pulmonary biopsy showed that scar tissue replaced the normal pulmonary parenchyma, which was also used as a standard for the diagnosis of PF (Solomon et al., 2013). The occurrence and development of PF and the decline of pulmonary function are closely related to the survival rate. According to reports, the incidence of PF is increasing year by year and is positively correlated with age, with males higher than females (Hutchinson et al., 2015). With ageing, patients will inevitably experience the gradual loss of physiological integrity, the decrease of steady-state controlling ability and the increase of vulnerability to death. If not taking corresponding treatment measures after diagnosis, most patients' pulmonary function, if not all, will be progressively and irreversibly worsening, and their survival time is within 3–5 years (Lederer and Martinez, 2018) **(Figure 1)**.

Currently, only two anti-fibrosis drugs, named pirfenidone and nintedanib, have been approved by the US Food and Drug Administration to treat PF, but, due to their side effects (headache, nausea, diarrhea, skin rash, and impaired liver function) and high cost, they cannot meet the medical needs (Galli et al., 2017). Lung transplantation can improve the survival rate, but the limited organ supply and the complexity of the surgery and medical treatment make it affordable for only a small number of patients (Ryu et al., 2014). Colchicine, prednisone, and cyclophosphamide were also used to reduce the incidence and mortality of PF, studies on PF reported (Miniati and Matucci Cerinic, 2007; Fiorucci et al., 2008). In the case of acute exacerbations, international guidelines recommend high-dose glucocorticoids, but there are no data to prove its safety and effectiveness (Song et al., 2011). It has also been suggested that the therapeutic effects of prednisolone, cyclophosphamide, interferon-1b, and N-acetylcysteine have no obvious advantages, but various adverse reactions and increase the economic burden of patients (Datta et al., 2011; Canestaro et al., 2016; Raimundo et al., 2016). Therefore, it is critical to developing new therapies and new drugs for PF. Many traditional Chinese medicines (TCM) have played a certain role in the treatment of various systems of diseases (Huang et al., 2018). Chinese herbal extracts also have many effective pharmacological ingredients to treat PF (Ji et al., 2016; Huo et al., 2020). In the past 30 years, the pharmacological activity of polysaccharides has attracted increasing attention (Layek and Mandal, 2020). Japanese scholar, Chihara Hiroro, firstly discovered that lentinan has an anti-tumor effect in 1968, thus striking the research boom of natural active polysaccharides (Chihara et al., 1969). Polysaccharides are natural macromolecular compounds composed of monosaccharides. They, with abundant biological activities and obviously low toxicity, are one of the main active components of Chinese medicine. Polysaccharides have received wide attention thanks to their effective biological activities and multiple molecular targets

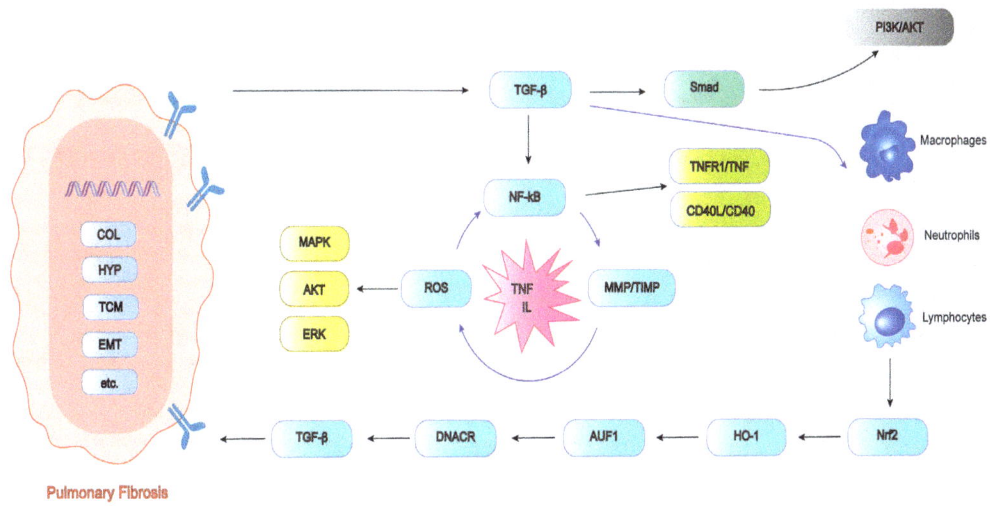

FIGURE 2 | The occurrence and development of PF can be related to these pathways.

(Muhamad et al., 2019; Cao et al., 2020; Mohammed et al., 2021). Studies have shown that polysaccharides have a variety of biological activities, such as anti-tumor, anti-oxidation, anti-radiation, anti-virus, and hypoglycemic effects (Mu et al., 2021; Niu et al., 2021). The development and application of polysaccharides in Chinese herbal medicine have enriched the treatment methods of modern medicine. Nowadays, TCM polysaccharides have been widely used clinically to treat related diseases, such as astragalus polysaccharide injection, ganoderma polysaccharide injection, ginseng polysaccharide injection, etc. (Li et al., 2019b). As expected, TCM polysaccharides have protective effects on PF. For example, astragalus polysaccharides (APS) can reduce the degree of PF by inhibiting transforming growth factor-β1 (TGF-β1) *in vitro* and *in vivo* (Zhang, Xu, 2020). Ganoderma lucidum polysaccharides (GIP) inhibit bleomycin (BLM)-induced adult male SD rats by improving lung antioxidant capacity (Chen et al., 2016). Therefore, Chinese herbal polysaccharides provide a new way to discover and develop anti-PF.

Repeated local micro-injuries play a fatal role in the aging alveolar epithelium, these micro-injuries start the connection of abnormal epithelial cell with fibroblast, induce myofibroblasts that produce matrix, and remodel a large amount of ECM accumulation and lung interstitial. There are many sources of myofibroblasts, including resident mesenchymal cell proliferatsion, pulmonary interstitial cells, circulating fibroblasts, epithelial-mesenchymal transition (EMT) and endothelial-mesenchymal transition (Todd et al., 2012). The histological characteristics of PF are excessive deposition of matrix collagen, increased fibrosis area and increased hydroxyproline (HYP) content, which can damage the normal structure and function of the lung. Activated alveolar epithelial cells secrete large amounts of fibrogenic growth factors and cytokines, including TGF-β1 and platelet-derived growth factors. TGF-β1 is an important regulator of fibrogenesis, which can activate fibroblasts and transform them into myofibroblasts (Organ et al., 2015), the initiation and regression of myofibroblasts herald disease progression. TGF-β1 not only promotes ECM deposition, but also concentrates it in the accumulated matrix, thereby accelerating it the pro-fibrotic reaction. The current pathogenesis of PF presumably includes abnormal accumulation of TGF-β, cell recruitment, apoptosis, inflammatory factors, oxidative stress, and the imbalance of matrix metalloproteinase/ tissue inhibitor of metalloproteinase (MMP/TIMP) (Ryu et al., 2014; Spagnolo et al., 2021) (**Figure 2**). Therefore, the use of various activities of Chinese herbal polysaccharides brings hope to the treatment of PF through these targets. Chinese herbal polysaccharides can participate in reversing the down-regulation of TGF-β and protecting PF, and have broad prospects in the field of anti-PF research.

Polysaccharides

Ginseng Polysaccharide (GPS)

GPS is a polysaccharide isolated from ginseng roots, with an average molecular weight (Mw) of 1.5 × 10^6 Da, mainly composed of Glc and Gal (over 90%, w/w) and 5–8% Man and Ara (Chen et al., 2020; Ahn et al., 2011; Ahn et al., 2011; Chen et al., 2020). It makes a variety of immunomodulatory functions, such as anti-oxidation, anti-tumor, anti-cancer and

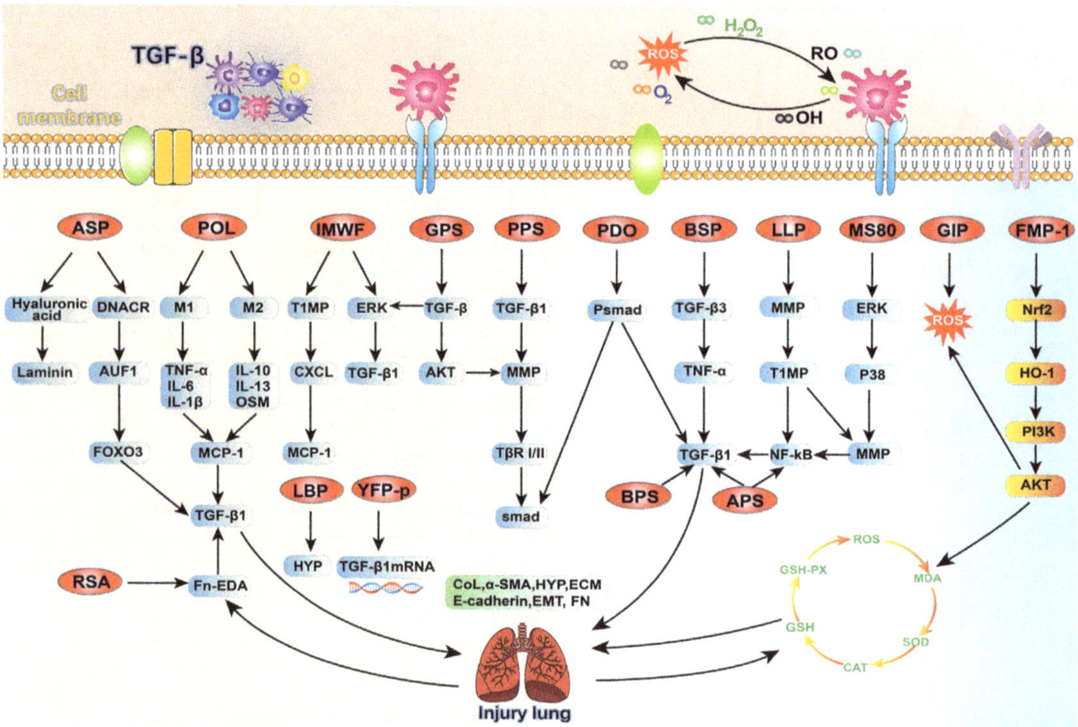

FIGURE 3 | An overview of the target signaling pathways of 16 Chinese herbal polysaccharides that antagonize PF, mainly by reversing TGF-β and improving ROS to treat pulmonary fibrosis, and further linking the relationship with these related pathways.

anti-adhesion (Akhter et al., 2018; Xiong et al., 2019). The Smad pathway is essential for TGF-β mediated signal transduction (Wilkes et al., 2005). Studies have shown that GPS inhibits the phosphorylation of Smad2 and Smad3 in fibroblasts through TGF-β, but has no response to the levels of Smad6 and Smad7, weakens the phosphorylation level of extracellular signal-regulated kinase/protein kinase B (ERK/AKT) and reverses the synthesis of collagen (COL)-1 and fibronectin (FN) also significantly reduces the protein expression of TGF-β1 receptor (TβRI) and TβRII in NIH/3T3 cells, preventing TβRII from its known that the protein expression of receptor TβRIII decreases, and it also inhibits the expression of a-smooth muscle actin (a-SMA) in IMR-90 and WI-38 cells (Ahn et al., 2011). Later, studies reported that ginsenosides can reduce EMT of lung tissue by inhibiting TGF-β1/Smad pathway (Guan et al., 2017). There are further reports that ginsenosides can prevent renal fibrosis (Li et al, 2018b). Recent observers have shown that ginseng can prevent liver, lung, kidney and myocardial fibrosis through TGF-β (Liu et al., 2020a). Therefore, the possible mechanism of GPS anti-PF is that the downstream Smad2 and Smad3 signals of TGF-β1 and its TβRI and TβRII can achieve the treatment purpose, and reduce the phosphorylation of ERK and AKT, and reduce the level of MMPs, which is beneficial to lung tissue damage (**Figure 3** and **Table 1**).

Basil Polysaccharide (BPS)

BPS is extracted from the Chinese herbal medicine basil, basil is a daily dish prepared in summer. BPS is a compound polysaccharide composed of fructose. It is mainly composed of Man, Rha, Glc, Fru, and Ara, the Mw is (8–10)×10^4 Da (Zhan et al., 2020). It has anti-tumor, anti-oxidation, anti-inflammatory, hypolipidemic, anti-diabetic and anti-liver cancer effects (Lv et al., 2013; Feng et al., 2018). Proves have shown that BPS has a potential inhibitory effect on the PF of human A549 cells induced by TGF-β, and down-regulates the expression of a-SMA and COL-1, up-regulates E-cadherin levels, and reduces HYP content (Yan et al., 2017), and proposed that BPS has an inhibitory effect on EMT (Feng et al., 2019). Therefore, BPS can reduce the inflammation of A549 cells by down-regulating TGF-β signaling to combat PF.

Astragalus polysaccharide (APS)

Astragalus as a medicinal and tonic food can keep fit and improve health. APS is a water-soluble polysaccharide isolated and purified from astragalus, the Mw is 1,334 kDa, composed of Rha, Ara, Glc, Gal, and GalA, the molar ratio is 0.03:1.00:0.27:0.36:0.30. The backbone of APS consisted of 1,2,4-linked Rhap, α-1, 4-linked Glcp, α-1, 4-linked GalAp6Me, β-1, 3, 6-linked Galp, with it branched at O-4 of the 1,2,4-linked Rhap and O-3 or O-4 of β-1, 3, 6-linked Galp. The side chains mainly consisted of α-T-Araf and α-1, 5-linked Araf with O-3 as branching points, having trace Glc and Gal, the terminal residues were T-linked Araf, T-linked Glcp, and T-linked Galp (Bao et al., 2018), its chemical structure is 2-(chloromethyl)-4-(4-nitrophenyl)-1,3-thiazole (Liu et al., 2019a). APS has been reported that have a variety of biological activities, including anti-inflammatory,

TABLE 1 | Overview of the research progress of Chinese herbal medicine polysaccharides in the treatment of PF.

Name	Monosaccharides composition	Mw (kDa)	Molecular structure	Experimental model	Anti-PF effect	References
GPS	Glc and Gla (over 90%, w/w) and 5–8% Man and Ara	1.5×10^6 Da	–	*In vivo*: BLM induced male C57BL/6 mice. *In vitro*: TGF-β1 induced NIH/3T3 cells and IMR-90 and WI-38 cells	Through the downstream Smad2 and Smad3 signals of TGF-β1 and its TβR I and TβRII, the treatment is achieved, which the levels of COL and α-SMA decreased, weaken the phosphorylation of ERK and AKT, reduce the level of MMPs to reduce lung tissue damage	(Ahn et al., 2011; Akhter et al., 2018; Xiong et al., 2019; Chen et al., 2020)
BPS	Man, Rha, Glc, Fru, Ara	$(8–10) \times 10^4$ Da	–	*In vitro*: TGF-β induced A549 cells	BPS can reduce the inflammation of A549 cells by down-regulating TGF-β signaling to combat PF.it can reduce HYP and COL content, down-regulate the expression of a-SMA, and up-regulate the level of E-cadherin	(Lv et al., 2013; Yan et al., 2017; Feng et al., 2018; Zhan et al., 2020)
APS	Rha:Ara: Glc:Gal:GalA = 0.03:1.00:0.27: 0.36:0.30	1,334 kDa	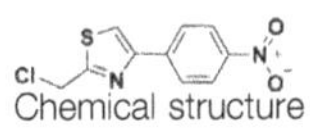 Chemical structure of APS: 2 -(Chloromethyl)-4-(4-nitrophenyl)-1,3-thiazole	*In vivo*: BLM induced male C57BL/6 mice. *In vitro*: TGF-β1 induced A549 cells	Regulate EMT and HYP content through the TGF-β1/NF-kB pathway, and reduce the area of a-SMA, COL deposition and fibrosis, and increase E-cadherin	(Bao et al., 2018; Ren et al., 2018; Jia et al., 2019; Liu et al., 2019a; Zhang et al., 2020)
PPS	Component consisting of (1 → 3)-β-glucan backbone and (1 → 6)-β-glucopyranose side chains	1.6×10^5 Da	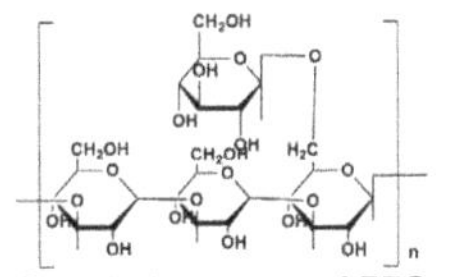 Chemical structure of PPS.	*In vivo*: BLM induced male C57BL/6 mice. *In vitro*: TGF-β1 induced in HLFs cells	The further deterioration of PF was prevented by TGF-β1/Smad2/3/TβRI and TβRII/MMP signaling, resulting in the decrease of α-SMA, MMP2/9, FN, COL-1/3 and ECM.	(Li et al., 2010; Zong et al., 2012; Guo et al., 2019; Jiang et al., 2020)
RSA	Ara:Rha:Xyl: Glc:Gal: GalA = 1.00:3.23:0.26: 0.34:0.84:10.24	50,000 Da	–	*In vitro*: TGF-β1 induced A549 cells	RSA inhibits the process of TGF-β1 inducing A549 cells and down-regulates the expression of Fn-EDA.	(Han et al., 2002; Li et al., 2016; Yang et al., 2016; Song et al., 2019)
PDO	Man:Glc = 5.9:1, it is composed of (1→4)-linked Man and (1→4)-linked Glc	1.78×10^5 Da	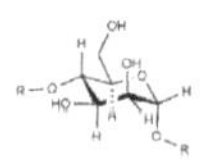 (1→4)-linked Man 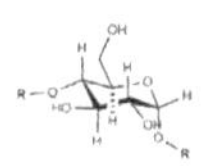 (1→4)-connected Glc	*In vivo*: BLM induced adult male Sprague Dawley rats. *In vitro*: TGF-β1 induced type II alveolar epithelial cells (RLE-6TN, CRL-2300)	PDO can reduce the number of neutrophils in rat lung tissue induced by BLM, improve inflammation and fibrosis, enhance Smad2/3 and inhibit the expression of pSmad2/3 protein through TGFβ1, thereby inhibiting the type II rat alveolar epithelial cells (RLE-6TN, CRL-2300) induced by TGF-β1 fibronectin and COL-1	(He et al., 2016; Wang et al., 2017a; Chen et al., 2018, Yu et al., 2018c; Liu et al., 2019b)
BSP	BSP-1:Man:Glc = 4.0: 1.0, BSP-2: Man:Glc = 3.0:1.0, the backbone of BSP-1 and BSP-2 were consisted of β-1,4-linked D-Man residues and β-1,4-linked D-Glc residues	BSP: 2.23×10^5 kDa, BSP-1:8.354×10^4 Da, BSP-2:1.26×10^4 Da	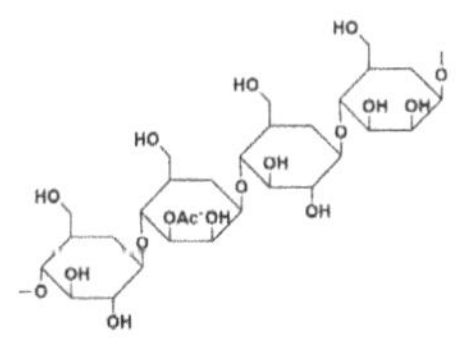 The main residues sequence of BSP-1 was deduced to be: →4)-β-D-Glcp (1→4)-β-D-Manp (1→4)-β-D-Manp (1→4)-β-D-Manp (1→4)-β-D-Manp (1→. The O-acetyl group position was also attached to C-3 of residue B (Man). 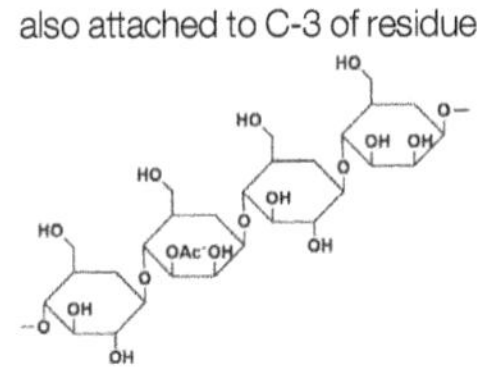 The residues sequence of BSP-2 was deduced to be: →4)-β-D-Glcp (1→4)-β-D-Manp (1→4)-β-D-Manp (1→4)-β-D-Manp (1→	*In vivo*: BLM induced male SD rats	BSP can reduce cell recruitment to protect lung tissue inflammation, HYP, a-SMA content is significantly reduced, and it also improves TGF-β3 and TNF-β1	(Guo et al., 2016; He et al., 2017; Wang et al., 2019b; Liu et al., 2020b)

(Continued on following page)

TABLE 1 | *(Continued)* Overview of the research progress of Chinese herbal medicine polysaccharides in the treatment of PF.

Name	Monosaccharides composition	Mw (kDa)	Molecular structure	Experimental model	Anti-PF effect	References
MS80	New type of sulfated oligosaccharide (1→4α-d-Glc)	8,000 Da	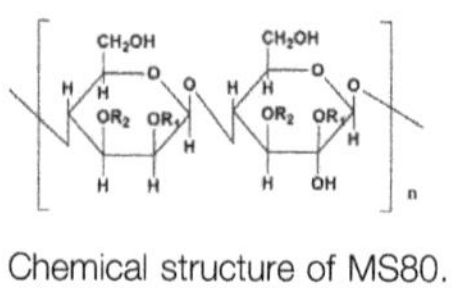 Chemical structure of MS80. R1 = SO3Na, R2 = SO3Na or H, n = 10~15	*In vivo*: BLM induced pathogen-free adult Wistar rats. *In vitro*: TGF-β1 induced HEPF cells	MS80 can improve PF through TGF-β1/MMP/ERK/NF-kB/p38, prevent COL deposition, and reduce COL and EMT content	(Jiang and Guan, 2009; Zhou et al., 2016; Chen et al., 2020)
LMWF	Rha, Fuc, Xly, Man, Glc, Gal, GlcA, Gala, the linkage is backbone →3)-Galp-(1→, →6)-Glcp-(1→, →6)-Galp-(1→, →3,6)-manp-(1→ with →3)-Fucp-(1→, →4)-Glcp-(1→ and sulfated end units. Consists of (1→3)-linked α-thiopropionyl residues or alternating (13→)- and (→14)-linked α-thiophosphoryl residues	8–10 kDa	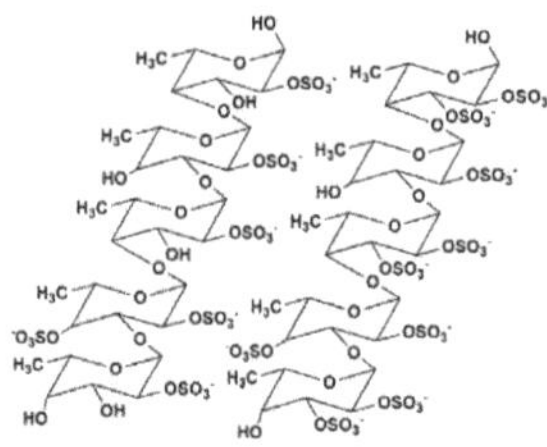 The overview of fucoidan regulation on signaling molecules	*In vivo*: BLM-induced male C57BL/6 mice. *In vitro*: TGF-β1 induced A549 cells	LMWF treats PF through TGF-β1/ERK signaling and improving inflammatory cytokines in pathological lung tissue, attenuates the expression of lung EMT phenotype a-SMA and HYP.	(Senthilkumar and Kim, 2014; Haddad et al., 2015; Wang et al., 2019a; Wang et al., 2018; Yu et al., 2018a; Zheng et al., 2018; Chen et al., 2020)
ASP	GalA:Glc:Ara:Gal = 1.00:1.70:1.85:5.02, its main chain is composed of (1→3)-connected Galp, (1→6)-connected Galp and 2-OMe-(1→6)-connected Galp, with three branches connected to 2-OMe-(-1→6) link Galp and terminate with GlcpA and Araf	80 kDa, 85 kDa	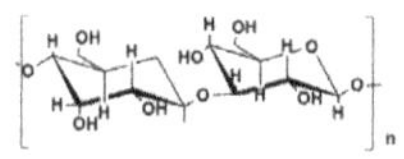 Chemically modified with branched LMW PEI (1,200 Da) to obtain cationic ASP.	*In vivo*: BLM induced healthy Wistar rats and Sprague-Dawley rats. *in vitro*: TGF-β1 induced alveolar type II epithelial (RLE-6TN) cells	ASP can inhibit EMT and PF through the TGF-β1/DANCR/AUF-1/FOXO3 regulatory axis, reduce and reverse the expression levels of α-SMA, COL and E-cadherin	(Deng et al., 2013a; Zhang et al., 2016; Li et al., 2020a; Qian et al., 2020; Wang et al., 2010; Xu et al., 2021)
POL	Gal: Man:Glc = 5.30: 13.38:81.31	3.2×10^5 Da	–	*In vivo*: BLM induced male C57BL/6 mice	Improve lung inflammation by inhibiting the excessive recruitment of M1 and M2 under TGF-β1 to achieve a therapeutic effect, reducing the levels of MCP-1, TNF-α, IL-1β, IL-6, IL-10,IL-13, and OSM.	(Zhang et al., 2017; Ying-Mei et al., 2020; Zhou et al., 2020)
LBP	Glycan backbone is mainly represented by α-(1→4)-GalA, α-(1→6)-Glc, β-(1→3)-Galp (typical arabinogalactan protein) and β-(1→6)-Giap, other structures that are less representative are α-(1→5)-Ara and β-(1→4)-Galp	10–2,300 kDa	–	*In vivo*: BLM induced C57BL/6 mice	Inhibit the increase of HYP content in lung tissue when PF occurs, inhibit the increase of ECM, and reduce the expression levels of α-SMA and COL-1	(Liu et al., 2016b; Masci et al., 2018; Huang et al., 2019; Tian et al., 2019)
FMP-1	Man:Glc:Gal = 1.00: 7.84:1.24, the main chain is 1,4-linked Glcp and 1,6-connected Galp composition	4.7×10^3 Da	–	*In vitro*: H202 induced human alveolar epithelial cells (A549)	FMP-1 can be used as a natural potential antioxidant to treat PF through the Nrf2/HO-1/PI3K/AKT signaling pathway, which can weaken MDA and ROS levels, increase SOD enzyme activity and total antioxidant capacity	(Liu et al., 2016a; Li et al., 2017; Cai et al., 2018; Li et al., 2018c)

(Continued on following page)

TABLE 1 | *(Continued)* Overview of the research progress of Chinese herbal medicine polysaccharides in the treatment of PF.

Name	Monosaccharides composition	Mw (kDa)	Molecular structure	Experimental model	Anti-PF effect	References
GIP	Gal:Rha:Glc = 1.00: 1.15:3.22, backbone structure is mainly composed of 1,2-linked β-L Rhap, 1,3,6-linked aD-Galp, 1,2,6-linked aD-Glcp and 1-link aD-Glcp	78 kDa	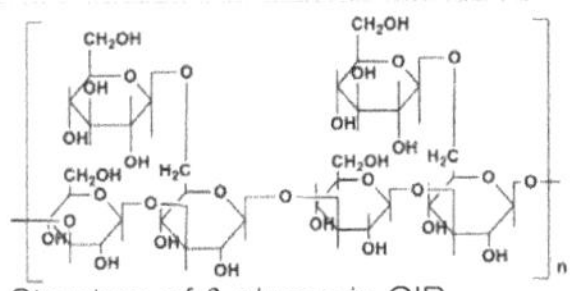 Structure of β-glucan in GIP.	*In vivo*: BLM induced adult male SD rats	Improve the status of PF by improving the antioxidant capacity of the lung, reducing inflammatory cell infiltration and collagen deposition, improving the content of CAT and SOD, increasing the levels of GSH, GSH-Px, and reducing the content of MDA and HYP in lung tissue	(Pan et al., 2012; Chen et al., 2016; Wang et al., 2017b; Sohretoglu and Huang, 2018; Zeng et al., 2018; Zeng et al., 2019)
LLP	LLP-1:Glc:Man = 1:2, LLP-2:Glc:Man = 1:1, LLP-3:Ara:Gal: Glc: Man = 2:2:2:1	LLP-1:2.25 × 10^6 Da, LLP-2: 2.02 × 10^6 Da, LLP-3:2.08 × 10^6 Da	—	*In vivo*: BLM induced SPF Kunming mice	Inhibit MMP-9 and TIMP-2 in lung tissue of BLM pulmonary fibrosis mice, reduce HYP content and COL level, and inhibit the expression of TNF-a, NF-kB in lung tissue of pulmonary fibrosis	(Chen et al., 2014; Hou et al., 2016; Li et al., 2020b; Luo et al., 2013a)
YPF-p	-	—	—	*In vivo*: pingyangmycin hydrochloride induced Wistar rats and BLM induced healthy adult female Sprague-Dawley rats	YPF-p treats PF by down-regulating the expression of TGF-β1 mRNA and improving the excessive aggregation of fibroblasts induced by TGF-β1, which reduces the expression of HYP, COL and a-SMA in lung tissue	(Wang et al., 2009; Xu et al., 2014; Sun et al., 2016; Fan et al., 2017)

anti-tumor, anti-diabetic and anti-oxidant (Ren et al., 2018; Jia et al., 2019). Previous reports suggested that astragalus injection and astragaloside IV have therapeutic effects on fibrosis (Qian et al., 2018). APS can protect renal fibrosis (Ren et al., 2019). *Astragalus* can improve EMT through β-catenin (Yu et al., 2018b). The overproduction of TGF-β1 is always closely related to PF, and TGF-β1 plays a key role in inducing EMT (Walton et al., 2017), nuclear factor-kB (NF-kB) regulates the expression of a variety of cytokines and inflammatory mediators, by inhibiting the expression of TGF-β1/NF-kB to block related signal pathways and prevent inflammation and reduce liver fibrosis (Li et al., 2018a). A recent observation proposed that APS can reduce PF through the TGF-β1/NF-kB pathway, which can effectively improve the deposition of COL-1, COL-3, and FN *in vivo*, APS reduce the area of fibrosis and HYP content in the matrix, and reduce the expression of a-SMA neutralizes E-cadherin, it significantly reduces the activation of the EMT and NF-kB pathways of TGF-β1 *in vitro* (Zhang et al., 2020). Therefore, the mechanism of APS protecting PF is the regulation of TGF-β1/NF-kB pathway.

Polyporus Polysaccharide (PPS)

The pharmaceutical ingredients of polyporus umbellatus include polysaccharides, ergosterol, biotin, protein and other molecules, among which PPS is one of the main biologically active substances of polyporus umbellatus, the main components of PPS are (1–3)-β-Glc main chain and (1–6)-β-Glc side chain β-glucan, the Mw is about 1.6 × 10^5 Da (Zong et al., 2012). Previous studies have reported various pharmacological activities of PPS, such as anti-tumor, anti-cancer, anti-oxidation and anti-inflammatory (Li et al., 2010; Guo et al., 2019). In renal fibrosis, PPS can improve the accumulation of TGF-β1, restore the balance of MMP/TIMP factors and improve renal fibrosis (Li et al., 2019a). PPS can significantly inhibit the ECM components in human lung fibrosis (HLFs) cells treated with TGF-β1, and inhibit Smad2/3 phosphorylation even reduce TβRI and TβRII, but it has no effect on TβRIV and can also inhibit medium MMP-2/MMP-9 expression (Jiang et al., 2020). Therefore, PPS prevented the further deterioration of PF through TGF-β1/Smad2/3/TβRI, and TβR II/MMP level signals.

Rhodiolasachalinensis Polysaccharide A (RSA)

RSA is an acidic heteropolysaccharide isolated from rhodiola alpina, its mainly composed of Ara, Rha, Xyl, Glc, Gal, and GalA, the molar ratio is 1.00:3.23:0.26:0.34:0.84:10.24, and the relative Mw is about 50,000 Da (Han et al., 2002), has anti-oxidant, anti-viral, anti-oxidant and anti-tumor effects (Yang et al., 2016; Song et al., 2019). Previous evaluations have reported that salidroside protects mice from acute lung injury through the NF-kB pathway by controlling the production of inflammatory cytokines, and is very effective in preventing oxidative stress after exercise in mice (Guan et al., 2012). Studies have suggested that RSA can significantly inhibit the death rate of A549 cells induced by TGF-β1 and the expression of the mesenchymal marker Fibronection-EDA (Fn-EDA) (Li, et al., 2016). Rhodiola rosea significantly reduced the expression levels of MMP-9 and α-SMA in PF in a dose-dependent manner (Zhang et al., 2016). Therefore, RSA can improve the abnormality of Fn-EDA through TGF-β1 to achieve the purpose of treating PF.

Polysaccharides From Dendrobium Officinale (PDO)

Dendrobium officinale is an epiphytic herb of the orchid family with mainly grows on semi-shaded moist rocks at an altitude of about 1,600 m in the Nanshan mountains of china. PDO is a neutral heteropolysaccharide isolated from the Chinese medicinal material dendrobium candidum, with composed of (1→4)-linked Man and (1→4)-linked Glc, the molar ratio is 5.9:1 and the Mw is 1.78×10^5 Da (He et al., 2016; Yu W. et al., 2018). It has the effects of anti-oxidation, anti-tumor, anti-viral, anti-aging, lowering blood sugar and promoting hair growth (Wang J.-H. et al., 2017; Liu et al., 2019b), and is often valued in the field of dermatology. Dendrobium nobile polysaccharides can improve the antioxidant capacity of rats and reduce liver inflammation, so it has an antagonistic effect on liver fibrosis (Sibinska et al., 2017). Early studies on dendrobium candidum can treat myocardial fibrosis (Zhang et al., 2016b; Zeng et al., 2020). PDO can reduce the number of neutrophils in lung tissue induced by BLM, improve inflammation and fibrosis, enhance Smad2/3 and inhibit the expression of pSmad2/3 protein through TGFβ1, thereby inhibiting the type II rat alveolar epithelial cells (RLE-6TN, CRL-2300) induced by TGF-β1 fibronectin and COL-1 (Chen et al., 2018). Therefore, PDO treatment of PF lies in the regulation of TGF-β1/Smad2, Smad3/pSmad2/3.

Bletilla Striata Polysaccharide (BSP)

Two water-soluble polysaccharides, BSP-1 and BSP-2, were extracted and purified from *bacillus* striata tuber, and their Mw are 8.354×10^4 and 1.26×10^4 Da, both BSP-1 and BSP-2 are composed of Man and Glc, and the molar ratio are 4.0:1.0 and 3.0: 1.0. The backbone is mainly composed of repeated β-1,4-linked d-Man residues and β-1, 4-linked d-Glc residue composition. It has anti-ulcer, anti-oxidation, anti-inflammatory, anti-tumor and immunomodulatory activities (He et al., 2017; Liu et al., 2020). BSP can protect renal fibrosis through the down-regulation of TβRI, TβRII and a-SMA mediated by TGF-β (Wang et al., 2014). Some researchers have confirmed that a Mw of 2.23×10^5 kDa, BSP can reduce cell recruitment to protect lung tissue inflammation, the content of HYP is significantly reduced, TGF-β3 and TNF-β1 are also improved, they also proved that bletilla striata extract also has a certain degree of resistance the role of fibrosis (Guo et al., 2016). Therefore, BSP improves lung inflammation and abnormal cell recruitment through TGF-β/TNF to improve lung tissue fibrosis.

Seaweed Sulfated Oligosaccharide (MS80)

Marine macroalgae are mainly divided into four parts, green algae, cyanobacteria, brown algae and red algae. MS80 is a new type of sulfated oligosaccharide (1→4α-d-Glc) extracted from seaweed, with the Mw is 8,000 Da, MS80 can anti-cancer, anti-inflammatory and anti-tumor (Chen et al., 2020). MS80 inhibits BLM-induced PF *in vivo*, antagonizes TGF-β1-induced human embryo pulmonary fibroblast (HEPF) cells proliferation *in vitro*, prevents COL deposition and MMP activity, and inactivates ERK and p38 signaling pathways (Jiang and Guan, 2009). In addition, the MS80 targeting protein is receptor interacting protein 2 (a key component of CD40 signal transduction). MS80 inhibits the activation of NF-kB induced by CD40 linkage, thereby inhibiting the secretion of inflammatory cytokines, COL synthesis and fibrogenesis the excessive proliferatsion of cells confirms that MS80 has anti-fibrosis effects both *in vivo* and *in vitro* (Du et al., 2010). MS80 can also effectively inhibit standardized TGF-β1/Smad signaling, thereby improving the changes in EMT marker levels (Zhou et al., 2016). Therefore, MS80 can improve PF through TGF-β1/MMP/ERK/NF-kB/p38.

Low Molecular Weight Fucoidan (LMWF)

LMWF is a sulfated polysaccharide extracted from brown algae, the Mw is 8–10 kDa, containing Rha, Fuc, Xly, Man, Glc, Gal, GlcA and Gala, the linkage is backbone →3)-Galp-(1→, →6)-Glcp-(1→, →6)-Galp-(1→, →3,6)-manp-(1→ with →3)-Fucp-(1→, →4)-Glcp-(1→ and sulfated end units (Chen et al., 2020), consists of (1→3)-linked α-thiopropionyl residues or alternating (13→)- and (→14)-linked α-thiophosphoryl residues. Depending on previous studies, LMWF can lower blood sugar, anti-inflammatory, and promote angiogenesis (Haddad et al., 2015; Wang et al., 2018; Zheng et al., 2018). LMWF has an antagonistic effect on liver fibrosis through the TGF-β1/Smad3 pathway (Hayashi et al., 2008). Its also lnhibit the proliferatsion of breast cancer cells and the expression of EMT biomarkers (Hsu et al., 2013). In addition, LMWF can reduce inflammation of the inflammatory cytokines TIMP-1, chemokine ligand 1 (CXCL1), monocyte chemotactic protein-1 (MCP-1), and macrophage inflammation protein-2 (MIP-2) of lung tissue, TNF content to improve radiation-induced pneumonia in mice and further PF (Yu H.-H. et al., 2018). LMWF inhibits the morphological changes and proliferatsion of A549 cells induced by TGF-β1. In the male C57BL/6 mice model, LMWF attenuates the lung EMT phenotype. LMWF down-regulates TGF-β1/ERK signals *in vivo* and *in vitro* to regulate PF (Wang et al., 2019a). Therefore, LMWF treats PF through TGF-β1/ERK signal and improves inflammatory cytokines in pathological lung tissue.

Angelica Sinensis Polysaccharide (ASP)

ASP is an acidic heteropolysaccharide extracted from the root of angelica sinensis, its composed of GalA, Glc, Ara and Gal with the molar ratio of 1.00:1.70:1.85:5.02, the Mw is 80 kDa. Its main chain is composed of (1→3)-connected Galp, (1→6)-connected Galp and 2-OMe-(1→6)-connected Galp, with three branches connected to 2-OMe-(- 1→6) link Galp and terminate with GlcpA and Araf (Zhang et al., 2016a). ASP has immune regulation, anti-tumor, anti-oxidation and anti-proliferatsion functions (Li M. M. et al., 2020; Xu et al., 2021). There is also the ability of the compound Danggui Buxue Decoction total glycosides (containing astragalus and angelica) to inhibit abnormal lung tissue ECM and reverse the expression of MMP/TIMP (Gao et al., 2012). ASP can improve the content of hyaluronic acid and laminin in the lung tissue of rats with PF induced by BLM (Wang et al., 2010). The latest report points out that ASP inhibits PF by down-regulating the expression of differentiation-antagonizing non-protein coding RNA (DANCR), which inactivates FOXO3 translation after transcription in an AU binding factor 1 (AUF1)-dependent manner (Qian et al., 2020). Therefore, ASP can inhibit EMT and PF through the TGF-β1/DANCR/AUF-1/FOXO3 regulatory axis.

Total Polysaccharide From O, Lanpingensis (POL)

POL is an insect fungal polysaccharide isolated from cordyceps Lanping. It is mainly distributed in northwestern Yunnan, china as a new species reported in recent years, which is closely a relative species of cordyceps sinensis. POL Mw is 3.2×10^5 Da, composed of Gal, Man and Glc, and the molar ratio is 5.30:13.38: 81.31 (Zhou et al., 2020). It was reported earlier that POL has an anti-inflammatory effect, which can improve liver fibrosis by alleviating the body's oxidative stress, reduce inflammation and anti-apoptosis of liver cells (Zhang et al., 2017). POL can Treat renal insufficiency by enhancing antioxidant capacity and improving immune regulation ability (Ying-Mei et al., 2020). Ophiocordyceps lanpingensis can treat respiratory diseases. POL can significantly reduce the content of collagen in lung tissue and inflammation of lung tissue by inhibiting classically activated macrophages 1 (M1) and alternately activated M2 in lung tissue The recruitment of PF inhibits the occurrence of PF (Zhou et al., 2020). Therefore, POL can improve lung inflammation by inhibiting the excessive recruitment of M1 and M2 under TGF-β1 to achieve a therapeutic effect.

Lycium Barbarum Polysaccharide (LBP)

In the wolfberry extract, LBP isolated from the fruit of lycium barbarum caused the biological activity of the wolfberry. LBP is a group of water-soluble sugar conjugates with a Mw is 10–2,300 kDa, accounting for 5–8% of dried fruit. LBP glycan backbone is mainly represented by α-(1→4)-galA, α-(1→6)-glc, β-(1→3)-galp (typical arabinogalactan protein) and β-(1→6)-giap, other structures that are less representative are α-(1→5)-ara and β-(1→4)-galp, which have different branching and terminal sites (Tian et al., 2019). LBP has the effects of lowering blood sugar, lowering blood lipid, anti-oxidation and anti-tumor effect (Masci et al., 2018; Huang et al., 2019). LBP possibly inhibit the expression of genes such as COL-1 and α-SMA in inflamed lung tissues, weaken the excessive proliferatsion of fibroblasts and prevent their differentiation into myofibroblasts, thereby reducing the content of HYP in lung tissues to inhibit the development of PF in C57BL/6 mice (Liu et al., 2016b). Therefore, LBP inhibits PF by improving the degree of fibers in the lung tissue.

Morel Polysaccharide-1 (FMP-1)

Morels belong to the category of mushrooms, with high nutritional value and delicious taste, both the flavor and the pharmacological effects have been highly regarded (Tietel and Masaphy, 2018). FMP-1 is a heteropolysaccharide in morchella fruiting body, the Mw is 4.7×10^3 Da, composed of Man, Glc, and Gal with the molar ratio of 1.00:7.84:1.24, the main chain is 1,4-linked Glcp and 1,6-connected Galp composition (Cai et al., 2018). Previous studies have shown that morel contains many biologically active ingredients, such as polysaccharides, protein, dietary fiber and vitamins. FMP-1 has immunomodulatory, anti-oxidant, anti-value-added and anti-tumor effects (C. Liu et al., 2016a; Li et al., 2017). Controlling oxidative stress after lung injury has been shown to be effective in inhibiting fibrosis, it is proposed that polysaccharides can activate antioxidant defenses and improve oxidative stress damage (Hao et al., 2016; Chen et al., 2017). The phosphatidylinositol 3-kinase (PI3K)/AKT pathway is one of the effective ways to fight oxidative stress (Mozaffari et al., 2010), and it has a protective effect on lung epithelial cell death induced by oxidative stress (Deng et al., 2013b). Many examines have confirmed that the up-regulation of heme oxidase-1 (HO-1) is involved in the cells defense mechanism against the results of oxidation (Lee et al., 2012; Jang et al., 2016). Related1 research reports that FMP-1 can promote nuclear factor erythroid 2-related factor 2 (Nrf2) phosphorylation and nuclear translocation, and up-regulate downstream protein HO-1 through the PI3K/AKT-Nrf2 signaling pathway, thereby protecting human alveolar epithelial cells (A549) from hydrogen peroxide oxidative stress (Li et al., 2018c). Therefore, FMP-1 can be used as a natural potential antioxidant to treat PF through the Nrf2/HO-1/PI3K/AKT signaling pathway.

Ganoderma Lucidum Polysaccharide (GIP)

Ganoderma is an edible medicinal mushroom, which has been praised for 2000 years. It can enhance human vitality. GIP is a neutral heteropolysaccharide isolated from ganoderma lucidum. It is composed of Gal, Rha and Glc with the molar ratio of 1.00: 1.15:3.22, the Mw is 78 kDa, and the backbone structure is mainly composed of 1,2-linked bL- Rhap, 1,3,6-linked aD-Galp, 1,2,6-linked aD-Glcp, and 1-link aD-Glcpconsisted mainly of 1,2-linked-β-L-Rhap, 1,3,6-linked-a-D-Galp, 1,2,6-linked-a-D-Glcp, and1-linked a-D-Glcp. (Pan et al., 2012). It is reported that a pure Glc polymer named β-glucan is considered to be one of the active ingredients of GIP (Zeng et al., 2019). GIP has many therapeutic effects on human diseases, including anti-oxidation, anti-inflammatory, anti-tumor, lowering blood sugar, lowering blood lipids, and anti-aging (Wang et al., 2017b; Sohretoglu and Huang, 2018; Zeng et al., 2018). In addition, it has been reported in the literatsure that GIP 100–300 mg/kg can reverse PF after 28 days. The main mechanism is related to the increase of lung antioxidant capacity. GIP can increase pathological lung tissue CAT (catalase), SOD (superoxide dismutation), GSH (glutathione), and GSH-Px (glutathione peroxidase) levels, simultaneously, reduce the content of MDA (malondialdehyde) and HYP in lung tissue (Chen et al., 2016). Later reports confirmed that ganoderma lucidum has obvious protective effect on oxidative damage caused by oxidants (Laçin et al., 2019; Lin and Deng, 2019). Ganoderic acid can treat renal fibrosis through TGF-β/Smad and MAPK signaling (Geng et al., 2020). Therefore, GIP improves the status of PF by improving the lung's antioxidant capacity.

Lily Polysaccharide (LLP)

LLP-1, LLP-2 and LLP-3 are the three new polysaccharide components in lily, their Mw are estimated to be 2.25×10^6, 2.02×10^6, and 2.08×10^6 Da, LLP-1 and LLP-2 are mainly composed of Glc and Man, with the molar ratio of 1:2 and 1:1, respectively, LLP-3 is mainly composed of Ara, Gal, Glc, and Man, with the molar ratio is 2:2:2:1 (Chen et al., 2014; Hou et al., 2016). LLP has a variety of activities, such as hypoglycemic, anti-oxidant and anti-cancer effects (Li et al., 2020b). LLP can improve the PF alveolar compartment and reduce the infiltratsion of inflammatory cells. The mechanism is to inhibit the protein expression of MMP-9 and TIMP-2 in the fibrosis model (Luo, et al., 2013a). LLP combined with bone marrow mesenchymal stem cell transplantation inhibits the expression of TNF-α and NF-kB in the lung tissue of PF mice, improves the recruitment of COL and reduces the content of HYP. LLP can reduce the pathological damage of PF (Luo, et al., 2013b). Therefore, LLP treats PF by adjusting the balance of MMP/TIMP in rats, improving the NF-kB signaling pathway and inflammatory TNF-a abnormalities in lung tissue.

Yupingfeng–Polysaccharide (YPF–p)

Yupingfeng powder is a well-known TCM compound consisting of *Astragalus*, Atractylodes and Fangfeng. There are many compounds in Yupingfeng powder, including total polysaccharides, total saponins and volatile oil. Among them, YPF-p is one of the important components extracted from Yupingfeng powder, it has anti-inflammatory, anti-allergic, immune-regulating and alleviating effects of lung qi deficiency (Sun et al., 2016; Fan et al., 2017). Anti-fibrosis studies have found that YPF-p can improve the level of HYP in Wistar rats induced by pingyangmycin hydrochloride and the content of COL-3, COL-4, laminin, and hyaluronic acid in serum, and can down-regulate Wistar rats lungs. TGF-β1 mRNA expression in tissues (Wang et al., 2009). The mechanism presumably is that inhibit the increase of TGF-β1 mediated fibroblast activation and thus reduce synthesis (Xu et al., 2014). In addition, the total glycosides of Yupingfeng reduced the protein expression of box1 in the high mobility group, and reversed TGF-β1 to improve PF (Cui et al., 2015; Li et al., 2015). Therefore, YPF-p treats PF by down-regulating the expression of TGF-β1 mRNA and improving the excessive aggregation of fibroblasts induced by TGF-β1.

CONCLUSION AND FUTURE PROSPECTS

These polysaccharides can significantly improve the abnormal recruitment and apoptosis of various cells in the lung tissue induced by the TGF-β signaling pathway, regulate the imbalance of the body caused by lung inflammation, and can control lung tissue damage through oxidative stress, thus confirming these polysaccharides can stabilize PF lung function and prevent further damage.

Our understanding of this evolving deadly disease is constantly improving, but effective treatments are still elusive. PF is also one of the main complications of COVID-19. Studying the properties of polysaccharides and combining polysaccharides with other drugs may provide medical help for PF patients with COVID-19. The epidemiological risk factors and biological process of PF and COVID-19 are similar. After severe acute respiratory syndrome coronavirus 2 (SARS-CoV-2) induced pneumonia may cause idiopathic PF related to its physical damage. Hence, modulating the mechanism of fibrosis in SARS-CoV-2 infection to exert a therapeutic effect may be acceptable. The chemical structure of Chinese herbal medicine polysaccharides is the basis of biological activity. Using the hydroxyl, carboxyl, amino, and other groups of sugar residues to modify the structure of polysaccharide molecules on the surface of polysaccharide molecules, For example, the GIP isolated from Fudan-Yueyang-G. lucidu has undergone methylation analysis, periodate oxidation, Smith degradation, and NMR characterization analysis to obtain a neutral polysaccharide with four residues A, B, C, and D which is significantly enhanced improve the lung's antioxidant capacity to achieve the purpose of treating PF, The structure determines the activity, can makes the multiple structure of the plant clearer, and seeks the regularity between the nanostructure and the biological activity to improve the immune activity of polysaccharides and reduce toxic effects. Chemical polysaccharides with different structures have great differences in biological activity. Further explore the relationship between the biological effects and efficacy of Chinese herbal medicine polysaccharides to explain the therapeutic mechanism of polysaccharides in PF. It is very important to provide a certain reference for the in-depth study and exploration of the structure-activity relationship of Chinese herbal medicine polysaccharides and the development and application of carbohydrate products. This provides important medical theory and economic value for the development of Chinese herbal polysaccharides to treat fibrotic diseases, and has a very important society. Polysaccharides can be a new type of anti-fibrosis treatment drugs. While, the structure of traditional Chinese medicine polysaccharides is complex and diverse, and its special active mechanism needs to be further studied. The establishment of specific, efficient and practical methods for the stability of polysaccharides is of great significance to the research and development of modern medicine.

AUTHOR CONTRIBUTIONS

JS guided the experiment. XW and JH collected supporting evidence and wrote the paper. All authors read and approved the final article.

Hospital (2021LZ03), the National Key Research and Development Program of China (2020YFC2005500), and the Key Research and

Development Program of Science and Technology Department of Sichuan Province (2019YFS0514).

REFERENCES

Ahn, J.-Y., Kim, M.-H., Lim, M.-J., Park, S., Lee, S.-l. -o., Yun, Y.-S., et al. (2011). The Inhibitory Effect of Ginsan on TGF-β Mediated Fibrotic Process. *J. Cel. Physiol.* 226 (5), 1241–1247. doi:10.1002/jcp.22452

Akhter, K. F., Mumin, M. A., Lui, E. M. K., and Charpentier, P. A. (2018). Fabrication of Fluorescent Labeled Ginseng Polysaccharide Nanoparticles for Bioimaging and Their Immunomodulatory Activity on Macrophage Cell Lines. *Int. J. Biol. Macromolecules* 109, 254–262. doi:10.1016/j.ijbiomac.2017.12.050

Bao, W.-R., Li, Z.-P., Zhang, Q.-W., Li, L.-F., Liu, H.-B., Ma, D.-L., et al. (2018). Astragalus Polysaccharide RAP Selectively Attenuates Paclitaxel-Induced Cytotoxicity toward RAW 264.7 Cells by Reversing Cell Cycle Arrest and Apoptosis. *Front. Pharmacol.* 9, 1580. doi:10.3389/fphar.2018.01580

Cai, Z.-N., Li, W., Mehmood, S., Pan, W.-J., Wang, Y., Meng, F.-J., et al. (2018). Structural Characterization, *In Vitro* and *In Vivo* Antioxidant Activities of a Heteropolysaccharide from the Fruiting Bodies of Morchella Esculenta. *Carbohydr. Polym.* 195, 29–38. doi:10.1016/j.carbpol.2018.04.069

Canestaro, W. J., Forrester, S. H., Raghu, G., Ho, L., and Devine, B. E. (2016). Drug Treatment of Idiopathic Pulmonary Fibrosis. *Chest* 149 (3), 756–766. doi:10.1016/j.chest.2015.11.013

Cao, P., Wu, S., Wu, T., Deng, Y., Zhang, Q., Wang, K., et al. (2020). The Important Role of Polysaccharides from a Traditional Chinese Medicine-Lung Cleansing and Detoxifying Decoction against the COVID-19 Pandemic. *Carbohydr. Polym.* 240, 116346. doi:10.1016/j.carbpol.2020.116346

Chen, J., Lu, J., Wang, B., Zhang, X., Huang, Q., Yuan, J., et al. (2018). Polysaccharides from Dendrobium Officinale Inhibit Bleomycin-Induced Pulmonary Fibrosis via the TGFβ1-Smad2/3 axis. *Int. J. Biol. Macromol.* 118 (Pt B), 2163–2175. doi:10.1016/j.ijbiomac.2018.07.056

Chen, J., Shi, Y., He, L., Hao, H., Wang, B., Zheng, Y., et al. (2016). Protective Roles of Polysaccharides from Ganoderma Lucidum on Bleomycin-Induced Pulmonary Fibrosis in Rats. *Int. J. Biol. Macromolecules* 92, 278–281. doi:10.1016/j.ijbiomac.2016.07.005

Chen, L., Liu, L., Li, C., Hu, C., Su, F., Liu, R., et al. (2017). A Mix of Apple Pomace Polysaccharide Improves Mitochondrial Function and Reduces Oxidative Stress in the Liver of High-Fat Diet-Induced Obese Mice. *Mol. Nutr. Food Res.* 61 (3), 1600433. doi:10.1002/mnfr.201600433

Chen, R.-r., Li, Y.-j., Chen, J.-j., and Lu, C.-l. (2020). A Review for Natural Polysaccharides with Anti-pulmonary Fibrosis Properties, Which May Benefit to Patients Infected by 2019-nCoV. *Carbohydr. Polym.* 247, 116740. doi:10.1016/j.carbpol.2020.116740

Chen, Z.-G., Zhang, D.-N., Zhu, Q., Yang, Q.-H., and Han, Y.-B. (2014). Purification, Preliminary Characterization and *In Vitro* Immunomodulatory Activity of Tiger Lily Polysaccharide. *Carbohydr. Polym.* 106, 217–222. doi:10.1016/j.carbpol.2014.02.004

Chihara, G., Maeda, Y., Hamuro, J., Sasaki, T., and Fukuoka, F. (1969). Inhibition of Mouse Sarcoma 180 by Polysaccharides from Lentinus Edodes (Berk.) Sing. *Nature* 222 (5194), 687–688. doi:10.1038/222687a0

Cui, W., Li, L., Li, D., Mo, X., Zhou, W., Zhang, Z., et al. (2015). Total Glycosides of Yupingfeng Protects against Bleomycin-Induced Pulmonary Fibrosis in Rats Associated with Reduced High Mobility Group Box 1 Activation and Epithelial-Mesenchymal Transition. *Inflamm. Res.* 64 (12), 953–961. doi:10.1007/s00011-015-0878-x

Datta, A., Scotton, C. J., and Chambers, R. C. (2011). Novel Therapeutic Approaches for Pulmonary Fibrosis. *Br. J. Pharmacol.* 163 (1), 141–172. doi:10.1111/j.1476-5381.2011.01247.x

Deng, W., Fu, M., Cao, Y., Cao, X., Wang, M., Yang, Y., et al. (2013a). Angelica Sinensis Polysaccharide Nanoparticles as Novel Non-viral Carriers for Gene Delivery to Mesenchymal Stem Cells. *Nanomedicine: Nanotechnology, Biol. Med.* 9 (8), 1181–1191. doi:10.1016/j.nano.2013.05.008

Deng, X., Rui, W., Zhang, F., and Ding, W. (2013b). PM2.5 Induces Nrf2-Mediated Defense Mechanisms against Oxidative Stress by Activating PIK3/AKT Signaling Pathway in Human Lung Alveolar Epithelial A549 Cells. *Cell. Biol. Toxicol.* 29 (3), 143–157. doi:10.1007/s10565-013-9242-5

Du, X., Jiang, S., Liu, H., Xin, X., Li, J., Geng, M., et al. (2010). MS80, a Novel Sulfated Polysaccharide, Inhibits CD40-NF-kappaB Pathway via Targeting RIP2. *Mol. Cel. Biochem.* 337 (1-2), 277–285. doi:10.1007/s11010-009-0309-9

Fan, W., Zheng, P., Wang, Y., Hao, P., Liu, J., and Zhao, X. (2017). Analysis of Immunostimulatory Activity of Polysaccharide Extracted from Yu-Ping-Feng *In Vitro* and *In Vivo*. *Biomed. Pharmacother.* 93, 146–155. doi:10.1016/j.biopha.2017.05.138

Feng, B., Zhu, Y., Su, Z., Tang, L., Sun, C., Li, C., et al. (2018). Basil Polysaccharide Attenuates Hepatocellular Carcinoma Metastasis in Rat by Suppressing H3K9me2 Histone Methylation under Hepatic Artery Ligation-Induced Hypoxia. *Int. J. Biol. Macromolecules* 107, 2171–2179. doi:10.1016/j.ijbiomac.2017.10.088

Feng, B., Zhu, Y., Sun, C., Su, Z., Tang, L., Li, C., et al. (2019). Basil Polysaccharide Inhibits Hypoxia-Induced Hepatocellular Carcinoma Metastasis and Progression through Suppression of HIF-1α-Mediated Epithelial-Mesenchymal Transition. *Int. J. Biol. Macromolecules* 137, 32–44. doi:10.1016/j.ijbiomac.2019.06.189

Fiorucci, E., Lucantoni, G., Paone, G., Zotti, M., Li, B. E., Serpilli, M., et al. (2008). Colchicine, Cyclophosphamide and Prednisone in the Treatment of Mild-Moderate Idiopathic Pulmonary Fibrosis: Comparison of Three Currently Available Therapeutic Regimens. *Eur. Rev. Med. Pharmacol. Sci.* 12 (2), 105–111. doi:10.1016/S0924-977X(08)70017-8

Galli, J. A., Pandya, A., Vega-Olivo, M., Dass, C., Zhao, H., and Criner, G. J. (2017). Pirfenidone and Nintedanib for Pulmonary Fibrosis in Clinical Practice: Tolerability and Adverse Drug Reactions. *Respirology* 22 (6), 1171–1178. doi:10.1111/resp.13024

Gao, J., Feng, L.-j., Huang, Y., Li, P., Xu, D.-j., Li, J., et al. (2012). Total Glucosides of Danggui Buxue Tang Attenuates Bleomycin-Induced Pulmonary Fibrosis via Inhibition of Extracellular Matrix Remodelling. *J. Pharm. Pharmacol.* 64 (6), 811–820. doi:10.1111/j.2042-7158.2012.01490.x

Geng, X.-q., Ma, A., He, J.-z., Wang, L., Jia, Y.-l., Shao, G.-y., et al. (2020). Ganoderic Acid Hinders Renal Fibrosis via Suppressing the TGF-β/Smad and MAPK Signaling Pathways. *Acta Pharmacol. Sin.* 41 (5), 670–677. doi:10.1038/s41401-019-0324-7

Guan, S., Liu, Q., Han, F., Gu, W., Song, L., Zhang, Y., et al. (2017). Ginsenoside Rg1 Ameliorates Cigarette Smoke-Induced Airway Fibrosis by Suppressing the TGF-β1/Smad Pathway *In Vivo* and *In Vitro*. *Biomed. Res. Int.* 2017, 1–12. doi:10.1155/2017/6510198

Guan, S., Xiong, Y., Song, B., Song, Y., Wang, D., Chu, X., et al. (2012). Protective Effects of Salidroside fromRhodiola Roseaon LPS-Induced Acute Lung Injury in Mice. *Immunopharmacology and Immunotoxicology* 34 (4), 667–672. doi:10.3109/08923973.2011.650175

Guo, N., Bai, Z., Jia, W., Sun, J., Wang, W., Chen, S., et al. (2019). Quantitative Analysis of Polysaccharide Composition in Polyporus Umbellatus by HPLC-ESI-TOF-MS. *Molecules* 24 (14), 2526. doi:10.3390/molecules24142526

Guo, Q., Meng, Y., Zhao, Y., Cheng, X. C., Lu, Y. X., and Zhang, Q. L. (2016). Therapeutic Effect of Baiji Extract on Pulmonary Fibrosis Induced by Bleomycin in Rats. *J. Int. Pharm. Res.* 43 (3), 518–523. doi:10.13220/j.cnki.jipr.2016.03.022

Haddad, O., Guyot, E., Marinval, N., Chevalier, F., Maillard, L., Gadi, L., et al. (2015). Heparanase and Syndecan-4 Are Involved in Low Molecular Weight Fucoidan-Induced Angiogenesis. *Mar. Drugs* 13 (11), 6588–6608. doi:10.3390/md13116588

Han, L. P., Liang, Z. Y., Han, L. M., Gong, R. C., and Ma, X. H. (2002). Isolation, Purification and Composition Analysis of the Polysaccharide RSA of Rhodiola Alpina. *Chi. Pharm. J.* 06, 19–22. doi:10.3321/j.issn:1001-2494.2002.06.00610.1142/s0219030302001933

Hao, L., Sheng, Z., Lu, J., Tao, R., and Jia, S. (2016). Characterization and Antioxidant Activities of Extracellular and Intracellular Polysaccharides from Fomitopsis Pinicola. *Carbohydr. Polym.* 141, 54–59. doi:10.1016/j.carbpol.2015.11.048

Hayashi, S., Itoh, A., Isoda, K., Kondoh, M., Kawase, M., and Yagi, K. (2008). Fucoidan Partly Prevents CCl4-Induced Liver Fibrosis. *Eur. J. Pharmacol.* 580 (3), 380–384. doi:10.1016/j.ejphar.2007.11.015

He, T.-B., Huang, Y.-P., Yang, L., Liu, T.-T., Gong, W.-Y., Wang, X.-J., et al. (2016). Structural Characterization and Immunomodulating Activity of Polysaccharide from Dendrobium Officinale. *Int. J. Biol. Macromolecules* 83, 34–41. doi:10.1016/j.ijbiomac.2015.11.038

He, X., Wang, X., Fang, J., Zhao, Z., Huang, L., Guo, H., et al. (2017). Bletilla Striata: Medicinal Uses, Phytochemistry and Pharmacological Activities. *J. Ethnopharmacology* 195, 20–38. doi:10.1016/j.jep.2016.11.026

Hou, R., Chen, J., Yue, C., Li, X., Liu, J., Gao, Z., et al. (2016). Modification of Lily Polysaccharide by Selenylation and the Immune-Enhancing Activity. *Carbohydr. Polym.* 142, 73–81. doi:10.1016/j.carbpol.2016.01.032

Hsu, H.-Y., Lin, T.-Y., Hwang, P.-A., Tseng, L.-M., Chen, R.-H., Tsao, S.-M., et al. (2013). Fucoidan Induces Changes in the Epithelial to Mesenchymal Transition and Decreases Metastasis by Enhancing Ubiquitin-dependent TGF Receptor Degradation in Breast Cancer. *Carcinogenesis* 34 (4), 874–884. doi:10.1093/carcin/bgs396

Huang, C., Yao, R., Zhu, Z., Pang, D., Cao, X., Feng, B., et al. (2019). A Pectic Polysaccharide from Water Decoction of Xinjiang Lycium Barbarum Fruit Protects against Intestinal Endoplasmic Reticulum Stress. *Int. J. Biol. Macromolecules* 130, 508–514. doi:10.1016/j.ijbiomac.2019.02.157

Huang, K.-C., Su, Y.-C., Sun, M.-F., and Huang, S.-T. (2018). Chinese Herbal Medicine Improves the Long-Term Survival Rate of Patients with Chronic Kidney Disease in Taiwan: A Nationwide Retrospective Population-Based Cohort Study. *Front. Pharmacol.* 9, 1117. doi:10.3389/fphar.2018.01117

Huo, J., Lu, Y., Xia, L., and Chen, D. (2020). Structural Characterization and Anticomplement Activities of Three Acidic Homogeneous Polysaccharides from Artemisia Annua. *J. Ethnopharmacology* 247, 112281. doi:10.1016/j.jep.2019.112281

Hutchinson, J., Fogarty, A., Hubbard, R., and McKeever, T. (2015). Global Incidence and Mortality of Idiopathic Pulmonary Fibrosis: a Systematic Review. *Eur. Respir. J.* 46 (3), 795–806. doi:10.1183/09031936.00185114

Jang, H. J., Hong, E. M., Kim, M., Kim, J. H., Jang, J., Park, S. W., et al. (2016). Simvastatin Induces Heme Oxygenase-1 via NF-E2-Related Factor 2 (Nrf2) Activation through ERK and PI3K/Akt Pathway in colon Cancer. *Oncotarget* 7 (29), 46219–46229. doi:10.18632/oncotarget.10078

Ji, S., Li, Z., Song, W., Wang, Y., Liang, W., Li, K., et al. (2016). Bioactive Constituents ofGlycyrrhiza uralensis(Licorice): Discovery of the Effective Components of a Traditional Herbal Medicine. *J. Nat. Prod.* 79 (2), 281–292. doi:10.1021/acs.jnatprod.5b00877

Jia, N., Qiao, H., Zhu, W., Zhu, M., Meng, Q., Lu, Q., et al. (2019). Antioxidant, Immunomodulatory, Oxidative Stress Inhibitory and Iron Supplementation Effect of Astragalus Membranaceus Polysaccharide-Iron (III) Complex on Iron-Deficiency Anemia Mouse Model. *Int. J. Biol. Macromolecules* 132, 213–221. doi:10.1016/j.ijbiomac.2019.03.196

Jiang, H.-d., and Guan, H.-s. (2009). MS80, a Novel Sulfated Oligosaccharide, Inhibits Pulmonary Fibrosis by Targeting TGF-B1 Both *In Vitro* and *In Vivo*. *Acta Pharmacol. Sin.* 30 (7), 973–979. doi:10.1038/aps.2009.86

Jiang, J., Wang, F., Luo, A., Lin, S., Feng, X., Yan, W., et al. (2020). Polyporus Polysaccharide Ameliorates Bleomycin-Induced Pulmonary Fibrosis by Suppressing Myofibroblast Differentiation via TGF-β/Smad2/3 Pathway. *Front. Pharmacol.* 11, 767. doi:10.3389/fphar.2020.00767

Layek, B., and Mandal, S. (2020). Natural Polysaccharides for Controlled Delivery of Oral Therapeutics: a Recent Update. *Carbohydr. Polym.* 230, 115617. doi:10.1016/j.carbpol.2019.115617

Laçin, N., İzol, S. B., İpek, F., and Tuncer, M. C. (2019). Ganoderma Lucidum, a Promising Agent Possessing Antioxidant and Anti-inflammatory Effects for Treating Calvarial Defects with Graft Application in Rats. *Acta Cir. Bras.* 34 (9), e201900904. doi:10.1590/s0102-865020190090000004

Lederer, D. J., and Martinez, F. J. (2018). Idiopathic Pulmonary Fibrosis. *N. Engl. J. Med.* 378 (19), 1811–1823. doi:10.1056/NEJMra1705751

Lee, Y.-J., Jeong, H.-Y., Kim, Y.-B., Lee, Y.-J., Won, S. Y., Shim, J.-H., et al. (2012). Reactive Oxygen Species and PI3K/Akt Signaling Play Key Roles in the Induction of Nrf2-Driven Heme Oxygenase-1 Expression in Sulforaphane-Treated Human Mesothelioma MSTO-211H Cells. *Food Chem. Toxicol.* 50 (2), 116–123. doi:10.1016/j.fct.2011.10.035

Li, D., Li, W., Chen, Y., Liu, L., Ma, D., Wang, H., et al. (2018a). Anti-fibrotic Role and Mechanism of *Periplaneta americana* Extracts in CCl4-Induced Hepatic Fibrosis in Rats. *Acta Biochim. Biophys. Sin.* 50 (5), 491–498. doi:10.1093/abbs/gmy024

Li, H., Yan, Z., Xiong, Q., Chen, X., Lin, Y., Xu, Y., et al. (2019a). Renoprotective Effect and Mechanism of Polysaccharide from Polyporus Umbellatus Sclerotia on Renal Fibrosis. *Carbohydr. Polym.* 212, 1–10. doi:10.1016/j.carbpol.2019.02.026

Li, L., Li, D., Xu, L., Zhao, P., Deng, Z., Mo, X., et al. (2015). Total Extract of Yupingfeng Attenuates Bleomycin-Induced Pulmonary Fibrosis in Rats. *Phytomedicine* 22 (1), 111–119. doi:10.1016/j.phymed.2014.10.011

Li, M. M., Zhang, Y., Wu, J., and Wang, K. P. (2020a). Polysaccharide from Angelica Sinensis Suppresses Inflammation and Reverses Anemia in Complete Freund's Adjuvant-Induced Rats. *Curr. Med. Sci.* 40 (2), 265–274. doi:10.1007/s11596-020-2183-3

Li, N., Yu, X., Yu, Q. H., and Wang, M. (2019b). Research Progress on Stability of Polysaccharides in Traditional Chinese Medicine. *Zhongguo Zhong Yao Za Zhi* 44 (22), 4793–4799. doi:10.19540/j.cnki.cjcmm.20190916.309

Li, S.-s., He, A.-l., Deng, Z.-y., and Liu, Q.-f. (2018b). Ginsenoside-Rg1 Protects against Renal Fibrosis by Regulating the Klotho/TGF-β1/Smad Signaling Pathway in Rats with Obstructive Nephropathy. *Biol. Pharm. Bull.* 41 (4), 585–591. doi:10.1248/bpb.b17-00934

Li, W., Cai, Z.-N., Mehmood, S., Wang, Y., Pan, W.-J., Zhang, W.-N., et al. (2018c). Polysaccharide FMP-1 from Morchella Esculenta Attenuates Cellular Oxidative Damage in Human Alveolar Epithelial A549 Cells through PI3K/AKT/Nrf2/HO-1 Pathway. *Int. J. Biol. Macromolecules* 120 (Pt A), 865–875. doi:10.1016/j.ijbiomac.2018.08.148

Li, W., Wang, Y., Wei, H., Zhang, Y., Guo, Z., Qiu, Y., et al. (2020b). Structural Characterization of Lanzhou Lily (Lilium Davidii Var. Unicolor) Polysaccharides and Determination of Their Associated Antioxidant Activity. *J. Sci. Food Agric.* 100 (15), 5603–5616. doi:10.1002/jsfa.10613

Li, X., Xu, W., and Chen, J. (2010). Polysaccharide Purified from Polyporus Umbellatus (Per) Fr Induces the Activation and Maturation of Murine Bone-Derived Dendritic Cells via Toll-like Receptor 4. *Cell Immunol.* 265 (1), 50–56. doi:10.1016/j.cellimm.2010.07.002

Li, Y., Yuan, Y., Lei, L., Li, F., Zhang, Y., Chen, J., et al. (2017). Carboxymethylation of Polysaccharide from Morchella Angusticepes Peck Enhances its Cholesterol-Lowering Activity in Rats. *Carbohydr. Polym.* 172, 85–92. doi:10.1016/j.carbpol.2017.05.033

Li, Z. L., Gao, Y., Zhao, L., and Hong, B. (2016). Study on Rhodiola Polysaccharide against Pulmonary Fibrosis. *J. Mol. Sci.* 32 (01), 34–39. doi:10.13563/j.cnki.jmolsci.2016.01.004

Lin, Z., and Deng, A. (2019). Antioxidative and Free Radical Scavenging Activity of Ganoderma (Lingzhi). *Adv. Exp. Med.* 1182, 271–297. doi:10.1007/978-981-32-9421-9_12

Liu, C., Li, H., Wang, K., Zhuang, J., Chu, F., Gao, C., et al. (2019a). Identifying the Antiproliferative Effect of Astragalus Polysaccharides on Breast Cancer: Coupling Network Pharmacology with Targetable Screening from the Cancer Genome Atlas. *Front. Oncol.* 9, 368. doi:10.3389/fonc.2019.00368

Liu, C., Sun, Y., Mao, Q., Guo, X., Li, P., Liu, Y., et al. (2016a). Characteristics and Antitumor Activity of Morchella Esculenta Polysaccharide Extracted by Pulsed Electric Field. *Ijms* 17 (6), 986. doi:10.3390/ijms17060986

Liu, D., Dong, L. J., Lei, T., and Ming, L. G. (2016b). The Interventional Effect and Mechanism ofLycium Barbarum Polysaccharides on Bleomycin-Induced Pulmonary Fibrosis in Mice. *J. Med. Postgraduates* 29 (09), 918–922. doi:10.16571/j.cnki.1008-8199.2016.09.006

Liu, H., Lv, C., and Lu, J. (2020a). Panax Ginseng C. A. Meyer as a Potential Therapeutic Agent for Organ Fibrosis Disease. *Chin. Med.* 15 (1), 124. doi:10.1186/s13020-020-00400-3

Liu, J., Li, Y., Liu, W., Qi, Q., Hu, X., Li, S., et al. (2019b). Extraction of Polysaccharide from Dendrobium Nobile Lindl. By Subcritical Water Extraction. *ACS. Omega.* 4 (24), 20586–20594. doi:10.1021/acsomega.9b02550

Liu, Y., Sun, C., Zhang, G., Wu, J., Huang, L., Qiao, J., et al. (2020b). Bio-responsive Bletilla Striata Polysaccharide-Based Micelles for Enhancing Intracellular Docetaxel Delivery. *Int. J. Biol. Macromolecules* 142, 277–287. doi:10.1016/j.ijbiomac.2019.09.099

Luo, Y. L., Cheng, X. L., Wang, Y. L., Li, N. L., She, Y. L., and Li, Y. (2013a). Lily Polysaccharide Inhibits the Expression of MMP-9 and TIMP-2 in Lung Tissue of Mice with Bleomycin-Induced Pulmonary Fibrosis. *Basic Clin. Med.* 3, 363–364. doi:10.16352/j.issn.1001-6325.2013.03.002

Luo, Y. L., Wang, Y. L., Pan, Z., Li, N. L., Li, Y., Yan, X., et al. (2013b). Effect of Lily Polysaccharides Combined with BMSCs Transplantation on Expression of TNF-Alpha and NF-kappaB in Bleomycin-Induced Pulmonary Fibrosis Mice. *J. Third Mil. Med. Univ.* 35 (5), 431–434. doi:10.16016/j.1000-5404.2013.05.004

Lv, J., Shao, Q., Wang, H., Shi, H., Wang, T., Gao, W., et al. (2013). Effects and Mechanisms of Curcumin and Basil Polysaccharide on the Invasion of SKOV3 Cells and Dendritic Cells. *Mol. Med. Rep.* 8 (5), 1580–1586. doi:10.3892/mmr.2013.1695

Majewski, S., and Piotrowski, W. J. (2020). Air Pollution-An Overlooked Risk Factor for Idiopathic Pulmonary Fibrosis. *Jcm* 10 (1), 77. doi:10.3390/jcm10010077

Masci, A., Carradori, S., Casadei, M. A., Paolicelli, P., Petralito, S., Ragno, R., et al. (2018). Lycium Barbarum Polysaccharides: Extraction, Purification, Structural Characterisation and Evidence about Hypoglycaemic and Hypolipidaemic Effects. A Review. *Food Chem.* 254, 377–389. doi:10.1016/j.foodchem.2018.01.176

Miniati, I., and Matucci Cerinic, M. (2007). Pulmonary Fibrosis in Systemic Sclerosis: Is Treatment with Cyclophosphamide More Effective Than Placebo?. *Nat. Rev. Rheumatol.* 3 (7), 372–373. doi:10.1038/ncprheum0507

Mohammed, A. S. A., Naveed, M., and Jost, N. (2021). Polysaccharides; Classification, Chemical Properties, and Future Perspective Applications in Fields of Pharmacology and Biological Medicine (A Review of Current Applications and Upcoming Potentialities). *J. Polym. Environ.* 29, 2359–2371. doi:10.1007/s10924-021-02052-2

Mozaffari, M. S., Liu, J. Y., and Schaffer, S. W. (2010). Effect of Pressure Overload on Cardioprotection via PI3K-Akt: Comparison of Postconditioning, Insulin, and Pressure Unloading. *Am. J. Hypertens.* 23 (6), 668–674. doi:10.1038/ajh.2010.43

Mu, S., Yang, W., and Huang, G. (2021). Antioxidant Activities and Mechanisms of Polysaccharides. *Chem. Biol. Drug Des.* 97 (3), 628–632. doi:10.1111/cbdd.13798

MuhamadII, Zulkifli, N., Selvakumaran, S. a. p., and Lazim, N. A. M. (2019). Bioactive Algal-Derived Polysaccharides: Multi-Functionalization, Therapeutic Potential and Biomedical Applications. *Cpd* 25 (11), 1147–1162. doi:10.2174/1381612825666190618152133

Niu, W., Chen, X., Xu, R., Dong, H., Yang, F., Wang, Y., et al. (2021). Polysaccharides from Natural Resources Exhibit Great Potential in the Treatment of Ulcerative Colitis: A Review. *Carbohydr. Polym.* 254, 117189. doi:10.1016/j.carbpol.2020.117189

Organ, L., Bacci, B., Koumoundouros, E., Barcham, G., Kimpton, W., Nowell, C. J., et al. (2015). A Novel Segmental challenge Model for Bleomycin-Induced Pulmonary Fibrosis in Sheep. *Exp. Lung Res.* 41 (3), 115–134. doi:10.3109/01902148.2014.985806

Pan, D., Wang, L., Chen, C., Teng, B., Wang, C., Xu, Z., et al. (2012). Structure Characterization of a Novel Neutral Polysaccharide Isolated from Ganoderma Lucidum Fruiting Bodies. *Food Chem.* 135 (3), 1097–1103. doi:10.1016/j.foodchem.2012.05.071

Phan, T. H. G., Paliogiannis, P., Nasrallah, G. K., Giordo, R., Eid, A. H., Fois, A. G., et al. (2021). Emerging Cellular and Molecular Determinants of Idiopathic Pulmonary Fibrosis. *Cell. Mol. Life Sci.* 78 (5), 2031–2057. doi:10.1007/s00018-020-03693 7

Qian, W., Cai, X., Qian, Q., Wang, D., and Zhang, L. (2020). Angelica Sinensis Polysaccharide Suppresses Epithelial-Mesenchymal Transition and Pulmonary Fibrosis via a DANCR/AUF-1/FOXO3 Regulatory Axis. *Aging Dis.* 11 (1), 17–30. doi:10.14336/ad.2019.0512

Qian, W., Cai, X., Qian, Q., Zhang, W., and Wang, D. (2018). Astragaloside IV Modulates TGF -β1-dependent Epithelial-mesenchymal Transition in Bleomycin-induced Pulmonary Fibrosis. *J. Cel. Mol. Med.* 22 (9), 4354–4365. doi:10.1111/jcmm.13725

Raimundo, K., Chang, E., Broder, M. S., Alexander, K., Zazzali, J., and Swigris, J. J. (2016). Clinical and Economic burden of Idiopathic Pulmonary Fibrosis: a Retrospective Cohort Study. *BMC. Pulm. Med.* 16, 2. doi:10.1186/s12890-015-0165-1

Ren, L., Guo, X.-Y., Gao, F., Jin, M.-L., and Song, X.-N. (2019). Identification of the Perturbed Metabolic Pathways Associating with Renal Fibrosis and Evaluating Metabolome Changes of Pretreatment with Astragalus Polysaccharide through Liquid Chromatography Quadrupole Time-Of-Flight Mass Spectrometry. *Front. Pharmacol.* 10, 1623. doi:10.3389/fphar.2019.01623

Ren, Q., Zhao, S., Ren, C., and Ma, Z. (2018). Astragalus Polysaccharide Alleviates LPS-Induced Inflammation Injury by Regulating miR-127 in H9c2 Cardiomyoblasts. *Int. J. Immunopathol. Pharmacol.* 31, 205873841875918. doi:10.1177/2058738418759180

Richeldi, L., Collard, H. R., and Jones, M. G. (2017). Idiopathic Pulmonary Fibrosis. *The Lancet* 389 (10082), 1941–1952. doi:10.1016/s0140-6736(17)30866-8

Ruigrok, M. J. R., Frijlink, H. W., Melgert, B. N., Olinga, P., and Hinrichs, W. L. J. (2021). Gene Therapy Strategies for Idiopathic Pulmonary Fibrosis: Recent Advances, Current Challenges, and Future Directions. *Mol. Ther. - Methods Clin. Dev.* 20, 483–496. doi:10.1016/j.omtm.2021.01.003

Ryu, J. H., Moua, T., Daniels, C. E., Hartman, T. E., Yi, E. S., Utz, J. P., et al. (2014). Idiopathic Pulmonary Fibrosis: Evolving Concepts. *Mayo Clinic Proc.* 89 (8), 1130–1142. doi:10.1016/j.mayocp.2014.03.016

Senthilkumar, K., and Kim, S.-K. (2014). Anticancer Effects of Fucoidan. *Adv. Food Nutr. Res.* 72, 195–213. doi:10.1016/b978-0-12-800269-8.00011-7

Sibinska, Z., Tian, X., Korfei, M., Kojonazarov, B., Kolb, J. S., Klepetko, W., et al. (2017). Amplified Canonical Transforming Growth Factor-β Signalling via Heat Shock Protein 90 in Pulmonary Fibrosis. *Eur. Respir. J.* 49 (2), 1501941. doi:10.1183/13993003.01941-2015

Sohretoglu, D., and Huang, S. (2018). Ganoderma Lucidum Polysaccharides as an Anti-cancer Agent. *Acamc* 18 (5), 667–674. doi:10.2174/1871520617666171113121246

Solomon, J. J., Olson, A. L., Fischer, A., Bull, T., Brown, K. K., and Raghu, G. (2013). Scleroderma Lung Disease. *Eur. Respir. Rev.* 22 (127), 6–19. doi:10.1183/09059180.00005512

Song, J. W., Hong, S.-B., Lim, C.-M., Koh, Y., and Kim, D. S. (2011). Acute Exacerbation of Idiopathic Pulmonary Fibrosis: Incidence, Risk Factors and Outcome. *Eur. Respir. J.* 37 (2), 356–363. doi:10.1183/09031936.00159709

Song, J., Wu, Y., Jiang, G., Feng, L., Wang, Z., Yuan, G., et al. (2019). Sulfated Polysaccharides from Rhodiola Sachalinensis Reduce D-Gal-Induced Oxidative Stress in NIH 3T3 Cells. *Int. J. Biol. Macromolecules* 140, 288–293. doi:10.1016/j.ijbiomac.2019.08.052

Spagnolo, P., Distler, O., Ryerson, C. J., Tzouvelekis, A., Lee, J. S., Bonella, F., et al. (2021). Mechanisms of Progressive Fibrosis in Connective Tissue Disease (CTD)-associated Interstitial Lung Diseases (ILDs). *Ann. Rheum. Dis.* 80 (2), 143–150. doi:10.1136/annrheumdis-2020-217230

Sun, H., Ni, X., Song, X., Wen, B., Zhou, Y., Zou, F., et al. (2016). Fermented Yupingfeng Polysaccharides Enhance Immunity by Improving the Foregut Microflora and Intestinal Barrier in Weaning rex Rabbits. *Appl. Microbiol. Biotechnol.* 100 (18), 8105–8120. doi:10.1007/s00253-016-7619-0

Tian, X., Liang, T., Liu, Y., Ding, G., Zhang, F., and Ma, Z. (2019). Extraction, Structural Characterization, and Biological Functions of Lycium Barbarum Polysaccharides: A Review. *Biomolecules* 9 (9), 389. doi:10.3390/biom9090389

Tietel, Z., and Masaphy, S. (2018). True Morels (Morchella)-Nutritional and Phytochemical Composition, Health Benefits and Flavor: A Review. *Crit. Rev. Food Sci. Nutr.* 58 (11), 1888–1901. doi:10.1080/10408398.2017.1285269

Todd, N. W., Luzina, I. G., and Atamas, S. P. (2012). Molecular and Cellular Mechanisms of Pulmonary Fibrosis. *Fibrogenesis. Tissue Repair* 5 (1), 11. doi:10.1186/1755-1536-5-11

Walton, K. L., Johnson, K. E., and Harrison, C. A. (2017). Targeting TGF-β Mediated SMAD Signaling for the Prevention of Fibrosis. *Front. Pharmacol.* 8, 461. doi:10.3389/fphar.2017.00461

Wang, J.-H., Zuo, S.-R., and Luo, J.-P. (2017a). Structural Analysis and Immuno-Stimulating Activity of an Acidic Polysaccharide from the Stems of Dendrobium Nobile Lindl. *Molecules* 22 (4), 611. doi:10.3390/molecules22040611

Wang, L., Zhang, P., Li, X., Zhang, Y., Zhan, Q., and Wang, C. (2019a). Low-molecular-weight Fucoidan Attenuates Bleomycin-Induced Pulmonary Fibrosis: Possible Role in Inhibiting TGF-Β1-Induced Epithelial-Mesenchymal Transition through ERK Pathway. *Am. J. Transl. Res.* 11 (4), 2590–2602.

Wang, S. X., Li, J., and Liu, Y. (2009). Interventional Effect of Yupingfeng Polysaccharide on Pulmonary Fibrosis in Rats and its Partial Mechanism. *J. Anhui Med. Univ.* 44 (05), 586–590. doi:10.3969/j.issn.1000-1492.2009.05.015

Wang, Y., Han, S., Li, R., Cui, B., Ma, X., Qi, X., et al. (2019b). Structural Characterization and Immunological Activity of Polysaccharides from the

Tuber of Bletilla Striata. *Int. J. Biol. Macromolecules* 122, 628–635. doi:10.1016/j.ijbiomac.2018.10.201

Wang, Y., Liu, D., Chen, S., Wang, Y., Jiang, H., and Yin, H. (2014). A New Glucomannan from Bletilla Striata: Structural and Anti-fibrosis Effects. *Fitoterapia* 92, 72–78. doi:10.1016/j.fitote.2013.10.008

Wang, Y., Liu, Y., Yu, H., Zhou, S., Zhang, Z., Wu, D., et al. (2017b). Structural Characterization and Immuno-Enhancing Activity of a Highly Branched Water-Soluble β-glucan from the Spores of Ganoderma Lucidum. *Carbohydr. Polym.* 167, 337–344. doi:10.1016/j.carbpol.2017.03.016

Wang, Y. Q., Wang, X. Q., Zhang, X. M., Lin, X. Y., Wang, X. H., and An, Y. F. (2010). Effects Ofangelica Polysaccharides on Lung Function and Lung Coefficient in Rats with Pulmonary Fibrosis. *Gansu Traditional Chin. Med.* 23 (011), 28–31. doi:10.3969/j.issn.1004-6852.2010.11.013

Wang, Z., Liu, T., Chen, X., You, H., Zhang, Q., Xue, J., et al. (2018). Low Molecular Weight Fucoidan Ameliorates Hindlimb Ischemic Injury in Type 2 Diabetic Rats. *J. Ethnopharmacology* 210, 434–442. doi:10.1016/j.jep.2017.09.014

Wilkes, M. C., Mitchell, H., Penheiter, S. G., Doré, J. J., Suzuki, K., Edens, M., et al. (2005). Transforming Growth Factor-β Activation of Phosphatidylinositol 3-Kinase Is Independent of Smad2 and Smad3 and Regulates Fibroblast Responses via P21-Activated Kinase-2. *Cancer Res.* 65 (22), 10431–10440. doi:10.1158/0008-5472.Can-05-1522

Xiong, X., Huang, G., and Huang, H. (2019). The Antioxidant Activities of Phosphorylated Polysaccharide from Native Ginseng. *Int. J. Biol. Macromolecules* 126, 842–845. doi:10.1016/j.ijbiomac.2018.12.266

Xu, C., Ni, S., Zhuang, C., Li, C., Zhao, G., Jiang, S., et al. (2021). Polysaccharide from Angelica Sinensis Attenuates SNP-Induced Apoptosis in Osteoarthritis Chondrocytes by Inducing Autophagy via the ERK1/2 Pathway. *Arthritis Res. Ther.* 23 (1), 47. doi:10.1186/s13075-020-02409-3

Xu, L., Li, L.-c., Zhao, P., Qi, L.-w., Li, P., Gao, J., et al. (2014). Total Polysaccharide of Yupingfeng Protects against Bleomycin-Induced Pulmonary Fibrosis via Inhibiting Transforming Growth Factor-B1-Mediated Type I Collagen Abnormal Deposition in Rats. *J. Pharm. Pharmacol.* 66 (12), 1786–1795. doi:10.1111/jphp.12308

Yan, D. D., Tian, J. Z., Zhang, D., Hou, L., Li, L., Zhang, C. H., et al. (2017). Inhibitory Effect of Basil Polysaccharide on TGF-Beta-Induced Epithelial-Mesenchymal Transition of A549 Cells. *Traditional Chin. Drug Res. Clin. Pharmacol.* 28 (02), 154–159.

Yang, S.-M., Wang, T., Wen, D.-G., Hou, J.-Q., and Li, H.-B. (2016). Protective Effect of Rhodiola Rosea Polysaccharides on Cryopreserved Boar Sperm. *Carbohydr. Polym.* 135, 44–47. doi:10.1016/j.carbpol.2015.08.081

Ying-Mei, K. E., Min, J., Shu-Bo, Z., Hong, Y. U., Juan, W., and Feng, G. E. (2020). Component Analysis of Ophiocordyceps Lanpingensis Polysaccharides and Study on Alleviation of Hepatic Fibrosis in Mice by Polysaccharides. *Zhongguo Zhong Yao Za Zhi* 45 (21), 5256–5264. doi:10.19540/j.cnki.cjcmm.20200628.401

Yu, H.-H., Chengchuan Ko, E., Chang, C.-L., Yuan, K., Wu, A., Shan, Y.-S., et al. (2018a). Fucoidan Inhibits Radiation-Induced Pneumonitis and Lung Fibrosis by Reducing Inflammatory Cytokine Expression in Lung Tissues. *Mar. Drugs* 16 (10), 392. doi:10.3390/md16100392

Yu, M., Shi, J., Sheng, M., Gao, K., Zhang, L., Liu, L., et al. (2018b). Astragalus Inhibits Epithelial-To-Mesenchymal Transition of Peritoneal Mesothelial Cells by Down-Regulating β-Catenin. *Cell. Physiol. Biochem.* 51 (6), 2794–2813. doi:10.1159/000495972

Yu, W., Ren, Z., Zhang, X., Xing, S., Tao, S., Liu, C., et al. (2018c). Structural Characterization of Polysaccharides from Dendrobium Officinale and Their Effects on Apoptosis of HeLa Cell Line. *Molecules* 23 (10), 2484. doi:10.3390/molecules23102484

Zeng, J., Li, D., Li, Z., Zhang, J., and Zhao, X. (2020). Dendrobium Officinale Attenuates Myocardial Fibrosis via Inhibiting EMT Signaling Pathway in HFD/STZ-Induced Diabetic Mice. *Biol. Pharm. Bull.* 43 (5), 864–872. doi:10.1248/bpb.b19-01073

Zeng, P., Chen, Y., Zhang, L., and Xing, M. (2019). Ganoderma Lucidum Polysaccharide Used for Treating Physical Frailty in China. *Prog. Mol. Biol. Transl. Sci.* 163, 179–219. doi:10.1016/bs.pmbts.2019.02.009

Zeng, P., Guo, Z., Zeng, X., Hao, C., Zhang, Y., Zhang, M., et al. (2018). Chemical, Biochemical, Preclinical and Clinical Studies of Ganoderma Lucidum Polysaccharide as an Approved Drug for Treating Myopathy and Other Diseases in China. *J. Cel. Mol. Med.* 22 (7), 3278–3297. doi:10.1111/jcmm.13613

Zhan, Y., An, X., Wang, S., Sun, M., and Zhou, H. (2020). Basil Polysaccharides: A Review on Extraction, Bioactivities and Pharmacological Applications. *Bioorg. Med. Chem.* 28 (1), 115179. doi:10.1016/j.bmc.2019.115179

Zhang, K., Si, X.-P., Huang, J., Han, J., Liang, X., Xu, X.-B., et al. (2016). Preventive Effects of Rhodiola Rosea L. On Bleomycin-Induced Pulmonary Fibrosis in Rats. *Ijms* 17 (6), 879. doi:10.3390/ijms17060879

Zhang, R., Xu, L., An, X., Sui, X., and Lin, S. (2020). Astragalus Polysaccharides Attenuate Pulmonary Fibrosis by Inhibiting the Epithelial-Mesenchymal transition and NF-Kb Pathway Activation. *Int. J. Mol. Med.* 46 (1), 331–339. doi:10.3892/ijmm.2020.4574

Zhang, Y., Du, Y., Yu, H., Zhou, Y., and Ge, F. (2017). Protective Effects of Ophiocordyceps Lanpingensis on Glycerol-Induced Acute Renal Failure in Mice. *J. Immunol. Res.* 2017, 1–8. doi:10.1155/2017/2012585

Zhang, Y., Zhou, T., Wang, H., Cui, Z., Cheng, F., and Wang, K.-p. (2016a). Structural Characterization and *In Vitro* Antitumor Activity of an Acidic Polysaccharide from Angelica Sinensis (Oliv.) Diels. *Carbohydr. Polym.* 147, 401–408. doi:10.1016/j.carbpol.2016.04.002

Zhang, Z., Zhang, D., Dou, M., Li, Z., Zhang, J., and Zhao, X. (2016b). Dendrobium officinale Kimura et Migo attenuates diabetic cardiomyopathy through inhibiting oxidative stress, inflammation and fibrosis in streptozotocin-induced mice. *Biomed. Pharmacother.* 84, 1350–1358. doi:10.1016/j.biopha.2016.10.074

Zheng, Y., Liu, T., Wang, Z., Xu, Y., Zhang, Q., and Luo, D. (2018). Low Molecular Weight Fucoidan Attenuates Liver Injury via SIRT1/AMPK/PGC1α axis in Db/db Mice. *Int. J. Biol. Macromolecules* 112, 929–936. doi:10.1016/j.ijbiomac.2018.02.072

Zhou, J., You, W., Sun, G., Li, Y., Chen, B., Ai, J., et al. (2016). The Marine-Derived Oligosaccharide Sulfate MS80, a Novel Transforming Growth Factor 1 Inhibitor, Reverses Epithelial Mesenchymal Transition Induced by Transforming Growth Factor- 1 and Suppresses Tumor Metastasis. *J. Pharmacol. Exp. Ther.* 359 (1), 54–61. doi:10.1124/jpet.116.234799

Zhou, S., Zhou, Y., Yu, J., Du, Y., Tan, Y., Ke, Y., et al. (2020). Ophiocordyceps Lanpingensis Polysaccharides Attenuate Pulmonary Fibrosis in Mice. *Biomed. Pharmacother.* 126, 110058. doi:10.1016/j.biopha.2020.110058

Zong, A., Cao, H., and Wang, F. (2012). Anticancer Polysaccharides from Natural Resources: a Review of Recent Research. *Carbohydr. Polym.* 90 (4), 1395–1410. doi:10.1016/j.carbpol.2012.07.026

15

High-Flow Nasal Cannula for COVID-19 Patients

Jun Duan[1†], Jia Zeng[2,3†], Puyu Deng[4†], Zhong Ni[5], Rongli Lu[6], Wenxi Xia[7], Guoqiang Jing[8], Xiaoping Su[9], Stephan Ehrmann[10], Wei Zhang[3,11] and Jie Li[12]**

[1]Department of Respiratory and Critical Care Medicine, First Affiliated Hospital of Chongqing Medical University, Chongqing, China, [2]Department of Aviation Disease, Naval Medical Center of PLA, Second Military Medical University, Shanghai, China, [3]Hubei Maternal and Child Health Hospital, Wuhan, China, [4]Department of Emergency and Critical Care Medicine, Shanghai General Hospital, Shanghai Jiao Tong University School of Medicine, Shanghai, China, [5]Department of Respiratory and Critical Care Medicine, West China Hospital, Sichuan University, Chengdu, China, [6]Department of Pulmonary and Critical Care Medicine, Xiangya Hospital, Central South University, Changsha, China, [7]Department of Critical Care Medicine, West China Hospital, Sichuan University, Chengdu, China, [8]Department of Pulmonary and Critical Care Medicine, Binzhou Medical University Hospital, Binzhou Medical University, Binzhou, China, [9]School of Basic Medicine, Wenzhou Medical University, Wenzhou Tea Mountain Higher Education Park, Wenzhou, China, [10]CHRU Tours, Médecine Intensive Réanimation, CIC INSERM 1415, CRICS-TriggerSep Network, Tours France, and INSERM, Centre D'étude des Pathologies Respiratoires, Université de Tours, Tours, France, [11]Department of Respiratory and Critical Care Medicine, First Affiliated Hospital, Second Military Medical University, Shanghai, China, [12]Department of Cardiopulmonary Sciences, Division of Respiratory Care, Rush University Medical Center, Chicago, IL, United States

***Correspondence:**
Wei Zhang
zhangweismmu@126.com
Jie Li
Jie_li@rush.edu

†These authors have contributed equally to this work

Background: High-flow nasal cannula (HFNC) may help avoid intubation of hypoxemic patients suffering from COVID-19; however, it may also contribute to delaying intubation, which may increase mortality. Here, we aimed to identify the predictors of HFNC failure among patients with COVID-19.

Methods: We performed a multicenter retrospective study in China from January 15 to March 31, 2020. Two centers in Wuhan (resource-limited centers) enrolled 32 patients, and four centers outside Wuhan enrolled 34 cases. HFNC failure was defined as the requirement of escalation therapy (NIV or intubation). The ROX index (the ratio of SpO_2/FiO_2 to the respiratory rate) was calculated.

Results: Among the 66 patients, 29 (44%) cases experienced HFNC failure. The ROX index was much lower in failing patients than in successful ones after 1, 2, 4, 8, 12, and 24 h of HFNC. The ROX index was independently associated with HFNC failure (OR = 0.65; 95% CI: 0.45–0.94) among the variables collected before and 1 h after HFNC. To predict HFNC failure tested by ROX index, the AUC was between 0.73 and 0.79 for the time points of measurement 1–24 h after HFNC initiation. The HFNC failure rate was not different between patients in and outside Wuhan (41% vs. 47%, $p = 0.63$). However, the time from HFNC initiation to intubation was longer in Wuhan than that outside Wuhan (median 63 vs. 22 h, $p = 0.02$). Four patients in Wuhan underwent intubation due to cardiac arrest; in contrast, none of the patients outside Wuhan received intubation (13 vs. 0%, $p = 0.05$). The mortality was higher in Wuhan than that out of Wuhan, but the difference did not reach statistical significance (31 vs. 12%, $p = 0.07$).

Conclusion: The ROX index can be used to predict HFNC failure among COVID-19 patients to avoid delayed intubation, which may occur in the resource-limited area.

Keywords: coronavirus, high-flow nasal cannula, ROX index, risk factor, delay intubation

INTRODUCTION

As of January 17, 2021, more than ninety million cases were confirmed with 2019 novel coronavirus disease (COVID-19) worldwide, with a fatality rate of approximately 2% (WHO Coronavirus Disease Dashboard, 2021). Nearly 20% of patients experienced hypoxemia, which was the primary reason for hospitalization (Wu and McGoogan, 2020). Oxygen therapy is the primary treatment for those hypoxemic patients. In recent years, high-flow nasal cannula (HFNC) has been proven to improve oxygenation and ultimately reduce intubation rates for hypoxemic respiratory failure patients of various etiologies (Li et al., 2020a). HFNC provides gas flow higher than the patient's inspiratory flow demand, which enables the delivery of a constant fraction of inspired oxygen (FiO_2) without dilution by room air. It also washes out the dead space and provides, to some extent, positive expiratory pressure (Nishimura, 2016).

Two retrospective studies with a small sample size from China reported that HFNC could improve oxygenation for COVID-19 patients, particularly among patients with PaO_2/FiO_2 > 200 mmHg (Geng et al., 2020; Wang et al., 2020). Among moderate-to-severe hypoxemic patients treated with HFNC, 36% of them did not require therapy escalation, such as intubation or noninvasive ventilation (NIV) (Wang et al., 2020). In Wuhan, China, 63.5% of ICU patients suffering from COVID-19 used HFNC (Yang et al., 2020). In Jiangsu, China, HFNC became the standard of care for hypoxemic COVID-19 patients (Sun et al., 2020). In the Seattle region, United States, 42% of critically ill patients received HFNC (Bhatraju et al., 2020). As the risk of virus transmission associated with HFNC is relatively low (Hui et al., 2019; Li et al., 2020b), current Surviving Sepsis Campaign COVID-19 subcommittee guidelines recommend using HFNC in hypoxemic patients with COVID-19 (Alhazzani et al., 2020). However, delayed intubation after HFNC failure is associated with increased mortality (Kang et al., 2015). Therefore, early identification of HFNC failure is essential, particularly in a resource-limited area, where the number of life-saving devices, such as ventilators, is limited; the use of those devices should be prioritized; early decision on the distribution of ventilators, instead of using a ventilator at the last minute, to patients with high possibility of HFNC failure might help reduce mortality (Kang et al., 2015).

The ROX index, the ratio of pulse oximetry (SpO_2)/FiO_2 to the respiratory rate, has been shown to effectively predict HFNC failure in patients with hypoxemia caused by bacterial pneumonia (Roca et al., 2016). However, its value for predicting HFNC failure in COVID-19 patients remains unknown. Albeit not fully elucidated so far, the pathophysiology of COVID-19–associated hypoxemia may differ from that of other diseases, such as bacterial pneumonia (Gattinoni et al., 2020a; Gattinoni et al., 2020b; Ziehr et al., 2020). In addition, the place where the device, such as the invasive ventilator, was unavailable when the patient required intubation was considered as a resource-limited area. Delayed intubation may occur in this area. As such, we aimed to identify the risk factors associated with HFNC failure in COVID-19 patients, and further explore the relationship between HFNC therapy and delayed intubation in a resource-limited area compared to a normal setting.

METHODS

A retrospective study was conducted in six Chinese hospitals, after approval by the institutional review board [approval No. FYGG(L)-2020-017], in the central institution (Guanggu, Wuhan). Adult patients with a laboratory-confirmed diagnosis of COVID-19 and treated by HFNC from January 15 to March 31, 2020 were enrolled. Exclusion criteria included 1) use of HFNC as palliative care and 2) use of HFNC for less than 30 min. Patients were identified by the medical record system in each hospital.

HFNC (Fisher & Paykel, Auckland, New Zealand; OH-70B/70C, Micomme Medical Technology, Hunan, China; and HiFent TM, Respircae Medical, Liaoning, China) was implemented according to the current consensus and experts' suggestions (Respiratory and Critical Care Medicine Group of Chinese Thoracic Society, 2019; Critical care committee of Chinese Association of Chest Physician, 2020; Yuan et al., 2020). Flow and FiO_2 were adjusted to maintain SpO_2 above 93% and the respiratory rate below 30 breaths/min, while favoring patients' tolerance. Withdrawal of HFNC was considered if FiO_2 was less than 0.4. In case of respiratory failure worsening, escalation therapy consisting of NIV or intubation was initiated based on the attending physicians' decision.

Patients' demographic data, including age, gender, preexisting chronic diseases such as hypertension, diabetes mellitus, chronic pulmonary diseases, coronary artery disease, and cerebral infarction, and admission comorbidities, were collected. Chronic pulmonary disease included asthma, COPD, and bronchiectasis. Laboratory tests including white blood cell counts, cluster of differentiation 4 (CD4), lymphocyte counts, procalcitonin, IL-6, C-reactive protein, lactate dehydrogenase, lactic acid, and arterial blood gas analysis were also recorded, if available. The data of HFNC utilization including flow and F_iO_2 settings, patients' changes in vital signs, and SpO_2 at 1, 2, 4, 8, 12, and 24 h of HFNC were extracted from patients' medical records. At the same time, the ROX index was calculated (Roca et al., 2016).

All the patients were followed up until discharge or death in the hospital. Data on HFNC duration, use of NIV as rescue therapy, intubation, survival, and length of stay in the ICU and hospital were collected. HFNC failure was defined as the

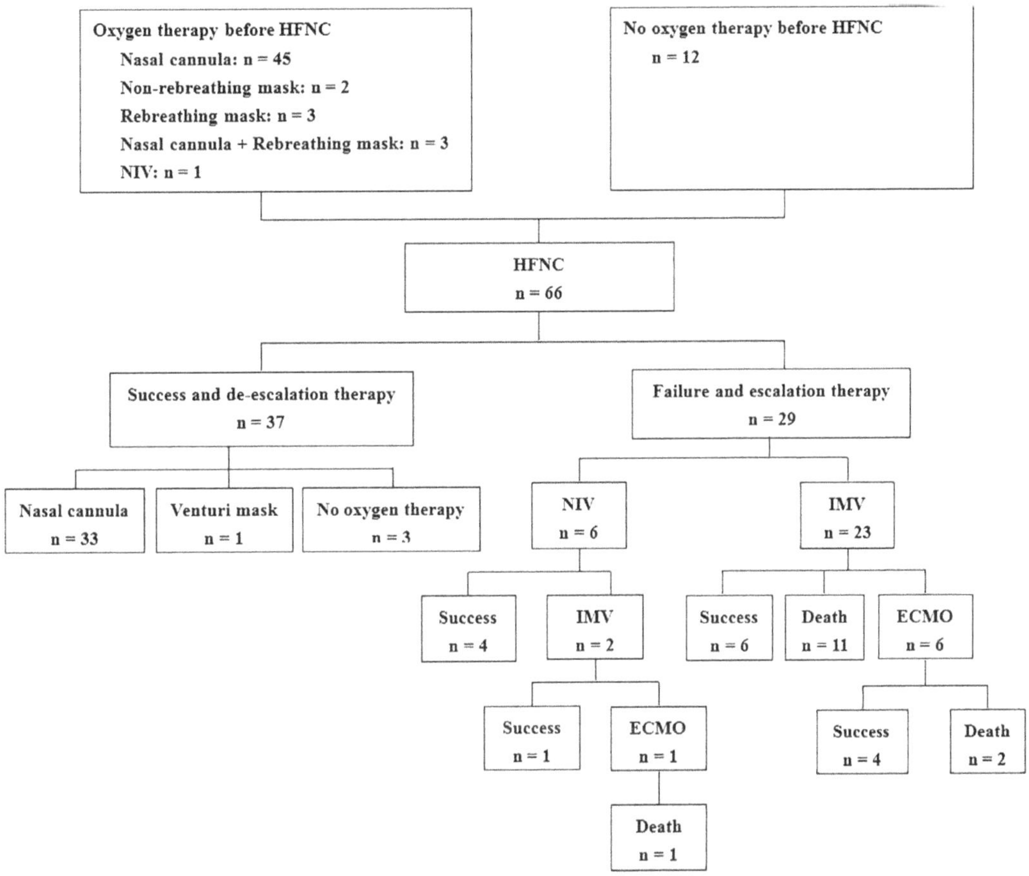

FIGURE 1 | Flowchart of the enrolled patients. HFNC, high-flow nasal cannula; NIV, noninvasive ventilation; IMV, invasive mechanical ventilation; ECMO, extracorporeal membranous oxygenation.

requirement of escalation therapy (NIV or intubation) (Geng et al., 2020); HFNC failure in 28 days was recorded.

Among the six centers, two were in Wuhan and four were out of Wuhan. As many COVID-19 patients crowded into hospitals in Wuhan within a short period, the healthcare workers were overwhelmed and a severe shortage of medical devices occurred. Compared to the hospitals outside Wuhan, the resources in Wuhan were relatively inadequate. Thus, we defined the two centers in Wuhan as resource-limited areas, which probably impacted intubation decisions in patients who underwent HFNC.

Statistical Analysis

Normally distributed continuous variables were reported as mean and standard deviation, and non-normally distributed continuous variables were reported as median and interquartile range (IQR). Differences between the groups of HFNC success and failure were analyzed using the Student's *t*-test or Mann–Whitney *U* test when appropriate. Categorical variables were reported as number and percentage, and differences between groups were analyzed with using chi-square test or Fisher's exact test when appropriate.

The area under the curve (AUC) of receiver operating characteristics was calculated to identify the predictive power of HFNC failure. The optimal cutoff value was determined at the maximal Youden index (Youden, 1950). Variables with a p value less than 0.1 in the univariate analysis were entered in a stepwise multivariate logistic regression analysis to identify independent risk factors associated with HFNC failure. As the respiratory rate, SpO_2, and PaO_2/FiO_2 were collinear with the ROX index, they were not included in the regression analysis. A p value less than 0.05 was considered to be significant.

RESULTS

Data Collected From Hospital Admission to Termination of High-Flow Nasal Cannula

We enrolled 66 patients with COVID-19 (32 in Wuhan and 34 outside Wuhan) in this study (**Figure 1**). Of them, 29 (44%) patients experienced HFNC failure and required escalation therapy within 28 days. Univariate comparisons of patients with HFNC success and failure are presented in **Table 1**. HFNC success was associated with younger age, lack of chronic respiratory disease, lower illness severity measured by the sequential organ failure score (SOFA), better oxygenation, less inflammation (lower procalcitonin levels), and immune

TABLE 1 | Baseline data collected before the use of HFNC.

	HFNC success (*N* = 37)	HFNC failure (*N* = 29)	*P* value
Age, years	63 ± 16	73 ± 14	0.01
Male, n (%)	14 (38)	11 (38)	> 0.99
Oxygen therapy before HFNC, n %	8 (22)	4 (14)	0.53
SOFA score	3.4 ± 2.1	4.5 ± 1.7	0.047
Underlying disease, n %			
Hypertension	21 (57)	19 (66)	0.61
Diabetes mellitus	13 (35)	6 (21)	0.28
Coronary heart disease	4 (11)	4 (14)	0.72
Cerebral infarction	4 (11)	4 (14)	0.72
Chronic respiratory disease	3 (8)	8 (28)	0.048
Hypoproteinemia	6 (16)	7 (24)	0.54
Anemia	5 (14)	4 (14)	> 0.99
Chronic renal dysfunction	2 (5)	3 (10)	0.65
Gastrointestinal bleeding	1 (3)	3 (10)	0.31
Airway secretions, n %			
None	20 (54)	12 (41)	0.33
Mild	16 (43)	17 (59)	0.32
Moderate to abundant	1 (3)	0 (0)	> 0.99
Laboratory tests			
White blood cell counts, × 10^9/L	8.5 ± 4.6	8.6 ± 3.5	0.94
Lymphocyte counts, × 10^9/L	1.12 ± 0.95	0.59 ± 0.30	0.02
PCT, ng/mL	0.10 (0.05–0.14)	0.42 (0.10–2.37)	< 0.01
IL-6	8 (1–76)	73 (24–192)	0.13
C-reactive protein, mg/L	65 ± 53	96 ± 67	0.08
LDH, U/L	365 ± 114	429 ± 144	0.18
CD4, counts/μL	335 ± 183	152 ± 113	0.06
pH	7.42 ± 0.06	7.42 ± 0.08	0.77
$PaCO_2$, mmHg	42 ± 9	37 ± 9	0.06
PaO_2/F_iO_2, mmHg	214 ± 110	168 ± 108	0.15
Lactate, mmol/L	2.6 ± 1.2	2.8 ± 1.5	0.57
Vital signs			
Heart rate, beats/min	90 ± 11	93 ± 21	0.50
Respiratory rate, breaths/min	24 ± 4	26 ± 7	0.17
Systolic blood pressure, mmHg	122 ± 18	132 ± 22	0.07
Diastolic blood pressure, mmHg	70 ± 9	73 ± 10	0.33
SpO_2, %	94 (92–96)	89 (85–93)	< 0.01
ROX index	9.4 ± 3.1	8.4 ± 4.7	0.32

HFNC, high-flow nasal cannula; SOFA, Sequential Organ Failure Assessment; PCT, procalcitonin; LDH, lactate dehydrogenase; ROX, the ratio of SpO_2/F_iO_2 to the respiratory rate. HFNC failure was defined as the requirement of escalation therapy (noninvasive ventilation or intubation).

dysfunction (higher lymphocyte count). However, the PaO_2/FiO_2 and ROX index did not differ between the two groups at hospital admission and before the use of HFNC (**Table 1**; **Supplementary Table S1**).

Outcomes

As the medical resources and staff were exhausted in the early stage of COVID-19, the data in ROX were missed in 5 patients before HFNC, 8 at 1, 24 at 2, 25 at 4, 25 at 8, 20 at 12, and 14 at 24 h. At 1, 2, 4, 8, 12, and 24 h and HFNC termination, the ROX index was much lower in patients experiencing HFNC failure than in those experiencing success (**Figure 2A**; **Supplementary Table S2**). In the multivariate analysis, we observed that the ROX index was independently associated with HFNC failure (odds ratio [OR] = 0.65; 95% confidence interval [CI]: 0.45–0.94) among the variables collected before and at 1 h of HFNC (**Table 2**). The AUC of the ROX index to predict HFNC failure was 0.74, 0.73, 0.73, 0.77, 0.75, and 0.79 at 1, 2, 4, 8, 12, and 24 h of HFNC, respectively (**Figure 2B**). Other variables to predict HFNC failure were summarized in **Supplementary Table S3**.

The median duration of HFNC therapy was 242 h (IQR: 144–295) in the HFNC success group and 39 h (IQR: 15–117) in the group experiencing HFNC failure (**Table 3**). Among the patients with HFNC failure, six cases used NIV as a rescue therapy (21%), and 23 cases (79%) were directly intubated for invasive mechanical ventilation (IMV). Among the six NIV patients, two were intubated after NIV failure. Cardiac arrest occurred during HFNC therapy in four patients (6%), and all occurred in the resource-limited setting of Wuhan. Among the intubated patients, seven underwent extracorporeal membranous oxygenation (ECMO). The median time from HFNC initiation to intubation was 41 h (IQR: 19–152). Mortality was higher in patients with HFNC failure than in those with HFNC success (28 vs. 0%, $p < 0.01$).

A

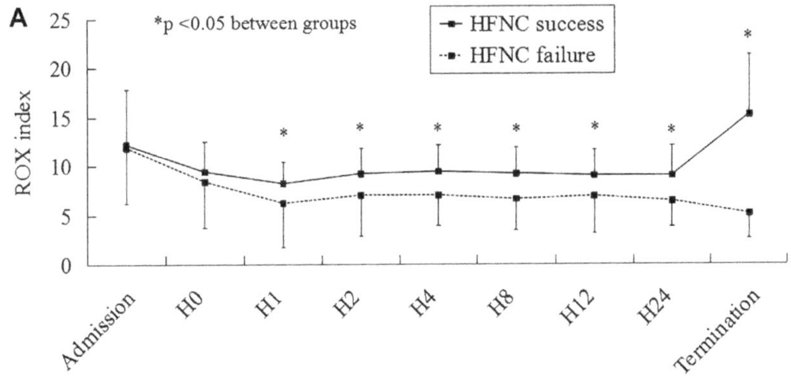

B

Prediction of HFNC failure tested by ROX index

	AUC (95%CI)	Cutoff value	Sensitivity, %	Specificity,%
1 h of HFNC	0.74 (0.61-0.85)	≤7.17	71%	70%
2 h of HFNC	0.73 (0.57-0.85)	≤7.93	75%	73%
4 h of HFNC	0.73 (0.57-0.86)	≤6.25	63%	86%
8 h of HFNC	0.77 (0.61-0.88)	≤5.63	50%	100%
12 h of HFNC	0.75 (0.60-0.86)	≤5.49	55%	100%
24 h of HFNC	0.79 (0.65-0.89)	≤5.94	57%	94%

FIGURE 2 | ROX index as a risk factor to predict HFNC failure. H0, H1, H2, H4, H8, H12, and H24 mean the data collected before and at 1, 2, 4, 8, 12, and 24 h HFNC, respectively. ROX, the ratio of SpO_2/F_iO_2 to the respiratory rate; HFNC, high-flow nasal cannula; AUC, area under the curve of receiver operating characteristics; CI, confidence interval.

TABLE 2 | Univariate and multivariate analysis for HFNC failure.

	Univariate analysis OR (95%CI)	*P* value	Multivariate analysis[a] OR (95% CI)	*p* value
Age, years	1.05 (1.01–1.08)	0.02	–	–
SOFA score	1.39 (0.97–1.98)	0.07	2.16 (1.19–5.53)	0.02
Chronic respiratory disease	4.32 (1.03–18.12)	0.05	–	–
Systolic blood pressure before HFNC, mmHg	1.03 (1.00–1.06)	0.07	–	–
ROX index at 1 h of HFNC	0.68 (0.53–0.88)	<0.01	0.65 (0.45–0.94)	0.02

[a]Due to missing data in some variables, 43 patients (22 HFNC successes and 21 failures) were entered in multivariate analysis.
HFNC, high-flow nasal cannula; OR, odds ratio; CI, confidence interval; SOFA, Sequential Organ Failure Assessment; ROX, the ratio of SpO_2/F_iO_2 to the respiratory rate.
HFNC failure was defined as the requirement of escalation therapy (noninvasive ventilation or intubation).

TABLE 3 | Outcomes of patients with HFNC success and failure.

	HFNC success (*N* = 37)	HFNC failure (*N* = 29)	*P* value
Duration of HFNC therapy, h	242 (144–295)	39 (15–117)	<0.01
Duration of NIV, h	–	72 (21–192)	–
Duration of IMV, h	–	120 (48–576)	–
Length of ICU stay, d	16 (13–22)	15 (8–34)	0.92
Length of hospital stay, d	23 (17–33)	23 (8–42)	0.43
Cardiac arrest during HFNC, n %	–	4 (14)	–
NIV as a rescue therapy, n %	–	6 (21)	–
Intubation for IMV, n %	–	25 (86)	–
Time from initiation of HFNC to intubation, h	–	41 (19–152)	–
Use of ECMO, n %	–	7 (24)	–
Mortality, n %	0 (0)	14 (48)	<0.01

HFNC, high-flow nasal cannula; NIV, noninvasive ventilation; IMV, invasive mechanical ventilation; ECMO, extracorporeal membranous oxygenation.
HFNC failure was defined as the requirement of escalation therapy (noninvasive ventilation or intubation).

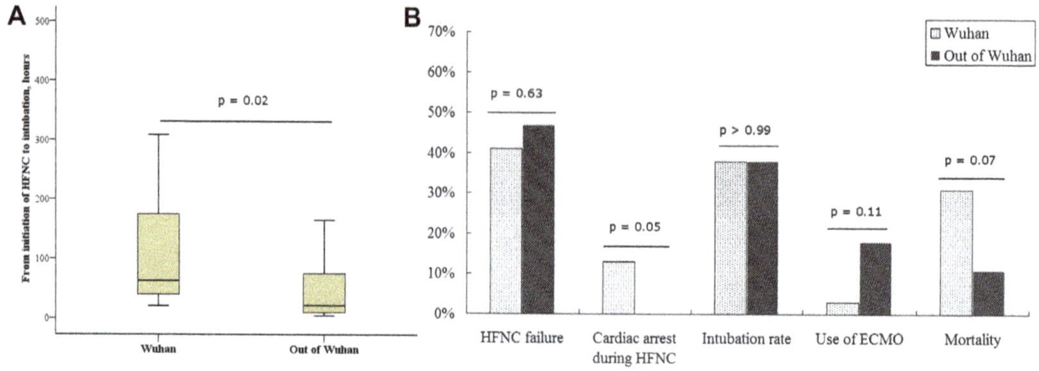

FIGURE 3 | The comparisons between patients in and out of Wuhan. HFNC, high-flow nasal cannula; ECMO, extracorporeal membranous oxygenation. In Wuhan, a very large number of patients crowded into hospitals, staff were overwhelmed, and a severe shortage of medical devices occurred; thus, Wuhan is to be considered as a resource-limited area.

Comparisons Between Patients Inside and Outside Wuhan, China

The rate of HFNC failure and intubation did not differ between patients inside and outside Wuhan (41 vs. 47% for HFNC failure, $p = 0.63$; 38 vs. 38% for intubation, $p > 0.99$). We also observed similar baseline characteristics of patients inside and outside Wuhan before HFNC initiation (**Supplementary Table S4**). However, the duration from HFNC initiation to intubation was longer in Wuhan than that outside Wuhan [63 (IQR: 39–179) vs. 22 (9–78) h, $p = 0.02$; **Figure 3A**]. Furthermore, all instances of cardiac arrests occurring under HFNC before intubation were in Wuhan, and all the cases died. Mortality trended higher in patients treated in Wuhan than in those treated outside Wuhan (31 vs. 12%, $p = 0.07$; **Figure 3B**).

DISCUSSION

In this study, we found the ROX index had a high predictive value to identify HFNC failure when it was measured within the first 24 h of HFNC therapy. Hospitals in Wuhan, as a resource-limited area, had similar HFNC failure rates but higher mortality than those centers outside Wuhan.

Several studies have reported the use of HFNC in COVID-19 patients (Geng et al., 2020; Wang et al., 2020; Chandel et al., 2020; Hu et al., 2020; Xu et al., 2020a). These studies showed that the rates of HFNC failure were between 38 and 45%, which agreed with the failure rate in our study (44%). We further explored if the resource limitation impacted the patients' outcomes and found that resource limitation was associated with increased mortality. Although HFNC appeared feasible and successful in about half of the patients in a setting with adequate resources, monitoring of the ROX index may enable early identification of patients who are likely to require intubation; conversely, the use of HFNC in resource-limited settings without sufficient monitoring and delayed intubation may be associated with poor outcome, especially among those patients who were intubated at the last minute.

Prior to the COVID-19 pandemic, the ROX index showed high discriminative power to predict HFNC failure in hypoxemic patients (Roca et al., 2016). Recently, this team validated the ROX index in five ICUs in Spain and France (Roca et al., 2019). In our study, we have confirmed that the efficacy of the ROX index can be served as a predictor of HFNC failure among patients with COVID-19. The ROX index showed high discriminative values to predict HFNC failure within 24 h of HFNC use (at 1, 2, 4, 8, 12, and 24 h after HFNC initiation). As the variables required to calculate the ROX index are easy to obtain, even in the resource-limited area, it may be helpful for the physicians to early identify patients with a high likelihood of success and those who will require escalation therapy. Apart from the ROX index, the advanced age, increased SOFA score, and decreased platelets were also reported to be associated with increased HFNC failure (Hu et al., 2020; Xu et al., 2020a). As such, the combined use of these variables and the ROX index might help improve the predictive accuracy.

The surge of patients largely overloaded the healthcare workers and challenged medical resources (Cesari and Proietti, 2020; Solnica et al., 2020; Vergano et al., 2020). In China, most of the COVID-19 patients were in Wuhan. The duration from HFNC initiation to intubation for cases in Wuhan was longer than that outside Wuhan, and four cases with cardiac arrest during HFNC therapy all occurred in Wuhan. The present study did not record the reasons for this difference in duration from HFNC initiation to intubation, but it may indicate that delayed intubation occurred in Wuhan possibly because of lack of life-saving device resources or the overwhelmed staff. This might have contributed to the increased mortality observed in Wuhan compared with the mortality in patients outside Wuhan. Intensive monitoring during HFNC therapy is needed to avoid such delay in escalation therapy, such as awake prone positioning, NIV, or IMV (Tu et al., 2020; Xu et al., 2020b). As the ROX is easily obtained, it can be used to improve the management of COVID-19 patients in resource-limited circumstances to rapidly identify patients who will require escalation therapy, and thus, anticipate the required resources or plan the patient transfer.

Among the patients with COVID-19, Chandel et al. explored the likelihood of death in hospitals among patients with early and late HFNC failure (Chandel et al., 2020). Although the sample size was larger than that of ours, it failed to find the difference between patients with early and late HFNC failure. In Chandel et al.'s study, the patients who required intubation within 48 h of HFNC were classified as early HFNC failure, in contrast to the late HFNC failure in which patients were intubated after 48 h of HFNC. This definition is unable to distinguish the duration of the hypoxemia, especially severe hypoxemia. A longer duration of hypoxemia was more likely to be associated with higher mortality. In our study, we classified the patients with and without resource limitation. The patients in resource-limited areas were bound to experience a longer duration of hypoxemia and delayed escalation care, which might explain the higher mortality in the resource-limited area.

This study has several limitations. First, only 43 patients (65%) were included in the multivariate analysis as some variables were missing due to retrospective design. And data imputation was not deemed feasible, given the small sample size. Consequently, it was not possible to combine several variables to predict HFNC failure with greater accuracy. Second, even though all the centers had built HFNC protocol and keeping SpO_2 above 93% was the goal, it is impossible to guarantee that the goal would be achieved all the time for all the patients, as the data points were not recorded minute by minute in the medical records. Third, delayed therapy may occur due to the bedside treating physician. Fourth, a lack of power may have resulted in the lack of statistically significant mortality between the patients with delayed intubation in Wuhan compared to those promptly intubated in the absence of resource limitation outside Wuhan. Last, HFNC gas flow settings were found to affect the ROX index (Mauri et al., 2019), due to room air entrainment when the gas flow is set below the patient inspiratory flow demand. As such, a constant gas flow setting might enable a more precise ROX index measurement but might not be feasible in a clinical study.

CONCLUSION

ROX index, calculated by the ratio of SpO_2/FiO_2 to the respiratory rate, is easily obtained at bedside and can be used to predict HFNC failure among the patients with COVID-19. It may be used to avoid delayed escalation care, which may otherwise occur in resource-limited areas.

AUTHOR CONTRIBUTIONS

JL and WZ conceived the study, and joined in study design, study management, data analysis, and manuscript preparation. JD participated in study design, study management, data analysis, data interpretation, and manuscript drafting. JZ, PD, ZN, RL, WX, GJ, and XS joined in study design and data collection. SE joined in data interpretation and manuscript preparation. All authors revised and approved the final version of the manuscript.

ACKNOWLEDGMENTS

We thank all the staff for participating in data collection.

REFERENCES

Alhazzani, W., Møller, M. H., Arabi, Y. M., Loeb, M., Gong, M. N., Fan, E., et al. (2020). Surviving sepsis campaign: guidelines on the management of critically ill adults with coronavirus disease 2019 (COVID-19). *Intensive Care Med.* 46, 854–887. doi:10.1007/s00134-020-06022-5

Bhatraju, P. K., Ghassemieh, B. J., Nichols, M., Kim, R., Jerome, K. R., Nalla, A. K., et al. (2020). Covid-19 in critically ill patients in the seattle region–case series. *N. Engl. J. Med.* 382, 2012. doi:10.1056/NEJMoa2004500

Cesari, M., and Proietti, M. (2020). COVID-19 in Italy: ageism and decision making in a pandemic. *J. Am. Med. Dir. Assoc.* 21, 576–577. doi:10.1016/j.jamda.2020.03.025

Chandel, A., Patolia, S., Brown, A. W., Collins, A. C., Sahjwani, D., Khangoora, V., et al. (2020). High-flow nasal cannula in COVID-19: outcomes of application and examination of the ROX index to predict success. *Respir. Care* 66, respcare.08631. doi:10.4187/respcare.08631

Critical care committee of Chinese Association of Chest Physician (2020). [Conventional respiratory support therapy for severe acute respiratory infections (SARI): clinical indications and nosocomial infection prevention and control]. *Zhonghua Jie He He Hu Xi Za Zhi* 43, 189–194. doi:10.3760/cma.j.issn.1001-0939.2020.03.010

Gattinoni, L., Coppola, S., Cressoni, M., Busana, M., Rossi, S., and Chiumello, D. (2020a). Covid-19 does not lead to a "typical" acute respiratory distress syndrome. *Am. J. Respir. Crit. Care Med.* 201, 1299. doi:10.1164/rccm.202003-0817LE

Gattinoni, L., Chiumello, D., Caironi, P., Busana, M., Romitti, F., Brazzi, L., et al. (2020b). COVID-19 pneumonia: different respiratory treatments for different phenotypes?. *Intensive Care Med.* 46, 1099. doi:10.1007/s00134-020-06033-2

Geng, S., Mei, Q., Zhu, C., Yang, T., Yang, Y., Fang, X., et al. (2020). High flow nasal cannula is a good treatment option for COVID-19. *Heart Lung* 49 (5), 444–445. doi:10.1016/j.hrtlng.2020.03.018

Hu, M., Zhou, Q., Zheng, R., Li, X., Ling, J., Chen, Y., et al. (2020). Application of high-flow nasal cannula in hypoxemic patients with COVID-19: a retrospective cohort study. *BMC Pulm. Med.* 20, 324. doi:10.1186/s12890-020-01354-w

Hui, D. S., Chow, B. K., Lo, T., Tsang, O. T. Y., Ko, F. W., Ng, S. S., et al. (2019). Exhaled air dispersion during high-flow nasal cannula therapy versus CPAP via different masks. *Eur. Respir. J.* 53. doi:10.1183/13993003.02339-2018

Kang, B. J., Koh, Y., Lim, C. M., Huh, J. W., Baek, S., Han, M., et al. (2015). Failure of high-flow nasal cannula therapy may delay intubation and increase mortality. *Intensive Care Med.* 41, 623–632. doi:10.1007/s00134-015-3693-5

Li, J., Fink, J. B., and Ehrmann, S. (2020a). High-flow nasal cannula for COVID-19 patients: low risk of bio-aerosol dispersion. *Eur. Respir. J.* 55, 2000892. doi:10.1183/13993003.00892-2020

Li, J., Jing, G., and Scott, J. B. (2020b). Year in review 2019: high-flow nasal cannula oxygen therapy for adult subjects. *Respir. Care* 65, 545–557. doi:10.4187/respcare.07663

Mauri, T., Carlesso, E., Spinelli, E., Turrini, C., Corte, F. D., Russo, R., et al. (2019). Increasing support by nasal high flow acutely modifies the rox index in hypoxemic patients: a physiologic study. *J. Crit. Care* 53, 183–185. doi:10.1016/j.jcrc.2019.06.020

Nishimura, M. (2016). High-flow nasal cannula oxygen therapy in adults: physiological benefits, indication, clinical benefits, and adverse effects. *Respir. Care* 61, 529–541. doi:10.4187/respcare.04577

Respiratory and Critical Care Medicine Group of Chinese Thoracic Society (2019). [Expert consensus of high flow nasal cannula oxygen therapy on clinical application regularity]. *Zhonghua Jie He He Hu Xi Za Zhi* 42, 83–91. doi:10.3760/cma.j.issn.1001-0939.2019.02.003

Roca, O., Caralt, B., Messika, J., Samper, M., Sztrymf, B., Hernández, G., et al. (2019). An index combining respiratory rate and oxygenation to predict outcome of nasal high-flow therapy. *Am. J. Respir. Crit. Care Med.* 199, 1368–1376. doi:10.1164/rccm.201803-0589OC

Roca, O., Messika, J., Caralt, B., García-de-Acilu, M., Sztrymf, B., Ricard, J. D., et al. (2016). Predicting success of high-flow nasal cannula in pneumonia patients with hypoxemic respiratory failure: the utility of the ROX index. *J. Crit. Care* 35, 200–205. doi:10.1016/j.jcrc.2016.05.022

Solnica, A., Barski, L., and Jotkowitz, A. (2020). Allocation of scarce resources during the COVID-19 pandemic: a Jewish ethical perspective. *J. Med. Ethics* 46, 444. doi:10.1136/medethics-2020-106242

Sun, Q., Qiu, H., Huang, M., and Yang, Y. (2020). Lower mortality of COVID-19 by early recognition and intervention: experience from Jiangsu Province. *Ann. Intensive Care* 10, 33. doi:10.1186/s13613-020-00650-2

Tu, G. W., Liao, Y. X., Li, Q. Y., Dong, H., Yang, L. Y., Zhang, X. Y., et al. (2020). Prone positioning in high-flow nasal cannula for COVID-19 patients with severe hypoxemia: a pilot study. *Ann. Transl. Med.* 8, 598. doi:10.21037/atm-20-3005

Vergano, M., Bertolini, G., Giannini, A., Gristina, G. R., Livigni, S., Mistraletti, G., et al. (2020). Clinical ethics recommendations for the allocation of intensive care treatments in exceptional, resource-limited circumstances: the Italian perspective during the COVID-19 epidemic. *Crit. Care* 24, 165. doi:10.1186/s13054-020-02891-w

Wang, K., Zhao, W., Li, J., Shu, W., and Duan, J. (2020). The experience of high-flow nasal cannula in hospitalized patients with 2019 novel coronavirus-infected pneumonia in two hospitals of Chongqing, China. *Ann. Intensive Care* 10, 37. doi:10.1186/s13613-020-00653-z

WHO Coronavirus Disease Dashboard (2021). WHO Coronavirus Disease Dashboard. Available at: https://arcg.is/XvuSX (Accessed January 17, 2021).

Wu, Z., and McGoogan, J. M. (2020). Characteristics of and important lessons from the coronavirus disease 2019 (COVID-19) outbreak in China. *JAMA* 323, 1239. doi:10.1001/jama.2020.2648

Xu, J., Yang, X., Huang, C., Zou, X., Zhou, T., Pan, S., et al. (2020a). A novel risk-stratification models of the high-flow nasal cannula therapy in COVID-19 patients with hypoxemic respiratory failure. *Front. Med.* 7, 607821. doi:10.3389/fmed.2020.607821

Xu, Q., Wang, T., Qin, X., Jie, Y., Zha, L., and Lu, W. (2020b). Early awake prone position combined with high-flow nasal oxygen therapy in severe COVID-19: a case series. *Crit. Care* 24, 250. doi:10.1186/s13054-020-02991-7

Yang, X., Yu, Y., Xu, J., Shu, H., Xia, J., Liu, H., et al. (2020). Clinical course and outcomes of critically ill patients with SARS-CoV-2 pneumonia in Wuhan, China: a single-centered, retrospective, observational study. *Lancet Respir. Med.* 8 (5), 475–481. doi:10.1016/S2213-2600(20)30079-5

Youden, W. J. (1950). Index for rating diagnostic tests. *Cancer* 3 (1), 32–35. doi:10.1002/1097-0142(1950)3:1<32::aid-cncr2820030106>3.0.co;2-3

Yuan, X., Mu, J. S., Mo, G. X., Hu, X. S., Yan, P., and Xie, L. X. (2020). [Respiratory support for severe 2019-nCoV pneumonia suffering from acute respiratory failure: time and strategy]. *Zhonghua Jie He He Hu Xi Za Zhi* 43, 177–180. doi:10.3760/cma.j.issn.1001-0939.2020.03.006

Ziehr, D. R., Alladina, J., Petri, C. R., Maley, J. H., Moskowitz, A., Medoff, B. D., et al. (2020). Respiratory pathophysiology of mechanically ventilated patients with COVID-19: a cohort study. *Am. J. Respir. Crit. Care. Med.* 201, 1560. doi:10.1164/rccm.202004-1163LE

16

Pemetrexed-Platinum with or without Bevacizumab for Chinese Chemo-Naive Advanced Lung Adenocarcinoma Patients

Xin Li[1†], Jie Huang[2†], Yao Qiu[3], Qianyun Zhang[3], Shaoyu Yang[1], Kan Wu[2], Jiaoli Wang[4], Limin Wang[4], Jian Ye[4], Shenglin Ma[2,5], Bing Xia[2] and Xueqin Chen[1,3]**

[1]Department of Thoracic Oncology, Key Laboratory of Clinical Cancer Pharmacology and Toxicology Research of Zhejiang Province, Affiliated Hangzhou First People's Hospital, Zhejiang University School of Medicine, Hangzhou, China, [2]Department of Thoracic Oncology, Hangzhou Cancer Hospital, Zhejiang University School of Medicine, Hangzhou, China, [3]Department of Thoracic Oncology, Nanjing Medical University Affiliated Hangzhou Hospital, Hangzhou, China, [4]Department of Respiratory Disease, Affiliated Hangzhou First People's Hospital, Zhejiang University School of Medicine, Hangzhou, China, [5]Cancer Center, Zhejiang University, Hangzhou, China

***Correspondence:**
Bing Xia
bingxia_hzch@163.com
Xueqin Chen
chenxueqin@zju.edu.cn

[†]These authors have contributed equally to this work

Despite recent advances in the treatment of advanced non–small-cell lung cancer (NSCLC), bevacizumab plus platinum–based doublet chemotherapy remains a commonly used first-line regimen. This study was conducted to compare the efficacy and safety of pemetrexed–platinum with or without bevacizumab in Chinese chemo-naive advanced lung adenocarcinoma patients in a real-world setting. We retrospectively collected 100 patients who received pemetrexed–platinum with or without bevacizumab (PP, n = 46; Bev+PP, n = 54) until disease progression or unacceptable toxicity. Clinical characteristics of patients were balanced, except for the proportion of stage IV b+c (Bev+PP and PP: 67.4 vs. 37.0%, p = 0.0066). Bev+PP significantly improved the objective response rate (ORR, 65 vs. 30%, p = 0.0004) and progression-free survival (PFS, 7.4 vs. 6.8 months, p = 0.009), but not overall survival (OS, 17.5 vs. 15.0 months, p = 0.553) compared with PP. Treatment (p = 0.001), gender (p = 0.008), adrenal metastasis (p = 0.001), and liver metastasis (p = 0.013) were independent risk factors for PFS. Patients with adrenal metastasis tended to be at the highest risk of not benefiting from bevacizumab addition (HR [95% CI]: 2.244 [0.6495–7.753]). The safety profile was acceptable, and grade ≥3 toxicity occurred similarly. This study showed that pemetrexed–platinum plus bevacizumab was effective compared to chemotherapy alone in Chinese patients with advanced NSCLC.

Keywords: bevacizumab, pemetrexed, platinum, lung adenocarcinoma, adrenal metastasis

INTRODUCTION

Lung cancer is the most common cancer in the world (Ferlay et al., 2019), and China is also faced with a heavy burden of lung cancer (Cao et al., 2020; Yang et al., 2020) which is linked to tobacco smoking, outdoor air pollution, household air pollution, etc. (Vermeulen et al., 2019; Guan et al., 2020). The rapid development of the pharmaceutical industry and molecular biology research, especially on the tumor-associated immune microenvironment, has resulted in a variety of treatment options for lung adenocarcinoma patients including small-molecule tyrosine kinase inhibitors (TKIs) that target the EGFR/ALK/ROS1 (EAR) gene (Pakkala and Ramalingam, 2018) and immune checkpoint inhibitors that block the PD1/PD-L1 and B7/CTLA4 pathways (Bansal et al., 2016). However, for patients lacking the EAR mutations and PD-L1 expression, or in patients where these therapeutic strategies fail, platinum-based chemotherapy regimens have been commonly used in clinical practice.

Bevacizumab is a widely researched monoclonal antibody that inhibits VEGF-A and has been approved in combination with chemotherapy for the treatment of chemo-naive non–small-cell lung cancer patients (Assoun et al., 2017; Garcia et al., 2020). Previous studies have shown that VEGF-A functions as a high-risk factor dampening the prognosis of lung cancer patients (Hu et al., 2013). Serum VEGF attenuates the efficacy of platinum-based chemotherapy in non–small-cell lung cancer (NSCLC) patients (Zang et al., 2017). Blockade of VEGF-A by bevacizumab decreases the microvessel structure density in tumors, reduces tumor volumes (Zhao et al., 2012), and reprograms the tumor immune microenvironment (Tamura et al., 2019), thus providing a rationale for combination strategies.

Previous observational cohort studies mainly explored the use of paclitaxel/platinum plus bevacizumab versus paclitaxel/platinum therapy in advanced NSCLC and demonstrated improved response and survival benefits of bevacizumab (Sandler et al., 2006; Zhou et al., 2015). A pointbreak study directly compared pemetrexed or paclitaxel combined with carboplatin and bevacizumab in patients with previously untreated stage IIIB or IV non-squamous NSCLC and reported significantly improved progression-free survival (PFS) but not overall survival (OS) (Patel et al., 2013). However, studies on pemetrexed-based chemotherapy with or without bevacizumab mostly focus on the maintenance therapy (Barlesi et al., 2013; Paz-Ares et al., 2013). The association between clinicopathologic characteristics and treatment outcomes of patients receiving pemetrexed-platinum doublet plus bevacizumab and specific populations which might or might not achieve tumor remission remains unclear.

Therefore, studies on whether pemetrexed-based chemotherapy plus antiangiogenesis agents can indeed prolong patients' survival with tolerable safety profiles in real-world settings are needed. In this study, we conducted a retrospective real-world study comparing pemetrexed-platinum doublet plus bevacizumab (Bev+PP) with doublet alone (PP) in Chinese chemo-naive advanced lung adenocarcinoma patients.

MATERIALS AND METHODS

Study Design and Patient Enrollment

This retrospective study collected clinical data from patients with advanced lung adenocarcinoma who received at least one cycle of first-line pemetrexed–platinum chemotherapy with or without bevacizumab between April 2014 and June 2020 in our own hospital. The study was approved by the Hangzhou Cancer Hospital Ethics Review Board. This study is observational and presents no more than minimal risk of harm to subjects and involves no procedures for which written consent is normally required outside the research context. The Hangzhou Cancer Hospital Ethics Review Board approved the waiver of informed consents for this study according to section 39 of Measures for the Ethical Review of Biomedical Research Involving Humans published by the National Health Commission of the People's Republic of China (CLI.4.282697). The inclusion criteria were as follows: 1) pathologic and radiographic confirmation of stage IIIb-IV (AJCC 7th edition) lung adenocarcinoma patients; 2) patients with no history of prior chemotherapy or antiangiogenesis drugs administration; 3) recipients of Bev+PP or PP; 4) recipients of ≥1 cycles of chemotherapy; and 5) complete medical records. Patients were excluded if they 1) were receiving other categories of antitumor therapy during the indicated treatments, 2) were given bevacizumab after the progression of pemetrexed–platinum–based chemotherapy, or 3) were lost to follow-up.

Data Collection

Patients' private information remained confidential; however, the characteristics including age, gender, smoking history, baseline Eastern Cooperative Oncology Group Performance Score (ECOG PS), pathological diagnosis and staging, medical history, and imaging data were captured from the electronic health system. The follow-up was conducted using both outpatient and telephone appointments. Treatment responses were assessed as complete response (CR), partial response (PR), stable disease (SD), or progressive disease (PD), by comparing the imaging data before and after treatment using the Response Evaluation Criteria in Solid Tumors (RECIST) version 1.1. The objective response rate (ORR) was calculated as CR + PR/total cases, while the disease control rate (DCR) was calculated as CR + PR + SD/total cases. PFS was defined as the time from treatment initiation to the first confirmation of disease progression or death, while OS was defined as the time from treatment initiation until death. Adverse events were graded according to the National Cancer Institute—Common Toxicity Criteria for Adverse Events version 4.0. Two professional oncologists performed the grading of the treatment responses and adverse events independently, which were later recorded in the database.

Statistical Analysis

A chi-square test or Fisher's exact test was used to assess for independence between the categorical variables in the two treatment groups with or without bevacizumab. The Kaplan–Meier method and log-rank test were used to compare the efficacy of combination therapy with chemotherapy alone. Multivariate Cox analyses were employed to estimate the factors affecting the efficacy of treatment (PFS and OS). For matched factors affecting PFS, the patients were divided on that factor and further analyzed whether the strength of one treatment could still be present in the subgroup. All analyses were performed with IBM SPSS Statistics 26.0. Survival curves were drawn using Prism GraphPad 8.0.

TABLE 1 | Clinical characteristics of lung adenocarcinoma patients.

Characteristic	Bev+PP (*n* = 46)		PP (*n* = 54)		*p*-value
	N	%	N	%	
Age (years)	62 [38–75]		63 [18–83]		
≥60	28	60.9	34	63.0	0.8298
<60	18	39.1	20	37.0	
Gender					
Male	33	71.7	32	59.3	0.2133
Female	13	28.3	22	40.7	
Smoking					
Never	20	43.5	11	20.4	0.08
Ever	26	56.5	43	79.6	
ECOG PS					
0	3	6.5	3	5.6	0.9648
1	41	89.1	49	90.7	
2	2	4.3	2	3.7	
Tumor stage					
III_b	2	4.3	9	16.7	0.0066*
IV_a	13	28.3	25	46.3	
IV_{b+c}	31	67.4	20	37.0	
Site of metastasis					
Lung	17	37.0	20	37.0	0.5052
Bone	20	43.5	21	38.9	
Pleura	11	23.9	15	27.8	
Brain	14	30.4	13	24.1	
Adrenal glands	9	19.6	3	5.6	
Liver	6	13.0	4	7.4	
Driver gene status					
EAR negative	26	56.5	37	68.5	0.3418
EGFR mutation	12	26.1	13	24.1	
ALK or ROS1 fusion	2	4.3	2	3.7	
Unknown	6	13.0	2	3.7	

RESULTS

Clinicopathologic Characteristics

Between April 2014 and June 2020, a total of 100 chemotherapy-naive patients with advanced lung adenocarcinoma at our institute met the inclusion criteria and were enrolled on our retrospective real-world study comparing the efficacy and safety of pemetrexed platinum with or without bevacizumab (46 patients in the Bev+PP group and 54 patients in the PP group).

The median age was 62 (38–75) years in the Bev+PP group and 63 (18–83) years in the PP group. Bev+PP and PP groups enrolled similar proportions of male (71.7 vs. 59.3%, p = 0.2133), elder (60.9 vs. 63.0%, p = 0.8298), ever smoking (56.5 vs. 79.6%, p = 0.08), ECOG PS = 1 (89.1 vs. 90.7%, p = 0.9648), and EAR-negative (56.5 vs. 68.5%, p = 0.3418) patients. The occurrence rates of metastasis in organs including the lung, bone, pleural, brain, adrenal glands, and liver, and the EAR gene mutation status were distributed evenly between the two groups (p = 0.5052, 0.3418, respectively). However, the Bev+PP group reported more later stage lung adenocarcinoma patients than PP group (IV_{b+c} 67.4 vs. 37.0%, p = 0.0066). (Detailed data are shown in **Table 1**.) The pre- and post-line treatment history information are presented in **Supplementary Table S1**; in brief, the Bev+PP group enrolled a higher number of patients reporting failed prior TKI treatments than the PP group (26.1 vs. 14.8%, p = 0.160).

Treatment and Efficacy

In brief, patients were intravenously injected with 500 mg/m2 pemetrexed on d1, 37.5 mg/m2 cisplatin on d1-2, or carboplatin (area under the curve, 4–5) on d1, with or without 7.5 mg/kg bevacizumab on d1 during induction therapy. Pemetrexed plus bevacizumab or pemetrexed monotherapy was administered during maintenance therapy. Patients in the two groups received similar cycles of induction therapy (mean cycle 4.1 [2–7] vs. 4.2 [1–6] for PP and Bev+PP groups, respectively, p = 0.9740). However, patients receiving Bev+PP were more likely to receive more cycles of maintenance therapy than patients in the PP group (5.3 [0–22] vs. 2.5 [0–18], p = 0.0015). Although none of the patients achieved complete clearance of cancer, 65% of patients in the Bev+PP group had PR, obviously higher than only 30% in the PP group (same with ORR, p = 0.0004). And surprisingly, only one patient experienced PD after administration of bevacizumab and pemetrexed–platinum, with the DCR of the Bev+PP group reaching 98% (45/46), compared with 87% in the PP group (p = 0.0663) (**Table 2**). Patients in the Bev+PP group achieved superior PFS than those in the PP group (median PFS, 7.4 vs. 6.8 months; HR [95% CI]: 0.59 [0.39–0.90], p = 0.0093) (**Figure 1A**). However, addition of bevacizumab did not cause any significant improvement in OS (median OS for Bev+PP and PP, 17.5 vs. 15.0 months; HR [95% CI]: 0.86 [0.50–1.47], p = 0.5531) (**Figure 1B**). When we merely looked at EAR-negative patients, bevacizumab addition also tended to improve PFS (median PFS, 8.9 vs. 7.0 months; HR [95% CI]: 0.63 [0.37–1.07], p = 0.0836), but not OS (median OS, 17.5 vs. 16.2 months; HR [95% CI]: 0.99 [0.51–1.91], p = 0.9638) (**Supplementary Figures S1A,B**). Multivariate Cox regression analysis showed that treatment with or without bevacizumab (p = 0.001), gender (p = 0.008), and adrenal metastasis (p = 0.001) as well as liver metastasis (p = 0.013) were independent risk factors for the PFS in lung adenocarcinoma patients (**Table 3**), reaffirming that bevacizumab addition improved the PFS of chemo-naive lung adenocarcinoma patients.

The relationship between the baseline clinicopathologic characteristics of enrolled patients and PFS or OS was further analyzed by multivariate Cox analyses to screen out a specific population of patients who could optimally benefit from Bev+PP treatment and risk factors that reduced the efficacy. As listed in **Table 4**, female patients had superior OS than male patients (Bev+PP, HR [95% CI]: 0.18 [0.04–0.87]; PP, HR [95% CI]: 0.08 [0.01–0.53]). EGFR or ALK/ROS1 status did not affect the efficacy of Bev+PP (p = 0.899 and 0.984) on OS. Additionally, adrenal metastasis severely reduce the PFS of patients receiving Bev+PP (HR [95% CI]: 10.17 [2.99–34.62]).

Subgroup Analysis

To further confirm whether adrenal metastasis or other characteristics may favor Bev+PP or PP on PFS, we conducted a subgroup analysis of hazard ratios for progression of enrolled patients after Bev+PP or PP administration using the Kaplan–Meier method. As shown in

TABLE 2 | Efficacy profile and treatment cycles of the two groups.

	Bev+PP (*n* = 46) N (%)	PP (*n* = 54) N (%)	*p*-value
Best response			
CR	0 (0)	0 (0)	
PR	30 (65)	16 (30)	
SD	15 (33)	31 (57)	
PD	1 (2)	7 (13)	
ORR	30 (65)	16 (30)	0.0004*
DCR	45 (98)	47 (87)	0.0663
Induction cycle mean (range)	4.1 [2–7]	4.2 [1–6]	0.9740
Maintenance cycle mean (range)	5.3 [0–22]	2.5 [0–18]	0.0015*

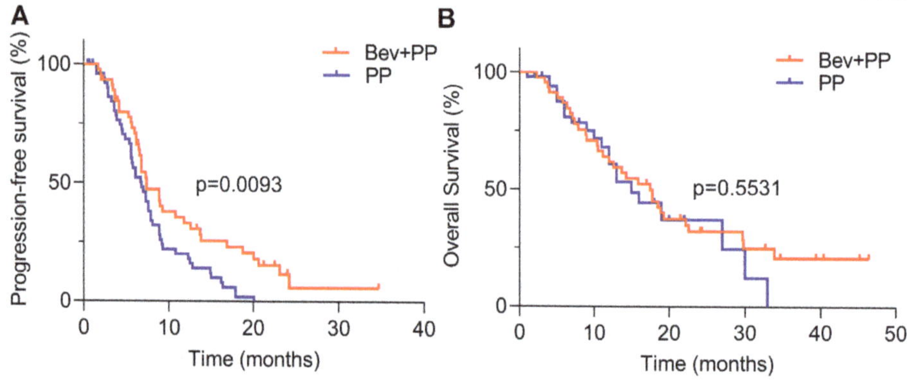

FIGURE 1 | PFS and OS curves of Bev+PP (red) and PP (blue) groups. **(A)** Kaplan–Meier survival curves showing the PFS of patients in the Bev+PP group (*n* = 46) and PP group (*n* = 54) (median PFS, 7.4 vs. 6.8 months; HR [95% CI]: 0.59 [0.39–0.90], *p* = 0.0093); **(B)** Kaplan–Meier survival curves showing the OS of patients in the Bev+PP group (*n* = 46) and PP group (*n* = 54) (median OS, 17.5 vs. 15 months; HR [95% CI]: 0.86 [0.50–1.47], *p* = 0.5531).

TABLE 3 | Multivariate analysis of PFS in all patients.

Characteristic	*p*-value	HR	95% CI Lower limit	95% CI Upper limit
Bev+PP	0.001*	0.42	0.25	0.71
Gender = female	0.008*	0.43	0.23	0.80
Age (years)	0.746	1.00	0.97	1.02
Smoking	0.750	0.89	0.44	1.79
Lung metastasis	0.671	0.89	0.52	1.52
Pleura metastasis	0.488	1.24	0.67	2.30
Adrenal metastasis	0.001*	3.80	1.77	8.18
Bone metastasis	0.981	0.99	0.55	1.81
Brain metastasis	0.188	1.49	0.82	2.71
Liver metastasis	0.013*	2.67	1.23	5.77
Distant metastasis	0.118	0.47	0.18	1.21
ECOG ≥ 2	0.232	2.17	0.61	7.68
EGFR mutation	0.149	1.56	0.85	2.85
ALK/ROS1 fusion	0.998	1.00	0.30	3.36
Unknown status	0.882	0.93	0.38	2.30

Figure 2, the effect of bevacizumab on the pemetrexed-platinum chemotherapy was generally consistent in subgroups including gender, age, smoking, stage, distant metastasis, and EAR status. However, adrenal metastasis tended to be relatively in favor of pemetrexed–platinum doublet alone (HR [95% CI]: 2.244 [0.6495–7.753]).

Adverse Events

The prevalence of all adverse events (AEs), including grade ≥3 adverse events in the two groups was similar (all AEs, $p = 0.465$; all grade ≥3 AEs, $p = 0.652$). The top three frequent AEs of patients in Bev+PP and PP groups were leukopenia (63.0%, 59.3%), fatigue (45.7%, 38.9%), and nausea (37.0%, 33.3%) (**Table 5**). Grade 3–4 leukopenia was the most common grade ≥3 AE occurring in 19.6 and 18.5% of patients in Bev+PP and PP groups, respectively, while other grade ≥3 AEs were rare in the two groups. The safety profiles in both groups were acceptable, and no new unexpected AEs were observed.

DISCUSSION

In the current real-world study, the addition of bevacizumab in first-line pemetrexed–platinum (either cisplatin or carboplatin) doublet significantly improved PFS compared to doublet alone, with similar and tolerable adverse events, although no differences in OS was observed between the two groups. Multivariate Cox regression

TABLE 4 | Multivariate Cox regression analysis of OS and PFS in the Bev+PP group.

Category	OS		PFS	
	HR	*p*-value	HR	*p*-value
Gender = female	0.18 [0.04–0.87]	0.032*	0.25 [0.07–0.90]	0.034*
Age (years)	1.00 [0.95–1.06]	0.899	0.99 [0.95–1.04]	0.796
Smoking	0.81 [0.23–2.77]	0.731	0.85 [0.28–2.64]	0.784
Distant metastasis	0.95 [0.09–9.83]	0.65	0.82 [0.08–8.33]	0.65
Lung metastasis	2.23 [0.79–6.27]	0.130	1.57 [0.65–3.82]	0.318
Pleura metastasis	0.51 [0.17–1.58]	0.245	0.58 [0.22–1.54]	0.273
Adrenal metastasis	2.18 [0.70–6.82]	0.179	10.17 [2.99–34.62]	0.000*
Bone metastasis	0.90 [0.36–2.25]	0.813	0.77 [0.33–1.81]	0.551
Brain metastasis	0.62 [0.24–1.62]	0.329	1.50 [0.59–3.85]	0.395
Liver metastasis	4.34 [0.99–18.91]	0.051	3.04 [0.88–10.58]	0.080
ECOG ≥ 2	1.10 [0.16–7.49]	0.919	2.27 [0.33–15.39]	0.402
EGFR mutation	1.08 [0.33–3.56]	0.899	1.28 [0.43–3.78]	0.660
ALK/ROS1 fusion	0.00 [0.00-NA]	0.984	0.69 [0.09–5.38]	0.720
Unknown status	0.28 [0.06–1.25]	0.095	0.34 [0.09–1.32]	0.118

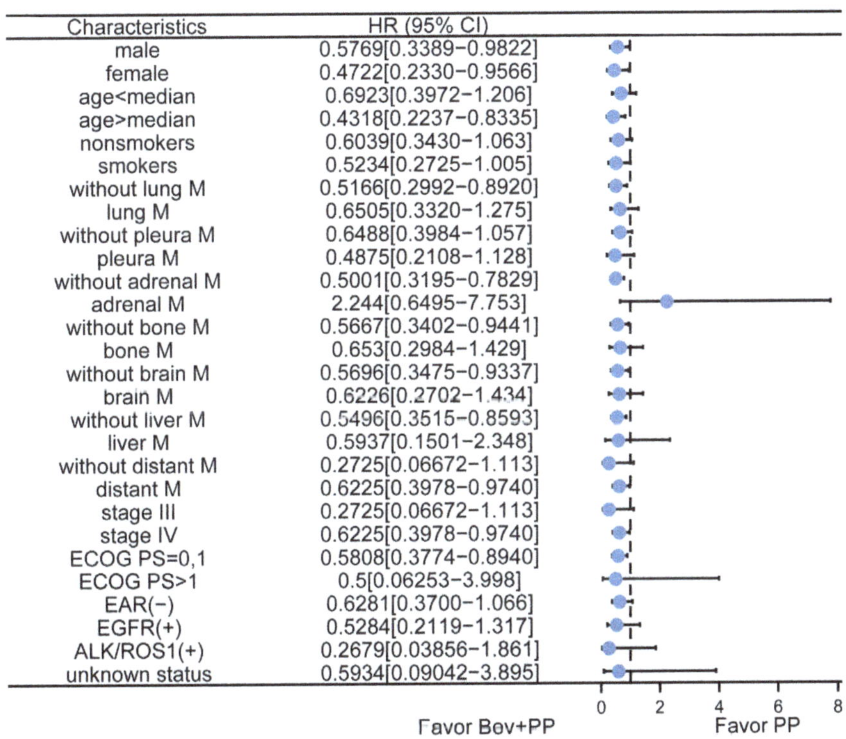

FIGURE 2 | Subgroup analysis of PFS in enrolled patients. Dots and horizontal lines represent the mean value and confidence intervals, respectively. Bev+PP denotes bevacizumab plus pemetrexed–platinum, and PP denotes pemetrexed–platinum.

analyses confirmed that pemetrexed–platinum doublet with bevacizumab was an independent favorable factor of PFS. This study confirmed that pemetrexed–platinum doublet combined with bevacizumab was safe and effective for Chinese chemo-naive lung adenocarcinoma patients.

Bevacizumab plus pemetrexed–platinum doublet chemotherapy has become a standard first-line treatment for advanced lung adenocarcinoma patients with negative results of detecting PD-L1 expression, EGFR mutations, and ALK/ROS1 gene fusions, or after the failure of targeted therapies for patients with EGFR mutations or ALK/ROS1 fusions, as recommended in NCCN NSCLC guidelines (Ettinger et al., 2019) and pan-Asian adapted ESMO NSCLC guideline (Wu et al., 2019), based on several large phase III clinical trials, including SAiL and ARIES (Crinò et al., 2010; Lynch Jr et al., 2014) and several other clinical trials comparing paclitaxel-based chemotherapy with or without bevacizumab. Consistent with the ORR and PFS benefits of bevacizumab addition found in these clinical trials, our study also demonstrated similar PFS and ORR improvements.

TABLE 5 | Safety profile of the two groups.

	All AEs			Grade ≥3 AEs		
	Bev+PP (n = 46)	PP (n = 54)	p-value	Bev+PP (n = 46)	PP (n = 54)	p-value
	N (%)	N (%)		N (%)	N (%)	
Leukopenia	29 (63.0)	32 (59.3)	0.837	9 (19.6)	10 (18.5)	0.999
Abnormal liver function	12 (26.1)	9 (16.7)	0.326	1 (2.2)	2 (3.7)	0.999
Fatigue	21 (45.7)	21 (38.9)	0.546	1 (2.2)	2 (3.7)	0.999
Nausea	17 (37.0)	18 (33.3)	0.834	0 (0.0)	1 (1.9)	0.999
Anemia	12 (26.1)	14 (25.9)	0.999	1 (2.2)	3 (5.6)	0.622
Thrombocytopenia	10 (21.7)	8 (14.8)	0.438	1 (2.2)	0 (0.0)	0.460
Thrombosis and hemorrhage	2 (4.3)	1 (1.9)	0.593	1 (2.2)	0 (0.0)	0.460
Hypertension	2 (4.3)	0 (0.0)	0.209	0 (0.0)	0 (0.0)	NA
Anorexia	2 (4.3)	5 (9.3)	0.447	0 (0.0)	0 (0.0)	NA
Headache	1 (2.2)	0 (0.0)	0.460	0 (0.0)	0 (0.0)	NA
Rash	1 (2.2)	1 (1.9)	0.999	0 (0.0)	0 (0.0)	NA
Increased creatinine	2 (4.3)	0 (0.0)	0.209	0 (0.0)	0 (0.0)	NA
Total	41 (89.1)	51 (94.4)	0.465	11 (23.9)	16 (29.6)	0.652

AVAPERL (Barlesi et al., 2013) and COMPASS (Seto et al., 2020) studies compared pemetrexed plus bevacizumab with single-agent bevacizumab in the maintenance and whole phases, respectively, which showed elevated PFS but not OS with bevacizumab addition. A Japanese clinical trial published in 2016 reported a nonsignificant beneficial PFS in the pemetrexed–platinum plus bevacizumab group compared with pemetrexed–platinum alone (mPFS 11.5 vs. 7.3 months, p = 0.198) (Karayama et al., 2016). The 2016 Japanese study and another Japanese study SAKK19_09 (Gautschi et al., 2015) all reported no significant improvement in OS when comparing Bev+Pem–platinum with chemo-monotherapy (24.4 vs. 21.3 months, p = 0.63; 14.7 vs. 14.6 months, p = 0.890; respectively). However, Stephen J et al. conducted a large sample retrospective cohort study including 4,724 patients with 58% receiving carboplatin–pemetrexed and 42% receiving carboplatin–pemetrexed–bevacizumab. The study demonstrated an OS benefit from 8.6 to 12.1 months (p < 0.001) and also showed that female patients had longer OS than male patients after the triple-reagent administration (Bagley et al., 2019). In our study, more patients received longer maintenance cycles of pemetrexed plus bevacizumab treatment, which might have contributed to the longer PFS and also indicated that the safety profile of combination therapy was tolerable in the real-world setting. Although the addition of bevacizumab or not was a constant factor in both induction and maintenance therapies, the final OS was not significantly altered in our study, which was consistent with findings from the abovementioned clinical studies but not the large-sample retrospective cohort study. We also found that female patients treated with pemetrexed–platinum with bevacizumab responded better than male patients. The limited PFS and insignificant OS improvement in our study might be due to a higher percent of patients with stage IV b+c lung adenocarcinoma. Besides, the limited population size may also cause the restricted application of our findings, and uncontrolled post-line treatments in the real-world may have an impact on the OS.

Several other studies have also reported the use of combination therapies in real-world settings. For instance, Katherine B. Winfree retrospectively compared maintenance therapies for non-squamous lung cancer patients in the United States and found that pemetrexed–bevacizumab treatment could improve patients' PFS compared to pemetrexed treatment alone (Winfree et al., 2019). However, the PFS was calculated from the first day of induction therapy, while the induction therapies included many different regimens such as platinum + bevacizumab, and platinum + other chemo-reagents. Thus, the improvement may be all attributed to the specific maintenance regimen. In our study, we specifically focused on pemetrexed–platinum doublet with or without bevacizumab, and the comparison was intended to investigate whether the addition of bevacizumab could benefit Chinese chemo-naive lung adenocarcinoma patients during the entire treatment, and we did observe an improvement in PFS but not in OS. Fei Qi et al. (Qi et al., 2019) and Xiaoyou Li et al. (Li et al., 2019) performed similar comparisons with ours and also found that the median PFS was significantly prolonged in the bevacizumab addition group compared with the chemo-only group (9.8 vs. 7.8 months, p = 0.006; 10.97 vs. 6.67 months, p = 0.0002), as well as ORR, which were consistent with our findings. More than 4 months of PFS improvement may not be all attributed to bevacizumab addition since the combination group enrolled significantly fewer patients with brain or pleural metastasis than the chemo-group, whereas in our study, a higher percent of patients enrolled in the pemetrexed–platinum treatment group were absent of distant metastasis, than the combination group.

The MAP study showed that when receiving platinum/pemetrexed/bevacizumab, patients with EGFR mutation had higher OS than patients with EGFR-negative status (NR vs. 20.7 months, p = 0.004). However, only 8 out of 23 patients had prior TKIs (Tsutani et al., 2018). The 2016 Japanese study also enrolled patients with failure from EGFR or ALK/ROS1 tyrosine kinase inhibitors; however, the authors failed to compare the survival difference between negative and positive patients (Karayama et al., 2016). EGFR-negative patients in the COMPASS study obtained a better OS with bevacizumab addition (HR [95% CI], 0.82 [0.68–0.99]) (Seto et al., 2020). In this study, we assessed the treatment efficacy in subgroups using outcome PFS, but not OS because the OS of the total samples did not show any significant tendency to either treatment. Bevacizumab addition tended to be beneficial to both EGFR-negative and -positive patients.

Our study also compared combination therapy with pemetrexed–platinum doublet in subgroup analysis, and surprisingly, the findings demonstrated that it tended to be favoring chemotherapy alone for patients with adrenal metastasis. However, to the best of our knowledge, no clinical trials or other retrospective studies analyzing such a specific population have been reported. Only the ECOG4599 study comparing paclitaxel–carboplatin doublet plus bevacizumab with chemotherapy alone in NSCLC reported the hazard ratio for OS (0.97 [0.65–1.46]) of patients with adrenal metastasis, with the largest value in analyses of all sites of metastasis, indicating the highest risk not benefiting from the addition of bevacizumab (Sandler et al., 2006). We have to admit that limited patients with adrenal metastasis were enrolled in our study, which might cause false discovery. However, to avoid the economic burden of bevacizumab addition, we cautiously suggest that clinical trials or retrospective studies with a large sample size be conducted to further investigate the effect of bevacizumab addition in patients with adrenal metastasis.

The combination treatment was well-tolerated, and no unexpected findings were reported in our real-world study. The two groups shared similar adverse effects, including severe adverse effects. Leukopenia (also categorized as neutropenia in clinical trials), fatigue, and nausea were found to be the most frequent AEs in the two groups, which are reported as common adverse effects of chemotherapy treatment (Zinner and Herbst, 2004), and bevacizumab addition in this study did not significantly augment those side effects. The ECOG-ACRIN 5508 study investigating the strategies for maintenance therapies revealed that the incidence of grade ≥3 AEs was obviously elevated in the combination regimen, from 37 to 51% (Ramalingam et al., 2019). However, such an increase in the incidence of grade ≥3 AEs was not demonstrated in the abovementioned clinical trials and retrospective studies and in the current study. Besides, patients in the ECOG-ACRIN 5508 study were administered with paclitaxel–carboplatin plus bevacizumab as induction therapy before randomization into pemetrexed or pemetrexed plus bevacizumab groups, which might cause late impact on grade ≥3 AEs during maintenance therapy.

In conclusion, although the survival benefit associated with bevacizumab addition is reported limited in our study, the overall response is increased and the safety profile is acceptable. The addition of bevacizumab is currently recommended and has been demonstrated to be a better treatment option in chemo-naive lung adenocarcinoma patients with PD-L1-negative scores in many clinical trials and real-world studies including this study. However, we carefully suggest that medical oncologists should be cautious with bevacizumab addition in patients with adrenal metastasis, unless large clinical studies focusing on this specific population are performed and show clear evidence.

AUTHOR CONTRIBUTIONS

Conceptualization: XC and BX; methodology: XL, JH, QZ, and YQ; validation: KW; formal analysis: JH; investigation: XL and YQ; resources: XL, SY, KW, JW, JY, and LW; data curation: JH; writing—original draft preparation: JH and QZ; writing—review and editing: JH and XC; visualization: JH; supervision: SM; project administration: XC; funding acquisition: XC and SM. All authors have read and agreed to the published version of the manuscript.

REFERENCES

Assoun, S., Brosseau, S., Steinmetz, C., Gounant, V., and Zalcman, G. (2017). Bevacizumab in Advanced Lung Cancer: State of the Art. *Future Oncol.* 13, 2515–2535. doi:10.2217/fon-2017-0302

Bagley, S. J., Talento, S., Mitra, N., Meropol, N. J., Cohen, R. B., Langer, C. J., et al. (2019). Comparative Effectiveness of Carboplatin/Pemetrexed with versus without Bevacizumab for Advanced Nonsquamous Nonsmall Cell Lung Cancer. *J. Natl. Compr. Cancer Netw.* 17, 469–477. doi:10.6004/jnccn.2018.7102

Bansal, P., Osman, D., Gan, G. N., Simon, G. R., and Boumber, Y. (2016). Recent Advances in Immunotherapy in Metastatic NSCLC. *Front. Oncol.* 6, 239. doi:10.3389/fonc.2016.00239

Barlesi, F., Scherpereel, A., Rittmeyer, A., Pazzola, A., Ferrer Tur, N., Kim, J.-H., et al. (2013). Randomized Phase III Trial of Maintenance Bevacizumab with or without Pemetrexed after First-Line Induction with Bevacizumab, Cisplatin, and Pemetrexed in Advanced Nonsquamous Nonsmall-cell Lung Cancer: AVAPERL (MO22089). *J Clin Oncol.* 31, 3004–3011. doi:10.1200/jco.2012.42.3749

Cao, M., Li, H., Sun, D., and Chen, W. (2020). *Cancer* Burden of Major Cancers in China: A Need for Sustainable Actions. *Cancer Commun.* 40, 205–210. doi:10.1002/cac2.12025

Crinò, L., Dansin, E., Garrido, P., Griesinger, F., Laskin, J., Pavlakis, N., et al. (2010). Safety and Efficacy of First-Line Bevacizumab-Based Therapy in Advanced Nonsquamous Nonsmall-cell Lung Cancer (SAiL, MO19390): a Phase 4 Study. *Lancet Oncol.* 11, 733–740. doi:10.1016/s1470-2045(10)70151-0

Ettinger, D. S., Wood, D. E., Aggarwal, C., Aisner, D. L., Akerley, W., Bauman, J. R., et al. (2019). NCCN Guidelines Insights: Nonsmall Cell Lung *Cancer*, Version 1.2020. *J. Natl. Compr. Cancer Netw.* 17, 1464–1472. doi:10.6004/jnccn.2019.0059

Ferlay, J., Colombet, M., Soerjomataram, I., Mathers, C., Parkin, D. M., Piñeros, M., et al. (2019). Estimating the Global Cancer Incidence and Mortality in 2018: GLOBOCAN Sources and Methods. *Int. J. Cancer* 144, 1941–1953. doi:10.1002/ijc.31937

Garcia, J., Hurwitz, H. I., Sandler, A. B., Miles, D., Coleman, R. L., Deurloo, R., et al. (2020). Bevacizumab (Avastin) in Cancer Treatment: A Review of 15 Years of Clinical Experience and Future Outlook. *Cancer Treat. Rev.* 86, 102017. doi:10.1016/j.ctrv.2020.102017

Gautschi, O., Mach, N., Rothschild, S. I., Li, Q., Stahel, R. A., Zippelius, A., et al. (2015). Bevacizumab, Pemetrexed, and Cisplatin, or Bevacizumab and Erlotinib for Patients with Advanced Nonsmall-cell Lung *Cancer* Stratified by Epidermal Growth Factor Receptor Mutation: Phase II Trial SAKK19/09. *Clin. Lung Cancer* 16, 358–365. doi:10.1016/j.cllc.2015.02.007

Guan, Y., Wang, G., Fails, D., Nagarajan, P., and Ge, Y. (2020). Unraveling Cancer Lineage Drivers in Squamous Cell Carcinomas. *Pharmacol. Ther.* 206, 107448. doi:10.1016/j.pharmthera.2019.107448

Hu, P., Liu, W., Wang, L., Yang, M., and Du, J. (2013). High Circulating VEGF Level Predicts Poor Overall Survival in Lung Cancer. *J. Cancer Res. Clin. Oncol.* 139, 1157–1167. doi:10.1007/s00432-013-1425-1

Karayama, M., Inui, N., Fujisawa, T., Enomoto, N., Nakamura, Y., Kuroishi, S., et al. (2016). Maintenance Therapy with Pemetrexed and Bevacizumab versus Pemetrexed Monotherapy after Induction Therapy with Carboplatin, Pemetrexed, and Bevacizumab in Patients with Advanced Nonsquamous Non Small Cell Lung Cancer. *Eur. J. Cancer* 58, 30–37. doi:10.1016/j.ejca.2016.01.013

Li, X., Abbas, M., Li, Y., Teng, Y., Fang, Y., Yu, S., et al. (2019). Comparative Effectiveness of Pemetrexed-Platinum Doublet Chemotherapy with or without Bevacizumab as First-Line Therapy for Treatment-Naive Patients with Advanced Nonsquamous Nonsmall-cell Lung *Cancer* in China. *Clin. Ther.* 41, 518–529. doi:10.1016/j.clinthera.2019.02.004

Lynch, T. J., Jr, Spigel, D. R., Brahmer, J., Fischbach, N., Garst, J., Jahanzeb, M., et al. (2014). Safety and Effectiveness of Bevacizumab-Containing Treatment for Nonsmall-cell Lung *Cancer*: Final Results of the ARIES Observational Cohort Study. *J. Thorac. Oncol.* 9, 1332–1339. doi:10.1097/jto.0000000000000257

Pakkala, S., and Ramalingam, S. S. (2018). Personalized Therapy for Lung Cancer: Striking a Moving Target. *JCI Insight* 3, e120858. doi:10.1172/jci.insight.120858

Patel, J. D., Socinski, M. A., Garon, E. B., Reynolds, C. H., Spigel, D. R., Olsen, M. R., et al. (2013). PointBreak: a Randomized Phase III Study of Pemetrexed Plus Carboplatin and Bevacizumab Followed by Maintenance Pemetrexed and Bevacizumab versus Paclitaxel Plus Carboplatin and Bevacizumab Followed by Maintenance Bevacizumab in Patients with Stage IIIB or IV Nonsquamous Nonsmall-cell Lung Cancer. *J Clin Oncol.* 31, 4349–4357. doi:10.1200/jco.2012.47.9626

Paz-Ares, L. G., de Marinis, F., Dediu, M., Thomas, M., Pujol, J.-L., Bidoli, P., et al. (2013). PARAMOUNT: Final Overall Survival Results of the Phase III Study of Maintenance Pemetrexed versus Placebo Immediately after Induction Treatment with Pemetrexed Plus Cisplatin for Advanced Nonsquamous Nonsmall-cell Lung Cancer. *J Clin Oncol.* 31, 2895–2902. doi:10.1200/jco.2012.47.1102

Qi, F., Hu, X., Hu, X., Liu, Y., Wang, Z., Duan, J., et al. (2019). First-line Pemetrexed-Platinum Doublet Chemotherapy with or without Bevacizumab in Nonsquamous Nonsmall Cell Lung Cancer: A Real-World Propensity Score-Matched Study in China. *Chin J Cancer Res.* 31, 749¯758. doi:10.21147/j.issn.1000-9604.2019.05.05

Ramalingam, S. S., Dahlberg, S. E., Belani, C. P., Saltzman, J. N., Pennell, N. A., Nambudiri, G. S., et al. (2019). Pemetrexed, Bevacizumab, or the Combination as Maintenance Therapy for Advanced Nonsquamous Nonsmall-cell Lung *Cancer*: ECOG-ACRIN 5508. *J Clin Oncol.* 37, 2360–2367. doi:10.1200/jco.19.01006

Sandler, A., Gray, R., Perry, M. C., Brahmer, J., Schiller, J. H., Dowlati, A., et al. (2006). Paclitaxel-carboplatin Alone or with Bevacizumab for Nonsmall-cell Lung Cancer. *N. Engl. J. Med.* 355, 2542–2550. doi:10.1056/nejmoa061884

Seto, T., Azuma, K., Yamanaka, T., Sugawara, S., Yoshioka, H., Wakuda, K., et al. (2020). Randomized Phase III Study of Continuation Maintenance Bevacizumab with or without Pemetrexed in Advanced Nonsquamous Nonsmall-cell Lung *Cancer*: COMPASS (WJOG5610L). *J Clin Oncol.* 38, 793–803. doi:10.1200/jco.19.01494

Tamura, R., Tanaka, T., Ohara, K., Miyake, K., Morimoto, Y., Yamamoto, Y., et al. (2019). Persistent Restoration to the Immunosupportive Tumor Microenvironment in Glioblastoma by Bevacizumab. *Cancer Sci.* 110, 499–508. doi:10.1111/cas.13889

Tsutani, Y., Miyata, Y., Masuda, T., Fujitaka, K., Doi, M., Awaya, Y., et al. (2018). Multicenter Phase II Study on Cisplatin, Pemetrexed, and Bevacizumab Followed by Maintenance with Pemetrexed and Bevacizumab for Patients with Advanced or Recurrent Nonsquamous Nonsmall Cell Lung Cancer: MAP Study. *BMC cancer* 18, 1231. doi:10.1186/s12885-018-5146-3

Vermeulen, R., Downward, G. S., Zhang, J., Hu, W., Portengen, L., Bassig, B. A., et al. (2019). Constituents of Household Air Pollution and Risk of Lung *Cancer* Among Never-Smoking Women in Xuanwei and Fuyuan, China. *Environ. Health Perspect.* 127, 097001. doi:10.1289/ehp4913

Winfree, K. B., Torres, A. Z., Zhu, Y. E., Muehlenbein, C., Aggarwal, H., Woods, S., et al. (2019). Treatment Patterns, Duration and Outcomes of Pemetrexed Maintenance Therapy in Patients with Advanced NSCLC in a Real-World Setting. *Curr. Med. Res. Opin.* 35, 817–827. doi:10.1080/03007995.2018.1547273

Wu, Y.-L., Planchard, D., Lu, S., Sun, H., Yamamoto, N., Kim, D.-W., et al. (2019). Pan-Asian Adapted Clinical Practice Guidelines for the Management of Patients with Metastatic Nonsmall-cell Lung Cancer: a CSCO-ESMO Initiative Endorsed by JSMO, KSMO, MOS, SSO and TOS. *Ann. Oncol.* 30, 171–210. doi:10.1093/annonc/mdy554

Yang, D., Liu, Y., Bai, C., Wang, X., and Powell, C. A. (2020). Epidemiology of Lung Cancer and Lung Cancer Screening Programs in China and the United States. *Cancer Lett.* 468, 82–87. doi:10.1016/j.canlet.2019.10.009

Zang, J., Hu, Y., Xu, X., Ni, J., Yan, D., Liu, S., et al. (2017). Elevated Serum Levels of Vascular Endothelial Growth Factor Predict a Poor Prognosis of Platinum-Based Chemotherapy in Nonsmall Cell Lung Cancer. *Onco Targets Ther.* 10, 409–415. doi:10.2147/ott.s124124

Zhao, Y.-Y., Xue, C., Jiang, W., Zhao, H.-Y., Huang, Y., Feenstra, K., et al. (2012). Predictive Value of Intratumoral Microvascular Density in Patients with Advanced Nonsmall Cell Lung *Cancer* Receiving Chemotherapy Plus Bevacizumab. *J. Thorac. Oncol.* 7, 71–75. doi:10.1097/jto.0b013e31823085f4

Zhou, C., Wu, Y.-L., Chen, G., Liu, X., Zhu, Y., Lu, S., et al. (2015). BEYOND: A Randomized, Double-Blind, Placebo-Controlled, Multicenter, Phase III Study of First-Line Carboplatin/Paclitaxel Plus Bevacizumab or Placebo in Chinese Patients with Advanced or Recurrent Nonsquamous Nonsmall-cell Lung *Cancer*. *J Clin Oncol.* 33, 2197–2204. doi:10.1200/jco.2014.59.4424

Zinner, R. G., and Herbst, R. S. (2004). Pemetrexed in the Treatment of Advanced Nonsmall-cell Lung *Cancer*: A Review of the Clinical Data. *Clin. Lung Cancer* 5, S67–S74. doi:10.3816/clc.2004.s.006

17

Deep Sequencing of T-Cell Receptors for Monitoring Peripheral CD8$^+$ T Cells in Chinese Advanced Non–Small-Cell Lung Cancer Patients Treated with the Anti–PD-L1 Antibody

Jin Sheng[1,2†], Huadi Wang[1,2†], Xiao Liu[3], Yunyun Deng[4], Yingying Yu[4], Pengfei Xu[4], Jiawei Shou[1,2], Hong Pan[1,2], Hongsen Li[1,2], Xiaoyun Zhou[1], Weidong Han[1,2], Tao Sun[4,5], Hongming Pan[1]* and Yong Fang[1]**

[1]*Department of Medical Oncology, School of Medicine, Sir Run Run Shaw Hospital, Zhejiang University, Hangzhou, China,* [2]*Laboratory of Cancer Biology, Institute of Clinical Science, School of Medicine, Sir Run Run Shaw Hospital, Zhejiang University, Hangzhou, China,* [3]*Department of Human Genetics, University of Chicago, Chicago, IL, United States,* [4]*Hangzhou ImmuQuad Biotechnologies, LLC, Hangzhou, China,* [5]*Zhejiang-California International Nano-Systems Institute, Zhejiang University, Hangzhou, China*

***Correspondence:**
Yong Fang
fangyong@zju.edu.cn
Hongming Pan
panhongming@zju.edu.cn
Tao Sun
taosun@immuquad.com

†*These authors have contributed equally to this work and share first authorship*

Background: Atezolizumab, a high-affinity engineered human anti–PD-L1 antibody, has produced a clinical benefit for patients with advanced non–small-cell lung cancer (NSCLC). However, associated with T-cell regulation, the immunomodulatory effect of PD-L1 blockade and its biomarker in peripheral immunity remains elusive.

Methods: In a prospective cohort with 12 Chinese advanced NSCLC patients who received atezolizumab 1,200 mg every 3 weeks as a second-line treatment, blood samples were obtained before and 6 weeks after atezolizumab initiation, and when disease progression was confirmed. Patients were classified into a response or progression group according to response evaluation criteria in solid tumors (RECIST) 1.1. Fresh peripheral blood mononuclear cells (PBMCs) from patients were stained with antihuman CD3, CD8, and PD-1 antibodies for flow cytometry analysis. T-cell receptor (TCR)-β chains of CD8$^+$ T cells were analyzed by next-generation sequencing (NGS) at the deep level. Diversity, clonality, and similarity of TCR have been calculated before and after treatment in both groups.

Results: Clonal expansion with high PD-1 expression was detected in all patients' peripheral CD8$^+$ T cells before the treatment of atezolizumab. Unlike the progression group, the diversity of TCR repertoire and singletons in the TCRβ pool increased over time with atezolizumab administration, and the TCR repertoire dynamically changes in the response group. The percentage of CD8$^+$ PD-1^{high} terminal exhausted T cells declined in the response group after the PD-L1 blockade. Two patterns of TCR changes among patients who received PD-L1–targeted immunotherapy were observed.

Conclusions: Deep sequencing of the T-cell receptors confirmed the existence of CD8$^+$ PD-1high T cells with an exhaustion phenotype in Chinese NSCLC patients. Our study demonstrated that efficient anti–PD-L1 therapy could reshape the TCR repertoire for antitumor patients. Furthermore, singleton frequency may help us select patients who are sensitive to anti–PD-L1 immunotherapy.

Keywords: next-generation sequencing, liquid biopsy, T-cell receptor repertoires, non–small cell lung cancer, anti–PD-L1 immunotherapy

INTRODUCTION

Non–small cell lung cancer (NSCLC) that accounts for almost 85 percent of total lung cancer patients is still the leading cause of cancer-related mortality, especially in those with advanced disease (Sui et al., 2018; Seigel et al., 2017). Over the past few years, the introduction of the epidermal growth factor receptor (EGFR), tyrosine kinase inhibitors (TKIs), and anaplastic lymphoma kinase (ALK)-based target therapy dramatically improved the therapeutic efficacy for lung cancer patients with specific gene mutations (Califano et al., 2017; Hida et al., 2017; Peters et al., 2017; Kiura et al., 2018; Novello et al., 2018). However, tumor heterogeneity inevitably leads to resistance of targeted therapies from multiple mechanisms (Tsui et al., 2018). Encouragingly, immune checkpoint blockade (ICB) immunotherapy had changed the landscape for treating advanced NSCLC, with a more durable response than targeted therapy and chemotherapy.

Several inhibitory immunoreceptors, including but not limited to CTLA-4, PD-1, TIM3, and LAG3, have been studied in some solid tumors in the past decades. Moreover, the most successfully developed ICB therapy is anti–PD-1/PD-L1 therapy, since atezolizumab, nivolumab, and pembrolizumab have been approved for NSCLC (Ribas and Wolchok, 2018). The PD-1/PD-L1 signaling pathway is one of the self-protection mechanisms of tumors against the endogenous immune response (Taube et al., 2012). Conventionally, the primary PD-1 ligand expressed on the surface of tumor cells or antigen-presenting cells is PD-L1, with PD-1 on T cells to trigger inhibitory signaling (Curiel et al., 2003, 2007; Keir et al., 2008; Lin et al., 2018). T cells respond highly specific to particular antigens as a consequence so that the gene encoding their adaptive immune receptors is generated somatically through a process that creates unique sequences when they encounter the cognate antigen. The generation process of adaptive immune receptor genes results in a tremendously diverse repertoire of distinct T-cell receptors (TCR) to bind the particular antigens (Robins et al., 2010; Warren et al., 2013; Zarnitsyna et al., 2013; Kaplinsky and Arnaout, 2016; Briney et al., 2019). A somatic recombination process of the variable (V), diversity (D, beta chain), and joining (J) exons generates a high degree of TCR diversity and defines the highly variable complementary determining region 3 (CDR3) (Lee and Prins, 2016). CDR3 characterizes the antigen recognition specificity of each T-cell clone. Therefore, deep sequencing data of the T-cell antigen receptor repertoire give us access to a better understanding of T lymphocyte population dynamics in response to therapy (Cowell, 2020).

The application of TCR repertoire deep sequencing to reveal lymphocyte responses in cancer or immunotherapy is widespread (Kirsch et al., 2015; Schrama et al., 2017). The majority of studies have focused on the T-cell receptor beta locus. Studies of clonal richness and diversity of T lymphocyte population have ranged from tumor-infiltrating T cells and sentinel lymph node T cells to T lymphocytes in peripheral blood. Tumor-infiltrating T cells are the front line of identifying tumor antigens in the tumor microenvironment, resulting in considerable heterogeneity. In NSCLC, abundant TCR sequences have been classified as ubiquitous or regional. As for peripheral blood TCR repertoires, despite that studies found little overlap (from 19 to 25%) between peripheral blood and TIL TCR repertoires so far, evidence confirmed the peripheral TCR repertoire correlated with TILs, and their alteration reflects various aspects of the disease. Moreover, a study (Liu et al., 2019) suggested that peripheral TCR diversity decreases as the disease progresses in lung cancer.

The blockade of PD-1:PD-L1 interactions contains two options: anti–PD-1 and anti–PD-L1. PD-1 is expressed by activated T cells that bind to PD-L1 in the tumor microenvironment. However, during chronic exposure of tumor antigen, T cells undergo exhaustion with upregulation of inhibitory checkpoints, typically PD-1, as one of the tumor escape mechanisms. Blocking of PD-1 is expected to change these exhausted T cells' behavior directly and hopefully reinvigorate them. In contrast, the blockade of PD-L1 produces more possibilities due to broad cell types expressing PD-L1 and the additional ligand B7-1. Intriguingly, the study from Fridman et al. (2017) has given us crucial evidence that anti–PD-L1 treatment during chronic lymphocytic choriomeningitis virus (LCMV) infection induced the interleukin-7 receptor (IL-7R or CD127) on exhausted T cells. IL-7 acts as a pivotal factor for the generation of memory T-cell phenotype (Schluns et al., 2000) and down regulates PD-1 expression on the $CD8^+$ T cells during chronic LCMV infection. To confirm if similar regulation happens in cancer anti–PD-L1 immunotherapy, monitoring PD-1 expression in peripheral blood could give us a preliminary insight into the invigoration of T-cell exhaustion of anti–PD-L1 in cancer patients.

Collectively, in the present prospective cohort study, the expression of PD-1 and TCR repertoire was analyzed through high-throughput sequencing in blood samples from Chinese advanced NSCLC patients who had received anti–PD-L1 checkpoint blockade immunotherapy, aiming at exploring predictive and monitoring biomarkers before treatment and selecting patients to exhibit better clinical outcomes.

MATERIALS AND METHODS

Study Design and Cohort

We performed a prospective cohort study of patients with metastatic lung cancer treated with atezolizumab (MPDL3280A), a PD-L1

TABLE 1 | Demographic and clinical characteristics of patients.

Patient ID	Gender	Age	Histology	Smoking history	Cycles	Best response	Efficacy group	PFS/months
1	Male	61	SCC	Previous smoker	3	PD	Progression	2.9
2	Male	63	SCC	Previous smoker	4	PD	Progression	2.7
3	Male	59	SCC	Smoker	2	PD	Progression	1.4
4	Male	51	SCC	Previous smoker	11	PR	Response	7.7
5	Male	58	ADN	Previous smoker	8	PD	Progression	5.6
6	Male	52	ADN	Smoker	9	SD	Response	6.3
7	Male	75	SCC	Smoker	6	PD	Progression	4.3
8	Male	45	SCC	Smoker	12	SD	Response	8.3
9	Male	49	SCC	Smoker	6	SD	Response	4.4
10	Male	73	ADN	Previous smoker	3	PD	Progression	2.1
11	Female	58	SCC	Nonsmoker	13	SD	Response	9.3
12	Female	60	ADN	Nonsmoker	8	SD	Response	5.6

SCC refers to squamous carcinoma; ADN refers to adenocarcinoma.
PD: progressive disease; SD: stable disease; PR: partial response.

inhibitor, at Sir Run Run Shaw Hospital, Zhejiang University. This study was approved by the Institutional Review Board (IRB) of the hospital. All patients received atezolizumab 1,200 mg intravenously every 3 weeks. Critical inclusion criteria for this study cohort were cytologically confirmed stage IIIB/IV squamous carcinoma or adenocarcinoma of NSCLC, Eastern Cooperative Oncology Group performance status (ECOG-PS) of 0–1, 18 years old or older measurable lesion confirmed by response evaluation criteria in solid tumors (RECIST) 1.1, and disease recurrence after one prior platinum-containing regimen. Patients with a known autoimmune disease, symptomatic interstitial lung disease, systemic immunosuppression, or prior immune-based therapies were excluded. Smoking status was classified as smokers and nonsmokers. Smokers have been referred to as those patients who smoke more than ten cigarettes per day and with cigarette withdrawal less than 2 years.

Therapeutic Efficacy Analysis in Response to Atezolizumab

Tumor responses to atezolizumab were evaluated by a CT scan every 6 months. Clinical responses such as complete response (CR), partial response (PR), stable disease (SD), and progressive disease (PD) were determined based on RECIST 1.1. Patients were further categorized into the response group based on tumor shrinkage, while the progression group included patients who achieved PD (**Table 1**). The median follow-up was 5.0 (IQR 2.75–7.35) months at the endpoint. The median PFS was 4.4 (95% CI: 2.9–5.9) months among all patients.

$$f(x) = a_0 + \sum_{n=1}^{\infty}\left(a_n \cos\frac{n\pi x}{L} + b_n \sin\frac{n\pi x}{L}\right).$$

PBMC Preparation and CD8$^+$ T-Cell Isolation

We collected 25 samples of peripheral blood mononuclear cells (PBMCs) from 12 Chinese advanced NSCLC patients. The samples were collected at baseline and 6 weeks after the initiation of treatment within a 3-day time window. PBMCs were immediately isolated from each sample using Ficoll-Hypaque 1077 (Sigma-Aldrich) gradient centrifugation. Total CD8$^+$ T cells were isolated from PBMCs with the BD IMag™ Anti-Human CD8 Magnetic Particles kit (catalog no. 557766).

Flow Cytometry

For the flow cytometry analysis, all antibodies were purchased from BioLegend (San Diego, CA). Cells were stained with antihuman CD3 (HIT3a), CD8 (SK1), and PD-1 (EH12.2H7), and analyzed on a BD LSRFortessa™ flow cytometer (Becton Dickinson) using FlowJo vX.0.7 software. Gates were set on CD3$^+$ cells with forward and side scatter, and doublets were gated out (**Supplementary Figure S1**).

TCR-β Full-Length Amplification and Sequencing

RNA extraction of pure CD8$^+$ T cells was performed following the RNeasy Plus Mini Kit (Qiagen). The samples were analyzed by high-throughput sequencing of TCR full length using the ImmuHub® TCR profiling system at the deep level (ImmuQuad Biotech, Hangzhou China). Briefly, a 5′ RACE unbiased amplification protocol was used. Sequencing was performed on an Illumina MiSeq® system with PE300 mode (Illumina), as previously described (Wang et al., 2019). A post-sequencing algorithm was applied to raw sequencing data for PCR and sequencing error correction and V, D, J, and C gene segments mapping with IMGT®. The resulting nucleotide and amino acid sequences of CDR3 of TCRβ were determined, and those with out-of-frame and stop codon sequences were removed from the identified TCR-β repertoire. We further defined each TCR-β clonotype's amounts by adding the numbers of TCR-β clones sharing the same nucleotide sequence of CDR3. The TCR-β repertoire analysis algorithm was based on R (version 3.5.1). The total-sequencing reads and the successfully aligned reads are listed in **Supplementary Table S1** in detail.

Diversity, Clonality, and Similarity Calculation

Pielou's evenness index (Pielou, 1966) was calculated to estimate the diversity of TCRβ repertoire, according to the equation:

$$\text{Pielou index} = \frac{\text{Shannon index H}}{\ln \text{N}} = \sum_{i=1}^{\text{N}} \frac{\text{p}_\text{i} (\ln \text{p}_\text{i})}{\ln \text{N}},$$

$$\text{Clonality index} = 1 - \text{Pielou index},$$

where p_i is the proportion of sequence, i is relative to the entire sequences, and N is the total quantity of clonotypes. The *Pielou index* describes the equability of a TCR repertoire and is positively related to the diversity represented by the *Shannon index.*

Singleton means one unique TCR clone, and the entire singletons in one patient TCR repertoire have shown a strong correlation with the percentage of naive T cells (Britanova et al., 2014), which are the backbone of immune repertoire diversity. *Singleton frequency*, which calculated the proportion of singletons in the total clonotypes, is an essential factor in estimating the total repertoire clonality. In this study, we illustrated *singleton frequency* in donut charts, where the inner layer includes the frequency of singleton ("1," T-cell clones that only had one sequence read) and high-order ("2+," T-cell clones that had more than two sequence reads) clonotypes. Repertoire clonality was depicted as the "2+" portion in the donut chart.

Last, to estimate the overlap of TCR-β clonotypes between time points or biological compartments, the *Baroni-Urbani and Buser overlap index* (BUB) (Zhang et al., 2017) was calculated according to the following formula:

$$BUB = \frac{n_{12}}{n_1 + n_2 - n_{12}},$$

where n_1 is the number of clonotypes present at time point 1, n_2 is the number of clonotypes present at time point 2, and n_{12} is the number of clonotypes presenting in both time points.

Statistical Analysis

The Student's t-test (two-tailed) was adopted to compare the Pielou's evenness index, singletons frequency, and BUB overlap index between data before and after treatment. Two-way ANOVA analyzed the differences between repeated-measures data during therapy. A p-value of 0.05 was considered statistically significant. The Student's t-test and two-way ANOVA were calculated by GraphPad Prism version 6.0 (La Jolla, CA, United States). The donut chart was made by R (version 3.4.0). A survival analysis was conducted using both Kaplan–Meier log-rank analysis and Cox proportional hazard models.

RESULTS

Patient Characteristics and Therapeutic Efficacy

The primary characteristics of the 12 enrolled patients in this study cohort are summarized in **Table 1**. Briefly, eight patients had squamous carcinoma, and the remaining had adenocarcinoma. 83.3 percent of the cohort were current (n = 2) or former smokers (n = 8). All patients had an ECOG performance status of 1. The response group had a significantly younger average age than the progression group (53.5 vs. 64.8 years, $p < 0.05$, **Supplementary Table S2**). In this study, patients received a median of seven cycles of PD-L1 blockade immunotherapy, while half of them progressed after six cycles of treatment (**Figure 1A**). Among the response group, one patient (Patient 4) presented PR (**Figure 1B**), and five patients reached SD as their best response to the treatment during follow-ups (**Table 1; Figure 1B**). One patient (Patient 11) in the response group continued to respond to atezolizumab for more than 12 months, although the target lesions did not shrink remarkably as evaluated by computed tomography (**Figure 1C**). Comparing with the progression group (median 2.7 months, 95% CI: 1.7–3.7), the PFS significantly prolonged in the response group (median 6.3 months, 95% CI: 3.8–8.8; Kaplan–Meier estimate $p < 0.005$, **Figure 1D**).

$CD8^+PD\text{-}1^{high}$ Terminal Exhausted T Cells Decreased in Response to PD-L1 Blockade

When tumor antigens persist in, exhausted T cells (T_{ex}) form with the growing levels of persistent PD-1 expression, inducing a less functional state of exhaustion among cognate antigen-specific T cells. T_{ex} cells in the early stage retain the capability of renewal and are characterized by intermediate expression of PD-1. Early T_{ex} cells as a progenitor population give rise to terminal T_{ex} cells with high expression of PD-L1, which loses the ability of proliferation upon tumor antigen stimulation (**Figure 2A**) (McLane et al., 2019). Among the enrolled NSCLC patients, we confirmed PD-1-positive $CD8^+$ T cells in peripheral blood and further classified them into $PD\text{-}1^{high}$, $PD\text{-}1^{low}$, and $PD\text{-}1^{neg}$ subsets by the expression level of PD-1 (**Figure 2B**). The $PD\text{-}1^{high}$ subsets were regarded as terminal T_{ex} cells.

The average number of sequencing reads was 851148 ± 120135 (range 69,600–1,892,801), and the average aligned reads were 638721 ± 84,218 (range 45,909–1,385,898). Details of the total sequencing reads and successfully aligned reads are listed in **Supplementary Table S1**. The number of $CD8^+PD\text{-}1^{high}$ terminal T_{ex} cells in the responders' circulation decreased after anti–PD-L1 antibody treatment, whereas there was almost no change of this subset in the progression group (**Figure 2C**). After initiation of atezolizumab, in the response group, the percentage of $PD\text{-}1^{high}CD8^+$ terminal T_{ex} in total $CD3^+$ T cells dropped from 12.5 ± 2.76 (95% CI: 5.38–19.6) to 6.38 ± 1.03 (95% CI: 3.73–9.02; $p = 0.0705$ posttreatment vs. pretreatment) after PD-L1 blockade treatment (**Figure 2D**). However, in the progression group, there was no significant difference in the percentage of $PD\text{-}1^+CD8^+$ T cells before and after treatment (**Figure 2D**; 8.86 ± 2.58 vs. 8.86 ± 2.84, $p > 0.999$).

PD-L1 Blockade Changes TCR Repertoire Diversity

For a given total number of distinct clonotypes in the repertoire, the maximally diverse repertoire consists of uniformly distributed adaptive immune receptors (*pi* are all equal in the formula) (Cowell, 2020). The evenness of the TCR repertoire represented by Pielou's index increased in the response group after treatment ($p = 0.36$, paired t-test; **Figure 3A**); in contrast, those who did not respond to atezolizumab showed no change in the evenness of the TCR repertoire ($p = 0.98$, unpaired t-test). To

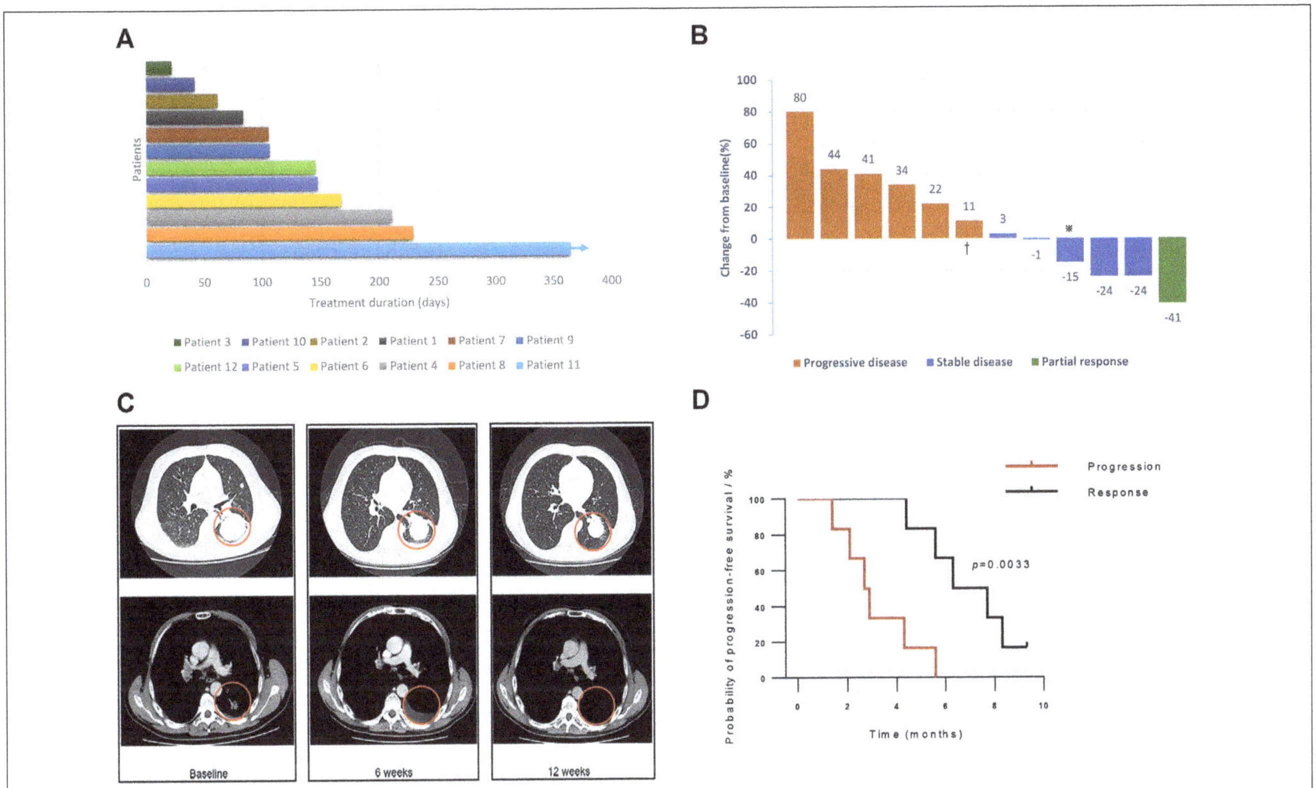

FIGURE 1 | Clinical efficacy of PD-L1 blockade. **(A)** Investigator-assessed duration of treatment. The arrow indicates censored patient with follow-up ongoing after one year. **(B)** The confirmed maximum reduction of target lesions, according to the investigator and authorized radiologist. Colors of bars representing the best response confirmed during follow-ups. Red bars represent progressive disease, blue bars represent stable disease, and green bars show partial response. Patient two was confirmed of nontarget lesion progression during the one-year follow-up. **(C)** Representative computed tomography (CT) scans of Patient 11, who achieved a partial response to atezolizumab. **(D)** Comparison of estimated progression-free survival of the response group and the progression group ($p < 0.005$). Note: ※: Patient 11, †: Patient 2.

assess the dynamic nature of the TCR repertoire diversity representing the whole course of effective anti–PD-L1 therapy, we collected blood samples from three patients in the response group with their consents when the progressive disease was confirmed. It is noticeable that the evenness of the TCR repertoire maintained or significantly elevated when the targeted lesions continued to respond to atezolizumab. However, Pielou's index dramatically dropped when the disease progressed ($p < 0.05$, 2-way ANOVA; **Figure 3B**).

The changes in the singleton frequency reflect the clonal proliferation of the TCR repertoire during anti–PD-L1 immunotherapy. Before treatment, the singleton frequency between the response and the progression group showed no significant difference (10.86 ± 3.67% vs. 5.22 ± 1.77%; p = 0.17, unpaired t-test; **Figure 3C**). Nevertheless, after the initiation of atezolizumab, the gap between the mean singleton frequency of the response and progression group grew (14.44 ± 2.25% vs. 7.51 ± 1.52%; $p < 0.05$, Welch's t-test; **Figure 3C**), which interpreted a better T-cell proliferative ability in patients who responded to PD-L1 blockade than in those who did not. Similarly, the singleton frequency of the same three patients in the response group was monitored during follow-ups. The clonal proliferation of the TCR repertoire dramatically elevated after the initiation of atezolizumab during stable disease. After progression, these three patients all had a decreased singleton frequency, indicating a lower level of richness of the TCR repertoire ($p < 0.05$, 2-way ANOVA; **Figure 3D**). There is not a clear correlation between the pretreatment singleton frequency and PFS (**Supplementary Figure S2**).

Also, we calculated the Baroni-Urbani and Buser index to measure the overlap among TCR-β clonotypes in the response and progression groups (**Supplementary Figure S3**). The average BUB index is moderately lower in the response group than that in the progression group (0.039 ± 0.0099 vs. 0.054 ± 0.017; p = 0.44, unpaired t-test), indicating the TCR similarity of patients in the response group is at a lower level than that of those in the progression group.

TCR Repertoire Changes due to anti–PD-L1 Treatment Had Typical Patterns Featured by Top Clonotype and Singleton Frequency

According to the clonotype and singleton frequency changes of the TCR repertoire before and after PD-L1 blockade immunotherapy, we summarized two patterns for every group, aiming at exploring a portable way to select proper patients for

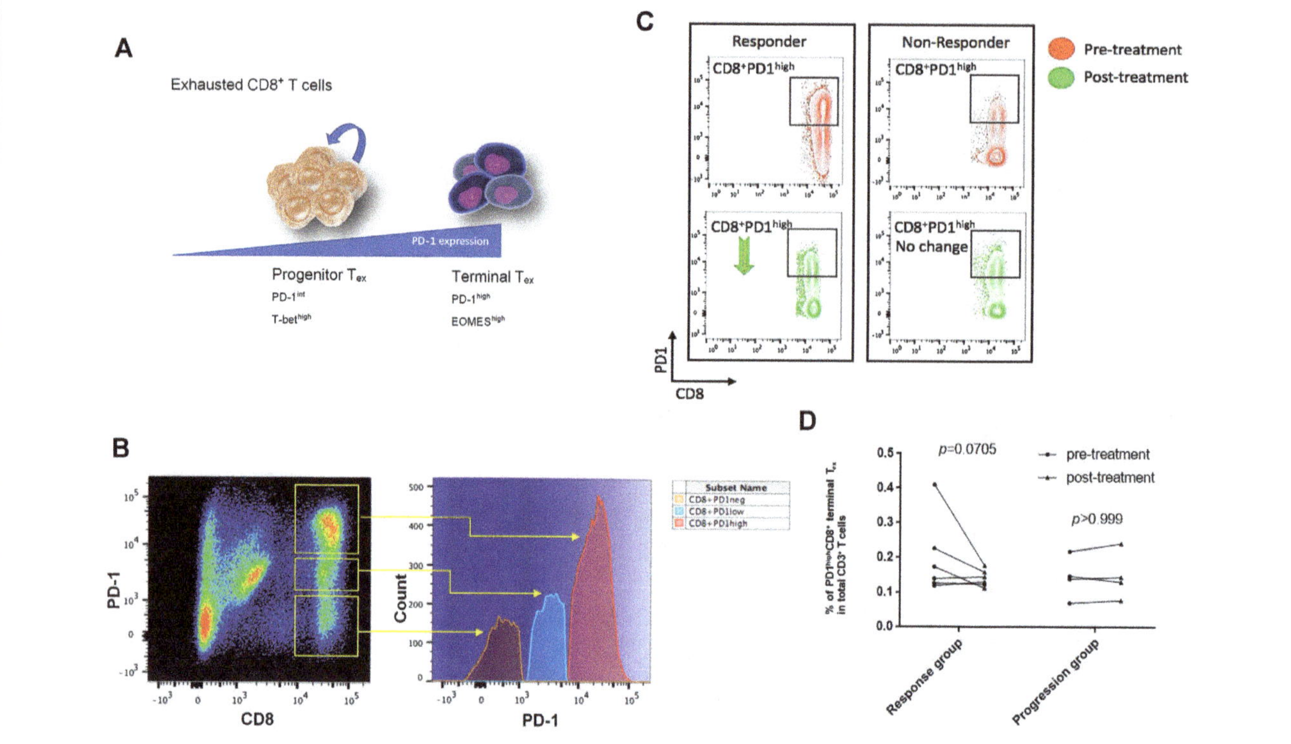

FIGURE 2 | CD8$^+$PD-1^{high} T cells decreased for responding to PD-L1 blockade treatment. **(A)** The CD8$^+$PD-1^{high} subset was identified as terminal exhausted T cells, which highly expressed the EOMES transcription factor, while CD8$^+$PD-1$^{int/low}$ population that expressed the T-bet transcription factor was known as progenitor exhausted T cells (Wherry and Kurachi, 2015). **(B)** According to the log-density plot of the PD-1 expression level, three subsets of CD8$^+$ T cells were found in Chinese non–small-cell lung cancer patients' peripheral blood. There were PD-1^{high}, PD-1^{low}, and PD-1^{neg} CD8 T$^+$ cells. **(C)** Two representatives illustrated that the percentage of CD8$^+$PD-1^{high} T cells in the response group decreased, whereas it did not have an apparent change in the progression cohort after PD-L1 blockade treatment. **(D)** The percentage of CD8$^+$PD-1^{high} T cells in each patient before and after treatment ($p = 0.0705$ in the response group; $p > 0.999$ in the progression group).

atezolizumab. In the first pattern of the response group, the singleton frequency of the TCR repertoire was increased primarily without variation of the top two clonotypes of CDR3 (**Figure 4A**). Pattern two had a decent percentage of singletons and was distinguished from the first pattern by the varied top two clones of the amino acid sequence of the CDR3 (**Figure 4A**). As for the progression group, pattern one had no change in neither singleton frequency nor top two clones of the TCR repertoire; in pattern two, the TCR repertoire of progressed patients maintained a small percentage of singletons in total clonotypes during treatment, but the top two clones changed (**Figure 4B**). The details of the top two clones of all patients before and after treatment are shown in **Table 2**. All information is given in **Supplementary Table S3**.

DISCUSSION

PD-L1 blockade immunotherapy has been proven to induce durable tumor remissions through T-cell response to cancer, and it remains unclear how these antibodies work in modulating T-cell immunity (Robert et al., 2014). Besides, serial monitoring of checkpoint inhibitors' efficacy needs easily accessible tumor biomarkers. Therefore, the TCR repertoire has become a focus in several studies since checkpoint inhibitor blockade dramatically changed the treatment for advanced cancer patients. However, exploratory studies of peripheral TCR diversity analysis among advanced cancer patients treated with different checkpoint inhibitors blockade have reached conflicting conclusions. So, we did this pilot study to continue illustrating PD-L1 blockade immunotherapy and exploring peripheral TCR repertoire in advanced NSCLC patients.

In this study, we confirmed the existence of PD-1^{high} terminal exhausted T cell and PD-1^{low} progenitor exhausted T cell in the enrolled Chinese NSCLC patients, and during treatment, effective anti–PD-L1 immunotherapy was correlated with decreased CD8$^+$ PD-1^{high} exhausted T cells. Multiple influencing factors function during the reform of antitumor immunity. Two main subsets constitute the CD8$^+$ PD-1–positive T cells: eomes^{high} PD-1^{high} CD8$^+$ T cells (terminal T$_{ex}$) respond poorly to the PD-1 pathway blockade; however, T-bet^{high} PD-1^{int} T cells can reverse exhaustion and produce protective immunity *in vivo* (Blackburn et al., 2008). Furthermore, atezolizumab is the inhibitor of both PD-1/PD-L1 and PD-L1/CD80 pathways (Syn et al., 2017), and CD80 on T cells delivered inhibitory signals as a receptor when engaged by PD-L1 (Butte et al., 2007). J. Park et al. demonstrated that by attenuation of the PD-L1/CD80 pathway through treatment with the anti–PD-L1 monoclonal antibody, blockade of PD-L1/CD80 could enhance T-cell expansion and restore response in the previously anergized

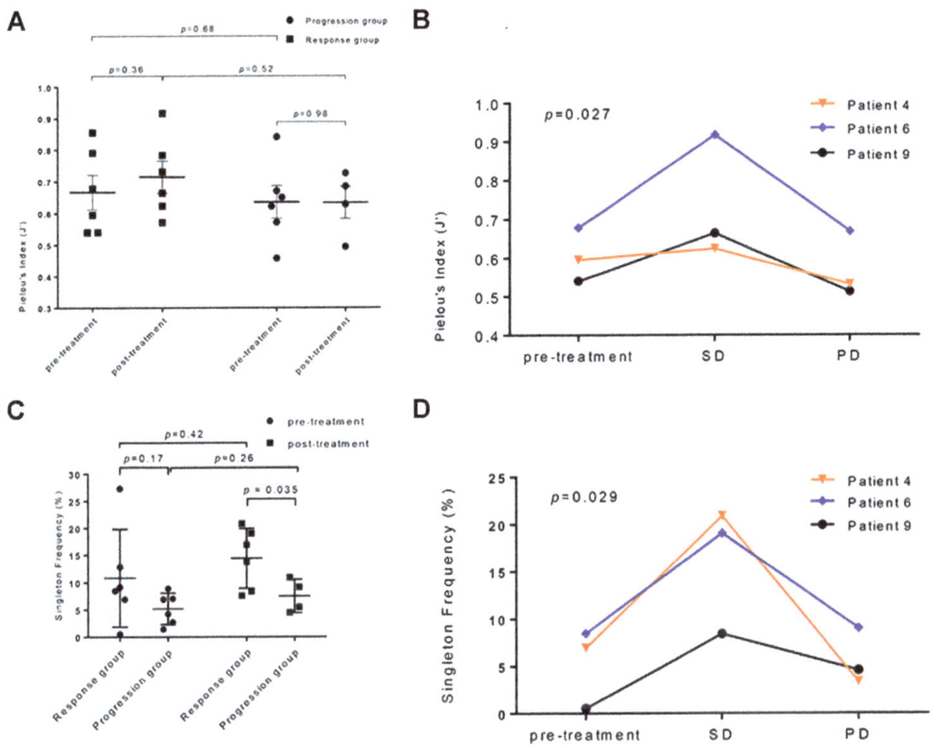

FIGURE 3 | The analysis of the T-cell receptor (TCR) repertoires diversity in anti–PD-L1–treated patients. **(A)** The comparison of TCR repertoire evenness changes in the progression and response groups calculated by Pielou's index (p = 0.36 in the response group; p = 0.98 in the progression group; response vs. progression: pretreatment p = 0.68, posttreatment p = 0.52). **(B)** The dynamic observation of TCR repertoire evenness at different disease statuses of three patients who responded to atezolizumab (p = 0.027). SD: stable disease; PD: progressive disease. **(C)** The singleton frequency in the response and progression groups before (p = 0.17) and after ($p < 0.05$) treatment. (pretreatment vs. posttreatment: p = 0.42 in the response group, p = 0.26 in the progression group). **(D)** The changes of the singleton frequency of the TCR repertoire in three patients responded to atezolizumab during treatment (p = 0.029).

T cells. So, we hypothesize that anti-PD-L1 antibodies protect the PD-1-positive T cells from apoptosis and T cells renewed from exhaustion without expression of PD-1, which leads to the decrease of $CD8^+$ PD-1^{high} T cell during effective atezolizumab treatment.

The blockade of PD-L1 makes more T cells survive from apoptosis, and therefore increases the diversity of T cells and TCR repertoires (**Figure 5**). Low TCR diversity indicates a severely impaired immune status of patients (Teng et al., 2015; Chen and Mellman, 2017; Snyder et al., 2017), and prospective studies in melanoma patients suggested that peripheral tumor-specific clones are likely to be concentrated in the $CD8^+PD\text{-}1^+$ subset (Gros et al., 2016). Therefore, the diversity of the TCR repertoire may reflect the immune status during treatment, and dynamic monitoring could improve its predictive power (Swanton and Govindan, 2016; Jamal-Hanjani et al., 2017). We dynamically analyzed peripheral TCR repertoire diversity in NSCLC patients, increased TCR repertoire diversity, and clonal proliferation that appeared under situations when patients responded to atezolizumab before progression. The TCR remained at a higher level during stable disease but dropped down after progression, which indicated the potential of peripheral TCR repertoire diversity to be a promising monitoring biomarker for checkpoint blockade immunotherapy. Similarly, Wieland et al. (2018) reported oligoclonal expansions in the peripheral $CD8^+$ TCR repertoire after pembrolizumab initiation in melanoma patients and identified the activation of tumor-infiltrating $CD8^+$ T-cell clones in peripheral blood after anti–PD-1 immunotherapy. In a study containing 29 advanced bladder cancer patients (Snyder et al., 2017), researchers noticed the expansion of circulating tumor-associated TCR 3 weeks after the initiation of atezolizumab, which is correlated with the durable clinical benefit. The further analysis helps us pick two characteristics of the TCR repertoire, the top two clones in CDR3, and singleton frequency (or its percentage), to summarize the changing pattern of the TCR repertoire. No matter the top two clones change or not, the response group always kept a decent or increased percentage of singleton frequency, which increases the possibility of more tumor-specific T cells to control tumor proliferation. Thus, we hypothesize that anti–PD-L1 leads to more tumor antigen presented to T cells, and more tumor-specific T cells survive. Nevertheless, unfortunately, pretreatment singleton frequency of the TCR repertoire could not predict the progression-free survival of NSCLC patients in our study. To further confirm the correlation between TCR repertoire diversity and PFS, a large-scale cohort study is needed.

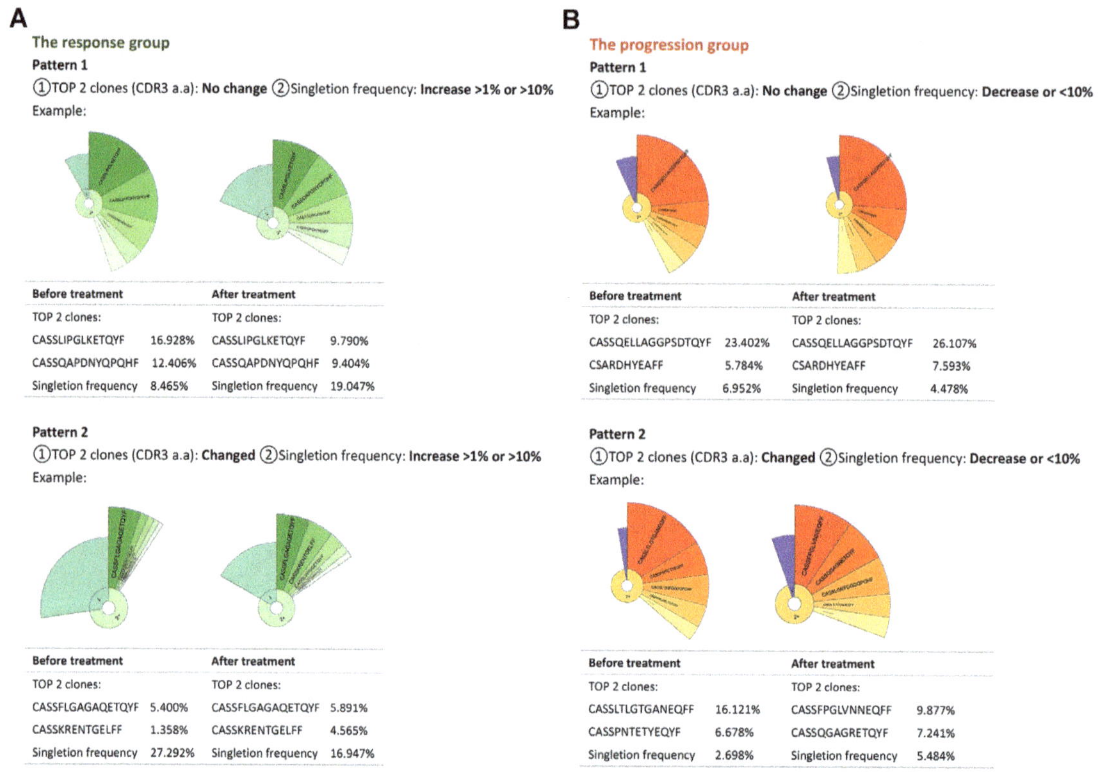

FIGURE 4 | Changing patterns of the TCR repertoire in the progression and response groups. Donut charts and tables summarized two patterns in each group. Each pattern took one patient as an example in either group. The fan-shaped area depicts the corresponding clonal frequency. The area of "1" in the donut chart represented the frequency of singletons. "2+" area was the TCR sequences whose reads were more than two. A larger radian meant a higher frequency. The top five clones' amino acid sequences of complementary determination region 3 (CDR3) of TCR were shown, and the frequencies of the top two clones were listed. The radian marked with the amino acid sequence displayed the frequency of the corresponding T-cell clones.

TABLE 2 | The Top two clones' amino acid sequences of complementary determination region 3 (CDR3) of TCR of each patient before and after treatment.

Group	Patient ID	Time point	Top 1 clone (CDR3)		Top 2 clone (CDR3)	
Progression	1	Pretreatment	11.80%	CASHRAGNEYEQYF	8.77%	CASSVAGTADYEQYF
		Posttreatment	NA	NA	NA	NA
	3	Pretreatment	43.09%	CASSFGTFGDGYT	4.45%	CASSLTSEHRFTDTQYF
		Posttreatment	NA	NA	NA	NA
	2	Pretreatment	16.12%	CASSLTLGTGANEQFF	6.68%	CASSPNTETYEQYF
		Posttreatment	9.88%	CASSFPGLVNNEQFF	7.24%	CASSQGAGRETQYF
	10	Pretreatment	8.45%	CASSEWGDTQYF	7.59%	CASRPSGTGGYNEQFF
		Posttreatment	9.04%	CASSEWGDTQYF	4.57%	CASRPSGTGGYNEQFF
	7	Pretreatment	23.40%	CASSQELLAGGPSDTQYF	5.78%	CSARDHYEAFF
		Posttreatment	26.11%	CASSQELLAGGPSDTQYF	7.59%	CSARDHYEAFF
	5	Pretreatment	9.33%	CASSEQGSGYEQYF	2.63%	CASSLNKGYGYTF
		Posttreatment	7.82%	CASSYSYEQYF	3.59%	CASSHPTGVEQYF
Response	9	Pretreatment	16.93%	CASSLIPGLKETQYF	12.41%	CASSQAPDNYQPQHF
		Posttreatment	9.79%	CASSLIPGLKETQYF	9.40%	CASSQAPDNYQPQHF
	12	Pretreatment	2.73%	CASSVKGSSGPLHF	2.08%	CATSSQDNTEAFF
		Posttreatment	9.94%	CASSVKGSSGPLHF	3.71%	CATSSQDNTEAFF
	6	Pretreatment	11.22%	CASSYSYEQYF	6.43%	CASSFGQGVYNEQFF
		Posttreatment	4.12%	CASRGTGLYNSPLHF	2.58%	CASSQPGQGTGELFF
	4	Pretreatment	19.50%	CSADGTSGNIQYF	14.21%	CASSQGQGGGQPQHF
		Posttreatment	14.00%	CSADGTSGNIQYF	7.16%	CASSQGQGGGQPQHF
	8	Pretreatment	5.40%	CASSFLGAGAQETQYF	1.36%	CASSKRENTGELFF
		Posttreatment	5.89%	CASSFLGAGAQETQYF	4.57%	CASSKRENTGELFF
	11	Pretreatment	14.07%	CATQWGQLALHF	12.58%	CATEDGRFRQYF
		Posttreatment	7.79%	CASSEGRGANGYTF	7.08%	CASSFTAGAETQYF

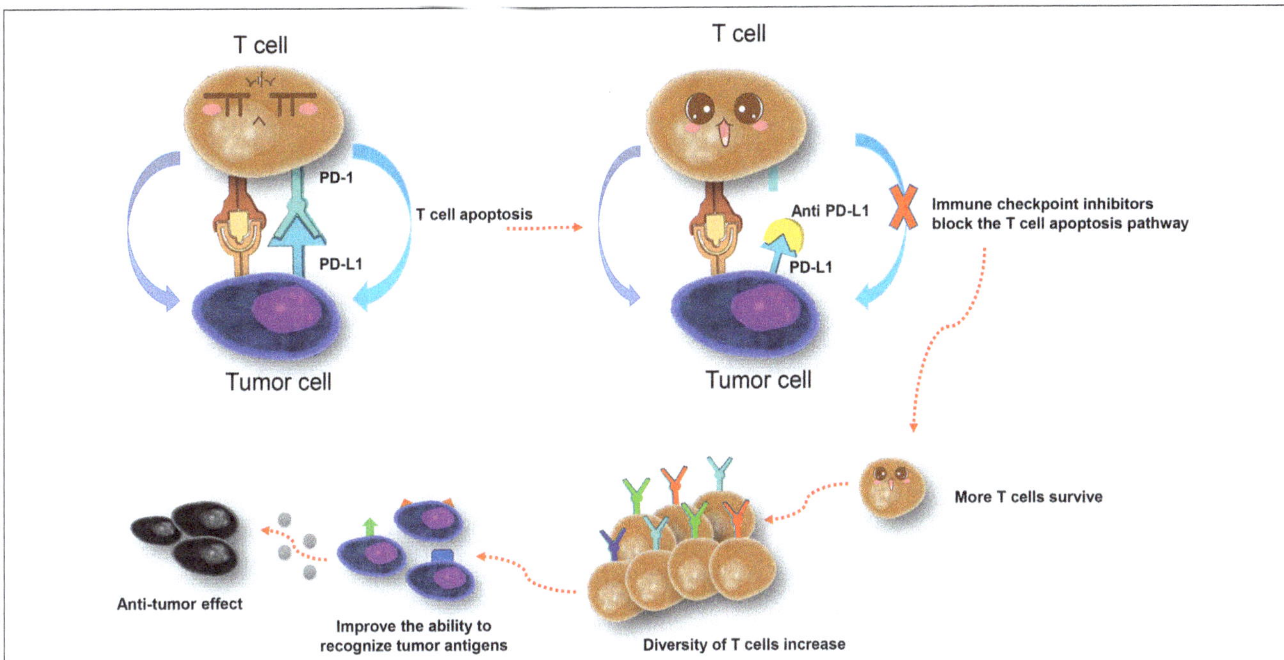

FIGURE 5 | One possible explanation of the increase of T cells and TCR repertoire diversity after PD-L1 blockade.

Targeting cancer immunity deficiency is not a single-factor control experiment; multiple factors and unknown events influence the final results of immunotherapy. Our study noticed that patients who responded to anti–PD-L1 therapy are younger than those who progressed (53.5 vs. 64.8 years, $p < 0.05$, **Supplementary Table S2**). The impact of age on the therapeutic efficacy of anti–PD-1/PD-L1 treatment is controversial, but phenotypic changes in the adaptive immune system with age certainly include less naïve T cells and more memory T cells, which result in decrease of the TCR repertoire (Nishijima et al., 2016; Daste et al., 2017; Marrone and Forde, 2017).

Several limitations of this study should be noticed. First, all of our patients were from a single institution, and the small cohort restricted the statistical power. So, we focused on describing the features of the TCR repertoire instead of making definite conclusions. Second, considering the patient's willingness and costs, the information of PD-L1 and other inhibitory receptors' expression levels were not recorded in every patient; therefore, more detailed analyses were lacking. Third, the percentage of overlap between tumor-infiltrating lymphocytes (TILs) and peripheral TCR repertoire is still in debate, but TILs are not tested. Further studies are needed to confirm whether circulating T cells can represent TILs. Finally, although we defined TCR repertoire changing patterns for early recognition of atezolizumab-sensitive patients, details of standards need large-scaled and well-organized research to confirm.

In conclusion, our study confirmed the existence of T cells with an exhaustion phenotype in Chinese advanced NSCLC patients, and TCR repertoire diversity is correlated with the efficacy of anti–PD-L1 therapy. Moreover, monitoring diversity index or patterns of reshaped TCR repertoires by effective PD-L1 blockade treatment may become the biomarkers during immunotherapy.

AUTHOR CONTRIBUTIONS

JS designed the analysis and collected the clinical follow-up data; HW contributed the data analysis, performed the data interpretation, and wrote the article; XL contributed analysis tools and performed the analysis of flow cytometry; YD, YY, and PX performed the analysis of sequencing; JS, HP, HL, and XZ collected the clinical follow-up data; WH contributed critical revision of the article; TS, HP, and YF approved the final version to be published.

REFERENCES

Blackburn, S. D., Shin, H., Freeman, G. J., and Wherry, E. J. (2008). Selective Expansion of a Subset of Exhausted CD8 T Cells by PD-L1 Blockade. *Proc. Natl. Acad. Sci.* 105, 15016–15021. doi:10.1073/pnas.0801497105

Briney, B., Inderbitzin, A., Joyce, C., and Burton, D. R. (2019). Commonality Despite Exceptional Diversity in the Baseline Human Antibody Repertoire. *Nature* 566, 393–397. doi:10.1038/s41586-019-0879-y

Britanova, O. V., Putintseva, E. V., Shugay, M., Merzlyak, E. M., Turchaninova, M. A., Staroverov, D. B., et al. (2014). Age-Related Decrease in TCR Repertoire Diversity Measured with Deep and Normalized Sequence Profiling. *J. Immunol.* 192, 2689–2698. doi:10.4049/jimmunol.1302064

Butte, M. J., Keir, M. E., Phamduy, T. B., Sharpe, A. H., and Freeman, G. J. (2007). Programmed Death-1 Ligand 1 Interacts Specifically with the B7-1 Costimulatory Molecule to Inhibit T Cell Responses. *Immunity* 27, 111–122. doi:10.1016/j.immuni.2007.05.016

Califano, R., Greystoke, A., Lal, R., Thompson, J., and Popat, S. (2017). Management of Ceritinib Therapy and Adverse Events in Patients with ALK -rearranged Non-small Cell Lung Cancer. *Lung Cancer* 111, 51–58. doi:10.1016/j.lungcan.2017.06.004

Chen, D. S., and Mellman, I. (2017). Elements of Cancer Immunity and the Cancer-Immune Set point. *Nature* 541, 321–330. doi:10.1038/nature21349

Cowell, L. G. (2020). The Diagnostic, Prognostic, and Therapeutic Potential of Adaptive Immune Receptor Repertoire Profiling in Cancer. *Cancer Res.* 80, 643–654. doi:10.1158/0008-5472.CAN-19-1457

Curiel, T. J., Wei, S., Dong, H., Alvarez, X., Cheng, P., Mottram, P., et al. (2003). Blockade of B7-H1 Improves Myeloid Dendritic Cell-Mediated Antitumor Immunity. *Nat. Med.* 9, 562–567. doi:10.1038/nm863

Curiel, T. J. (2007). Tregs and rethinking cancer immunotherapy. *J. Clin. Invest.* 117, 1167–1174. doi:10.1172/JCI31202

Daste, A., Domblides, C., Gross-goupil, M., Chakiba, C., Quivy, A., Cochin, V., et al. (2017). Immune Checkpoint Inhibitors and Elderly People: A Review. *Eur. J. Cancer* 82, 155–166. doi:10.1016/j.ejca.2017.05.044

Fridman, W. H., Zitvogel, L., Sautès–Fridman, C., and Kroemer, G. (2017). The Immune Contexture in Cancer Prognosis and Treatment. *Nat. Rev. Clin. Oncol.* 14, 717–734. doi:10.1038/nrclinonc.2017.101

Gros, A., Parkhurst, M. R., Tran, E., Pasetto, A., Robbins, P. F., Ilyas, S., et al. (2016). Prospective Identification of Neoantigen-specific Lymphocytes in the Peripheral Blood of Melanoma Patients. *Nat. Med.* 22, 433–438. doi:10.1038/nm.4051

Hida, T., Nokihara, H., Kondo, M., Kim, Y. H., Azuma, K., Seto, T., et al. (2017). Alectinib versus Crizotinib in Patients with ALK -positive Non-small-cell Lung Cancer (J-ALEX): an Open-Label, Randomised Phase 3 Trial. *The Lancet* 390, 29–39. doi:10.1016/S0140-6736(17)30565-2

Jamal-Hanjani, M., Wilson, G. A., McGranahan, N., Birkbak, N. J., Watkins, T. B. K., Veeriah, S., et al. (2017). Tracking the Evolution of Non-small-Cell Lung Cancer. *N. Engl. J. Med.* 376, 2109–2121. doi:10.1056/NEJMoa1616288

Kaplinsky, J., and Arnaout, R. (2016). Robust Estimates of Overall Immune-Repertoire Diversity from High-Throughput Measurements on Samples. *Nat. Commun.* 7, 11881. doi:10.1038/ncomms11881

Keir, M. E., Butte, M. J., Freeman, G. J., and Sharpe, A. H. (2008). PD-1 and Its Ligands in Tolerance and Immunity. *Annu. Rev. Immunol.* 26, 677–704. doi:10.1146/annurev.immunol.26.021607.090331

Kirsch, I., Vignali, M., and Robins, H. (2015). T-cell Receptor Profiling in Cancer. *Mol. Oncol.* 9, 2063–2070. doi:10.1016/j.molonc.2015.09.003

Kiura, K., Imamura, F., Kagamu, H., Matsumoto, S., Hida, T., Nakagawa, K., et al. (2018). Phase 3 Study of Ceritinib vs Chemotherapy in ALK-Rearranged NSCLC Patients Previously Treated with Chemotherapy and Crizotinib (ASCEND-5): Japanese Subset. *Jpn. J. Clin. Oncol.* 48, 367–375. doi:10.1093/jjco/hyy016

Lee, A. H., and Prins, R. M. (2016). New Applications for Deep Sequencing of the T Cell Receptor Repertoire in Cancer Patients. *Transl. Cancer Res.* 5, S842–S843. doi:10.21037/tcr.2016.10.10

Lin, H., Wei, S., Hurt, E. M., Green, M. D., Zhao, L., Vatan, L., et al. (2018). Host Expression of PD-L1 Determines Efficacy of PD-L1 Pathway Blockade-Mediated Tumor Regression. *J. Clin. Invest.* 128, 805–815. doi:10.1172/JCI96113

Liu, Y. Y., Yang, Q. F., Yang, J. S., Cao, R. B., Liang, J. Y., Liu, Y. T., et al. (2019). Characteristics and Prognostic Significance of Profiling the Peripheral Blood T-cell Receptor Repertoire in Patients with Advanced Lung Cancer. *Int. J. Cancer* 145, 1423–1431. doi:10.1002/ijc.32145

Marrone, K. A., and Forde, P. M. (2017). Cancer Immunotherapy in Older Patients. *Cancer J.* 23, 4. doi:10.1097/00130404-201707000-00005

McLane, L. M., Abdel-Hakeem, M. S., and Wherry, E. J. (2019). CD8 T Cell Exhaustion During Chronic Viral Infection and Cancer. *Annu. Rev. Immunol.* 37, 457–495. doi:10.1146/annurev-immunol-041015-055318

Nishijima, T. F., Muss, H. B., Shachar, S. S., and Moschos, S. J. (2016). Comparison of Efficacy of Immune Checkpoint Inhibitors (ICIs) between Younger and Older Patients: A Systematic Review and Meta-Analysis. *Cancer Treat. Rev.* 45, 30–37. doi:10.1016/j.ctrv.2016.02.006

Novello, S., Mazières, J., Oh, I.-J., de Castro, J., Migliorino, M. R., Helland, Å., et al. (2018). Alectinib versus Chemotherapy in Crizotinib-Pretreated Anaplastic Lymphoma Kinase (ALK)-positive Non-small-cell Lung Cancer: Results from the Phase III ALUR Study. *Ann. Oncol.* 29, 1409–1416. doi:10.1093/annonc/mdy121

Peters, S., Camidge, D. R., Shaw, A. T., Gadgeel, S., Ahn, J. S., Kim, D.-W., et al. (2017). Alectinib versus Crizotinib in Untreated ALK-Positive Non-small-Cell Lung Cancer. *N. Engl. J. Med.* 377, 829–838. doi:10.1056/NEJMoa1704795

Pielou, E. C. (1966). The Measurement of Diversity in Different Types of Biological Collections. *J. Theor. Biol.* 13, 131–144. doi:10.1016/0022-5193(66)90013-0

Ribas, A., and Wolchok, J. D. (2018). Cancer Immunotherapy Using Checkpoint Blockade. *Science* 359, 1350–1355. doi:10.1126/science.aar4060

Robert, L., Tsoi, J., Wang, X., Emerson, R., Homet, B., Chodon, T., et al. (2014). CTLA4 Blockade Broadens the Peripheral T-Cell Receptor Repertoire. *Clin. Cancer Res.* 20, 2424–2432. doi:10.1158/1078-0432.CCR-13-2648

Robins, H. S., Srivastava, S. K., Campregher, P. V., Turtle, C. J., Andriesen, J., Riddell, S. R., et al. (2010). Overlap and Effective Size of the Human CD8+ T Cell Receptor Repertoire. *Sci. Translational Med.* 2, 47ra64. doi:10.1126/scitranslmed.3001442

Schluns, K. S., Kieper, W. C., Jameson, S. C., and Lefrançois, L. (2000). Interleukin-7 Mediates the Homeostasis of Naïve and Memory CD8 T Cells *In Vivo*. *Nat. Immunol.* 1, 426–432. doi:10.1038/80868

Schrama, D., Ritter, C., and Becker, J. C. (2017). T Cell Receptor Repertoire Usage in Cancer as a Surrogate Marker for Immune Responses. *Semin. Immunopathol* 39, 255–268. doi:10.1007/s00281-016-0614-9

Siegel, R. L., Miller, K. D., and Jemal, A. (2017). Cancer statistics, 2017. *CA. Cancer J. Clin.* 67, 7–30. doi:10.3322/caac.21387

Snyder, A., Nathanson, T., Funt, S. A., Ahuja, A., Buros Novik, J., Hellmann, M. D., et al. (2017). Contribution of Systemic and Somatic Factors to Clinical Response and Resistance to PD-L1 Blockade in Urothelial Cancer: An Exploratory Multi-Omic Analysis. *PLOS Med.* 14, e1002309. doi:10.1371/journal.pmed.1002309

Sui, H., Ma, N., Wang, Y., Li, H., Liu, X., Yu, Y., et al. (2018). Anti-PD-1/PD-L1 Therapy for Non-Small Cell Lung Cancer: Toward Personalized Medicine and Combination Strategies. *J. Immunol. Res.* 2018, 1–17. doi:10.1155/2018/6984948

Swanton, C., and Govindan, R. (2016). Clinical Implications of Genomic Discoveries in Lung Cancer. *N. Engl. J. Med.* 374, 1864–1873. doi:10.1056/NEJMra1504688

Syn, N. L., Teng, M. W. L., Mok, T. S. K., and Soo, R. A. (2017). De-novo and Acquired Resistance to Immune Checkpoint Targeting. *Lancet Oncol.* 18, e731–e741. doi:10.1016/S1470-2045(17)30607-1

Taube, J. M., Anders, R. A., Young, G. D., Xu, H., Sharma, R., McMiller, T. L., et al. (2012). Colocalization of Inflammatory Response with B7-H1 Expression in Human Melanocytic Lesions Supports an Adaptive Resistance Mechanism of Immune Escape. *Sci. Translational Med.* 4, 127ra37. doi:10.1126/scitranslmed.3003689

Teng, M. W. L., Ngiow, S. F., Ribas, A., and Smyth, M. J. (2015). Classifying Cancers Based on T-Cell Infiltration and PD-L1. *Cancer Res.* 75, 2139–2145. doi:10.1158/0008-5472.CAN-15-0255

Tsui, D. W. Y., Murtaza, M., Wong, A. S. C., Rueda, O. M., Smith, C. G., Chandrananda, D., et al. (2018). Dynamics of Multiple Resistance Mechanisms in Plasma DNA during EGFR-Targeted Therapies in Non-small Cell Lung Cancer. *EMBO Mol. Med.* 10. doi:10.15252/emmm.201707945

Wang, X., Hu, Y., Liu, X., Yu, J., Xu, P., Wei, G., et al. (2019). Quantitative Characterization of T-Cell Repertoire Alteration in Chinese Patients with B-Cell Acute Lymphocyte Leukemia after CAR-T Therapy. *Bone Marrow Transpl.* 54, 2072–2080. doi:10.1038/s41409-019-0625-y

Warren, E. H., Iv, F. A. M., and Chou, J. (2013). High-throughput Sequencing of B- and T-Lymphocyte Antigen Receptors in Hematology. *Blood* 122, 5. doi:10.1182/blood-2013-03-453142

Wherry, E. J., and Kurachi, M. (2015). Molecular and Cellular Insights into T Cell Exhaustion. *Nat. Rev. Immunol.* 15, 486–499. doi:10.1038/nri3862

Wieland, A., Kamphorst, A. O., Adsay, N. V., Masor, J. J., Sarmiento, J., Nasti, T. H., et al. (2018). T Cell Receptor Sequencing of Activated CD8 T Cells in the Blood Identifies Tumor-Infiltrating Clones that Expand after PD-1 Therapy and Radiation in a Melanoma Patient. *Cancer Immunol. Immunother.* 67, 1767–1776. doi:10.1007/s00262-018-2228-7

Zarnitsyna, V. I., Evavold, B. D., Schoettle, L. N., Blattman, J. N., and Antia, R. (2013). Estimating the Diversity, Completeness, and Cross-Reactivity of the T Cell Repertoire. *Front. Immunol.* 4, 485. doi:10.3389/fimmu.2013.00485

Zhang, L., Cham, J., Paciorek, A., Trager, J., Sheikh, N., and Fong, L. (2017). 3D: Diversity, Dynamics, Differential Testing - a Proposed Pipeline for Analysis of Next-Generation Sequencing T Cell Repertoire Data. *BMC Bioinformatics* 18, 129. doi:10.1186/s12859-017-1544-9

18

Relationships Between Oral Microecosystem and Respiratory Diseases

Jiajia Dong[1†], Wei Li[2†], Qi Wang[2], Jiahao Chen[2], Yue Zu[2], Xuedong Zhou[2] and Qiang Guo[2]*

[1]Department of Pulmonary and Critical Care Medicine, West China Hospital, Sichuan University, Chengdu, China, [2]State Key Laboratory of Oral Diseases, National Clinical Research Center for Oral Diseases, West China Hospital of Stomatology, Sichuan University, Chengdu, China

***Correspondence:**
Qiang Guo
guoqiang2014@scu.edu.cn

†These authors have contributed equally to this work.

Oral microecosystem is a very complicated ecosystem that is located in the mouth and comprises oral microbiome, diverse anatomic structures of oral cavity, saliva and interactions between oral microbiota and between oral microbiota and the host. More and more evidence from studies of epidemiology, microbiology and molecular biology is establishing a significant link between oral microecosystem and respiratory diseases. Microbiota settling down in oral microecosystem is known as the main source of lung microbiome and has been associated with the occurrence and development of respiratory diseases like pneumonia, chronic obstructive pulmonary disease, lung cancer, cystic fibrosis lung disease and asthma. In fact, it is not only indigenous oral microbes promote or directly cause respiratory infection and inflammation when inhaled into the lower respiratory tract, but also internal environment of oral microecosystem serves as a reservoir for opportunistic respiratory pathogens. Moreover, poor oral health and oral diseases caused by oral microecological dysbiosis (especially periodontal disease) are related with risk of multiple respiratory diseases. Here, we review the research status on the respiratory diseases related with oral microecosystem. Potential mechanisms on how respiratory pathogens colonize oral microecosystem and the role of indigenous oral microbes in pathogenesis of respiratory diseases are also summarized and analyzed. Given the importance of oral plaque control and oral health interventions in controlling or preventing respiratory infection and diseases, we also summarize the oral health management measures and attentions, not only for populations susceptible to respiratory infection like the elderly and hospitalized patients, but also for dentist or oral hygienists who undertake oral health care. In conclusion, the relationship between respiratory diseases and oral microecosystem has been established and supported by growing body of literature. However, etiological evidence on the role of oral microecosystem in the development of respiratory diseases is still insufficient. Further detailed studies focusing on specific mechanisms on how oral microecosystem participate in the pathogenesis of respiratory diseases could be helpful to prevent and treat respiratory diseases.

Keywords: oral microecosystem, respiratory disease, respiratory pathogen, oral microorganism, dental plaque, oral health care

INTRODUCTION

Oral microecosystem is a very complicated ecosystem that is located in the mouth and comprises oral microbiome, anatomic structures of oral cavity (teeth, periodontium, tongue, oral mucosa, etc.), and saliva, in which also included interactions between oral microbiota and between oral microbiota and their hosts (Wang, 2019). As exposed to air, the mouth is in direct contact with the outside environment and is constantly challenged by microbial species present in the environment via breath and eating. The complex anatomical structure of oral cavity (as well as dental repairing materials), the presence of saliva, and other physical and chemical characteristics such as pH, oxygen content and temperature in the environment determine the organisms that settle down in oral microecosystem (Kilian, 2018). The oral microecosystem of human harbors a vast amount of highly diverse microorganisms, including bacteria, fungi, protozoa, mycoplasmas and viruses. ~700 bacterial species constitute the majority of a healthy oral microbiome and are further categorized into six major phyla by 16S rDNA profiling, viz, *Firmicutes, Actinobacteria, Proteobacteria, Fusobacteria, Bacteroidetes* and *Spirochaetes* (Verma et al., 2018). Besides, fungi (more than 100 species) also constitute the significant proportion of an oral microbiota, in which *Candida* spp. are one of the most common taxa (Seed, 2014). In oral microecosystem, microbes like bacteria and fungi attach to the tooth surface and form biofilms called dental plaques with surrounded extracellular matrix, in order to protect themselves from environmental fluctuation of oral cavity and external drug stimulations, and evade host defense mechanisms (Jhajharia et al., 2015). For the most common oral diseases, caries, the major pathogen of which is *Streptococcus mutans*, and periodontal disease, the major pathogens of which are red-complex bacteria (*Porphyromonas gingivalis, Treponema denticola and Tannerella forsythia*), dental plaques are the critical pathogenic basis (Kinane et al., 2008).

The balance of oral microecosystem not only contributes to the maintenance of oral health, but also has a potential impact on overall health. Through complicated interspecies interactions like mutualism, competition and antagonism, microbes living in oral microecosystem achieve the dynamic balance with each other, as well as with the host. However, in the condition of ecological disturbance or in occurrence of oral diseases, oral microorganisms have a chance to transfer into the circulatory system or the digestive system through oral cavity, thus affecting overall health (Hasan et al., 2014; Seedorf et al., 2014). The involvement of oral microorganisms has been observed in many diseases such as diabetes (Genco et al., 2005), bacteremia (Poveda-Roda et al., 2008), endocarditis (Parahitiyawa et al., 2009), rheumatoid arthritis (Ogrendik, 2009), atherosclerosis (Chhibber-Goel et al., 2016), preterm delivery (Teshome and Yitayeh, 2016), digestive system cancers (Seedorf et al., 2014) and other diseases.

In terms of anatomy, the oral cavity is also the gateway for the respiratory tract. In the cases of breathing with the mouth, accidentally inhaling and trachea cannula, saliva in oral microecosystem would enter the respiratory tract, and on the one hand, certain behaviors like cough could make the mucus of the respiratory tract and other substances enter the mouth, thereby achieving the mutual exchange between the oral cavity and the respiratory tract. Extensive evidence from studies of epidemiology, microbiology and molecular biology has established a significant link between oral microbes, dental plaque, oral health, oral diseases and respiratory diseases. Oral microbiota is known as the main source of lung microbiome (Bassis et al., 2015; Pragman et al., 2018; Maddi et al., 2019). Microbes indigenous to oral microecosystem are likely to be inhaled into lower respiratory tract (Tunney et al., 2008; Worlitzsch et al., 2009; Yamasaki et al., 2013; Tan et al., 2014; Coburn et al., 2015; Yan et al., 2015; Wu et al., 2017; Muhlebach MS. et al., 2018), and may infect the lung and trachea by pathogenic virulence factors or change respiratory mucosal microenvironment conducive to the colonization of respiratory pathogens. Besides, the diverse environment inside oral microecosystem could provide latent sites for the lodging of common respiratory pathogens (Sumi et al., 2007; Heo et al., 2008; Bensel et al., 2010; Tan et al., 2014; Rivas Caldas et al., 2015; To et al., 2020), which could further invade the respiratory tract and cause diseases under the condition of low host resistance. Many studies have observed an association between oral health, oral diseases and risk of respiratory diseases like pneumonia, chronic obstructive pulmonary disease (COPD) and lung cancer (Bágyi et al., 2006; Awano et al., 2008; Prasanna, 2011; Zeng et al., 2012; Yamasaki et al., 2013; Chrysanthakopoulos, 2016; Zeng et al., 2016; Qian et al., 2020). Therefore, it is pretty critical to understand the role of oral microecosystem in pathogenesis of respiratory diseases, which would contribute to the prevention and treatment of respiratory diseases.

Here, we review and analyze the research status on the respiratory diseases related with oral microecosystem and potential mechanisms on how respiratory pathogens colonize oral microecosystem and how indigenous oral microbes participate in pathogenesis of respiratory diseases. Oral health management strategies maintaining oral hygiene and oral microbiome symbiosis are also summarized to guide oral care interventions on populations susceptible to respiratory infection like the elderly and hospitalized patients and reduce their incidence of respiratory diseases.

THE RESPIRATORY DISEASES ASSOCIATED WITH ORAL MICROECOSYSTEM

Increasing evidence has linked oral microecosystem, as well as oral health and oral diseases, with respiratory diseases mainly pneumonia, COPD, lung cancer, cystic fibrosis (CF) lung disease and asthma (**Table 1**). Primary respiratory pathogens could be found in dental plaques, periodontal pockets and saliva, suggesting that oral microecosystem is a potential source of the respiratory infection and diseases (Sumi et al., 2007; Heo et al., 2008; Bensel et al., 2010; Tan et al., 2014; Rivas Caldas et al., 2015; To et al., 2020). On the other hand, the presence of orally derived bacteria in sputum and bronchoalveolar lavage (BAL) fluid have been observed by many studies (Tunney et al., 2008;

TABLE 1 | The relationship of oral microbes, oral infection and disease, oral health (care) with respiratory diseases.

Respiratory diseases	Oral microbes	Oral infection and disease	Oral health (care)	Respiratory pathogens detected in oral microecosystem
Pneumonia	BAL specimens (CAP patients): oral *streptococci*, *Neisseria* spp. and anaerobes (*Prevotella* spp., *Fusobacterium* spp., *Veillonella* spp., and *Clostridium* spp.) Yamasaki et al. (2013)	Dental infection as a risk factor for pneumonia Laurence et al. (2015)	Professional oral care reduces AP risk Quagliarello et al. (2005); Chebib et al. (2018); Khadka et al. (2021)	Pneumonia pathogens in dental plaques (dependent elderly): *S. pneumoniae*, *H. influenzae* and *K. pneumoniae* Sumi et al. (2007)
	Saliva bacteria counts as a risk factor for AP Kikutani et al. (2015); Nishizawa et al. (2019)	Periodontal disease as a risk factor for CAP Bágyi et al. (2006); Awano et al. (2008); Yamasaki et al. (2013)	Brushing teeth helps control the pneumopathogens (*staphylococci*, Enterobacteriaceae and yeasts) in resting saliva and reduce VAP risk Cecon et al. (2010); Stonecypher (2010) An increase in oral care frequency significantly reduces the NV-HAP incidence rate Giuliano et al. (2021) Preoperative oral hygiene interventions such as dental brushing and professional oral plaque control reduce incidence of POP Akutsu et al. (2010); Gonzalez-Rubio Aguilar et al. (2019); Jia et al. (2020) The elderly who wear denture during sleep are more likely to have tongue and denture plaque, gum inflammation, positive culture for *C. albicans*, higher levels of circulating IL-6, and an increased risk for incident pneumonia Iinuma et al. (2015)	VAP pathogens in dental plaques (VAP patients): *S. aureus*, *P. aeruginosa*, *Acinetobacter* species, and enteric species Heo et al. (2008) Saliva (COVID-19 patients): SARS-CoV-2 To et al. (2020)
CF lung disease	Sputum and BAL specimens (CF patients): oral anaerobic bacteria Tunney et al. (2008); Worlitzsch et al. (2009); Coburn et al. (2015); Muhlebach et al. (2018a) Lower respiratory tract is dominated by oral microbiome (CF children at age 2) Muhlebach et al. (2018b)	NA	NA	Periodontal pockets (CF patients): *P. aeruginosa, S. aureus* Bensel et al. (2010) Saliva and subgingival plaques (CF patients): *P. aeruginosa* Rivas Caldas et al. (2015)
COPD	Tracheal aspirate specimens (COPD patients with severe acute exacerbations): *P. gingivalis, Treponema denticola. Tannerella forsythia, A. actinomycetemcomitans* and *Capnocytophaga sputigena* Tan et al. (2014) Lung tissues specimens (mild-moderate COPD patients): the sources of the lung tissue microbiota were 21.1% (mean) oral microbiota, 8.7% nasal microbiota, and 70.1% unknown Pragman et al. (2018) Six genera and 15 species in subgingival plaques may be associated to COPD, especially the genera *Dysgonomonas, Desulfobulbus* and *Catonella* with much higher proportions (COPD patients) Wu et al. (2017)	Periodontal disease as a risk factor for COPD Prasanna (2011); Zeng et al. (2012); Qian et al. (2020)	Periodontal therapy reduces the frequency of the exacerbation of COPD Kucukcoskun et al. (2013); Zhou et al. (2014) COPD patients have significant fewer teeth, higher plaque index, poorer periodontal status and poorer oral health knowledge and behaviors, Wang et al. (2009); Gaeckle et al. (2018); Zhou et al. (2020)	Lung pathogens in subgingival plaque (COPD patients with severe acute exacerbations): *Acinetobacter baumannii, K. pneumoniae, P. aeruginosa* and *S. pneumoniae* Tan et al. (2014)
Asthma	A stronger shift in dental biofilm microbiome compared to healthy controls, with 14 different taxa (children	NA	NA	NA

(Continued on following page)

TABLE 1 | *(Continued)* The relationship of oral microbes, oral infection and disease, oral health (care) with respiratory diseases.

Respiratory diseases	Oral microbes	Oral infection and disease	Oral health (care)	Respiratory pathogens detected in oral microecosystem
	with allergic asthma) Arweiler et al. (2021)			
Lung cancer	Significant changes in saliva microbiome which are indicated by the significant increase of *Capnocytophaga* and *Veillonella* (lung cancer patients with SCC or AC) Yan et al. (2015) Lower microbial diversity and richness of salivary microbiome (non-smoking lung cancer patients) Yang et al. (2018); Hosgood et al. (2021) Salivary microbiome is related to cancer pathways, p53 signaling pathway, apoptosis and tuberculosis (non-smoking lung cancer patients) Yang et al. (2018)	Periodontal disease as a risk factor for lung cancer Chrysanthakopoulos (2016); Zeng et al. (2016)	NA	NA

BAL, bronchoalveolar lavage; CAP, community-acquired pneumonia; AP, aspiration pneumonia; VAP, ventilator-associated pneumonia; NV-HAP, nonventilator hospital-acquired pneumonia; POP, postoperative pneumonia; COVID-19, coronavirus disease 2019; SARS-CoV-2, severe acute respiratory syndrome coronavirus 2; CF, cystic fibrosis; NA, not applicable; COPD, chronic obstructive pulmonary disease; SCC, small cell carcinoma; AC, adenocarcinoma.

Worlitzsch et al., 2009; Yamasaki et al., 2013; Tan et al., 2014; Coburn et al., 2015; Yan et al., 2015; Wu et al., 2017; Muhlebach MS. et al., 2018). Oral diseases driven by dysbiosis of oral microecosystem, typically, periodontal disease (Bágyi et al., 2006; Awano et al., 2008; Prasanna, 2011; Zeng et al., 2012; Yamasaki et al., 2013; Chrysanthakopoulos, 2016; Zeng et al., 2016; Qian et al., 2020), and poor oral health status (Wang et al., 2009; Iinuma et al., 2015; Gaeckle et al., 2018; Zhou et al., 2020) are recognized as risk factors for the occurrence and progression of many respiratory diseases.

Infectious Pulmonary Diseases

Pneumonia

Pneumonia is a very common infection that inflames the air sacs in one or both lungs. Dental plaques are known to be a reservoir for common respiratory pathogens responsible for pneumonia (Sumi et al., 2007). Community-acquired pneumonia (CAP) occurs outside of hospitals or other health care facilities and the most commonly identified bacterial pathogens of CAP could be detected in dental plaques, including *Streptococcus pneumoniae (S. pneumoniae), Haemophilus influenzae* and *Klebsiella pneumoniae* (Sumi et al., 2007). In an etiology study of CAP, high rates of oral *streptococci* and anaerobes were found in the BAL specimens of CAP patients (Yamasaki et al., 2013). The level of periodontal disease has a significant association with the mortality of pneumonia and the anaerobic bacteria from the dental plaques of patients with periodontal disease could be causative agents of CAP (Bágyi et al., 2006; Awano et al., 2008; Yamasaki et al., 2013). Thus, it is suggested by a study that the presence of dental infections may worsen the symptoms of the patients who made a visit to the emergency departments because of pneumonia and increase the chance to be hospitalized (Laurence et al., 2015). In contrast to CAP, hospital-acquired pneumonia (HAP), which include ventilator-associated pneumonia (VAP) and healthcare-associated pneumonia (HCAP), refers in particular to pneumonia occurs in hospitals (including rehabilitation hospitals, nursing homes for the elderly, etc.). The pathogenic microbial spectrum of HAP contains gram-positive cocci, such as *Staphylococcus aureus (S. aureus)* and *S. pneumoniae*, but more gram-negative bacteria, such as *Pseudomonas aeruginosa, K. pneumoniae, enterococci* and *Enterobacter* spp. (Miyashita et al., 2005; Cilloniz et al., 2011; Koulenti et al., 2017; Leone et al., 2018). The increasing of dental plaque is also related to the incidence of nosocomial infections of the patients in the intensive care units (ICUs) (Fourrier et al., 1998). With the aid of the molecular methods, respiratory pathogens of VAP that are isolated from dental plaque and BAL fluid from patients in ICU are found to be genetically related (Heo et al., 2008). As a form of HCAP, aspiration pneumonia increases the mortality especially in old-age people (Feng et al., 2019). Oral bacteria are recognized as a source of infection for aspiration pneumonia and oral bacteria counts are a risk factor for aspiration pneumonia (Kikutani et al., 2015; Nishizawa et al., 2019). The observation that aspiration pneumonia occurred less in older people who received professional oral care compared with no such care, indicates the importance of oral health in reducing aspiration pneumonia risk (Quagliarello et al., 2005; Chebib et al., 2018; Khadka et al., 2021).

More and more researchers are focusing on viral pneumonia, especially in the context of the current pandemic of Coronavirus disease 2019 (COVID-19), which is caused by severe acute respiratory syndrome coronavirus 2 (SARS-CoV-2). The association of COVID-19 with oral microecosystem is becoming clear. Saliva has been shown to contain infective viral loads, indicating not only its role in SARS-CoV-2 transmission but also its diagnostic value for viral RNA testing as a more easily obtainable sample (To et al., 2020; Imai and

Tanaka, 2021). The finding that angiotensin-converting enzyme II, the main host cell receptor of SARS-CoV-2, is widely expressed in salivary glands, tongue and mucosa of oral cavity (Chen et al., 2020; Xu et al., 2020), also correlates oral microecosystem with the infection and transmission of SARS-CoV-2.

CF Lung Disease

CF lung disease is characterized by persistent airway infection with complex microbial communities which often consist of pathogens, including *S. aureus, H. influenzae* and *P. aeruginosa,* and endogenous microorganisms typically associated with the oral cavity (Salsgiver et al., 2016; Muhlebach M. S. et al., 2018). Oral microecosystem provides the habitats for the colonization of pathogens of CF lung disease. Identical facultative and obligate anaerobic strains, including *P. aeruginosa and S. aureus,* are found in CF periodontal pockets and sputum samples, suggesting that periodontal pockets is a potential source of the respiratory infection for CF patients (Bensel et al., 2010). The study of Caldas et al. also demonstrated that the primary CF pathogen *P. aeruginosa* is detected not only in the sputum samples of CF patients, but also in their saliva and subgingival plaque samples, with clonal relatedness (Rivas Caldas et al., 2015). The presence of orally derived anaerobic bacteria in sputum and BAL fluid from CF patients have been observed by many studies (Tunney et al., 2008; Worlitzsch et al., 2009; Coburn et al., 2015; Muhlebach MS. et al., 2018). Recently, a study on succession of the CF lung microbiome in early life further revealed the role of oral bacteria on the pathophysiology of CF lung disease. It was found that CF infants had relatively sterile lower airways with a progressive shift to a microbiome dominated by aerobic and anaerobic bacteria commonly associated with the oral cavity at age two, which was correlated with a significant increase in bacterial density and inflammation, and the lung microbiome was dominated by pathogens in the majority of CF children older than four, which was associated with a further increase in inflammation and the onset of structural lung disease (Muhlebach M. S. et al., 2018). These findings suggest that oral microbes may be associated with the progression of early CF lung disease and could potentially predispose subjects to subsequent infection by pathogens (Muhlebach M. S. et al., 2018). Considering the correlation between oral bacteria and CF lung disease, the impact of oral bacteria-driven diseases especially periodontal disease, as well as the oral health management measures, on the development of CF lung disease should be further investigated.

Obstructive Pulmonary Diseases

COPD

COPD is a chronic inflammatory lung disease that causes obstructed airflow from the lungs. Metagenomic analysis shows that both periodontal pathogens (the red-complex bacteria, *Aggregatibacter actinomycetemcomitans* and *Capnocytophaga sputigena*) and lung pathogens (*Acinetobacter baumannii, K. pneumoniae, P. aeruginosa* and *S. pneumoniae*) are present in subgingival plaque biofilm and tracheal aspirate of patients with severe acute exacerbations of COPD (Tan et al., 2014), indicating that not only oral microecosystem is a reservoir of respiratory pathogens but also periodontal pathogens may contribute to the pathology of COPD. The study of Wu et al. found that six genera and 15 species in subgingival plaques might be associated to COPD, among which the genera *Dysgonomonas, Desulfobulbus* and *Catonella* showed much higher proportions in COPD patients (Wu et al., 2017). To get rid of interference of upper airway microbes, a recent study surgically obtained the mild-moderate COPD lung tissues and found that the sources of the lung tissue microbiota were 21.1% (mean) oral microbiota, 8.7% nasal microbiota, and 70.1% unknown (Pragman et al., 2018). The association between oral disease and the incidence of COPD have been proved by many studies and periodontal disease is a significant risk factor for COPD (Prasanna, 2011; Zeng et al., 2012). A most recent study by Qian et al. provides substantial evidence that risks for COPD mortality increased significantly with increasing severity of periodontitis in the elderly (Qian et al., 2020). Moreover, the periodontal therapy could help COPD patients reduce the frequency of the exacerbation (Kucukcoskun et al., 2013; Zhou et al., 2014). The observations that compared with controls with normal pulmonary function, patients with COPD have significant fewer teeth, higher plaque index, poorer periodontal status and poorer oral health knowledge and behaviors, highlight the importance of oral health care and oral health knowledge in the prevention and treatment of COPD (Wang et al., 2009; Zhou et al., 2020).

Asthma

Asthma is a chronic respiratory disease involving intermittent wheezing and airway inflammation. Although there are numerous risk factors to trigger an asthma attack or exacerbate symptoms, the main risk factor is proposed to be a hereditary predisposition to allergic inflammation of the bronchial tree that develops in response to respiratory allergens (Cherkasov et al., 2019). The hygiene hypothesis contends that fewer opportunities for infections and microbial exposures contribute to the prevalence of asthma and other allergic diseases. Consistent with the hygiene hypothesis, the high serum level of immunoglobulin G (IgG) antibodies to *P. gingivalis* corresponded with the low prevalence of asthma and it was concluded that colonization of the oral cavity by bacteria and other microbes might play a protective role in the etiology of allergic disease (Arbes et al., 2006). In fact, there are only few reports regarding the relationship between oral microbes and asthma or other allergic diseases and the few clinical findings are controversially discussed (Arweiler et al., 2021). Most recently, Arweiler et al. for the first time reported the contribution of dental biofilm to allergic health or disease. Through analysis of dental biofilm microbiome by a 16s-rRNA gene-based next-generation sequencing, it was observed that children with allergic asthma showed a stronger microbial shift compared to healthy controls, with 14 different taxa, suggesting a correlation between allergic asthma and oral bacteria (Arweiler et al., 2021). Several studies report that asthmatics presented with greater risk for caries development, worse gingival health, as well as disorders of salivary flow, composition and pH (Stensson et al., 2008; Mehta et al., 2009; Arafa et al., 2017). However, there is no clear evidence clarifying the role of oral health status, oral diseases and specific oral pathogens on the pathophysiology of asthma. Thus, further in-depth studies on the association of asthma with oral microecosystem become necessary.

Lung Cancers

Lung cancer is one of the most common types of cancer, with the leading cancer mortality worldwide. Besides chemical carcinogens, bacterial and viral infections are involved in the development of lung cancer. It has been verified that the microbial factors may participate in the tumorigenesis of the lung cancer through production of bacteriotoxins and other proinflammatory factors (Littman et al., 2004; Moghaddam et al., 2011; Kovaleva et al., 2019). The lung has a distinct microbiome which may influence the development of lung cancer and more and more evidence suggests that oral microbiome is one of the main sources of lung microbiome (Maddi et al., 2019). Yan et al. for the first time demonstrated the association of saliva microbiota with lung cancer. It was observed that the saliva microbiome in lung cancer patients with small cell carcinoma or adenocarcinoma had significant changes compared to the controls, which was indicated by the significant increase of *Capnocytophaga* and *Veillonella* (Yan et al., 2015). Variations in oral microbiome have been associated with future risk of lung cancer among never-smokers. Lower microbial diversity and richness of salivary microbiota are found in non-smoking lung cancer patients and the abundance of certain specific taxa is associated with altered risk (Yang et al., 2018; Hosgood et al., 2021). More specifically, a greater abundance of the *Bacilli* class and *Lactobacillales* order in saliva was associated with an increased risk of lung cancer, while a greater abundance of *Spirochaetia* and *Bacteroidetes* in saliva was associated with a decreased risk of lung cancer (Hosgood et al., 2021). Furthermore, functional analysis indicates that salivary microbiome in non-smoking female lung cancer patients is related to cancer pathways, p53 signaling pathway, apoptosis and tuberculosis (Yang et al., 2018). The relevance of periodontal disease with lung cancer are also reported. A meta-analysis of cohort studies showed that patients with periodontal disease were at increased risk of developing lung cancer (Zeng et al., 2016). In addition, the association of periodontal disease indices, including probing pocket depth, clinical attachment loss and bleeding on probing, with the risk of lung cancer is demonstrated (Chrysanthakopoulos, 2016). Oral care intervention may have their roles in the prevention and treatment of lung cancer, but relevant research is needed to provide evidence.

COLONIZATION OF RESPIRATORY PATHOGENS IN ORAL MICROECOSYSTEM

Oral microecosystem is an important reservoir for respiratory pathogens. Various respiratory pathogens have been detected in dental plaques, periodontal pockets and saliva, including *S. pneumoniae*, *K. pneumoniae*, *S. aureus*, *P. aeruginosa*, *H. influenzae*, *Haemophilus parainfluenzae*, *Enterobacte cloacae*, *Proteus mirabilis*, *Escherichia coli*, *Acinetobacter species* and SARS-CoV-2 (Sumi et al., 2007; Heo et al., 2008; Bensel et al., 2010; Tan et al., 2014; Rivas Caldas et al., 2015; To et al., 2020). Colonization of the oral microecosystem by respiratory pathogens lays a foundation for subsequent invasion and infection by these pathogens in the lower respiratory tract while the body's immune system is weakened. Both the biological characteristics of respiratory pathogens and perturbations in oral microecosystem contribute to the adaptation and colonization of respiratory pathogens in oral microecosystem.

Adaptation of Respiratory Pathogens to Oral Environment

When exposed to invading pathogens, oral cavity releases reactive oxygen species (ROS) and nitric oxide (NO) from neutrophils and macrophages infiltrating, which are toxic metabolites to some bacteria due to the oxidative stress they elicit (Sato et al., 2008). However, pathogens such as *K. pneumoniae* and *S. aureus* develop hydrogen (H_2) generation to against oxidative environments in the human oral cavity (Kanazuru et al., 2010). *P. aeruginosa* is found to be killed by hydrogen peroxide (H_2O_2)-producing oral commensal *streptococci* in a nitrite-dependent manner through the production of reactive nitrogenous species (RNS) (Scoffield and Wu, 2015). The observation that the *P. aeruginosa* strain defective in the production of nitrite reductase, which is responsible for catalyzing the reduction of nitrite to NO, showed a reduced survival rate when co-cultured with oral commensal *Streptococcus parasanguinis* (Scoffield and Wu, 2016), suggests that nitrite reductase could play an important role in the interspecies interaction with oral microbes and the survival of *P. aeruginosa* in oral microecosystem. In addition to toxic metabolites from oral cavity, common oral antibacterial agents like chlorhexidine (CHX) are also challenge for respiratory pathogens. Nevertheless, it has been observed the adaptation of clinical *K. pneumoniae* isolates to CHX exposure, which is associated with mutations in the two-component regulator *phoPQ* and a putative Tet repressor gene *(smvR)*, could lead to not only stable resistance to CHX, but also cross-resistance to colistin (Wand et al., 2017). Duman et al. further demonstrated decreased susceptibility to the complement-mediated serum killing within the CHX adapted strain of *K. pneumoniae*, as well as increased efflux pump expression (*cepA and kdeA*) (Duman et al., 2019).

Given that oral microecosystem is a complex and open environment with saliva flow and other flowing liquids from the diet, adherence is an essential step in oral colonization and subsequent respiratory infection by a respiratory pathogen. Respiratory pathogens have developed some characteristics to facilitate their adherence capacity in oral cavity. Merghni et al. found that within the twenty-one *S. aureus* strains that were isolated from the oral cavity and detected the presence of adhesins, 76.2% of strains were *icaA* and *icaD* (encoding polysaccharide intercellular adhesins) positive and 90.5% harbored both the *fnbA* and *fnbB* genes encoding fibronectin-binding proteins. Besides, the *cna* gene encoding a collagen-binding protein and *hla* gene encoding α-toxin were found in 57.2 and 52.4% of the isolates, respectively, which both play an important role in the pathogenesis of staphylococcal diseases (Merghni et al., 2015). Moreover, Wang et al. reported that *S. aureus* could activate the COX-2/PGE2 pathway in oral epithelial cell and subsequently facilitate the growth and adherence of the pathogen (Wang et al., 2017). Proteins in human saliva could modulate bacterial colonization of the oral cavity. The study of Thamadilok et al. revealed that unencapsulated *S. pneumoniae* was able to bind to low molecular-weight salivary mucin-7, presumably through a glycan-mediated mechanism which could further mediate its adherence to saliva-covered surfaces in the oral cavity (Thamadilok et al., 2016).

Interactions of Respiratory Pathogens With Oral Microbes Facilitate Formation of Dental Plaque

Several respiratory pathogens are reported to interact with indigenous oral bacteria. Certain interspecies interactions like coaggregation would promote the formation of dental plaque biofilm. Compared with planktonically grown counterparts, microbes growing within biofilms often exhibit increased resistance to antimicrobial compounds and innate immune mechanisms. Thus, the participation of respiratory pathogens in formation of dental plaque would contribute to their oral colonization and subsequent respiratory infection. Komiyama et al. studied the interbacterial interaction between strains of *P. aeruginosa* and strains of indigenous oral bacteria, both of which were isolated from the oral cavity of CF patients, and observed coaggregation reactions between oral bacteria (*Streptococcus sanguis, Streptococcus mitis, Actinomyces naeslundii and Actinomyces viscosus*) and both the mucoid and nonmucoid variants of *P. aeruginosa* (Komiyama et al., 1987). These findings suggest that the diverse interbacterial interactions with indigenous oral bacteria may contribute to the oral colonization of *P. aeruginosa* in CF patients and affect the course and pathogenesis of CF. *S. aureus* is also reported to coaggregate with indigenous oral bacteria like *Streptococcus* spp., *A. naeslundii, A. viscosus, P. gingivalis and Fusobacterium nucleatum* (Kamaguchi et al., 2003). Further analysis of the interaction between *F. nucleatum* and *S. aureus* revealed that the outer-membrane adhesin RadD of *F. nucleatum* might partially participate in aggregation and increase the expression of the staphylococcal global regulator gene *sarA* (Lima et al., 2019). It is interesting to note that colonization of *S. aureus* also benefits other respiratory pathogens, since an interaction between the SpA protein secreted by *S. aureus* and the *P. aeruginosa* exopolysaccharide Psl has been identified, which causes aggregation of bacterial cells that leaves them resistant to tobramicin (Beaudoin et al., 2017). Complex communication and interaction within dental plaque biofilm also create a condition for further progression of virulence of pathogens. For example, *nanA*, a virulence determinant of *S. pneumoniae* that is important for colonization and infection, could be evolved by recombination of the pathogen with oral *streptococci* (King et al., 2005).

Perturbation in Oral Microecosystem Favor Colonization of Respiratory Pathogens

Disturbance of Oral Microecology

Normal oral microbiota plays important roles in preventing the invasion of pathogenic bacteria like *P. aeruginosa*, which is showed to fail to integrate into salivary microbial community when co-cultivated in saliva medium and whose growth is inhibited by the oral microflora via producing lactic acid (He et al., 2011). However, disturbance of oral microecology gives opportunistic respiratory pathogens chances to invade and colonize. It has widely reported that oral microbial dysbiosis or changes in oral microecosystem, such as the progression of periodontitis and denture stomatitis or the presence of dentures, promote oral colonization by *S. aureus, P. aeruginosa, Enterococcus faecalis* and *Acinetobacter* spp. and may favor the spread of more pathogenic strains (Baena-Monroy et al., 2005; Passariello et al., 2012; Colombo et al., 2013; Souto et al., 2014). Moreover, smoking is found to benefit early acquisition and colonization of respiratory pathogens including *Haemophilus* and *Pseudomonas* in dental plaque biofilms (Kumar et al., 2011).

One potential mechanism is that in the condition of oral microflora dysbiosis, the increase of some oral pathogens enhance their interaction with certain respiratory pathogens, as aforementioned, and further facilitate the oral colonization of these non-indigenous pathogens. Another mechanism could refer to the decrease of oral commensal bacteria, the function of which is to inhibit the invasion and colonization of external microorganism as well as to maintain balance of oral microecology (Tada and Hanada, 2010). Plenty of oral commensal bacteria are found to exhibit antagonistic effects against respiratory pathogens. The majority of oral *lactobacilli* strains are reported to suppress the growth of common respiratory pathogens including *S. pneumoniae, P. aeruginosa,* as well as clinical isolates of Methicillin-resistant *staphylococcus aureus* (MRSA) (Busarcevic et al., 2008; Sikorska and Smoragiewicz, 2013; Alexandre et al., 2014; Mahdi et al., 2019). Take *Lactobacillus salivarius* for example, studies revealed that it could produce LS1 against the growth of *S. aureus* and *S. pneumoniae*, and salivaricin LHM against the activity of *P. aeruginosa* (Busarcevic et al., 2008; Mahdi et al., 2019). *Streptococci* are another main source of oral commensal bacteria to antagonize respiratory pathogens, particularly *Streptococcus salivarius,* which produces a variety of bacteriocins antagonizing *S. pneumoniae* (Tagg, 2004) and *Streptococcus pyogenes* (Walls et al., 2003; Tagg, 2009; Wescombe et al., 2009; Santagati et al., 2012), and block the adherence sites to reduce *S. pneumoniae* colonization (Manning et al., 2016).

Impairment of Oral Immunity

Oral immune system functions as the foremost barrier and defense against pathogens, which depends on efficient function of oral mucosa, salivary glands and saliva, and gingival crevice. Saliva plays a key role in host defense against invading respiratory pathogens via antibody production (Aanaes et al., 2013; Mauch et al., 2017), blocking oral adherence (Lerrer et al., 2005), bacteriostatic or bactericidal activities (Geetha et al., 2003; Prokopovic et al., 2014), interfering with their interactions with oral bacteria

(Komiyama and Gibbons, 1984). Internal and external factors such as aging, dysplasia, disease progression and treatment which influence salivary function or oral immunity have potential impacts on oral colonization of respiratory pathogens. Oral radiotherapy and chemotherapy, except for direct mucosal damage, both lead to decreased salivary flow and increased colonization of opportunistic pathogens such as *S. aureus* and *Candida* (Main et al., 1984; Jain et al., 2016). Natural aging, parotid and submandibular salivary gland aplasia or agenesis, medication (including anticholinergic drugs, diuretics, alpha-adrenergic agents, and antihypertensive agents) are able to change the saliva composition or affect the secretion or flow rate of saliva, and subsequently result in dry mouth and poor oral hygiene (Mathews et al., 2008), which may cause shifts form the normal oral microflora to a community that harbors a higher number of pathogens (Scannapieco, 1999).

What is noteworthy is that immunocompromise and general immunodepression also raise the risk of oral colonization by potential respiratory pathogens. Higher level of *S. aureus* in oral cavity of the elderly and institutionalized individuals was reported, including hospitalized and nursing home patients (Scannapieco et al., 1992; Tada and Hanada, 2010). Diaz et al. also found a higher prevalence of potentially opportunistic *Gammaproteobacteria* including *K. pneumoniae, Pseudomonas fluorescens, Acinetobacter* species, *Vibrio* species, *Enterobacteriaceae* species, *Staphylococcus* species, and *Enterococcus* species in the salivary bacterial microbiome of transplant recipients who were constantly on pharmacological immunosuppression (Diaz et al., 2013).

PARTICIPATION OF INDIGENOUS ORAL MICROBES IN PATHOGENESIS OF RESPIRATORY DISEASES

The presence of oral microbes with high detectable rates in sputum and BAL specimens of patients with multiple respiratory diseases suggests a potential association of oral microbes with respiratory diseases, including oral *streptococci, Neisseria* spp. and anaerobes (*P. gingivalis, Treponema denticola. Tannerella forsythia, A. actinomycetemcomitans, Capnocytophaga sputigena, Prevotella* spp., *Fusobacterium* spp., *Veillonella* spp., and *Clostridium* spp.) (Tunney et al., 2008; Worlitzsch et al., 2009; Yamasaki et al., 2013; Tan et al., 2014; Coburn et al., 2015; Yan et al., 2015; Wu et al., 2017; Muhlebach MS. et al., 2018) In fact, common oral microbes such as *P. gingivalis, F. nucleatum, A. actinomycetemcomitans and* oral *streptococci* have been reported to be involved in the pathogenesis of respiratory diseases (Petelin et al., 2004; Pan et al., 2009; Nagaoka et al., 2013; Yamasaki et al., 2013; Whiley et al., 2014; Hayata et al., 2019). Various mechanisms have been developed to help explain how indigenous oral microorganisms may participate in the occurrence and development of respiratory diseases, based on the understanding of their virulence factors or their effects on pathogenicity of respiratory pathogens.

Oral Microbes Inhaled Into the Lower Respiratory Tract Cause Infection and Regulate Immune Responses

Oral microbiome is one of the primary sources of respiratory infection and indigenous oral microbes in dental plaques, periodontal pockets or saliva could be inhaled into the lower respiratory tract to cause or aggravate respiratory infections and diseases such as aspiration pneumonia and COPD. The pathogenicity of oral microorganisms invading the lower respiratory tract is involved in different mechanisms, within which the critical one is the immunoregulation on respiratory system, including T-helper 1 (Th1) and T-helper 2 (Th2) immune responses. Regulation of the Th1/Th2 balance is a typical way by which infections of microbes influence the host immune response (Schaub et al., 2006). Effects of oral microbes on inflammatory process have been widely reported, which is characterized by Th1 immune response. The data of Scannapieco et al. revealed the potential effect of oral bacteria on inducing the release of proinflammatory cytokines from epithelial cell lines to an extent similar to that seen for respiratory pathogens (Scannapieco et al., 2001). Significantly increased production of soluble TNF receptors, TNF-α, IL-1β and IL-6 are also observed in *P. gingivalis*-infected pneumonia model (Petelin et al., 2004) (**Figure 1**). Recently, it was showed that some periodontopathic bacteria, especially *F. nucleatum*, strongly induced IL-6 and IL-8 production by bronchial epithelial cells, which might trigger exacerbation of COPD (Hayata et al., 2019) (**Figure 1**).

In addition of inflammatory reactions, oral microbes are observed to impact allergy reactions. The first direct evidence on regulatory effects of oral pathogens on allergic airway inflammation and responsiveness was reported by Card et al. Their study underlined the temporal importance of the establishment of infection since *P. gingivalis* infection established before ovalbumin (OVA) sensitization reduced airway levels of Th2 cytokines (IL-4, IL-5, IL-13) and granulocyte-macrophage colony-stimulating factor, and decreased histological inflammation, without the alteration of serum levels of OVA-specific immunoglobulin E (IgE) and airway responsiveness. Conversely, a subcutaneous infection with *P. gingivalis* initiated after allergen sensitization did not alter inflammatory end points but did reduce airway responsiveness in spite of increased serum IgE levels (Card et al., 2010). Card et al. observed a reduction of the inflammatory migrated cells in the BAL fluid (eosinophils, lymphocytes, macrophages), as well as the levels of the IL-4 and tumor necrosis factor (TNF)-α cytokines, in mice with asthma and periodontitis, accompanied by a decreased mucus production (Card et al., 2010). Oral microbes also have the capacity to induce Th2 immune responses. Some studies reported that *Candida albicans*, an opportunistic pathogen that colonizes oral cavity, and its extract were able to induce IL-5 production by Th2 cells which is related with eosinophilic airway inflammation (Kimura et al., 1999; Mori et al., 2001) (**Figure 1**).

Apoptosis, which plays an important role in immune response and tumorigenesis, is also proposed to be affected

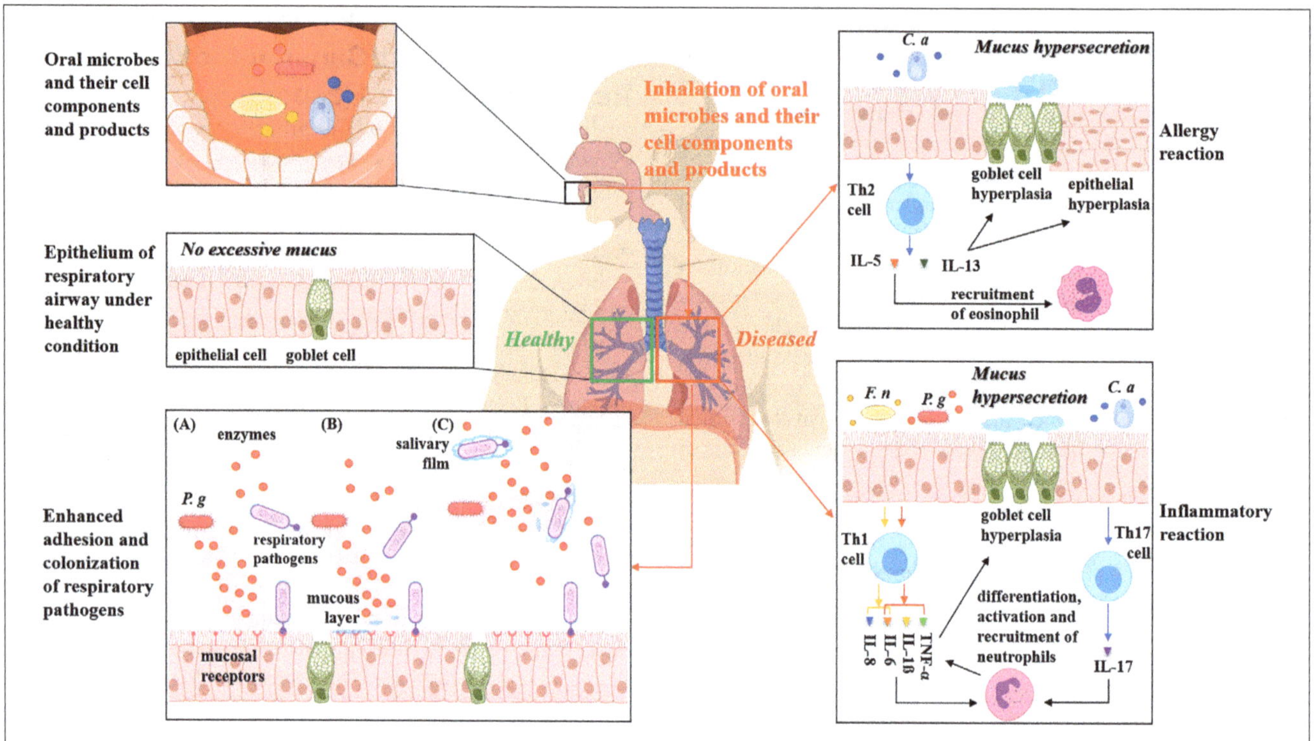

FIGURE 1 | Potential mechanisms on aspiration of oral microorganisms and their cell components and products into the lower respiratory tract to modulate immunoreaction and facilitate adherence and colonization of respiratory pathogens. Indigenous oral microorganisms, as well as their cell components and products such as lipopolysaccharide, peptidoglycans, enzymes and toxins in saliva, may be inhaled into the lower respiratory tract including the lung. Here, we classify the reactions of the lower respiratory tract to invaded oral microbes and their cell components and products into allergy and inflammation. In allergy reaction mode, take *C. albicans* (*C. a*) for example, the fungus and its lysates are reported to induce IL-5 and IL-13 production by Th2 cells. IL-5 activates eosinophils which is related with airway eosinophilic inflammation. IL-13 induces goblet cell hyperplasia resulting in increased mucus production and smooth muscle cell hyperplasia and hyperactivity which are prominent pathological features of allergic reaction. In inflammatory reaction mode, typical oral microbes such as *F. nucleatum* (*F. n*) and *P. gingivalis* (*P. g*) could induce IL-8 and IL-6 production, or soluble TNF receptors, TNF-α, IL-1ß and IL-6 production, respectively, both contributing to inflammation because of the subsequent differentiation, activation and recruitment of neutrophils. TNF-α also induce goblet cell hyperplasia and mucus hypersecretion. Moreover, *C. albicans* (*C. a*) infection could induce Th17 $CD4^+$ occurrence, whose main functions are the differentiation, activation and recruitment of neutrophils, which contribute to the inflammation and destruction of the lung tissue. In addition of effects on immunoreaction and inflammation, inhaled cell components and products of oral microbes (for example, *P. gingivalis*) may enhance adherence and colonization of respiratory pathogens on respiratory mucosa, mainly via three ways: **(A)** modification or upregulating expression of the mucosal epithelium receptors by specific enzymes or by other cell components and products. **(B)** clearance of the mucous layer that covers the receptors resulting in exposure of surface receptors. **(C)** the salivary film that protects against the colonization of pathogenic bacteria is destroyed by hydrolytic enzymes.

by oral bacteria. Potential regulation of lung cancer cell apoptosis by oral microbiome through p53 pathway is observed (Yang et al., 2018). Other possible mechanisms, for example, infertile defense function of tracheal mucosa causing by the invasion of oral bacteria to surface protein (fibronectin, etc.), still need exploration and evidence (Woods, 1987; Mamani et al., 2012).

Aspiration of Oral Microbial Components and Products Alters Respiratory Mucosal Surfaces and Modulates Immune Responses

Enzymes, cytokines and other biologically active substances in saliva which are released by oral microorganisms and inflammatory periodontal tissues could be inhaled into the lower respiratory tract and potentially influence respiratory tract mucosal epithelium. In the human airway, proteases released by invading pathogens have been associated with the regulation of the airway surface liquid layer, host defense, pathogenic infection and inflammation (Thibodeau and Butterworth, 2013). Besides proteases, it is possible for specific enzymes such as mannosidase, fucosidase, hexosaminidase and sialidase released from oral microecosystem to alter respiratory tract mucosal surfaces via modification of the mucosal epithelium or exposure of adhesion receptors located on mucosal surfaces, which would contribute to adherence and colonization by respiratory pathogens and consequent respiratory infection (Scannapieco, 1999; Gomes-Filho et al., 2010) (**Figure 1**). Moreover, hydrolytic enzymes from periodontal pathogens are proposed to destroy the salivary film that protects against pathogenic bacteria and leave respiratory pathogens free to enter respiratory tract, which would benefit their adherence to mucosal receptors (Scannapieco, 1999; Gomes-Filho et al., 2010) (**Figure 1**). Through oropharyngeal aspiration, other cell components and products of oral microbes, such as

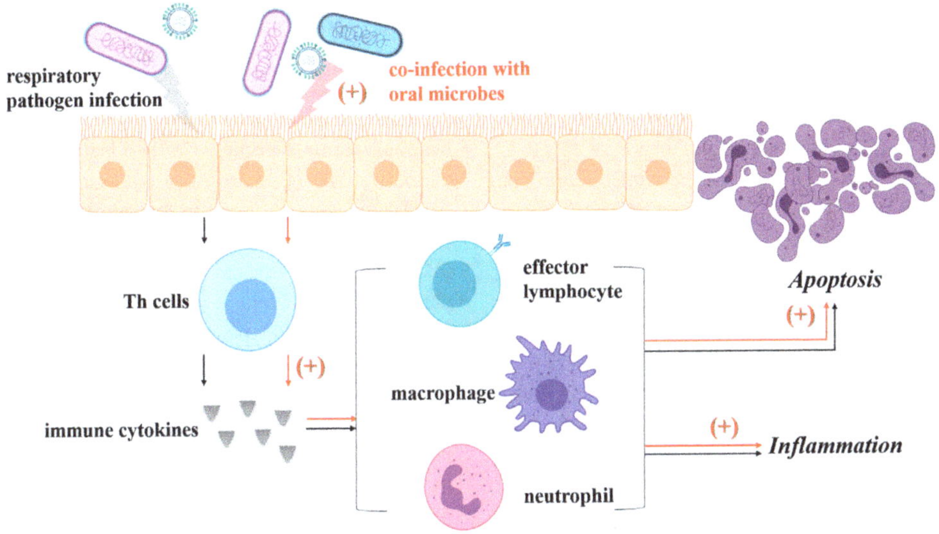

FIGURE 2 | Co-infection with oral microbes strengths the pathogenicity of respiratory pathogens. Usually, respiratory pathogen infection (black arrow) could induce the Th cells to produce cytokines, then lead to the differentiation, activation and recruitment of effector lymphocytes, neutrophils and macrophages. These immune cells not only bring about inflammation, but also activate the death receptor apoptotic pathway and finally lead to apoptosis. Once oral microbes (including oral *streptococci*, *P. gingivalis*, *F. nucleatum* and *A. actinomycetemcomitans*, *Prevotella intermedia*, *C. albicans*) inhaled into airways co-infect respiratory epithelium with respiratory pathogens (red arrow), the levels of multiple cytokines are elevated including TNF-α, IL-1β, IL-6, as well as those signaling pathway related with apoptosis of respiratory epithelial cells. Besides, some oral microbes can promote the virulence of respiratory pathogens, for example, via increasing the virulence factor production or forming pathogenic partnerships. As a result, aggravated inflammation and expanded apoptosis is observed.

lipopolysaccharide (LPS), peptidoglycans, lipoteichoic acids, fimbriae and toxins, as well as the cytokines released from inflammatory periodontal tissues, may also alter the respiratory epithelium and promote colonization by respiratory pathogens via the upregulation of adhesion receptor expression on the mucosal surfaces or stimulate cytokine production from respiratory epithelial cells, resulting in recruitment of inflammatory cells and inflamed epithelium that is more susceptible to respiratory infection (Scannapieco et al., 2001; Gomes-Filho et al., 2010) (**Figure 1**).

Effects of oral microbial components and products on modulating immune responses have been revealed by many studies. Take *C. albicans* for example, oropharyngeal aspiration of fungal lysates from *C. albicans* promotes the Th2 immune response, including airway eosinophilia, secretion of Th2 cytokines and mucus cell metaplasia (Allard et al., 2009) (**Figure 1**). Interestingly, oropharyngeal aspiration of *C. albicans* lysates together with *P. aeruginosa* is found to result in the shift of immune response from Th2 to Th1 in an LPS/TLR4 independent but MyD88 dependent mechanism (Allard et al., 2009). Furthermore, a soluble cell-wall β-glucan from *C. albicans* could facilitate OVA-induced allergic airway inflammation in mice (Inoue et al., 2009a) and induce apoptosis and oxidative stress in the lung that enhance lung inflammation and injury (Inoue et al., 2009b).

As a hallmark of chronic airway diseases including asthma, CF and COPD, mucous hypersecretion is also related with oral microbial products. Nagaoka et al. found the products of *F. nucleatum* inhibited mucus production in high concentrations, while increased mucus production in low concentrations. Thus, aspiration of saliva containing low concentrations of *F. nucleatum* products, which is more common, might promote mucus hypersecretion in the related diseases (Nagaoka et al., 2013).

Interactions Between Oral Microbes and Respiratory Pathogens Strengthen Respiratory Pathogenicity

Indigenous oral microbes are likely to be inhaled into the lower respiratory tract and may interact with respiratory pathogens, further modulating the pathogenicity of respiratory pathogens or both (The main mechanisms are summarized in **Figure 2**). Previous studies have reported the potential interactions between oral *streptococci* and *P. aeruginosa* which result in increased virulence and strengthened pathopoiesis of the latter (Duan et al., 2003; Parkins et al., 2008; Sibley et al., 2008). Recently, Whiley et al. demonstrated that pathogenic potential of the high-virulence *P. aeruginosa* CF Liverpool Epidemic Strain (LES) could be enhanced by the presence of anginosus-group of *streptococci* (AGS) and some other viridans *streptococci* (*S. mitis*, *Streptococcus oralis*, *Streptococcus gordonii* and *Streptococcus sanguinis*), and the pathogenic partnerships between the LES and AGS were verified in the *Galleria mellonella* infection model (Whiley et al., 2014; Whiley et al., 2015). However, it should be noticed that they also pointed out the negative modulation of these oral *streptococci* to *P. aeruginosa* virulence, which was found to be dependent on inoculation sequence and environment. Instead of air cooperation within a high cell density co-culture biofilm, when co-cultured in an atmosphere containing added CO_2, *S. oralis* antagonized *P. aeruginosa* LES growth via H_2O_2 production. *S. mitis*, *S. gordonii* and *S. sanguinis* showed similar H_2O_2 mediated inhibitory effect when inoculated as a primary colonizer prior to introduction of the LES (Whiley et al., 2015).

There is evidence showing that co-infection of multiple periodontal pathogens and respiratory pathogens in lung epithelial cells promote the production of inflammatory cytokines and apoptosis (Pan et al., 2009; Li et al., 2014; Chen et al., 2018; Li et al., 2018). *P. gingivalis, F. nucleatum*, and *A. actinomycetemcomitans* are reported to foster *P. aeruginosa* invasion into HEp-2 respiratory epithelial cells and enhance host cell cytokine release and apoptosis (Pan et al., 2009). Further study showed that *P. gingivalis* modulated *P. aeruginosa*-induced apoptosis of respiratory epithelial cells through the signal transducer and activator of transcription 3 (STAT3) signaling pathway and their co-invasion led to greater cell death compared with *P. aeruginosa* challenge alone (Li et al., 2014). Recently, the study by Chen et al. revealed that co-infection of *P. gingivalis* and influenza A virus (IAV) subtype H1N1 in lung epithelial cells could induce the production of inflammatory cytokines including TNF-α, IL-1β and IL-6, as well as the production of NO, consequently promoting apoptosis in lung epithelial cells via the Bcl-2/Bax/caspase-3 signaling pathway (Chen et al., 2018). It was also observed that infection by *P. gingivalis* combined with IAV temporarily inhibited apoptosis in respiratory epithelial cells, possibly related to the initiation of autophagy (Li et al., 2018). Besides, the supernatant of *Prevotella intermedia* was found to promote pneumococcal adherence to human alveolar cells, elevate inflammatory cytokine levels in the BAL fluid, and increase platelet-activating factor receptor transcription (Nagaoka et al., 2014).

ORAL HEALTH MANAGEMENT STRATEGIES FOR CONTROLLING RESPIRATORY DISEASES

The relationships between oral microecosystem, oral health and respiratory diseases highlight the importance of oral health management in prevention and treatment of respiratory diseases (especially pneumonia and COPD). Effective oral self-health management as well as professional oral health care, not only improve oral health, but also benefit controlling the progression or occurrence of respiratory diseases. Currently, it is clear that oral care measures maintaining oral health and oral microbiome symbiosis could reduce the incidence of pneumonia and COPD (**Table 1**).

Professional Oral Health Care

Providing oral health care, including tooth, tongues and dentures, is helpful to reduce the number of microorganisms inhalable in the lower respiratory tract and control subsequent respiratory infections (Scannapieco and Shay, 2014). Professional oral health care by dentist or oral hygienists significantly benefits the populations susceptible to respiratory infection, particularly the elderly and the comatose patients. Oral health condition has been recognized as one important risk factor in the incidence of aspiration pneumonia (Quagliarello et al., 2005; Chebib et al., 2018). A systematic review conducted by Khadka et al. analyzed the articles addressing aspiration pneumonia, oral microorganisms, oral health and treatment and their results showed that professional oral hygiene care that reduces bacteria is useful in reducing aspiration pneumonia risk (Khadka et al., 2021). For nursing home residents, a weekly professional oral care leads to a significantly lower annual prevalence of pneumonia hospitalization, especially in residents whose salivary bacterial concentration exceeded the median (Chiang et al., 2020). Brushing teeth is found to be an effective way to control the pneumopathogens (*staphylococci*, Enterobacteriaceae and yeasts) in resting saliva for reducing pulmonary infection of comatose patients and brushing twice-a-day can reduce respiratory tract infections by 69 percent in VAP (Cecon et al., 2010; Stonecypher, 2010). Most recently, a Four-Unit Cluster Randomized Study assessing the effectiveness of a standardized oral care protocol in preventing nonventilator hospital-acquired pneumonia (NV-HAP) in the acute care setting found that an increase in oral care frequency significantly reduced the NV-HAP incidence rate, suggesting that daily oral care can play a crucial role in NV-HAP prevention (Giuliano et al., 2021). Many studies also reported that preoperative oral hygiene interventions such as dental brushing and professional oral plaque control are associated with a lower incidence of postoperative pneumonia (POP) (Akutsu et al., 2010; Gonzalez-Rubio Aguilar et al., 2019; Jia et al., 2020). Therefore, oral health management is a favorable factor for preventing POP, and it could be carried out before surgery. In addition, professional oral cleansing once a week for 6 months during winter could reduce influenza infection in the elderly (Okuda et al., 2005).

Based on the current understanding of the relationship between oral microecosystem, oral health and aspiration pneumonia, it has been recommended by some scholars to use oral bacterial counts and the Oral Health Assessment Tool which assesses oral hygiene as a tool to assess the requirement of taking oral care and other preventive procedures in patients at high risk of aspiration pneumonia (Nishizawa et al., 2019). Such an oral health and oral hygiene assessment tool could be developed into a standardized oral assessment procedure and applied in the treatment of respiratory diseases related to oral bacteria and oral health.

Personal Oral Health Care

Common oral care, such as tooth brushing, flossing and regular dental visits, has been shown to be beneficial to controlling respiratory diseases. Through comparing 20 COPD individuals with 10 healthy individuals as control, Gaeckle et al. found that the healthy controls flossed frequently as their regular dental care while COPD patients not, and the control group also visited dental clinic more regularly (Gaeckle et al., 2018). Further analysis on the observation that COPD patients have fewer teeth and higher plaque index than the controls with normal pulmonary function revealed that inappropriate tooth brushing method, lower regular supra-gingival scaling and poorer oral health knowledge were significantly associated with the risk of COPD, indicating the importance of promoting dental care and oral health knowledge that can be integrated into the prevention and treatment of COPD (Wang et al., 2009). Oral health behaviors are also related to the incidence of pneumonia. It was found that denture wearing during sleep would increase the risk of incident pneumonia in the elderly and the elderly having this behavior were more likely to have tongue and denture plaque, gum inflammation, positive culture for *C. albicans*, and higher levels of circulating IL-6 as compared with those who remove their dentures at night, suggesting potential implications of oral hygiene programs for pneumonia prevention in the community (Iinuma et al., 2015).

Utilization of Antimicrobial Agents and Probiotics

There has been evidence showing that mechanical oral care combined with povidone iodine (PVP-I) significantly reduced the risk of pneumonia in nursing home residents. A concentration of 0.23% PVP-I was showed rapid bactericidal activity and virucidal efficacy against *K. pneumoniae*, *S. pneumoniae*, severe acute respiratory syndrome associated coronavirus, Middle East respiratory syndrome associated coronavirus, H1N1 and rotavirus (Eggers et al., 2018). It could provide a protective oropharyngeal hygiene measure for individuals at high risk of exposure to oral and respiratory pathogens (Eggers et al., 2018). For ICU nursing, using 0.2% CHX gel three times a day to clean gingiva and dental plaque significantly decreases the colonization rate of oropharyngeal aerobic pathogens in artificially ventilated patients (Fourrier et al., 2005). A recent study showed application of oral care protocol based on the removal of secretions from the oral cavity with 0. 12% CHX gluconate solution for brushing could significantly reduce the risk of development of VAP and *S. aureus* infection (Galhardo et al., 2020) . In addition to the use of CHX, specific antibiotics against *P. gingivalis*, *F. nucleatum*, *A. actinomycetemcomitans or streptococci* (including *S. oralis*, *S. pyogenes*, *S. agalactiae*, *S. intermedius*, and *S. mitis*) are pointed out as a further direction in controlling respiratory infections, since these bacteria are reported to promote the colonization or virulence of respiratory pathogens (King et al., 2005; Pan et al., 2009; Li et al., 2014).

Utilization of probiotics is also proposed as a strategy to fight against respiratory infections. Multiple studies have demonstrated the negative effect of oral *lactobacilli*, *streptococci* on respiratory pathogens and the potential of these bacteria as probiotics in the future to combat various lung infections (Alexandre et al., 2014; Scoffield and Wu, 2015; Kang et al., 2017; Scoffield et al., 2017; Mahdi et al., 2019).

Attentions in Dental Treatment

Patients with COPD have large amounts of mucous secretions (chronic bronchitis) with repeated coughing or dyspnea (emphysema) caused by airway destruction. If possible, it is recommended that during dental treatment, severely affected COPD patients be treated by sitting upright in dental chairs because they may experience difficulties in breathing while lying flat. At the same time, taking into account the important role of dental care and oral health knowledge in the prevention and treatment of COPD, attention should be paid to their oral hygiene guidance (Devlin, 2014).

Since an asthma attack could be triggered or exacerbated by a lot of risk factors, asthma patients should receive greater attention in dental treatment. It is suggested to assess the risk level of an asthma patient by a dental professional to decide whether the patient's health is stable enough to proceed with treatment and make sure that the patient has his or her own rescue inhaler on hand and on the bracket table (Little et al., 2017). All dental operations as well as dental instruments and materials used during dental treatment should not trigger an asthma attack and prolonged supine positioning should be avoided (Khalifa et al., 2014; Harrington et al., 2016).

Although the number of reported cases of infection or respiratory symptoms caused by dental waterway pollution is limited, the American Dental Association requires that the routine dental treatment output water used in dental unit waterlines should meet the quality standard for drinking water (i.e., ≤500 CFU/ml of heterotrophic water bacteria) and it is recommended to use sterile saline or sterile water as a coolant or irrigant when performing surgical procedures (Kohn et al., 2003).

CONCLUSIONS AND FURTHER DIRECTIONS

The relationship between oral microecosystem and respiratory diseases have been proved by plenty of studies. On the one hand, indigenous oral microorganisms take a part in the occurrence and development of respiratory diseases via their pathogenicity and virulence factors when inhaled into respiratory tract or interact with respiratory pathogens. On the other hand, many respiratory pathogens are found to adapt to the fluctuational oral environment with the help of their biological characteristics and their interspecies interactions with oral residents. Although we are making continuous progresses on understanding the role of oral microecosystem in development of respiratory diseases, etiological evidence that relates respiratory diseases with oral microecosystem is still insufficient. There are a lot of aspects to be explored and studied, including: (1) the specific oral microorganisms related to different respiratory diseases, and the potential mechanisms involved in the pathogenic process; (2) the adaptation and colonization mechanisms of respiratory pathogens in oral microecosystem, influence factors and available intervention measures; (3) the specific oral health management and treatment measures for patients or susceptible populations of respiratory diseases; (4) the potential oral biomarkers or indexes such as the abundance of specific microbes to predict the progress of respiratory diseases.

AUTHOR CONTRIBUTIONS

All authors listed have made a substantial, direct, and intellectual contribution to the work and approved it for publication.

REFERENCES

Aanaes, K., Johansen, H. K., Poulsen, S. S., Pressler, T., Buchwald, C., and Høiby, N. (2013). Secretory IgA as a Diagnostic Tool for *Pseudomonas aeruginosa* Respiratory Colonization. *J. Cystic Fibrosis* 12, 81–87. doi:10.1016/j.jcf.2012.07.001

Akutsu, Y., Matsubara, H., Shuto, K., Shiratori, T., Uesato, M., Miyazawa, Y., et al. (2010). Pre-operative Dental Brushing Can Reduce the Risk of Postoperative Pneumonia in Esophageal Cancer Patients. *Surgery* 147, 497–502. doi:10.1016/j.surg.2009.10.048

Alexandre, Y., Le Berre, R., Barbier, G., and Le Blay, G. (2014). Screening of Lactobacillus Spp. For the Prevention of *Pseudomonas aeruginosa* Pulmonary Infections. *BMC Microbiol.* 14, 107. doi:10.1186/1471-2180-14-107

Allard, J. B., Rinaldi, L., Wargo, M. J., Allen, G., Akira, S., Uematsu, S., et al. (2009). Th2 Allergic Immune Response to Inhaled Fungal Antigens Is Modulated by TLR-4-independent Bacterial Products. *Eur. J. Immunol.* 39, 776–788. doi:10.1002/eji.200838932

Arafa, A., Aldahlawi, S., and Fathi, A. (2017). Assessment of the Oral Health Status of Asthmatic Children. *Eur. J. Dent* 11, 357–363. doi:10.4103/ejd.ejd_65_17

Arbesjr, S., Jr., Sever, M., Vaughn, B., Cohen, E., and Zeldin, D. (2006). Oral Pathogens and Allergic Disease: Results from the Third National Health and Nutrition Examination Survey. *J. Allergy Clin. Immunol.* 118, 1169–1175. doi:10.1016/j.jaci.2006.07.029

Arweiler, N. B., Rahmel, V., Alhamwe, B. A., Alhamdan, F., Zemlin, M., Boutin, S., et al. (2021). Dental Biofilm and Saliva Microbiome and its Interplay with Pediatric Allergies. *Microorganisms* 9, 1. doi:10.3390/microorganisms9061330

Awano, S., Ansai, T., Takata, Y., Soh, I., Akifusa, S., Hamasaki, T., et al. (2008). Oral Health and Mortality Risk from Pneumonia in the Elderly. *J. Dent Res.* 87, 334–339. doi:10.1177/154405910808700418

Baena-Monroy, T., Moreno-Maldonado, V., Franco-Martínez, F., Aldape-Barrios, B., Quindós, G., and Sánchez-Vargas, L. O. (2005). Candida Albicans, *Staphylococcus aureus* and Streptococcus Mutans Colonization in Patients Wearing Dental Prosthesis. *Med. Oral Patol Oral Cir Bucal* 10 (Suppl. 1), E27–E39.

Bágyi, K., Klekner, A., Hutóczki, G., and Márton, I. (2006). The Role of the Oral flora in the Pathogenesis of Aspiration Pneumonia. *Fogorv Sz* 99, 205–212.

Bassis, C. M., Erb-Downward, J. R., Dickson, R. P., Freeman, C. M., Schmidt, T. M., Young, V. B., et al. (2015). Analysis of the Upper Respiratory Tract Microbiotas as the Source of the Lung and Gastric Microbiotas in Healthy Individuals. *mBio* 6, e00037. doi:10.1128/mBio.00037-15

Beaudoin, T., Yau, Y. C. W., Stapleton, P. J., Gong, Y., Wang, P. W., Guttman, D. S., et al. (2017). *Staphylococcus aureus* Interaction with *Pseudomonas aeruginosa* Biofilm Enhances Tobramycin Resistance. *NPJ Biofilms Microbiomes* 3, 25. doi:10.1038/s41522-017-0035-0

Bensel, T., Huse, A., Borneff-Lipp, M., Wollschläger, B., Bekes, K., Setz, J., et al. (2010). Periodontal Pockets as Potential Sources of Cystic Fibrosis Lung Infection. *J. Cystic Fibrosis* 9, S38. doi:10.1016/s1569-1993(10)60147-6

Busarcevic, M., Kojic, M., Dalgalarrondo, M., Chobert, J.-M., Haertlé, T., and Topisirovic, L. (2008). Purification of Bacteriocin LS1 Produced by Human Oral Isolate Lactobacillus Salivarius BGHO1. *Oral Microbiol. Immunol.* 23, 254–258. doi:10.1111/j.1399-302x.2007.00420.x

Card, J. W., Carey, M. A., Voltz, J. W., Bradbury, J. A., Ferguson, C. D., Cohen, E. A., et al. (2010). Modulation of Allergic Airway Inflammation by the Oral Pathogen Porphyromonas Gingivalis. *Infect. Immun.* 78, 2488–2496. doi:10.1128/iai.01270-09

Cecon, F., Ferreira, L. E. N., Rosa, R. T., Gursky, L. C., De Paula E Carvalho, A., Samaranayake, L. P., et al. (2010). Time-related Increase of Staphylococci, Enterobacteriaceae and Yeasts in the Oral Cavities of Comatose Patients. *J. Microbiol. Immunol. Infect.* 43, 457–463. doi:10.1016/s1684-1182(10)60071-0

Chebib, N., Müller, F., and Prendki, V. (2018). Pneumonia of the Elderly and its Link to Oral Health. *Rev. Med. Suisse* 14, 2007–2011.

Chen, L., Zhao, J., Peng, J., Li, X., Deng, X., Geng, Z., et al. (2020). Detection of SARS-CoV-2 in Saliva and Characterization of Oral Symptoms in COVID-19 Patients. *Cell Prolif* 53, e12923. doi:10.1111/cpr.12923

Chen, Y., Zhou, R., Yi, Z., Li, Y., Fu, Y., Zhang, Y., et al. (2018). Porphyromonas Gingivalis Induced Inflammatory Responses and Promoted Apoptosis in Lung Epithelial Cells Infected with H1N1 via the Bcl-2/Bax/Caspase-3 S-ignaling P-athway. *Mol. Med. Rep.* 18, 97–104. doi:10.3892/mmr.2018.8983

Cherkasov, S. V., Popova, L. Y., Vivtanenko, T. V., Demina, R. R., Khlopko, Y. A., Balkin, A. S., et al. (2019). Oral Microbiomes in Children with Asthma and Dental Caries. *Oral Dis.* 25, 898–910. doi:10.1111/odi.13020

Chhibber-Goel, J., Singhal, V., Bhowmik, D., Vivek, R., Parakh, N., Bhargava, B., et al. (2016). Linkages between Oral Commensal Bacteria and Atherosclerotic Plaques in Coronary Artery Disease Patients. *NPJ Biofilms Microbiomes* 2, 7. doi:10.1038/s41522-016-0009-7

Chiang, T.-C., Huang, M.-S., Lu, P.-L., Huang, S.-T., and Lin, Y.-C. (2020). The Effect of Oral Care Intervention on Pneumonia Hospitalization, *Staphylococcus aureus* Distribution, and Salivary Bacterial Concentration in Taiwan Nursing home Residents: a Pilot Study. *BMC Infect. Dis.* 20, 374. doi:10.1186/s12879-020-05061-z

Chrysanthakopoulos, N. A. (2016). Correlation between Periodontal Disease Indices and Lung Cancer in Greek Adults: a Case - Control Study. *Exp. Onc.* 38, 49–53. doi:10.31768/2312-8852.2016.38(1):49-53

Cilloniz, C., Ewig, S., Polverino, E., Marcos, M. A., Esquinas, C., Gabarrus, A., et al. (2011). Microbial Aetiology of Community-Acquired Pneumonia and its Relation to Severity. *Thorax* 66, 340–346. doi:10.1136/thx.2010.143982

Coburn, B., Wang, P. W., Diaz Caballero, J., Clark, S. T., Brahma, V., Donaldson, S., et al. (2015). Lung Microbiota across Age and Disease Stage in Cystic Fibrosis. *Sci. Rep.* 5, 10241. doi:10.1038/srep10241

Colombo, A. V., Barbosa, G. M., Higashi, D., Di Micheli, G., Rodrigues, P. H., and Simionato, M. R. L. (2013). Quantitative Detection of *Staphylococcus aureus*, *Enterococcus faecalis* and *Pseudomonas aeruginosa* in Human Oral Epithelial Cells from Subjects with Periodontitis and Periodontal Health. *J. Med. Microbiol.* 62, 1592–1600. doi:10.1099/jmm.0.055830-0

Devlin, J. (2014). Patients with Chronic Obstructive Pulmonary Disease: Management Considerations for the Dental Team. *Br. Dent J.* 217, 235–237. doi:10.1038/sj.bdj.2014.756

Diaz, P. I., Hong, B.-Y., Frias-Lopez, J., Dupuy, A. K., Angeloni, M., Abusleme, L., et al. (2013). Transplantation-associated Long-Term Immunosuppression Promotes Oral Colonization by Potentially Opportunistic Pathogens without Impacting Other Members of the Salivary Bacteriome. *Clin. Vaccin. Immunol* 20, 920–930. doi:10.1128/cvi.00734-12

Duan, K., Dammel, C., Stein, J., Rabin, H., and Surette, M. G. (2003). Modulation of *Pseudomonas aeruginosa* Gene Expression by Host Microflora through Interspecies Communication. *Mol. Microbiol.* 50, 1477–1491. doi:10.1046/j.1365-2958.2003.03803.x

Duman, G. G., Çuhadar, T., Yamak, A. S., Albakkour, K., Çağlar, K., and Kalkanci, A. (2019). Düşük Düzeyde Klorhekzidin Ile Karşılaştırılmış *Klebsiella pneumoniae* İzolatlarının Karakterizasyonu. *Mikrobiyol Bul* 53, 114–117. doi:10.5578/mb.67793

Eggers, M., Koburger-Janssen, T., Eickmann, M., and Zorn, J. (2018). *In Vitro* Bactericidal and Virucidal Efficacy of Povidone-Iodine Gargle/Mouthwash against Respiratory and Oral Tract Pathogens. *Infect. Dis. Ther.* 7, 249–259. doi:10.1007/s40121-018-0200-7

Feng, M.-C., Lin, Y.-C., Chang, Y.-H., Chen, C.-H., Chiang, H.-C., Huang, L.-C., et al. (2019). The Mortality and the Risk of Aspiration Pneumonia Related with Dysphagia in Stroke Patients. *J. Stroke Cerebrovasc. Dis.* 28, 1381–1387. doi:10.1016/j.jstrokecerebrovasdis.2019.02.011

Fourrier, F., Dubois, D., Pronnier, P., Herbecq, P., Leroy, O., Desmettre, T., et al. (2005). Effect of Gingival and Dental Plaque Antiseptic Decontamination on Nosocomial Infections Acquired in the Intensive Care Unit: A Double-Blind Placebo-Controlled Multicenter Study*. *Crit. Care Med.* 33, 1728–1735. doi:10.1097/01.ccm.0000171537.03493.b0

Fourrier, F., Duvivier, B., Boutigny, H., Roussel-Delvallez, M., and Chopin, C. (1998). Colonization of Dental Plaque: a Source of Nosocomial Infections in Intensive Care Unit Patients. *Crit. Care Med.* 26, 301–308. doi:10.1097/00003246-199802000-00032

F. Sato, E., Choudhury, T., Nishikawa, T., and Inoue, M. (2008). Dynamic Aspect of Reactive Oxygen and Nitric Oxide in Oral Cavity. *J. Clin. Biochem. Nutr.* 42, 8–13. doi:10.3164/jcbn.2008002

Gaeckle, N. T., Heyman, B., Criner, A. J., and Criner, G. J. (2018). Markers of Dental Health Correlate with Daily Respiratory Symptoms in COPD. *J. Copd F* 5, 97–105. doi:10.15326/jcopdf.5.2.2017.0159

Galhardo, L. F., Ruivo, G. F., Santos, F. O., Ferreira, T. T., Santos, J., L Eão, M. V., et al. (2020). Impact of Oral Care and Antisepsis on the Prevalence of Ventilator-Associated Pneumonia. *Oral Health Prev. Dent* 18, 331–336. doi:10.3290/j.ohpd.a44443

Geetha, C., Venkatesh, S. G., Fasciotto Dunn, B. H., and Gorr, S.-U. (2003). Expression and Anti-bacterial Activity of Human Parotid Secretory Protein (PSP). *Biochem. Soc. Trans.* 31, 815–818. doi:10.1042/bst0310815

Genco, R. J., Grossi, S. G., Ho, A., Nishimura, F., and Murayama, Y. (2005). A Proposed Model Linking Inflammation to Obesity, Diabetes, and Periodontal Infections. *J. Periodontol.* 76 (Suppl. 11S), 2075–2084. doi:10.1902/jop.2005.76.11-S.2075

Giuliano, K. K., Penoyer, D., Middleton, A., and Baker, D. (2021). Original Research: Oral Care as Prevention for Nonventilator Hospital-Acquired Pneumonia. *Am. J. Nurs.* 121, 24–33. doi:10.1097/01.naj.0000753468.99321.93

Gomes-Filho, I. S., Passos, J. S., and Seixas Da Cruz, S. (2010). Respiratory Disease and the Role of Oral Bacteria. *J. Oral Microbiol.* 2, 1. doi:10.3402/jom.v2i0.5811

González-Rubio Aguilar, P., Ávalos Arenas, V., Vega Gudiño, N. A., Moreno Herrera, S. D., Villa Guillén, M., Moyao-García, D., et al. (2019). The Impact of Tooth Brushing versus Tooth Brushing and Chlorhexidine Application to Avoid Postoperative Pneumonia in Children. *Am. J. Infect. Control.* 47, 1340–1345. doi:10.1016/j.ajic.2019.05.018

Harrington, N., Prado, N., and Barry, S. (2016). Dental Treatment in Children with Asthma - a Review. *Br. Dent J.* 220, 299–302. doi:10.1038/sj.bdj.2016.220

Hasan, N. A., Young, B. A., Minard-Smith, A. T., Saeed, K., Li, H., Heizer, E. M., et al. (2014). Microbial Community Profiling of Human Saliva Using Shotgun Metagenomic Sequencing. *PLoS One* 9, e97699. doi:10.1371/journal.pone.0097699

Hayata, M., Watanabe, N., Tamura, M., Kamio, N., Tanaka, H., Nodomi, K., et al. (2019). The Periodontopathic Bacterium Fusobacterium Nucleatum Induced Proinflammatory Cytokine Production by Human Respiratory Epithelial Cell Lines and in the Lower Respiratory Organs in Mice. *Cell Physiol Biochem* 53, 49–61. doi:10.33594/000000120

He, X., Hu, W., He, J., Guo, L., Lux, R., and Shi, W. (2011). Community-based Interference against Integration of *Pseudomonas aeruginosa* into Human Salivary Microbial Biofilm. *Mol. Oral Microbiol.* 26, 337–352. doi:10.1111/j.2041-1014.2011.00622.x

Heo, S. M., Haase, E. M., Lesse, A. J., Gill, S. R., and Scannapieco, F. A. (2008). Genetic Relationships between Respiratory Pathogens Isolated from Dental Plaque and Bronchoalveolar Lavage Fluid from Patients in the Intensive Care Unit Undergoing Mechanical Ventilation. *Clin. Infect. Dis.* 47, 1562–1570. doi:10.1086/593193

Hosgood, H. D., Cai, Q., Hua, X., Long, J., Shi, J., Wan, Y., et al. (2021). Variation in Oral Microbiome Is Associated with Future Risk of Lung Cancer Among Never-Smokers. *Thorax* 76, 256–263. doi:10.1136/thoraxjnl-2020-215542

Iinuma, T., Arai, Y., Abe, Y., Takayama, M., Fukumoto, M., Fukui, Y., et al. (2015). Denture Wearing during Sleep Doubles the Risk of Pneumonia in the Very Elderly. *J. Dent Res.* 94, 28s–36s. doi:10.1177/0022034514552493

Imai, K., and Tanaka, H. (2021). SARS-CoV-2 Infection and Significance of Oral Health Management in the Era of "the New Normal with COVID-19. *Int. J. Mol. Sci.* 22, 1. doi:10.3390/ijms22126527

Inoue, K.-i., Takano, H., Koike, E., Yanagisawa, R., Oda, T., Tamura, H., et al. (2009a). Candida Soluble Cell wall β-glucan Facilitates Ovalbumin-Induced Allergic Airway Inflammation in Mice: Possible Role of Antigen-Presenting Cells. *Respir. Res.* 10, 68. doi:10.1186/1465-9921-10-68

Inoue, K.-i., Takano, H., Oda, T., Yanagisawa, R., Tamura, H., Adachi, Y., et al. (2009b). Soluble Cell wall β-glucan of candida Induces/enhances Apoptosis and Oxidative Stress in Murine Lung. *Immunopharmacology and Immunotoxicology* 31, 140–145. doi:10.1080/08923970802534678

Jain, M., Shah, R., Chandolia, B., Mathur, A., Chauhan, Y., Chawda, J., et al. (2016). The Oral Carriage of Candida in Oral Cancer Patients of Indian Origin Undergoing Radiotherapy And/or Chemotherapy. *J. Clin. Diagn. Res.* 10, Zc17–20. doi:10.7860/JCDR/2016/15702.7180

Jhajharia, K., Mehta, L., Parolia, A., and Shetty, K. (2015). Biofilm in Endodontics: A Review. *J. Int. Soc. Prevent Communit Dent* 5, 1–12. doi:10.4103/2231-0762.151956

Jia, C., Sun, M., Wang, W., Li, C., Li, X., and Zhang, X. (2020). Effect of Oral Plaque Control on Postoperative Pneumonia Following Lung Cancer Surgery. *Thorac. Cancer* 11, 1655–1660. doi:10.1111/1759-7714.13448

Kamaguchi, A., Nakayama, K., Ichiyama, S., Nakamura, R., Watanabe, T., Ohta, M., et al. (2003). Effect of Porphyromonas Gingivalis Vesicles on Coaggregation of *Staphylococcus aureus* to Oral Microorganisms. *Curr. Microbiol.* 47, 485–491. doi:10.1007/s00284-003-4069-6

Kanazuru, T., Sato, E. F., Nagata, K., Matsui, H., Watanabe, K., Kasahara, E., et al. (2010). Role of Hydrogen Generation by *Klebsiella pneumoniae* in the Oral Cavity. *J. Microbiol.* 48, 778–783. doi:10.1007/s12275-010-0149-z

Kang, M. S., Lim, H. S., Oh, J. S., Lim, Y. J., Wuertz-Kozak, K., Harro, J. M., et al. (2017). Antimicrobial Activity of Lactobacillus Salivarius and Lactobacillus Fermentum against *Staphylococcus aureus*. *Pathog. Dis.* 75, 1. doi:10.1093/femspd/ftx009

Khadka, S., Khan, S., King, A., Goldberg, L. R., Crocombe, L., and Bettiol, S. (2021). Poor Oral hygiene, Oral Microorganisms and Aspiration Pneumonia Risk in Older People in Residential Aged Care: a Systematic Review. *Age Ageing* 50, 81–87. doi:10.1093/ageing/afaa102

Khalifa, M. A. A. A., Abouelkheir, H. M., Khodiar, S. E.-F., and Mohamed, G. A. M. (2014). Salivary Composition and Dental Caries Among Children Controlled Asthmatics. *Egypt. J. Chest Dis. Tuberculosis* 63, 777–788. doi:10.1016/j.ejcdt.2014.05.003

Kikutani, T., Tamura, F., Tashiro, H., Yoshida, M., Konishi, K., and Hamada, R. (2015). Relationship between Oral Bacteria Count and Pneumonia Onset in Elderly Nursing home Residents. *Geriatr. Gerontol. Int.* 15, 417–421. doi:10.1111/ggi.12286

Kilian, M. (2018). The Oral Microbiome - Friend or Foe? *Eur. J. Oral Sci.* 126, 5–12. doi:10.1111/eos.12527

Kimura, M., Tsuruta, S., and Yoshida, T. (1999). Differences in Cytokine Production by Peripheral Blood Mononuclear Cells (PBMC) between Patients with Atopic Dermatitis and Bronchial Asthma. *Clin. Exp. Immunol.* 118, 192–196. doi:10.1046/j.1365-2249.1999.01055.x

Kinane, D. F., Galicia, J. C., Gorr, S. U., Stathopoulou, P. G., and Benakanakere, M. (2008). P. Gingivalis Interactions with Epithelial Cells. *Front. Biosci.* 13, 966–984. doi:10.2741/2736

King, S. J., Whatmore, A. M., and Dowson, C. G. (2005). NanA, a Neuraminidase from Streptococcus Pneumoniae , Shows High Levels of Sequence Diversity, at Least in Part through Recombination with Streptococcus Oralis. *J. Bacteriol.* 187, 5376–5386. doi:10.1128/jb.187.15.5376-5386.2005

Kohn, W. G., Collins, A. S., Cleveland, J. L., Harte, J. A., Eklund, K. J., and Malvitz, D. M. (2003). Guidelines for Infection Control in Dental Health-Care Settings--2003. *MMWR Recomm Rep.* 52, 1 61.

Komiyama, K., and Gibbons, R. J. (1984). Interbacterial Adherence between Actinomyces Viscosus and Strains of Streptococcus Pyogenes, Streptococcus Agalactiae, and *Pseudomonas aeruginosa*. *Infect. Immun.* 44, 86–90. doi:10.1128/iai.44.1.86-90.1984

Komiyama, K., Habbick, B. F., and Gibbons, R. J. (1987). Interbacterial Adhesion between *Pseudomonas aeruginosa* and Indigenous Oral Bacteria Isolated from Patients with Cystic Fibrosis. *Can. J. Microbiol.* 33, 27–32. doi:10.1139/m87-005

Koulenti, D., Tsigou, E., and Rello, J. (2017). Nosocomial Pneumonia in 27 ICUs in Europe: Perspectives from the EU-VAP/CAP Study. *Eur. J. Clin. Microbiol. Infect. Dis.* 36, 1999–2006. doi:10.1007/s10096-016-2703-z

Kovaleva, O. V., Romashin, D., Zborovskaya, I. B., Davydov, M. M., Shogenov, M. S., and Gratchev, A. (2019). Human Lung Microbiome on the Way to Cancer. *J. Immunol. Res.* 2019, 1394191. doi:10.1155/2019/1394191

Kucukcoskun, M., Baser, U., Oztekin, G., Kiyan, E., and Yalcin, F. (2013). Initial Periodontal Treatment for Prevention of Chronic Obstructive Pulmonary Disease Exacerbations. *J. Periodontol.* 84, 863–870. doi:10.1902/jop.2012.120399

Kumar, P. S., Matthews, C. R., Joshi, V., De Jager, M., and Aspiras, M. (2011). Tobacco Smoking Affects Bacterial Acquisition and Colonization in Oral Biofilms. *Infect. Immun.* 79, 4730–4738. doi:10.1128/iai.05371-11

Laurence, B., Mould-Millman, N.-K., Scannapieco, F. A., and Abron, A. (2015). Hospital Admissions for Pneumonia More Likely with Concomitant Dental Infections. *Clin. Oral Invest.* 19, 1261–1268. doi:10.1007/s00784-014-1342-y

Leone, M., Bouadma, L., Bouhemad, B., Brissaud, O., Dauger, S., Gibot, S., et al. (2018). Hospital-acquired Pneumonia in ICU. *Anaesth. Crit. Care Pain Med.* 37, 83–98. doi:10.1016/j.accpm.2017.11.006

Lerrer, B., Lesman-Movshovich, E., and Gilboa-Garber, N. (2005). Comparison of the Antimicrobial Adhesion Potential of Human Body Fluid Glycoconjugates Using Fucose-Binding Lectin (PA-IIL) of *Pseudomonas aeruginosa* and Ulex

Europaeus Lectin (UEA-I). *Curr. Microbiol.* 51, 202–206. doi:10.1007/s00284-005-4571-0

Li, Q., Pan, C., Teng, D., Lin, L., Kou, Y., Haase, E. M., et al. (2014). Porphyromonas Gingivalis Modulates Pseudomonas Aeruginosa-Induced Apoptosis of Respiratory Epithelial Cells through the STAT3 Signaling Pathway. *Microbes Infect.* 16, 17–27. doi:10.1016/j.micinf.2013.10.006

Li, X., Li, C., Liu, J.-c., Pan, Y.-p., and Li, Y.-g. (2018). *In Vitro* effect of Porphyromonas Gingivalis Combined with Influenza A Virus on Respiratory Epithelial Cells. *Arch. Oral Biol.* 95, 125–133. doi:10.1016/j.archoralbio.2018.04.003

Lima, B. P., Hu, L. I., Vreeman, G. W., Weibel, D. B., and Lux, R. (2019). The Oral Bacterium Fusobacterium Nucleatum Binds *Staphylococcus aureus* and Alters Expression of the Staphylococcal Accessory Regulator sarA. *Microb. Ecol.* 78, 336–347. doi:10.1007/s00248-018-1291-0

Little, J. W., Miller, C., and Rhodus, N. L. (2017). *Dental Management of the Medically Compromised Patient - E-Book.* Elsevier Health Sciences.

Littman, A. J., White, E., Jackson, L. A., Thornquist, M. D., Gaydos, C. A., Goodman, G. E., et al. (2004). Chlamydia Pneumoniae Infection and Risk of Lung Cancer. *Cancer Epidemiol. Biomarkers Prev.* 13, 1624–1630.

Maddi, A., Sabharwal, A., Violante, T., Manuballa, S., Genco, R., Patnaik, S., et al. (2019). The Microbiome and Lung Cancer. *J. Thorac. Dis.* 11, 280–291. doi:10.21037/jtd.2018.12.88

Mahdi, L. H., Jabbar, H. S., and Auda, I. G. (2019). Antibacterial Immunomodulatory and Antibiofilm Triple Effect of Salivaricin LHM against *Pseudomonas aeruginosa* Urinary Tract Infection Model. *Int. J. Biol. Macromolecules* 134, 1132–1144. doi:10.1016/j.ijbiomac.2019.05.181

Main, B. E., Calman, K. C., Ferguson, M. M., Kaye, S. B., Macfarlane, T. W., Mairs, R. J., et al. (1984). The Effect of Cytotoxic Therapy on Saliva and Oral flora. *Oral Surg. Oral Med. Oral Pathol.* 58, 545–548. doi:10.1016/0030-4220(84)90077-x

Mamani, M., Hashemi, S. H., Hajilooi, M., Saedi, F., Niayesh, A., and Fallah, M. (2012). Evaluation of Fibronectin and C-Reactive Protein Levels in Patients with Sepsis: a Case-Control Study. *Acta Med. Iran* 50, 404–410.

Manning, J., Dunne, E. M., Wescombe, P. A., Hale, J. D. F., Mulholland, E. K., Tagg, J. R., et al. (2016). Investigation of Streptococcus Salivarius-Mediated Inhibition of Pneumococcal Adherence to Pharyngeal Epithelial Cells. *BMC Microbiol.* 16, 225. doi:10.1186/s12866-016-0843-z

Mathews, S. A., Kurien, B. T., and Scofield, R. H. (2008). Oral Manifestations of Sjögren's Syndrome. *J. Dent Res.* 87, 308–318. doi:10.1177/154405910808700411

Mauch, R. M., Rossi, C. L., Aiello, T. B., Ribeiro, J. D., Ribeiro, A. F., Høiby, N., et al. (2017). Secretory IgA Response against *Pseudomonas aeruginosa* in the Upper Airways and the Link with Chronic Lung Infection in Cystic Fibrosis. *Pathog. Dis.* 75, 1. doi:10.1093/femspd/ftx069

Mehta, A., Sequeira, P. S., Sahoo, R. C., and Kaur, G. (2009). Is Bronchial Asthma a Risk Factor for Gingival Diseases? A Control Study. *N. Y State. Dent J.* 75, 44–46.

Merghni, A., Ben Nejma, M., Helali, I., Hentati, H., Bongiovanni, A., Lafont, F., et al. (2015). Assessment of Adhesion, Invasion and Cytotoxicity Potential of Oral *Staphylococcus aureus* Strains. *Microb. Pathogenesis* 86, 1–9. doi:10.1016/j.micpath.2015.05.010

Miyashita, N., Fukano, H., Mouri, K., Fukuda, M., Yoshida, K., Kobashi, Y., et al. (2005). Community-acquired Pneumonia in Japan: a Prospective Ambulatory and Hospitalized Patient Study. *J. Med. Microbiol.* 54, 395–400. doi:10.1099/jmm.0.45920-0

Moghaddam, S. J., Ochoa, C. E., Sethi, S., and Dickey, B. F. (2011). Nontypeable Haemophilus Influenzae in Chronic Obstructive Pulmonary Disease and Lung Cancer. *Copd* 6, 113–123. doi:10.2147/copd.s15417

Mori, A., Ikeda, Y., Taniguchi, M., Aoyama, C., Maeda, Y., Hasegawa, M., et al. (2001). IL-5 Production by Peripheral Blood Th Cells of Adult Asthma Patients in Response to Candida Albicans Allergen. *Int. Arch. Allergy Immunol.* 125 (Suppl. 1), 48–50. doi:10.1159/000053853

Muhlebach, M. S., Hatch, J. E., Einarsson, G. G., Mcgrath, S. J., Gilipin, D. F., Lavelle, G., et al. (2018a). Anaerobic Bacteria Cultured from Cystic Fibrosis Airways Correlate to Milder Disease: a Multisite Study. *Eur. Respir. J.* 52, 1. doi:10.1183/13993003.00242-2018

Muhlebach, M. S., Zorn, B. T., Esther, C. R., Hatch, J. E., Murray, C. P., Turkovic, L., et al. (2018b). Initial Acquisition and Succession of the Cystic Fibrosis Lung Microbiome Is Associated with Disease Progression in Infants and Preschool Children. *Plos Pathog.* 14, e1006798. doi:10.1371/journal.ppat.1006798

Nagaoka, K., Yanagihara, K., Harada, Y., Yamada, K., Migiyama, Y., Morinaga, Y., et al. (2013). Macrolides Inhibit Fusobacterium Nucleatum-Induced MUC5AC Production in Human Airway Epithelial Cells. *Antimicrob. Agents Chemother.* 57, 1844–1849. doi:10.1128/aac.02466-12

Nagaoka, K., Yanagihara, K., Morinaga, Y., Nakamura, S., Harada, T., Hasegawa, H., et al. (2014). Prevotella Intermedia Induces Severe Bacteremic Pneumococcal Pneumonia in Mice with Upregulated Platelet-Activating Factor Receptor Expression. *Infect. Immun.* 82, 587–593. doi:10.1128/iai.00943-13

Nishizawa, T., Niikura, Y., Akasaka, K., Watanabe, M., Kurai, D., Amano, M., et al. (2019). Pilot Study for Risk Assessment of Aspiration Pneumonia Based on Oral Bacteria Levels and Serum Biomarkers. *BMC Infect. Dis.* 19, 761. doi:10.1186/s12879-019-4327-2

Ogrendik, M. (2009). Rheumatoid Arthritis Is Linked to Oral Bacteria: Etiological Association. *Mod. Rheumatol.* 19, 453–456. doi:10.3109/s10165-009-0194-9

Okuda, K., Kimizuka, R., Abe, S., Kato, T., and Ishihara, K. (2005). Involvement of Periodontopathic Anaerobes in Aspiration Pneumonia. *J. Periodontol.* 76 (Suppl. 11S), 2154–2160. doi:10.1902/jop.2005.76.11-S.2154

Pan, Y., Teng, D., Burke, A. C., Haase, E. M., and Scannapieco, F. A. (2009). Oral Bacteria Modulate Invasion and Induction of Apoptosis in HEp-2 Cells by *Pseudomonas aeruginosa*. *Microb. Pathogenesis* 46, 73–79. doi:10.1016/j.micpath.2008.10.012

Parahitiyawa, N. B., Jin, L. J., Leung, W. K., Yam, W. C., and Samaranayake, L. P. (2009). Microbiology of Odontogenic Bacteremia: beyond Endocarditis. *Clin. Microbiol. Rev.* 22, 46–64. doi:10.1128/cmr.00028-08

Parkins, M. D., Sibley, C. D., Surette, M. G., and Rabin, H. R. (2008). TheStreptococcus Milleri Group-An Unrecognized Cause of Disease in Cystic Fibrosis: A Case Series and Literature Review. *Pediatr. Pulmonol.* 43, 490–497. doi:10.1002/ppul.20809

Passariello, C., Puttini, M., Iebba, V., Pera, P., and Gigola, P. (2012). Influence of Oral Conditions on Colonization by Highly Toxigenic *Staphylococcus aureus* Strains. *Oral Dis.* 18, 402–409. doi:10.1111/j.1601-0825.2011.01889.x

Petelin, M., Naruishi, K., Shiomi, N., Mineshiba, J., Arai, H., Nishimura, F., et al. (2004). Systemic Up-Regulation of sTNFR2 and IL-6 in Porphyromonas Gingivalis Pneumonia in Mice. *Exp. Mol. Pathol.* 76, 76–81. doi:10.1016/j.yexmp.2003.09.002

Poveda-Roda, R., Jiménez, Y., Carbonell, E., Gavaldá, C., Margaix-Muñoz, M. M., and Sarrión-Pérez, G. (2008). Bacteremia Originating in the Oral Cavity. A Review. *Med. Oral Patol Oral Cir Bucal* 13, E355–E362.

Pragman, A. A., Lyu, T., Baller, J. A., Gould, T. J., Kelly, R. F., Reilly, C. S., et al. (2018). The Lung Tissue Microbiota of Mild and Moderate Chronic Obstructive Pulmonary Disease. *Microbiome* 6, 7. doi:10.1186/s40168-017-0381-4

Prasanna, S. (2011). Causal Relationship between Periodontitis and Chronic Obstructive Pulmonary Disease. *J. Indian Soc. Periodontol.* 15, 359–365. doi:10.4103/0972-124x.92570

Prokopovic, V., Popovic, M., Andjelkovic, U., Marsavelski, A., Raskovic, B., Gavrovic-Jankulovic, M., et al. (2014). Isolation, Biochemical Characterization and Anti-bacterial Activity of BPIFA2 Protein. *Arch. Oral Biol.* 59, 302–309. doi:10.1016/j.archoralbio.2013.12.005

Qian, Y., Yuan, W., Mei, N., Wu, J., Xu, Q., Lu, H., et al. (2020). Periodontitis Increases the Risk of Respiratory Disease Mortality in Older Patients. *Exp. Gerontol.* 133, 110878. doi:10.1016/j.exger.2020.110878

Quagliarello, V., Ginter, S., Han, L., Van Ness, P., Allore, H., and Tinetti, M. (2005). Modifiable Risk Factors for Nursing home-acquired Pneumonia. *Clin. Infect. Dis.* 40, 1–6. doi:10.1086/426023

Rivas Caldas, R., Le Gall, F., Revert, K., Rault, G., Virmaux, M., Gouriou, S., et al. (2015). *Pseudomonas aeruginosa* and Periodontal Pathogens in the Oral Cavity and Lungs of Cystic Fibrosis Patients: a Case-Control Study. *J. Clin. Microbiol.* 53, 1898–1907. doi:10.1128/jcm.00368-15

Salsgiver, E. L., Fink, A. K., Knapp, E. A., Lipuma, J. J., Olivier, K. N., Marshall, B. C., et al. (2016). Changing Epidemiology of the Respiratory Bacteriology of Patients with Cystic Fibrosis. *Chest* 149, 390–400. doi:10.1378/chest.15-0676

Santagati, M., Scillato, M., Patanè, F., Aiello, C., and Stefani, S. (2012). Bacteriocin-producing Oral Streptococci and Inhibition of Respiratory Pathogens. *FEMS Immunol. Med. Microbiol.* 65, 23–31. doi:10.1111/j.1574-695x.2012.00928.x

Scannapieco, F. A. (1999). Role of Oral Bacteria in Respiratory Infection. *J. Periodontol.* 70, 793–802. doi:10.1902/jop.1999.70.7.793

Scannapieco, F. A., and Shay, K. (2014). Oral Health Disparities in Older Adults. *Dental Clin. North America* 58, 771–782. doi:10.1016/j.cden.2014.06.005

Scannapieco, F. A., Stewart, E. M., and Mylotte, J. M. (1992). Colonization of Dental Plaque by Respiratory Pathogens in Medical Intensive Care Patients. *Crit. Care Med.* 20, 740–745. doi:10.1097/00003246-199206000-00007

Scannapieco, F. A., Wang, B., and Shiau, H. J. (2001). Oral Bacteria and Respiratory Infection: Effects on Respiratory Pathogen Adhesion and Epithelial Cell Proinflammatory Cytokine Production. *Ann. Periodontol.* 6, 78–86. doi:10.1902/annals.2001.6.1.78

Schaub, B., Lauener, R., and Von Mutius, E. (2006). The many Faces of the hygiene Hypothesis. *J. Allergy Clin. Immunol.* 117, 969–977. quiz 978. doi:10.1016/j.jaci.2006.03.003

Scoffield, J. A., Duan, D., Zhu, F., and Wu, H. (2017). A Commensal streptococcus Hijacks a *Pseudomonas aeruginosa* Exopolysaccharide to Promote Biofilm Formation. *Plos Pathog.* 13, e1006300. doi:10.1371/journal.ppat.1006300

Scoffield, J. A., and Wu, H. (2016). Nitrite Reductase Is Critical for *Pseudomonas aeruginosa* Survival during Co-infection with the Oral Commensal Streptococcus Parasanguinis. *Microbiology (Reading)* 162, 376–383. doi:10.1099/mic.0.000226

Scoffield, J. A., and Wu, H. (2015). Oral Streptococci and Nitrite-Mediated Interference of *Pseudomonas aeruginosa. Infect. Immun.* 83, 101–107. doi:10.1128/iai.02396-14

Seed, P. C. (2014). The Human Mycobiome. *Cold Spring Harbor Perspect. Med.* 5, a019810. doi:10.1101/cshperspect.a019810

Seedorf, H., Griffin, N. W., Ridaura, V. K., Reyes, A., Cheng, J., Rey, F. E., et al. (2014). Bacteria from Diverse Habitats Colonize and Compete in the Mouse Gut. *Cell* 159, 253–266. doi:10.1016/j.cell.2014.09.008

Sibley, C. D., Parkins, M. D., Rabin, H. R., Duan, K., Norgaard, J. C., and Surette, M. G. (2008). A Polymicrobial Perspective of Pulmonary Infections Exposes an Enigmatic Pathogen in Cystic Fibrosis Patients. *Proc. Natl. Acad. Sci.* 105, 15070–15075. doi:10.1073/pnas.0804326105

Sikorska, H., and Smoragiewicz, W. (2013). Role of Probiotics in the Prevention and Treatment of Meticillin-Resistant *Staphylococcus aureus* Infections. *Int. J. Antimicrob. Agents* 42, 475–481. doi:10.1016/j.ijantimicag.2013.08.003

Souto, R., Silva-Boghossian, C. M., and Colombo, A. P. V. (2014). Prevalence of *Pseudomonas aeruginosa* and Acinetobacter Spp. In Subgingival Biofilm and Saliva of Subjects with Chronic Periodontal Infection. *Braz. J. Microbiol.* 45, 495–501. doi:10.1590/s1517-83822014000200017

Stensson, M., Wendt, L.-K., Koch, G., Oldaeus, G., and Birkhed, D. (2008). Oral Health in Preschool Children with Asthma. *Int. J. Paediatr. Dent* 18, 243–250. doi:10.1111/j.1365-263x.2008.00921.x

Stonecypher, K. (2010). Ventilator-Associated Pneumonia. *Crit. Care Nurs. Q.* 33, 339–347. doi:10.1097/cnq.0b013e3181f649a6

Sumi, Y., Miura, H., Michiwaki, Y., Nagaosa, S., and Nagaya, M. (2007). Colonization of Dental Plaque by Respiratory Pathogens in Dependent Elderly. *Arch. Gerontol. Geriatr.* 44, 119–124. doi:10.1016/j.archger.2006.04.004

Tada, A., and Hanada, N. (2010). Opportunistic Respiratory Pathogens in the Oral Cavity of the Elderly. *FEMS Immunol. Med. Microbiol.* 60, 1–17. doi:10.1111/j.1574-695x.2010.00709.x

Tagg, J. R. (2004). Prevention of Streptococcal Pharyngitis by Anti-Streptococcus Pyogenes Bacteriocin-like Inhibitory Substances (BLIS) Produced by Streptococcus Salivarius. *Indian J. Med. Res.* 119 (Suppl. l), 13–16.

Tagg, J. R. (2009). Streptococcal Bacteriocin-like Inhibitory Substances: Some Personal Insights into the Bacteriocin-like Activities Produced by Streptococci Good and Bad. *Probiotics Antimicro. Prot.* 1, 60–66. doi:10.1007/s12602-008-9002-7

Tan, L., Wang, H., Li, C., and Pan, Y. (2014). 16S rDNA-Based Metagenomic Analysis of Dental Plaque and Lung Bacteria in Patients with Severe Acute Exacerbations of Chronic Obstructive Pulmonary Disease. *J. Periodont Res.* 49, 760–769. doi:10.1111/jre.12159

Teshome, A., and Yitayeh, A. (2016). Relationship between Periodontal Disease and Preterm Low Birth Weight: Systematic Review. *Pan Afr. Med. J.* 24, 215. doi:10.11604/pamj.2016.24.215.8727

Thamadilok, S., Roche-Håkansson, H., Håkansson, A. P., and Ruhl, S. (2016). Absence of Capsule Reveals Glycan-Mediated Binding and Recognition of Salivary Mucin MUC7 byStreptococcus Pneumoniae. *Mol. Oral Microbiol.* 31, 175–188. doi:10.1111/omi.12113

Thibodeau, P. H., and Butterworth, M. B. (2013). Proteases, Cystic Fibrosis and the Epithelial Sodium Channel (ENaC). *Cell Tissue Res* 351, 309–323. doi:10.1007/s00441-012-1439-z

To, K. K., Tsang, O. T., Leung, W. S., Tam, A. R., Wu, T. C., Lung, D. C., et al. (2020). Temporal Profiles of Viral Load in Posterior Oropharyngeal Saliva Samples and Serum Antibody Responses during Infection by SARS-CoV-2: an Observational Cohort Study. *Lancet Infect. Dis.* 20, 565–574. doi:10.1016/S1473-3099(20)30196-1

Tunney, M. M., Field, T. R., Moriarty, T. F., Patrick, S., Doering, G., Muhlebach, M. S., et al. (2008). Detection of Anaerobic Bacteria in High Numbers in Sputum from Patients with Cystic Fibrosis. *Am. J. Respir. Crit. Care Med.* 177, 995–1001. doi:10.1164/rccm.200708-1151oc

Verma, D., Garg, P. K., and Dubey, A. K. (2018). Insights into the Human Oral Microbiome. *Arch. Microbiol.* 200, 525–540. doi:10.1007/s00203-018-1505-3

Walls, T., Power, D., and Tagg, J. (2003). Bacteriocin-like Inhibitory Substance (BLIS) Production by the normal flora of the Nasopharynx: Potential to Protect against Otitis media? *J. Med. Microbiol.* 52, 829–833. doi:10.1099/jmm.0.05259-0

Wand, M. E., Bock, L. J., Bonney, L. C., and Sutton, J. M. (2017). Mechanisms of Increased Resistance to Chlorhexidine and Cross-Resistance to Colistin Following Exposure of *Klebsiella pneumoniae* Clinical Isolates to Chlorhexidine. *Antimicrob. Agents Chemother.* 61, 16. doi:10.1128/AAC.01162-16

Wang, Y., Ren, B., Zhou, X., Liu, S., Zhou, Y., Li, B., et al. (2017). Growth and Adherence of *Staphylococcus aureus* Were Enhanced through the PGE2 Produced by the Activated COX-2/PGE2 Pathway of Infected Oral Epithelial Cells. *PLoS One* 12, e0177166. doi:10.1371/journal.pone.0177166

Wang, Z. M. (2019). Relationship between Oral Microecological Imbalance and General Health. *Zhonghua Kou Qiang Yi Xue Za Zhi* 54, 145–150. doi:10.3760/cma.j.issn.1002-0098.2019.03.001

Wang, Z., Zhou, X., Zhang, J., Zhang, L., Song, Y., Hu, F. B., et al. (2009). Periodontal Health, Oral Health Behaviours, and Chronic Obstructive Pulmonary Disease. *J. Clin. Periodontol.* 36, 750–755. doi:10.1111/j.1600-051x.2009.01448.x

Wescombe, P. A., Heng, N. C., Burton, J. P., Chilcott, C. N., and Tagg, J. R. (2009). Streptococcal Bacteriocins and the Case for Streptococcus Salivarius as Model Oral Probiotics. *Future Microbiol.* 4, 819–835. doi:10.2217/fmb.09.61

Whiley, R. A., Fleming, E. V., Makhija, R., and Waite, R. D. (2015). Environment and Colonisation Sequence Are Key Parameters Driving Cooperation and Competition between *Pseudomonas aeruginosa* Cystic Fibrosis Strains and Oral Commensal Streptococci. *PLoS One* 10, e0115513. doi:10.1371/journal.pone.0115513

Whiley, R. A., Sheikh, N. P., Mushtaq, N., Hagi-Pavli, E., Personne, Y., Javaid, D., et al. (2014). Differential Potentiation of the Virulence of the *Pseudomonas aeruginosa* Cystic Fibrosis liverpool Epidemic Strain by Oral Commensal Streptococci. *J. Infect. Dis.* 209, 769–780. doi:10.1093/infdis/jit568

Woods, D. E. (1987). Role of Fibronectin in the Pathogenesis of Gram-Negative Bacillary Pneumonia. *Rev. Infect. Dis.* 9 (Suppl. 4), S386–S390. doi:10.1093/clinids/9.supplement_4.s386

Worlitzsch, D., Rintelen, C., Böhm, K., Wollschläger, B., Merkel, N., Borneff-Lipp, M., et al. (2009). Antibiotic-resistant Obligate Anaerobes during Exacerbations of Cystic Fibrosis Patients. *Clin. Microbiol. Infect.* 15, 454–460. doi:10.1111/j.1469-0691.2008.02659.x

Wu, X., Chen, J., Xu, M., Zhu, D., Wang, X., Chen, Y., et al. (2017). 16S rDNA Analysis of Periodontal Plaque in Chronic Obstructive Pulmonary Disease and Periodontitis Patients. *J. Oral Microbiol.* 9, 1324725. doi:10.1080/20002297.2017.1324725

Xu, H., Zhong, L., Deng, J., Peng, J., Dan, H., Zeng, X., et al. (2020). High Expression of ACE2 Receptor of 2019-nCoV on the Epithelial Cells of Oral Mucosa. *Int. J. Oral Sci.* 12, 8. doi:10.1038/s41368-020-0074-x

Yamasaki, K., Kawanami, T., Yatera, K., Fukuda, K., Noguchi, S., Nagata, S., et al. (2013). Significance of Anaerobes and Oral Bacteria in Community-Acquired Pneumonia. *PLoS One* 8, e63103. doi:10.1371/journal.pone.0063103

Yan, X., Yang, M., Liu, J., Gao, R., Hu, J., Li, J., et al. (2015). Discovery and Validation of Potential Bacterial Biomarkers for Lung Cancer. *Am. J. Cancer Res.* 5, 3111–3122.

Yang, J., Mu, X., Wang, Y., Zhu, D., Zhang, J., Liang, C., et al. (2018). Dysbiosis of the Salivary Microbiome Is Associated with Non-smoking Female Lung Cancer and

Correlated with Immunocytochemistry Markers. *Front. Oncol.* 8, 520. doi:10.3389/fonc.2018.00520

Zeng, X.-T., Tu, M.-L., Liu, D.-Y., Zheng, D., Zhang, J., and Leng, W. (2012). Periodontal Disease and Risk of Chronic Obstructive Pulmonary Disease: a Meta-Analysis of Observational Studies. *PLoS One* 7, e46508. doi:10.1371/journal.pone.0046508

Zeng, X.-T., Xia, L.-Y., Zhang, Y.-G., Li, S., Leng, W.-D., and Kwong, J. S. W. (2016). Periodontal Disease and Incident Lung Cancer Risk: A Meta-Analysis of Cohort Studies. *J. Periodontol.* 87, 1158–1164. doi:10.1902/jop.2016.150597

Zhou, X., Han, J., Liu, Z., Song, Y., Wang, Z., and Sun, Z. (2014). Effects of Periodontal Treatment on Lung Function and Exacerbation Frequency in Patients with Chronic Obstructive Pulmonary Disease and Chronic Periodontitis: a 2-year Pilot Randomized Controlled Trial. *J. Clin. Periodontol.* 41, 564–572. doi:10.1111/jcpe.12247

Zhou, X., Wang, J., Liu, W., Huang, X., Song, Y., Wang, Z., et al. (2020). Periodontal Status and Microbiologic Pathogens in Patients with Chronic Obstructive Pulmonary Disease and Periodontitis: A Case-Control Study. *Copd* 15, 2071–2079. doi:10.2147/copd.s266612

19

Initial PCR Testing Negative, but Chest CT Suggesting for Viral Pneumonia Urges for Repeated Testing for COVID-19 Diagnosis

Lingwei Wang[1,2†], Danting Zhan[1,2†], Xiaodi Liu[3†], Kai Yang[1,2†], Shipin Wu[3], Heng Zhang[1,2], Min Yu[1,2], Yimin Zha[1,2], Weibin Huang[1,2], Lei Li[4], Rongchang Chen[1,2*] and Chen Qiu[1,2*]*

[1]The Department of Respiratory Diseases and Critic Care Unit, Shenzhen Institute of Respiratory Diseases, Shenzhen People's Hospital (The Second Clinical Medical College, Jinan University; The First Affiliated Hospital, Southern University of Science and Technology), Shenzhen, China, [2]Shenzhen Key Laboratory of Respiratory Diseases, Shenzhen Major Respiratory Diseases's Prevention and Treatment Center, Shenzhen, China, [3]Department of Infectious Diseases, Shenzhen People's Hospital (The Second Clinical Medical College, Jinan University; The First Affiliated Hospital, Southern University of Science and Technology), Shenzhen, China, [4]Guangdong Provincial Key Laboratory of Brain Connectome and Behavior, CAS Key Laboratory of Brain Connectome and Manipulation, The Brain Cognition and Brain Disease Institute (BCBDI), Shenzhen Institutes of Advanced Technology, Chinese Academy of Sciences, Shenzhen-Hong Kong Institute of Brain Science-Shenzhen Fundamental Research Institutions, Shenzhen, China

Keywords: COVID-19, chest CT, PCR test, pneumonia, diagnosis

***Correspondence:**
Lei Li
saralilei@siat.ac.cn
Rongchang Chen
chonrc@vip.163.com
Chen Qiu
szchester@163.com

[†]These authors have contributed equally to this work

INTRODUCTION

The COVID-19 pandemic has become one of the major health crises worldwide (Guan et al., 2020). PCR testing of SARS-CoV-2 is generally used as the gold standard of confirmation for diagnostics of COVID-19. With the growing awareness of the high false-negative rates of PCR testing (Ai et al., 2020; Yang et al., 2020b), whether and which subgroup of patients with initial negative results should be subjected to repeated testing is a matter that requires more clinical data.

Under this circumstance, the value of chest CT as a screening tool in COVID-19 has been vigorously discussed (Ai et al., 2020; Bao et al., 2020; ; Merkus and Klein, 2020). A recent report with 1,014 cases (Ai et al., 2020; Bao et al., 2020) proposed that chest CT has a high sensitivity for the diagnosis of COVID-19 and may be considered as a primary tool for COVID-19 screening. Others have called for caution regarding the usage of CT due to its ionizing radiation, and some have specified its unsuitability as a screening tool for pediatric patients (Merkus and Klein, 2020). After evaluation, our triaging procedure and diagnostic practice for a total of 358 outpatients (149 COVID-19–suspected cases including 13 confirmed) at Shenzhen People's Hospital, Shenzhen, China, we found that chest CT can distinguish COVID-19 patients from suspected cases (AUC = 0.85) much better than other indicators (AUCs < 0.65) without PCR testing, including epidemiological history, symptoms, white blood cell (WBC) count, and lymphocyte count. Therefore, we propose chest CT as a main tool in determining which subgroup of suspected patients should be subjected to repeated tests after their initial negative PCR testing for SARS-CoV-2.

The first COVID-19 patient was admitted on January 9, 2020 in Shenzhen, an international city with a population of 13.43 million. Different levels of responsive strategies were quickly developed under the pressure of the highly contagious pandemic (Yang et al., 2020a). We received 358 patients at the emergency department and fever clinic with fever or upper respiratory syndromes from January 2020 to March 2020 in our hospital. Among them, 149 were classified as COVID-19–suspected cases according to the criteria complying with the guidelines for the diagnosis and treatment of novel coronavirus pneumonia issued by the

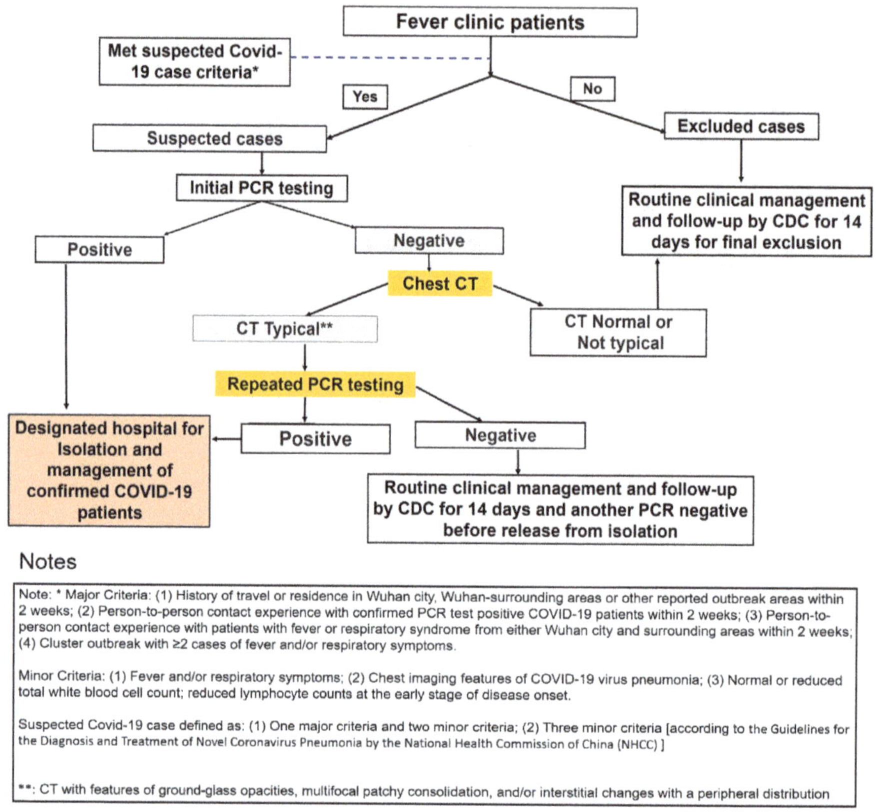

FIGURE 1 | Fever clinic patients were efficiently triaged and diagnosed for COVID-19. The false-negative rate for initial PCR testing is 30.8% (4 out of 13). A high percentage (8.9%) of the initial PCR testing–negative patients with typical CT signature were confirmed to be COVID-19 positive after repeated testing. Initial PCR testing–negative results but chest CT–positive results for viral pneumonia urges for repeated testing for COVID-19 diagnosis.

National Health Commission of China (NHCC) (National Health Commission and State Administration of Traditional Chinese Medicine, 2020) and required by at least two COVID-19 specialists, and they were subjected to our triaging procedure for suspected cases. Among all 149 patients, after tests and evaluation, 22 patients who were confirmed or highly suspected with COVID-19 were transferred to a special neighboring hospital in Shenzhen that has a special ward for the COVID-19 outbreak.

Our initial oropharyngeal swab PCR testing confirmed 9 SARS-CoV-2-positive patients and 140 negative patients. Expert consultation, chest CT scan, blood WBC counting, epidemiology investigation, and further repeated PCR tests revealed that four patients of the 140 with initial negative PCR tests were false-negative, making the final COVID-19 patient number up to 13. The false-negative initial PCR testing accounts for 30.8% (4 out of 13) of the total confirmed cases (**Figure 1**), with a true-positive rate of initial PCR test of 69.2% (9 out of 13). This is in line with the reported positive rate from 30 to 60% (Ai et al., 2020) and suggests that additional diagnostic procedures should be carried out after initial negative PCR testing before patients are being subjected to routine clinical follow-up.

SUBSECTIONS RELEVANT FOR THE SUBJECT

The Description of Four Patients With Positive Computed Tomography and Initial Negative Reverse-Transcription Polymerase Chain Reaction Test

Patient 1: A 35-year-old male with fever for 6 days, with a recent travel history to Wuhan, China, where the pandemic was going on at that time, visited the hospital. Although the initial PCR test for SARS-CoV-2 was negative, the chest CT (January 26, 2020) showed multifocal ground-glass opacity (GGO) and parenchyma consolidation, predominantly involving subpleural regions of both the lungs. A routine blood test showed that the WBC count was 5.24 × 10^9/L, and the absolute value of the lymphocyte count was 0.87 × 10^9/L. However, the patient met the diagnostic criteria for a suspected COVID-19 patient and was quarantined at the hospital. The PCR test was repeated with bronchoalveolar lavage fluid (BALF), and the result was positive.

Patient 2: A 76-year-old female with fatigue and drowsiness, and with no fever visited the hospital. She had a travel history to Wuhan during the COVID-19 outbreak period. Although the initial PCR test for SARS-CoV-2 was negative, the chest CT (January 23, 2020) showed multifocal parenchyma. A routine blood test showed that the WBC count was 6.96×10^9/L, while the absolute value of the lymphocyte count was 1.09×10^9/L. The second throat swab test was positive. Patient 3: A 66-year-old female appeared with cough and sputum but had no fever. She had a travel history from Wuhan in January 2020. The first swab test was negative. The chest CT (January 25, 2020) showed a bit of GGO. A routine blood test showed that the WBC count was 4.9×10^9/L, and the absolute value of the lymphocyte count was 1.27×10^9/L. A repeated nasopharyngeal swab for the PCR test was positive, and follow-up chest CT showed typical GGO consistent with COVID-19. Patient 4: A 78-year-old male with fever, cough, and sputum, and a recent travel history to Wuhan, China, visited the hospital in January 2020. The first throat swab test was negative. The chest CT (January 25, 2020) showed multifocal GGO. A routine blood test showed that the WBC count was 4.53×10^9/L, and the absolute value of the lymphocyte count was 0.96×10^9/L. However, the patient met the diagnostic criteria for suspected COVID-19 and was quarantined in the hospital. A repeated nasopharyngeal swab for the PCR test was positive.

Influence of Different Indexes on the Diagnosis of COVID-19

Variable positive rates of the PCR test may be associated with sample collection, PCR methodology, and developing stages of COVID-19 in patients (Ai et al., 2020). Two articles reported using specimens from nasopharyngeal swabs showed a higher positive PCR test rate than oropharyngeal swabs (Tan et al., 2020; Xiao et al., 2020). For the high false-negative rate of the initial PCR test (30.8%), it is necessary to do repeated tests. To avoid occupation of limited hospital resources and speed up the screening procedure, it is not practical to test all the initial PCR-negative patients repeatedly. One parameter or a cluster of test parameters would help in selecting the most possible COVID-19 patients among all the initial PCR test–negative cases.

Typical chest CT refers to ground-glass opacities, multifocal patchy consolidation, and/or interstitial changes with a peripheral distribution (National Health Commission and State Administration of Traditional Chinese Medicine, 2020). The sensitivity and the specificity of typical chest CT in suggesting COVID-19 among all 149 suspected cases are 100% (13/13) and 69.85% (95/136), respectively. A positive WBC parameter means a normal or decreased WBC count (National Health Commission and State Administration of Traditional Chinese Medicine, 2020; National Institutes of Health, 2020). The sensitivity and the specificity of WBC counting in suggesting COVID-19 among all 149 suspected cases are 100% (13/13) and 0.74% (1/136), respectively. The specificity of WBC counting is much lower than that of chest CT. The sensitivity and the specificity of the combination of chest CT positive and WBC counting are 100% (13/13) and 70.59% (96/136), respectively, with not much improvement compared with using chest CT alone as a parameter. When we used the strict parameter combinations in our study according to the guideline of the NHCC, which includes fever/cough, positive result of chest CT manifestations, and WBC counting, along with epidemiology characteristic (history of traveling to Wuhan or being in close contact with COVID-19 patients), the sensitivity and the specificity in suggesting COVID-19 among all suspected cases are 84.62% (11/13) and 88.24% (120/136), respectively. Although the specificity increases from 69.85 to 88.24%, the sensitivity decreases from 100 to 84.62% when compared with using chest CT alone as a parameter.

DISCUSSION

Among the 140 initial PCR test–negative patients, 95 showed normal chest CT, and they were excluded from the diagnosis of COVID-19 and released after another PCR test confirmation complying with the NHCC guideline. For the 45 cases with pneumonia CT features, 40 were classified as not typical COVID-19 CT presentation, and four were classified as typical COVID-19 CT presentation. In these four cases, repeated PCR tests revealed all positive results (**Figure 1**), which account for 8.9% (4 out of 45) of the "initial PCR testing negative but chest CT positive for viral pneumonia" group. This is quite a high percentage considering the high contagious nature of SARS-CoV-2. We strongly suggest that for patients with initial PCR testing–negative results but chest CT positive, repeated PCR tests should be carried out. Here we are not considering chest CT as an alternative screening tool to replace the PCR test for COVID-19 but rather proposing that chest CT serves well as a tool in determining which subgroup of suspected patients should be subjected to repeated tests after their negative initial PCR testing for SARS-CoV-2.

Among our 140 initial PCR-negative cases, the sensitivity and the specificity of chest CT in suggesting COVID-19 are 100% (4/4) and 69.85% (95/136), respectively; the sensitivity and the specificity of WBC counting are 100% (4/4) and 0.74% (1/136), respectively; and the sensitivity and the specificity of combined parameters (fever/cough, chest CT, WBC counting, and epidemiology characteristic) are 50.0% (2/4) and 88.24% (120/136), respectively. Considering both the sensitivity and the specificity, chest CT proves to be the most powerful parameter in suggesting COVID-19 among initial PCR-negative cases. In our study, upon using chest CT as a parameter, the repeated PCR testing pressure was reduced by 67.9% (95 out of 145) (**Figure 1**). All of the CT nontypical cases among the initial negative testing cases were excluded from COVID-19 diagnosis (confirmed by repeat PCR before releasing and then followed up). Altogether, in our study, chest CT serves well as a tool in determining what kind of suspected patients should be subjected to repeated tests after their negative initial PCR testing for SARS-CoV-2.

As demonstrated in **Figure 1**, our triage operation process showed a high performance, with a screening rate of 14.77% (22/149) in COVID-19–suspected patients to be sent to the special ward, while the screening rate was 0% (0/209) for non-suspected outpatients. For all 149 suspected cases, the top four diagnoses were upper respiratory tract infection (54/149), community-acquired pneumonia (53/149), COVID-19 (13/149), and gastroenteritis (5/149). This suggests that upper respiratory tract infection and community-acquired pneumonia should be emphasized and excluded from the COVID-19 diagnostic process to avoid the occupation of hospital resources. Till date, all 13 confirmed patients have recovered and were discharged.

Our clinical practice showed that with an initial PCR positive rate of 69.2% in those finally confirmed COVID-19 cases, further testing and repeated PCR testing for subgroups of the initial PCR test–negative patients should be emphasized. In a recently published article, it was stated that to compensate for the potential risk of false-negative PCR, chest CT should be applied for clinically suspected patients with negative initial RT-PCR (He et al., 2020), and repeated swab tests should be carried out (Xie et al., 2020). In terms of chest imaging findings, the less pulmonary consolidation found *via* CT scan, the greater the possibility of negative initial RT-PCR results (Chen et al., 2021).

Our study had limitations. First, the limitation of the hospital and the confirmed patient resources is an unavoidable problem for this study. However, from another perspective, as the vaccines are developed and applied, suspected or confirmed patients of COVID-19 infection will be reduced in number. The idea in this opinion article is to somehow provide clinical instruction. Second, the PCR result is affected by many factors, such as laboratory reagents, test methods, and subjective performance. However, at this time, the nucleic acid detection method is not mature yet, and our research results are more important. We try to provide evidence to support the importance of chest CT scan in "work protocol for fever clinic" in detection of COVID-19 patients. In our protocol, chest CT does not serve as a screening tool but as an important indicator for follow-up and repeated PCR testing after initial PCR-negative results. We provide more evidence to show that this work protocol could provide high sensitivity and acceptable specificity, which are better than other criteria and able to reduce the missed diagnosis of false-negative nucleic acid patients.

AUTHOR CONTRIBUTIONS

All authors listed have made a substantial, direct, and intellectual contribution to the work and approved it for publication.

REFERENCES

Ai, T., Yang, Z., Hou, H., Zhan, C., Chen, C., Chen, C., et al. (2020). Correlation of Chest CT and RT-PCR Testing in Coronavirus Disease 2019 (COVID-19) in China: A Report of 1014 Cases. *Radiology* 296, E32–E40. doi:10.1148/radiol.2020200642

Bao, C., Liu, X., Zhang, H., Li, Y., and Liu, J. (2020). Coronavirus Disease 2019 (COVID-19) CT Findings: A Systematic Review and Meta-Analysis. *J. Am. Coll. Radiol.* 17, 701–709. doi:10.1016/j.jacr.2020.03.006

Chen, D., Jiang, X., Hong, Y., Wen, Z., Wei, S., Peng, G., et al. (2021). Can Chest CT Features Distinguish Patients with Negative from Those with Positive Initial RT-PCR Results for Coronavirus Disease (COVID-19)? *AJR Am. J. Roentgenol* 216, 66–70. doi:10.2214/AJR.20.23012

Guan, W., Ni, Z., Hu, Y., Liang, W., Ou, C., He, J., et al. (2020). Clinical Characteristics of Coronavirus Disease 2019 in China. *N. Engl. J. Med.* 382, 1708–1720. doi:10.1056/NEJMoa2002032

He, J. L., Luo, L., Luo, Z. D., Lyu, J. X., Ng, M. Y., Shen, X. P., et al. (2020). Diagnostic Performance between CT and Initial Real-Time RT-PCR for Clinically Suspected 2019 Coronavirus Disease (COVID-19) Patients outside Wuhan, China. *Respir. Med.* 168, 105980. doi:10.1016/j.rmed.2020.105980

Merkus, P. J., and Klein, W. M. (2020). Value of Chest CT as COVID 19 Screening Tool in Children. *Eur. Respir. J.* 55, 2001241. doi:10.1183/13993003.01241-2020

National Health Commission and State Administration of Traditional Chinese Medicine (2020). Diagnosis and Treatment Protocol for Novel Coronavirus Pneumonia (Trial Version 7). Available online at: http://www.nhc.gov.cn/yzygj/s7653p/202003/46c9294a7dfe4cef80dc7f59 (Accessed March 3, 2020).

National Institutes of Health (2020). Coronavirus Disease 2019 (COVID-19) Treatment Guidelines. Available online at: https://www.covid19treatmentguidelines.nih.gov/ (Accessed March 3, 2020).

Tan, L., Wang, X., Liu, W., Lu, Y., Cheng, L., and Sun, Z. (2020). Comparison of Nasopharyngeal and Oropharyngeal Swabs for SARS-CoV-2 Detection in 353 Patients Received Tests with Both Specimens Simultaneously. *Int. J. Infect. Dis.* 94, 107–109. doi:10.1016/j.ijid.2020.04.023

Xiao, A., Tong, Y., Gao, C., Zhu, L., Zhang, Y., and Zhang, S. (2020). Dynamic Profile of RT-PCR Findings from 301 COVID-19 Patients in Wuhan, China: A Descriptive Study. *J. Clin. Virol.* 127, 104346. doi:10.1016/j.jcv.2020.104346

Xie, X., Zhong, Z., Zhao, W., Zheng, C., Wang, F., and Liu, J. J. R. (2020). Chest CT for Typical 2019-nCoV Pneumonia: Relationship to Negative RT-PCR Testing. *Radiology* 296, 200343. doi:10.1148/radiol.2020200343

Yang, K., Wang, L., Li, F., Chen, D., Li, X., Qiu, C., et al. (2020a). The Influence of Preventive Strategies on the COVID-2019 Epidemic in Shenzhen, China. *Eur. Respir. J.* 55, 2000599. doi:10.1183/13993003.00599-2020

Yang, Y., Yang, M., Shen, C., Wang, F., Yuan, J., Li, J., et al. (2020b). Evaluating the Accuracy of Different Respiratory Specimens in the Laboratory Diagnosis and Monitoring the Viral Shedding of 2019-nCoV Infections. doi:10.1101/2020.02.11.20021493

20

Development and Validation of the Prognostic Index based on Inflammation-Related Gene Analysis in Idiopathic Pulmonary Fibrosis

Yanjiao Lu[1], Jinkun Chen[2], Kun Tang[1], Shanshan Wang[1], Zhen Tian[1], Meijia Wang[1], Jianping Zhao[1] and Jungang Xie[1]**

[1]Department of Respiratory and Critical Care Medicine, National Clinical Research Center of Respiratory Disease, Tongji Hospital, Tongji Medical College, Huazhong University of Science and Technology, Wuhan, China, [2]Department of science, Western University, London, ON, Canada

***Correspondence:**
Jianping Zhao
Zhaojp88@126.com
Jungang Xie
xiejjgg@hotmail.com*

Background: Historically, idiopathic pulmonary fibrosis (IPF) was considered a chronic inflammation disorder, but this conception was reassessed in the past decades. Our understanding of the role of inflammation in IPF and its association with clinical significance remained incomplete.

Methods: We downloaded mRNA expression data of peripheral blood mononuclear cells (PBMCs) from the Gene Expression Omnibus (GEO) repository. Inflammation-related genes (IRGs) expressed differently between IPF and control (CTRL) were determined. In this study, we systemically analyzed the expression of differently expressed IRGs by comprehensive bioinformatic analysis, and then investigated their potential prognostic values. The related prognostic gene expressions were verified in our cohort.

Results: 110 differently expressed IRGs were identified in this study, including 64 upregulated and 46 downregulated IRGs. Three IRGs (*S100A12*, *CCR7*, and *TNFSF4*) were identified as potential hub genes for prognosis. Those genes were subsequently subjected to the construction of the prognostic models. In the results, IPF patients categorized as high risk demonstrated a poor overall survival rate compared to patients categorized as low risk. Based on this prognostic model, the area under the curve (AUC) of the survival-dependent receiver operator characteristic (ROC) for 1-year, 2-year, and 3-year survival rates was 0.611, 0.695, and 0.681, respectively, in the GSE28042 cohort. These observations were validated in the GSE27957 cohort, confirming the good prognostic effect of this model. The expression of the three genes was validated in our cohort. We also conducted a nomogram based on the three IRGs' mRNA for quantitative IPF prognosis.

Abbreviations: CCR7: C-C motif chemokine receptor 7, CTRL: control, FC: fold change, FDA: food and drug Administration, FDR: false discovery rate, GEO: gene expression omnibus, ILD: interstitial lung disease, IPF: idiopathic pulmonary fibrosis, IRGs: inflammation-related genes, PBMCs: peripheral blood mononuclear cells, PPT: protein-protein interaction, RA: rheumatoid arthritis, ROC: receiver operator characteristic, S100A12: S100 calcium binding protein A12, STRING: search tool for the retrieval of interacting genes, TOLLIP: toll-interacting protein, TNFSF4: TNF superfamily member 4.

Conclusion: Three IRGs (*S100A12*, *CCR7*, and *TNFSF4*) were identified as potential markers for the prognosis of IPF.

Keywords: idiopathic pulmonary fibrosis, inflammation, prognostic, interstitial lung disease, gene

INTRODUCTION

Idiopathic pulmonary fibrosis (IPF), caused by an unknown reason and characterized by poor clinical prognosis, is a progressive, chronic, and irreversible interstitial lung disease (ILD) (Raghu et al., 2011a; Raghu et al., 2015). IPF occurs in elderly and middle-aged adults, and the median survival time from diagnosis is 2–4 years (Ley et al., 2011). Due to the recent advantages in the development of new therapies, the prognosis of IPF has been improved. However, it remains incurable partly due to the complexity and incomprehension of the etiology (Nathan et al., 2016; Richeldi et al., 2016). Therefore, better understandings of the molecular mechanisms of IPF are vital for the improvement of the prognosis of patients with IPF, early screening, and diagnosis.

Historically, IPF is assumed to be caused by chronic inflammation. However, the significance of inflammation in the onset and development of IPF has been strongly challenged. Evidenced by poor response to anti-inflammatory therapy, inflammation has demonstrated to be a nonessential pathogenic event in IPF (Selman et al., 2001; Richeldi, 2013). However, inflammation presents at different stages of IPF as a secondary event due to the activation of the innate and adaptive immune system and participates in IPF development (Mura et al., 2005; Heukels et al., 2019). Gene variants in *TOLLIP* (Toll-interacting protein), directly involved in inflammatory processes, resulted in reduced protein expression, which possibly contributes to an increased pro-inflammatory response observed in IPF patients (Noth et al., 2013). So far, the pathogenic role of inflammation in IPF remains controversial.

Regarding the changes in the understanding of inflammation, some researchers suggest that glucocorticoid treatment, a classic anti-inflammation therapy, is potentially effective in selected IPF patients (Heukels et al., 2019; Khor et al., 2019). Recent advances in precision treatment and increasing awareness of patient subgroup classification indicate a fundamental role of inflammation in IPF (Zhang et al., 2015). Macrophage-targeted lung delivery of dexamethasone improves pulmonary fibrosis therapy *via* regulating the immune microenvironment (Sang et al., 2021). More understanding of inflammation in IPF provides more evidence for the anti-inflammation treatment of IPF patients. Therefore, a systematic functional study of inflammation-related genes (IRGs) in IPF is of critical importance in understanding the roles of inflammation in IPF.

The blood components, including peripheral blood mononuclear cells (PBMCs) and white blood cells, are indicative factors of disease onset, progress, and prognosis of IPF (Richards et al., 2012; Scott et al., 2019). Maya et al. identified a 52-gene signature in PBMCs to stratify IPF patients to different risk levels and validated this signature in a prospective cohort (Herazo-Maya et al., 2013; Herazo-Maya et al., 2017). Studies using large-scale IRG expression profiles of patients are critically important for stratifying IPF patients and predicting the prognosis of IPF with different inflammation degrees.

The subject of this study was to investigate the roles of inflammation played in IPF and explore the potential clinical utility of IRGs for prognostic stratifications. Therefore, we downloaded the mRNA expression data of PBMCs and the clinicopathological data from the Gene Expression Omnibus (GEO) repository. We identified abnormally expressed IRGs between IPF and control (CTRL) using bioinformatic analysis, and systematically investigated their potential molecular mechanisms and functions. Finally, we analyzed the potential impact of IRGs on prognosis by combining the IRG expression data with clinical information.

METHODS

Data Acquisition and Processing

A total of 569 inflammation-related genes were extracted from the Gene Ontology and GO Annotations (https://www.ebi.ac.uk/QuickGO/), which provides detailed annotations of genes. We downloaded the microarray expression matrix dataset of 75 IPF and 19 CTRL PBMCs with corresponding clinical data from GSE28042 (https://www.ncbi.nlm.nih.gov/geo/query/acc.cgi?acc=GSE28042). To identify differently expressed inflammation-related genes between IPF and CTRL PBMCs, and the limma R package (http://www. bioconductor.org/packages) was used to perform the negative binomial distribution method according to the absolute value of fold change (FC) (>1.3) and false discovery rate (FDR) <0.05.

Protein–Protein Interaction Network and Hub Inflammation-Related Gene Screening

The differently expressed IRGs were submitted to the Search Tool for the Retrieval of Interacting Genes (STRING) (http://string-db.org) (version 10.5) for the prediction of the PPI network. Meanwhile, Cytoscape (version 3.8.0) was applied to visualize the PPI networks. The hub genes were identified in the PPI network according to the prediction of cytoHubba plug-in with Nodes' Scores. p values less than 0.05 were considered statistically significant.

Inflammation-Related Prognostic Model Construction

Univariate Cox regression analysis and log-rank tests were applied to analyze the significant risk factors in all hub IRGs using the survival R package. Afterward, we set up a multivariate Cox regression model for the calculation of the risk scores to

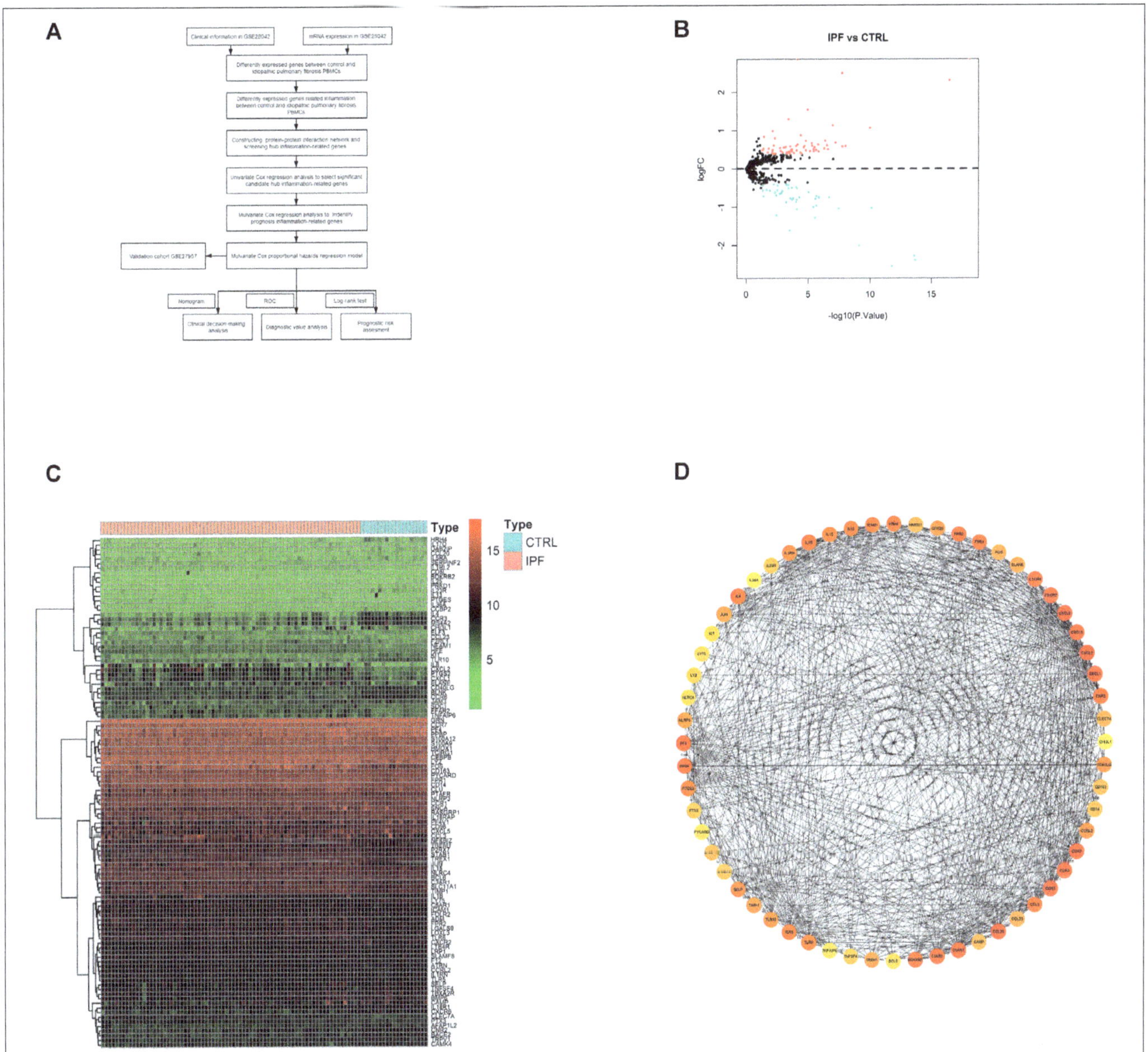

FIGURE 1 | The differentially expressed inflammation-related genes (IRGs) in idiopathic pulmonary fibrosis. **(A)** Flowchart for analyzing inflammation signature associated with idiopathic pulmonary fibrosis. **(B)** Volcano plot and **(C)** heatmap of differentially expressed IRGs. **(D)** Top 60 hub genes from protein–protein interaction (PPI) network. Blue circles: downregulated genes with a fold change over 1.3, and red circles: upregulated genes with fold change over 1.3. Red circle: higher correlation, and orange circle: lower correlation.

estimate the prognosis outcomes of IPF patients. Based on the above significant candidate hub genes, the risk scoring formula for each sample was as follows:

$$\text{Risk Score} = \beta 1 * \text{Exp1} + \beta 2 * \text{Exp2} + \beta 3 * \text{Exp3},$$

where β represented the coefficient value, while Exp represented the gene expression level.

Based on the median estimated risk score, IPF patients were categorized as high-risk and low-risk subgroups. The log-rank test was carried out for the comparison of the prognostic outcomes between the two subgroups. Further, the receiver operating characteristic (ROC) analysis was applied to assess the prognostic capabilities of the above model by the SurvivalROC R package.

Validation of the Prognostic Model

45 samples of IPF patients with the corresponding prognosis from the GSE27957 dataset were used to validate the estimating results to evaluate the accuracy of the model prediction. We also performed expression validation of the three prognostic genes in our cohort by real-time PCR. We collected PBMC samples and

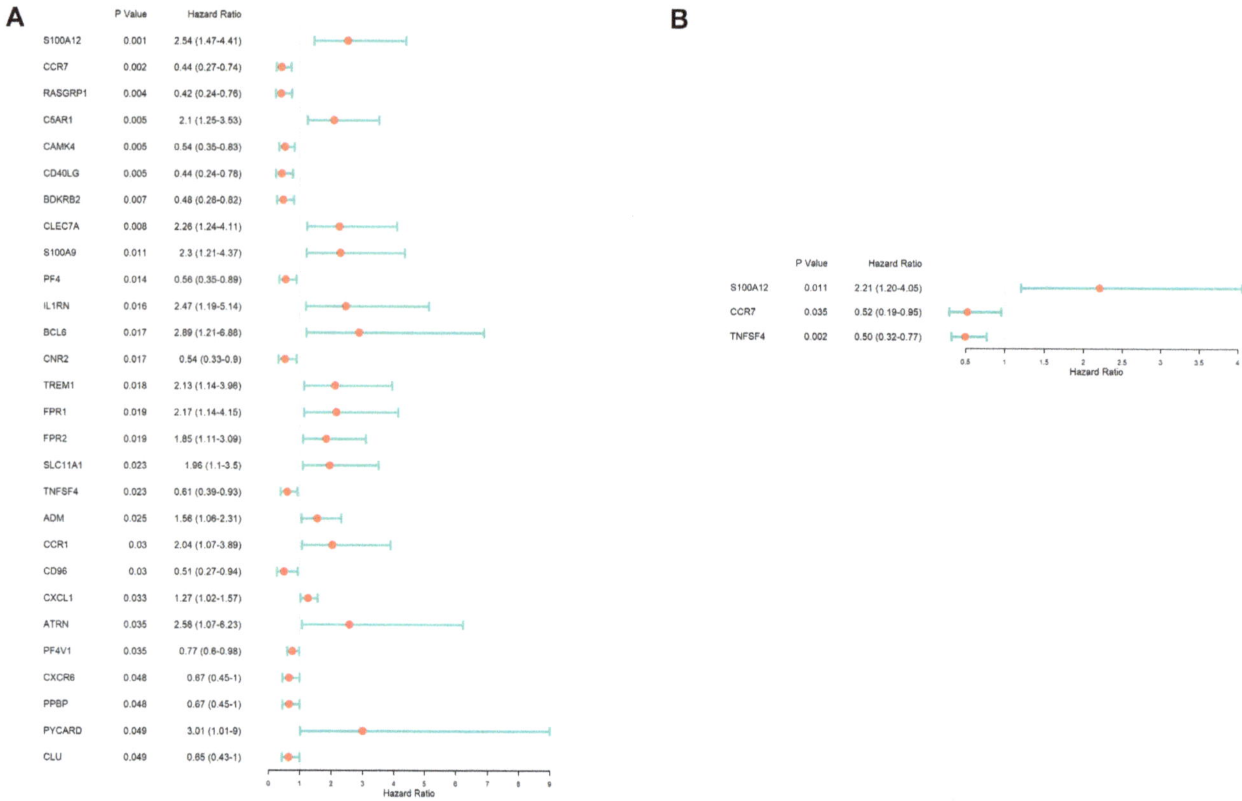

FIGURE 2 | Identification of prognosis-associated inflammation-related genes according to Cox regression analysis. **(A)** Univariate Cox regression analysis. **(B)** Multivariate Cox regression analysis.

clinical information of IPF patients in Tongji Hospital in Wuhan, China, from July 2020 to November 2020. Adult patients with clinical IPF diagnosis according to the American Thoracic Society/European Respiratory Society guideline (2011) were eligible for this study (Raghu et al., 2011b). This study was approved by the Ethics Committee of Tongji Hospital (IRB ID: 20150503). Results were presented as median with interquartile range (IQR), and nonparametric tests (Kruskal–Wallis or Mann–Whitney test) were used to compare across groups. Finally, a nomogram was conducted using the rms R package to predict the likelihood of a prognostic outcome in IPF patients. p values lower than 0.05 were set as statistical significance.

RESULTS

Differentially Expressed Inflammation-Related Genes Identification

A systematic analysis was carried out for the critical roles and the potential prognostic values of IRGs played in IPF. As shown in **Figure 1A**, the study was carried out according to the design. The databases of IPF patients were obtained from GEO-contained 75 IPF and 19 CTRL PBMCs samples. The R packages were used to process the data and discover differently expressed IRGs. According to the screening criteria, 110 IRGs were identified as differentially expressed between IPF and CTRL, containing 64 upregulated IRGs and 46 downregulated IRGs. The results were illustrated in the heatmap and volcano plot as in **Figures 1B,C**; details of the results were listed as in **Supplementary Table S1**.

Protein–Protein Interaction Network Construction and Hub Gene Analysis

Gene network complexes were generated by STRING according to the results of differently expressed IRGs. The PPI network contained 110 nodes and 470 edges (**Supplementary Figure S1**). The interaction network was operated using cytoHubba tools in Cytoscape to identify top 60 hub IRGs (**Figure 1D**).

Prognosis-Related Inflammation–Related Gene Selecting

To identify IRGs of significant correlation with the overall survival, a univariate Cox regression analysis was established based on hub IRGs. As shown in the forest map of the hazard ratio (**Figure 2A**), 28 IRGs were significantly associated with the prognosis of IPF patients. To estimate the impact of prognostic-associated hub IRGs on the clinical outcomes and survival time, the 28 hub IRGs were further analyzed by multiple stepwise Cox regression. As shown in **Figure 2B**, S100 calcium binding protein A12 (*S100A12*), C-C motif chemokine receptor 7 (*CCR7*), and

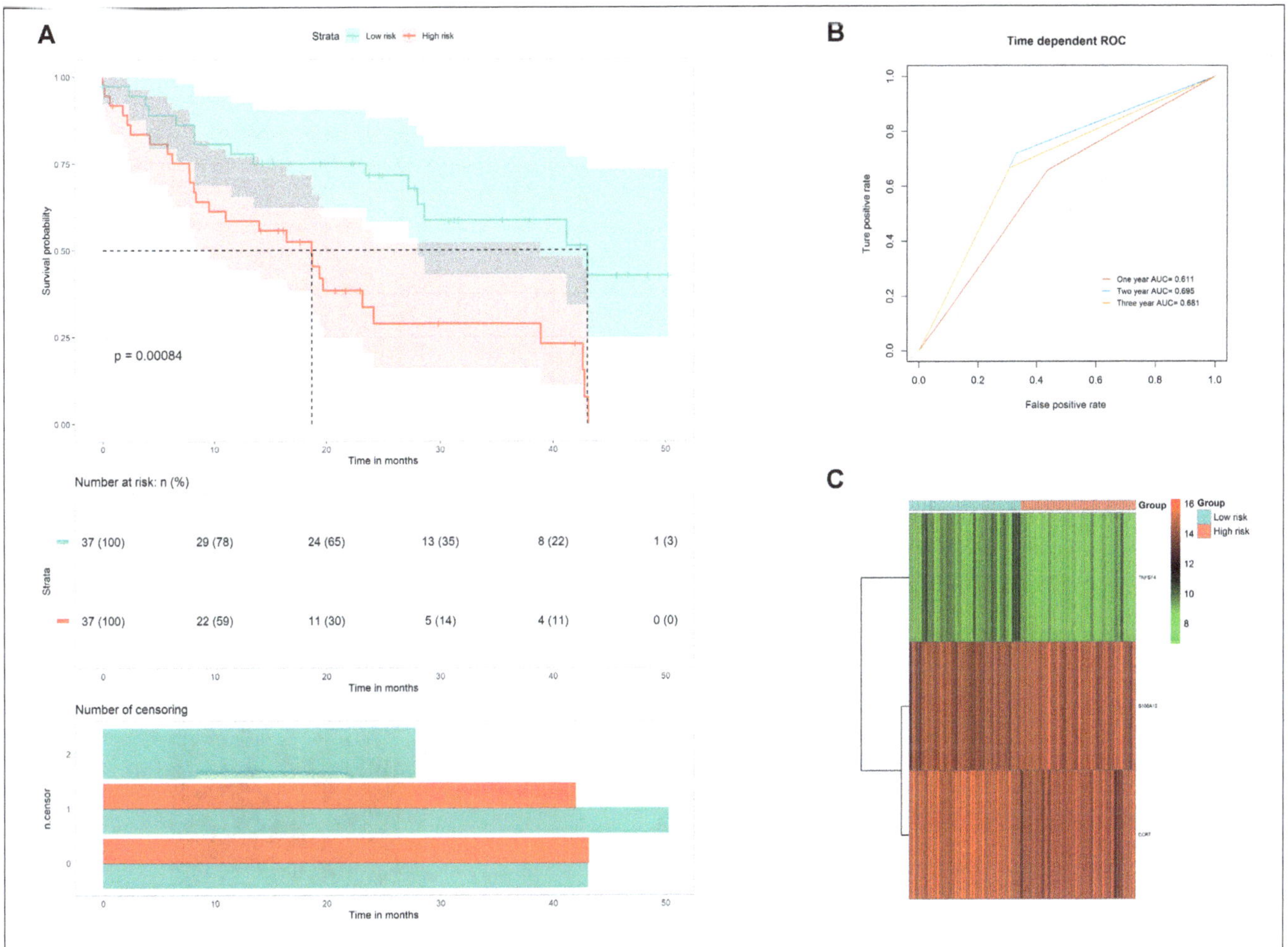

FIGURE 3 | Risk score analysis of the three-gene prognostic model in the GSE28042 training cohort. **(A)** Survival curve for patients with low- or high-risk scores. **(B)** ROC curves for forecasting overall survival. **(C)** Heat map for gene expressions.

TNF superfamily member 4 (*TNFSF4*) were identified as independent predictors for IPF patients.

Model Construction and Analysis for Prognosis-Related Genetic Risk Score

The three hub IRGs identified from the above analysis were used for the construction of the inflammation predictive model. The risk score of each IPF patient was calculated as

$$\text{Risk Score} = (0.792 * \text{ExpS100A12}) + (-0.645 * \text{ExpCCR7}) + (-0.704 * \text{ExpTNFSF4}).$$

Then, we performed a survival analysis to evaluate the predictive effect of this model. As the result, 75 IPF patients were categorized as high-risk or low-risk according to the median of risk scores. As revealed by the result, IPF patients with high-risk scores were associated with poor prognosis compared with those with low-risk scores (**Figure 3A**). A survival-dependent ROC analysis was carried out for the assessment of the prognostic abilities (**Figure 3B**). The area under the ROC curve for 1 year, 2 years, and 3 years survival rates were 0.611, 0.695, and 0.681 respectively, indicating a moderate prognostic potential of IRGs in the survival prediction of the patients. The expressions heatmap of IRGs between subgroups are shown in **Figure 3C**.

Validation of the Prognostic Model

On the one hand, to evaluate the prognostic accuracies of the three IRGs' predictive model in IPF cohorts, this formula was applied to GSE27957 datasets. We discovered that high-risk patients had poorer overall survival than low-risk patients in GSE27957 cohorts (**Figure 4**). These results revealed that this prognostic model based on IRGs had better sensitivity and specificity. On the other hand, we performed verification of the three core genes expression in our cohort. As predicted, *S100A12* was significantly increased in IPF patients, while *CCR7* and *TNFSF4* were decreased (**Figure 5**).

Construction of a Nomogram Based on Three Hub Inflammation-Related Genes

For the establishment of quantitative methods for IPF prognosis, a nomogram was established according to the three hub IRGs (**Figure 6**). Points were distributed to each

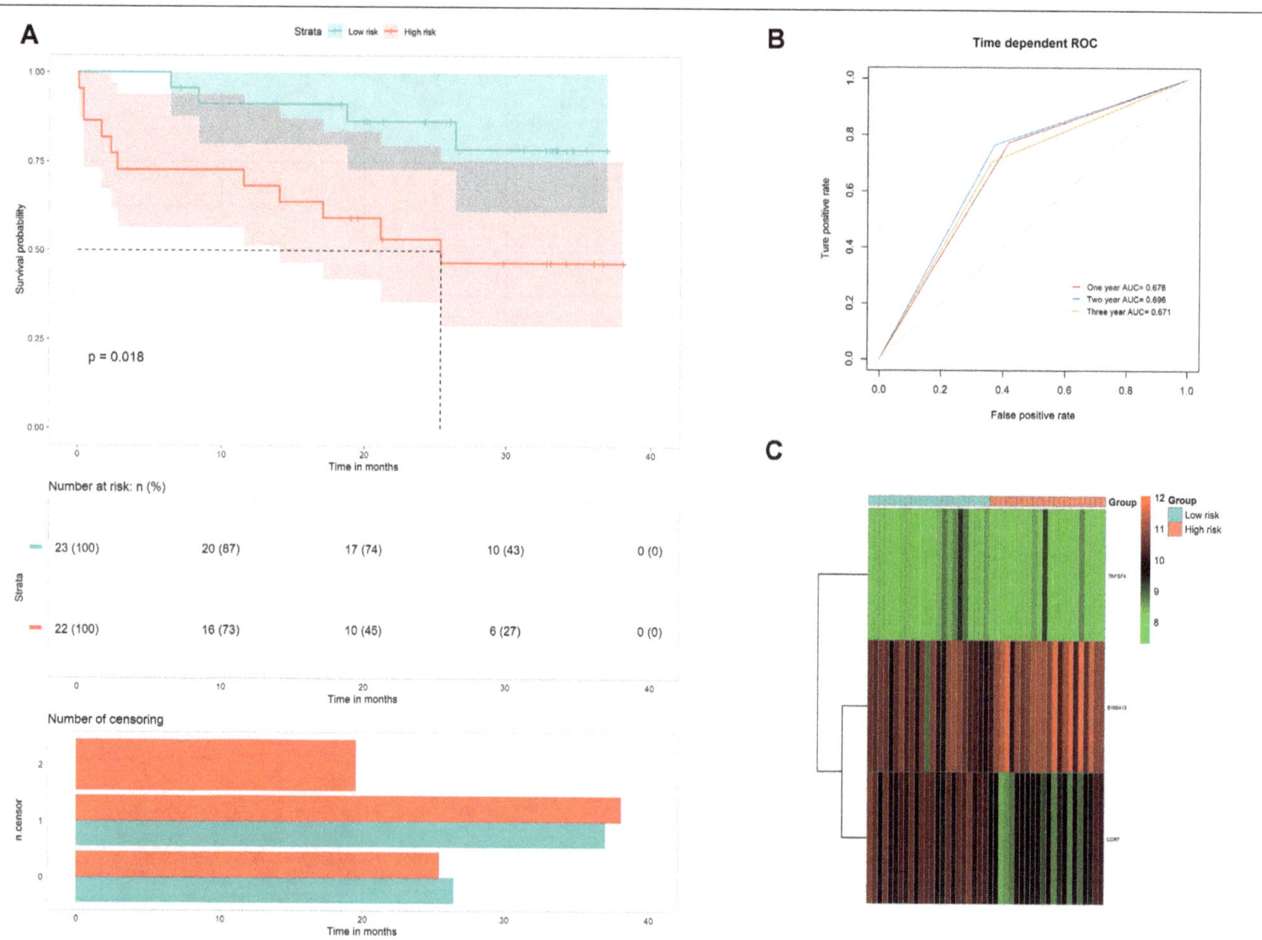

FIGURE 4 | Risk score analysis of the three-gene prognostic model in the GSE27957 cohort. **(A)** Survival curve for patients with low- or high-risk scores **(B)** ROC curves for forecasting overall survival based on the risk score. **(C)** heat map for gene expressions.

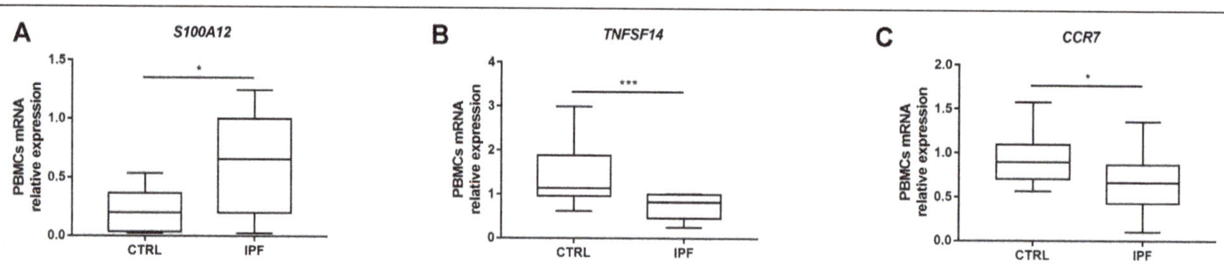

FIGURE 5 | Changes in the expression of three prognostic genes in the peripheral blood mononuclear cells (PBMCs) of idiopathic pulmonary fibrosis (IPF) patients. Quantitative real-time polymerase chain reaction (qRT-PCR) was conducted to quantify the relative expression of the three prognostic genes in the PBMCs in healthy control (CTRL) (n = 16) and IPF (n = 14) patients. **(A)** SA100A12, **(B)** TNFSF4, and **(C)** CCR7. 18s RNA was used as an internal control gene. The data are presented as median with interquartile range (IQR) (Mann–Whitney test). $^{***}p < 0.001$, $^{**}p < 0.01$, and $^{*}p < 0.05$ were considered statistically significant.

variable by the point scale in this nomogram based on the multivariable stepwise Cox regression analysis. We calculated the total points of each IPF patient by summing points of three variables. Next, we could infer the survival rate for IPF patients at 1 and 3 years by matching the total points with below survival rate in our nomogram.

DISCUSSION

As the contributions of inflammation in the development of IPF were complicated and controversial, a comprehensive analysis of IRGs has not been conducted to explore its clinical significance. From the perspective of inflammation, we identified and

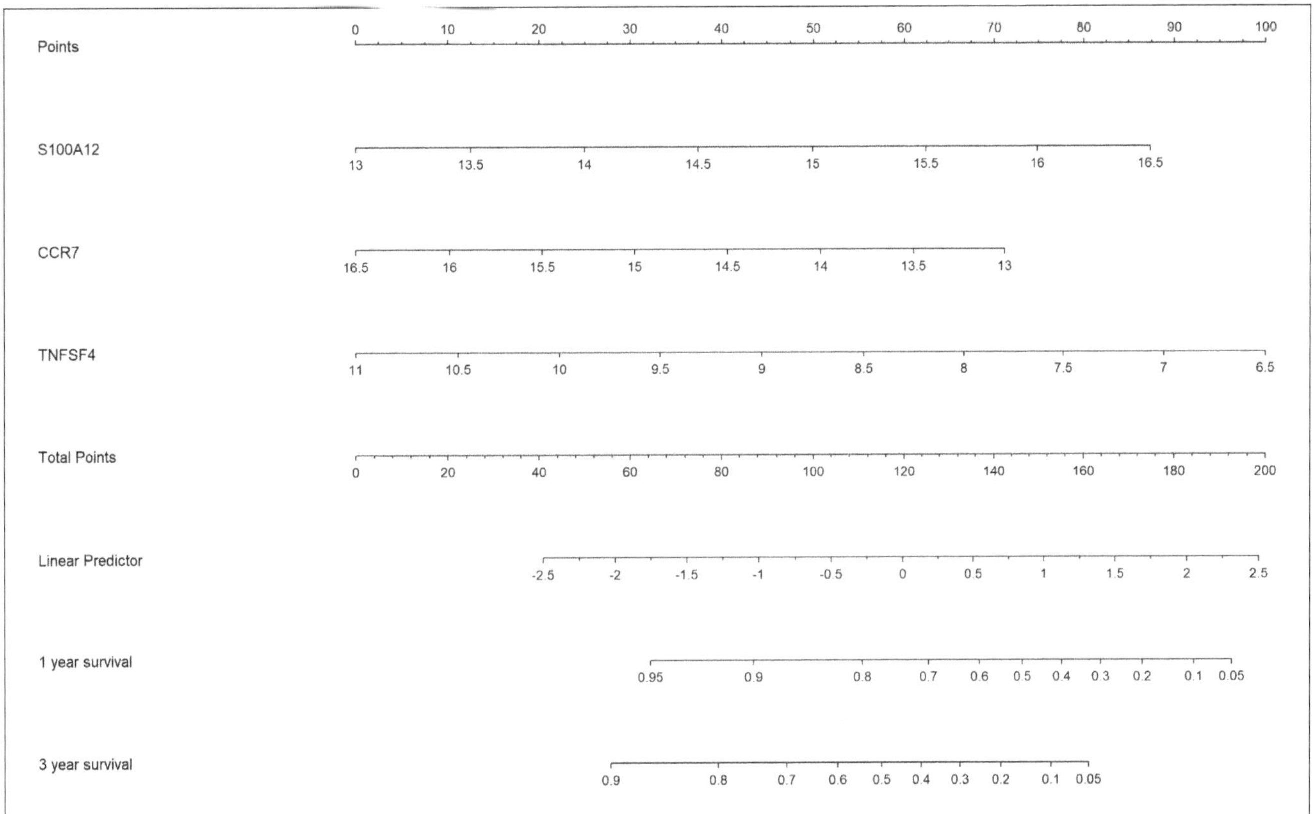

FIGURE 6 | Nomogram for predicting 1- and 3-year overall survival of idiopathic pulmonary fibrosis (IPF) patients in the GSE28042 cohort.

validated three prognostic IRGs. The results indicated that a prognostic model based on three IRGs can be applied for prognostic stratification in IPF patients, helping to provide individualized treatment based on patient risk.

In this study, we identified 110 differently expressed IRGs between IPF and CTRL PBMCs based on GSE28042 from GEO dataset, and constructed a PPI network and co-expression network of these IRGs. As a result, up to 60 hub IRGs were obtained. Many of the hub IRGs had been demonstrated to associate with the development and progression of IPF (Keane et al., 1997; Kowal-Bielecka et al., 2005; Okuda et al., 2015; Yang et al., 2018; Cui et al., 2020). Three IRGs were identified to associate with the prognosis of IPF, including *S100A12, CCR7,* and *TNFSF4.*

The increased expression level of *S100A12,* related to neutrophil recruitment and activation, was associated with significantly worse outcomes in IPF. A previous study has reported that *S100A12* levels in the lung, bronchoalveolar lavage fluid (BALF), and serum were increased in acute respiratory distress syndrome (ARDS) patients compared to healthy controls (Lorenz et al., 2008; Kikkawa et al., 2010). Thomas et al. have demonstrated that a high *S100A12* protein level in serum was associated with poor prognosis in the overall survival, transplant-free survival, and progression-free survival in IPF patients (Richards et al., 2012), which was consistent with our findings. *S100A12* could promote inflammation and cell apoptosis in sepsis-induced ARDS while inhibiting fibroblast migration *via* the receptor for advanced glycation end products (Tanaka et al., 2019; Zhang et al., 2020). The role of *S100A12* in pulmonary fibrosis is still worth investigating.

The decreased level of *CCR7* was related to IPF poor prognosis in this study. But Choi et al. (2006) reported that *CCR7* expression was significantly raised in usual interstitial pneumonia (UIP) relative to biopsies from patients diagnosed with nonspecific interstitial pneumonia (NSIP) or respiratory bronchiolitis/ interstitial lung disease (RBILD). *CCR7* was expressed by IPF fibroblasts but not normal fibroblasts and could promote migration and proliferation of IPF fibroblasts (Pierce et al., 2007a; Habiel and Hogaboam, 2014). Therapeutic targeting *CCR7* abrogates pulmonary fibrosis induced by the adoptive transfer of human pulmonary fibroblasts to immunodeficient mice (Pierce et al., 2007b). The discrepancy between our result and the previous study might result from the important but opposing roles of *CCR7* in disease. The *CCR7* axis could combat the spread of cancer by trafficking of effecter cells involved in mounting an immune response to a growing tumor, while contribute to the expansion of cancer *via* controlling the migration of tumor cells towards the lymphatic system and metastasis (Salem et al., 2021).

The lower level of *TNFSF14* of PBMCs was associated with a worse IPF prognosis. The cytokine *TNFSF14* was demonstrated to be an important factor in the development of lung tissue remodeling in the murine model, which is associated with asthma, IPF, and systemic sclerosis (da Silva Antunes et al.,

2018). Rana Herro et al. demonstrated that *TNFSF14* was upregulated in bleomycin-induced pulmonary fibrosis and is a profibrogenic cytokine (Herro et al., 2015). Considering that *TNFSF14* as an inflammatory indicator was increased in different diseases (Hsu et al., 2019; Fan et al., 2020), the serum protein level of *TNFSF14* should be validated in IPF patients.

Subsequently, a risk model was established for the prediction of IPF prognosis according to multiple stepwise Cox regression analysis of hub IRGs, validated using the GSE27957 cohort. In this study, the ROC curve analysis demonstrated that the IRG signature was better fitted for diagnosis rather than predicting poor prognosis in IPF patients. A nomogram was constructed for intuitively predicting the 1- and 3-year overall survival. This prognostic model based on these three IRGs is financially cost-less and efficient for clinical use.

Nonetheless, limitations were found in this prediction system. First, this prognostic model was constructed according to the GEO database; therefore, further validation in the clinical patient cohort was needed. Second, as a retrospective study, further prospective studies were needed for verification of the outcomes. Finally, functional experiments were needed to further reveal the potential mechanisms of IRGs in the future.

Conclusively, this study identified three IPF prognostic IRGs based on comprehensive bioinformatic analyses in GSE datasets. Our results contributed to the understanding of the roles inflammation played in IPF pathogenesis, and therefore potentially promoted the development of markers for prognosis assessment.

patients/participants provided their written informed consent to participate in this study.

AUTHOR CONTRIBUTIONS

YL: conceptualization, investigation, formal analysis, and writing–original draft. JC: conceptualization, investigation, formal analysis, and writing–original draft. KT: conceptualization, investigation, formal analysis, and writing–original draft. SW: conceptualization, investigation, formal analysis, and writing–original draft. ZT: formal analysis. MW: formal analysis. Chengfeng Xiao: visualization, writing-review, and editing. JZ: conceptualization and supervision. JX: conceptualization and supervision.

ACKNOWLEDGMENTS

We thank all the IPF patients and healthy controls involved in our study.

REFERENCES

Choi, E. S., Pierce, E. M., Jakubzick, C., Carpenter, K. J., Kunkel, S. L., Evanoff, H., et al. (2006). Focal Interstitial CC Chemokine Receptor 7 (CCR7) Expression in Idiopathic Interstitial Pneumonia. *J. Clin. Pathol.* 59 (1), 28–39. doi:10.1136/jcp.2005.026872

Cui, L., Chen, S. Y., Lerbs, T., Lee, J. W., Domizi, P., Gordon, S., et al. (2020). Activation of JUN in Fibroblasts Promotes Pro-fibrotic Programme and Modulates Protective Immunity. *Nat. Commun.* 11 (1), 2795. doi:10.1038/s41467-020-16466-4

da Silva Antunes, R., Mehta, A. K., Madge, L., Tocker, J., and Croft, M. (2018). TNFSF14 (LIGHT) Exhibits Inflammatory Activities in Lung Fibroblasts Complementary to IL-13 and TGF-β. *Front. Immunol.* 9, 576. doi:10.3389/fimmu.2018.00576

Fan, H., Lu, B., Cao, C., Li, H., Yang, D., Huang, L., et al. (2020). Plasma TNFSF13B and TNFSF14 Function as Inflammatory Indicators of Severe Adenovirus Pneumonia in Pediatric Patients. *Front. Immunol.* 11, 614781. doi:10.3389/fimmu.2020.614781

Habiel, D. M., and Hogaboam, C. (2014). Heterogeneity in Fibroblast Proliferation and Survival in Idiopathic Pulmonary Fibrosis. *Front. Pharmacol.* 5, 2. doi:10.3389/fphar.2014.00002

Herazo-Maya, J. D., Noth, I., Duncan, S. R., Kim, S., Ma, S. F., Tseng, G. C., et al. (2013). Peripheral Blood Mononuclear Cell Gene Expression Profiles Predict Poor Outcome in Idiopathic Pulmonary Fibrosis. *Sci. translational Med.* 5 (205), 205ra136. doi:10.1126/scitranslmed.3005964

Herazo-Maya, J. D., Sun, J., Molyneaux, P. L., Li, Q., Villalba, J. A., Tzouvelekis, A., et al. (2017). Validation of a 52-gene Risk Profile for Outcome Prediction in Patients with Idiopathic Pulmonary Fibrosis: an International, Multicentre, Cohort Study. *Lancet Respir. Med.* 5 (11), 857–868. doi:10.1016/s2213-2600(17)30349-1

Herro, R., Da Silva Antunes, R., Aguilera, A. R., Tamada, K., and Croft, M. (2015). Tumor Necrosis Factor Superfamily 14 (LIGHT) Controls Thymic Stromal Lymphopoietin to Drive Pulmonary Fibrosis. *J. Allergy Clin. Immunol.* 136 (3), 757–768. doi:10.1016/j.jaci.2014.12.1936

Heukels, P., Moor, C. C., von der Thüsen, J. H., Wijsenbeek, M. S., and Kool, M. (2019). Inflammation and Immunity in IPF Pathogenesis and Treatment. *Respir. Med.* 147, 79–91. doi:10.1016/j.rmed.2018.12.015

Hsu, C.-Y., Tseng, W.-K., Wu, Y.-W., Lin, T.-H., Yeh, H.-I., Chang, K.-C., et al. (2019). Circulating TNFSF14 (Tumor Necrosis Factor Superfamily 14) Predicts Clinical Outcome in Patients with Stable Coronary Artery Disease. *Atvb* 39 (6), 1240–1252. doi:10.1161/atvbaha.118.312166

Keane, M. P., Arenberg, D. A., Lynch, J. P., 3rd, Whyte, R. I., Iannettoni, M. D., Burdick, M. D., et al. (1997). The CXC Chemokines, IL-8 and IP-10, Regulate Angiogenic Activity in Idiopathic Pulmonary Fibrosis. *J. Immunol. (Baltimore, Md* 159 (3), 1437–1443.

Khor, Y. H., Glaspole, I., and Goh, N. S. L. (2019). Therapeutic burden in Interstitial Lung Disease: Lessons to Learn. *Respirology* 24 (6), 566–571. doi:10.1111/resp.13480

Kikkawa, T., Sato, N., Kojika, M., Takahashi, G., Aoki, K., Hoshikawa, K., et al. (2010). Significance of Measuring S100A12 and sRAGE in the Serum of Sepsis Patients with Postoperative Acute Lung Injury. *Dig. Surg.* 27 (4), 307–312. doi:10.1159/000313687

Kowal-Bielecka, O., Kowal, K., Lewszuk, A., Bodzenta-Lukaszyk, A., Walecki, J., and Sierakowski, S. (2005). Beta Thromboglobulin and Platelet Factor 4 in Bronchoalveolar Lavage Fluid of Patients with Systemic Sclerosis. *Ann. Rheum. Dis.* 64 (3), 484–486. doi:10.1136/ard.2004.022970

Ley, B., Collard, H. R., and King, T. E., Jr (2011). Clinical Course and Prediction of Survival in Idiopathic Pulmonary Fibrosis. *Am. J. Respir. Crit. Care Med.* 183 (4), 431–440. doi:10.1164/rccm.201006-0894ci

Lorenz, E., Muhlebach, M. S., Tessier, P. A., Alexis, N. E., Duncan Hite, R., Seeds, M. C., et al. (2008). Different Expression Ratio of S100A8/A9 and S100A12 in Acute and Chronic Lung Diseases. *Respir. Med.* 102 (4), 567–573. doi:10.1016/j.rmed.2007.11.011

Mura, M., Belmonte, G., Fanti, S., Contini, P., Pacilli, A. M. G., Fasano, L., et al. (2005). Inflammatory Activity Is Still Present in the Advanced Stages of Idiopathic Pulmonary Fibrosis. *Respirology* 10 (5), 609–614. doi:10.1111/j.1440-1843.2005.00757.x

Nathan, S. D., Albera, C., Bradford, W. Z., Costabel, U., du Bois, R. M., Fagan, E. A., et al. (2016). Effect of Continued Treatment with Pirfenidone Following Clinically Meaningful Declines in Forced Vital Capacity: Analysis of Data from Three Phase 3 Trials in Patients with Idiopathic Pulmonary Fibrosis. *Thorax* 71 (5), 429–435. doi:10.1136/thoraxjnl-2015-207011

Noth, I., Zhang, Y., Ma, S.-F., Flores, C., Barber, M., Huang, Y., et al. (2013). Genetic Variants Associated with Idiopathic Pulmonary Fibrosis Susceptibility and Mortality: a Genome-wide Association Study. *Lancet Respir. Med.* 1 (4), 309–317. doi:10.1016/s2213-2600(13)70045-6

Okuda, R., Matsushima, H., Aoshiba, K., Oba, T., Kawabe, R., Honda, K., et al. (2015). Soluble Intercellular Adhesion Molecule-1 for Stable and Acute Phases of Idiopathic Pulmonary Fibrosis. *SpringerPlus* 4, 657. doi:10.1186/s40064-015-1455-z

Pierce, E. M., Carpenter, K., Jakubzick, C., Kunkel, S. L., Evanoff, H., Flaherty, K. R., et al. (2007). Idiopathic Pulmonary Fibrosis Fibroblasts Migrate and Proliferate to CC Chemokine Ligand 21. *Eur. Respir. J.* 29 (6), 1082–1093. doi:10.1183/09031936.00122806

Pierce, E. M., Carpenter, K., Jakubzick, C., Kunkel, S. L., Flaherty, K. R., Martinez, F. J., et al. (2007). Therapeutic Targeting of CC Ligand 21 or CC Chemokine Receptor 7 Abrogates Pulmonary Fibrosis Induced by the Adoptive Transfer of Human Pulmonary Fibroblasts to Immunodeficient Mice. *Am. J. Pathol.* 170 (4), 1152–1164. doi:10.2353/ajpath.2007.060649

Raghu, G., Collard, H. R., Egan, J. J., Martinez, F. J., Behr, J., Brown, K. K., et al. (2011). An Official ATS/ERS/JRS/ALAT Statement: Idiopathic Pulmonary Fibrosis: Evidence-Based Guidelines for Diagnosis and Management. *Am. J. Respir. Crit. Care Med.* 183 (6), 788–824. doi:10.1164/rccm.2009-040gl

Raghu, G., Collard, H. R., Egan, J. J., Martinez, F. J., Behr, J., Brown, K. K., et al. (2011). An Official ATS/ERS/JRS/ALAT Statement: Idiopathic Pulmonary Fibrosis: Evidence-Based Guidelines for Diagnosis and Management. *Am. J. Respir. Crit. Care Med.* 183 (6), 788–824. doi:10.1164/rccm.2009-040gl

Raghu, G., Rochwerg, B., Zhang, Y., Garcia, C. A. C., Azuma, A., Behr, J., et al. (2015). An Official ATS/ERS/JRS/ALAT Clinical Practice Guideline: Treatment of Idiopathic Pulmonary Fibrosis. An Update of the 2011 Clinical Practice Guideline. *Am. J. Respir. Crit. Care Med.* 192 (2), E3–E19. doi:10.1164/rccm.201506-1063st

Richards, T. J., Kaminski, N., Baribaud, F., Flavin, S., Brodmerkel, C., Horowitz, D., et al. (2012). Peripheral Blood Proteins Predict Mortality in Idiopathic Pulmonary Fibrosis. *Am. J. Respir. Crit. Care Med.* 185 (1), 67–76. doi:10.1164/rccm.201101-0058oc

Richeldi, L. (2013). Clinical Trials of Investigational Agents for IPF: a Review of a Cochrane Report. *Respir. Res.* 14 (Suppl. 1), S4. doi:10.1186/1465-9921-14-s1-s4

Richeldi, L., Cottin, V., du Bois, R. M., Selman, M., Kimura, T., Bailes, Z., et al. (2016). Nintedanib in Patients with Idiopathic Pulmonary Fibrosis: Combined Evidence from the TOMORROW and INPULSIS Trials. *Respir. Med.* 113, 71–79. doi:10.1016/j.rmed.2016.02.001

Salem, A., Alotaibi, M., Mroueh, R., Basheer, H. A., and Afarinkia, K. (2021). CCR7 as a Therapeutic Target in Cancer. *Biochim. Biophys. Acta (Bba) - Rev. Cancer* 1875 (1), 188499. doi:10.1016/j.bbcan.2020.188499

Sang, X., Wang, Y., Xue, Z., Qi, D., Fan, G., Tian, F., et al. (2021). Macrophage-Targeted Lung Delivery of Dexamethasone Improves Pulmonary Fibrosis Therapy via Regulating the Immune Microenvironment. *Front. Immunol.* 12, 613907. doi:10.3389/fimmu.2021.613907

Scott, M. K. D., Quinn, K., Li, Q., Carroll, R., Warsinske, H., Vallania, F., et al. (2019). Increased Monocyte Count as a Cellular Biomarker for Poor Outcomes in Fibrotic Diseases: a Retrospective, Multicentre Cohort Study. *Lancet Respir. Med.* 7 (6), 497–508. doi:10.1016/s2213-2600(18)30508-3

Selman, M., King, T. E., and Pardo, A. (2001). Idiopathic Pulmonary Fibrosis: Prevailing and Evolving Hypotheses about its Pathogenesis and Implications for Therapy. *Ann. Intern. Med.* 134 (2), 136–151. doi:10.7326/0003-4819-134-2-200101160-00015

Tanaka, N., Ikari, J., Anazawa, R., Suzuki, M., Katsumata, Y., Shimada, A., et al. (2019). S100A12 Inhibits Fibroblast Migration via the Receptor for Advanced Glycation End Products and P38 MAPK Signaling. In Vitro *Cell.Dev.Biol.-Animal* 55 (8), 656–664. doi:10.1007/s11626-019-00384-x

Yang, L., Herrera, J., Gilbertsen, A., Xia, H., Smith, K., Benyumov, A., et al. (2018). IL-8 Mediates Idiopathic Pulmonary Fibrosis Mesenchymal Progenitor Cell Fibrogenicity. *Am. J. Physiology-Lung Cell Mol. Physiol.* 314 (1), L127–L136. doi:10.1152/ajplung.00200.2017

Zhang, H.-T., Fang, S.-C., Wang, C.-Y., Wang, W., Wu, J., Wang, C., et al. (2015). MMP-9 1562C>T Gene Polymorphism and Efficacy of Glucocorticoid Therapy in Idiopathic Pulmonary Fibrosis Patients. *Genet. Test. Mol. biomarkers* 19 (11), 591–597. doi:10.1089/gtmb.2015.0057

Zhang, Z., Han, N., and Shen, Y. (2020). S100A12 Promotes Inflammation and Cell Apoptosis in Sepsis-Induced ARDS via Activation of NLRP3 Inflammasome Signalingflammasome Signaling. *Mol. Immunol.* 122, 38–48. doi:10.1016/j.molimm.2020.03.022

Permissions

All chapters in this book were first published by Frontiers; hereby published with permission under the Creative Commons Attribution License or equivalent. Every chapter published in this book has been scrutinized by our experts. Their significance has been extensively debated. The topics covered herein carry significant findings which will fuel the growth of the discipline. They may even be implemented as practical applications or may be referred to as a beginning point for another development.

The contributors of this book come from diverse backgrounds, making this book a truly international effort. This book will bring forth new frontiers with its revolutionizing research information and detailed analysis of the nascent developments around the world.

We would like to thank all the contributing authors for lending their expertise to make the book truly unique. They have played a crucial role in the development of this book. Without their invaluable contributions this book wouldn't have been possible. They have made vital efforts to compile up to date information on the varied aspects of this subject to make this book a valuable addition to the collection of many professionals and students.

This book was conceptualized with the vision of imparting up-to-date information and advanced data in this field. To ensure the same, a matchless editorial board was set up. Every individual on the board went through rigorous rounds of assessment to prove their worth. After which they invested a large part of their time researching and compiling the most relevant data for our readers.

The editorial board has been involved in producing this book since its inception. They have spent rigorous hours researching and exploring the diverse topics which have resulted in the successful publishing of this book. They have passed on their knowledge of decades through this book. To expedite this challenging task, the publisher supported the team at every step. A small team of assistant editors was also appointed to further simplify the editing procedure and attain best results for the readers.

Apart from the editorial board, the designing team has also invested a significant amount of their time in understanding the subject and creating the most relevant covers. They scrutinized every image to scout for the most suitable representation of the subject and create an appropriate cover for the book.

The publishing team has been an ardent support to the editorial, designing and production team. Their endless efforts to recruit the best for this project, has resulted in the accomplishment of this book. They are a veteran in the field of academics and their pool of knowledge is as vast as their experience in printing. Their expertise and guidance has proved useful at every step. Their uncompromising quality standards have made this book an exceptional effort. Their encouragement from time to time has been an inspiration for everyone.

The publisher and the editorial board hope that this book will prove to be a valuable piece of knowledge for researchers, students, practitioners and scholars across the globe.

List of Contributors

Lihua Wang, Yeerfan Jiaerken, Qian Li, Peiyu Huang, Zhujing Shen and Minming Zhang
Department of Radiology, Second Affiliated Hospital, School of Medicine, Zhejiang University, Hangzhou, China

Tongtong Zhao
Fuyang Second People's Hospital, Fuyang, China

Hanpeng Zheng
Yueqing People's Hospital, Yueqing, China

Wenbin Ji
Zhejiang Taizhou Hospital, Taizhou, China

Yuantong Gao
Radiology Department, Third Affiliated Hospital of Wenzhou Medical University, Wenzhou, China

Junli Xia
Bozhou Bone Trauma Hospital Image Center, Bozhou, China

Jianmin Cheng
Department of Radiology, Second Affiliated Hospital and Yuying Children's Hospital of Wenzhou Medical University, Wenzhou, China

Jianbing Ma
First Hospital of Jiaxing, Jiaxing, China

Jun Liu
Second Xiangya Hospital, Central South University, Changsha, China

Yongqiang Liu
Quzhou Kecheng People's Hospital, Quzhou, China

Miaoguang Su
Pingyang County People's Hospital, Wenzhou, China

Guixiang Ruan
Yuhang First People's Hospital, Hangzhou, China

Jiner Shu
Jinhua Central Hospital, Jinhua, China

Dawei Ren
Ningbo First Hospital, Ningbo, China

Zhenhua Zhao
Shaoxing People's Hospital, Shaoxing, China

Weigen Yao
Yuyao People's Hospital, Yuyao, China

Yunjun Yang
Radiology Department, First Affiliated Hospital of Wenzhou Medical University, Wenzhou, China

Caijuan Huan, Wangting Xu, Kexin Ruan and Jianying Zhou
Department of Respiratory Medicine, The First Affiliated Hospital, Zhejiang University School of Medicine, Hangzhou, China

Hongqiang Cheng, Yuehai Ke and Yaru Liu
Department of Pathology and Pathophysiology, Zhejiang University School of Medicine, Hangzhou, China

Yueli Shi
The Fourth Affiliated Hospital, Zhejiang University School of Medicine, Yiwu, China

Yan-yan Yan, Fu-xi Zhao, Zhuang-yan Zhu, Yan-xia Xing and Hai-yan Zhang
School of Medicine, Shanxi Datong University, Datong, China

Wen-min Zhou, Yu-qing Wang and Jian-ye Zhang
Key Laboratory of Molecular Target and Clinical Pharmacology and the State Key Laboratory of Respiratory Disease, School of Pharmaceutical Sciences and the Fifth Affiliated Hospital, Guangzhou Medical University, Guangzhou, China

Qiao-ru Guo
Key Laboratory of Molecular Target and Clinical Pharmacology and the State Key Laboratory of Respiratory Disease, School of Pharmaceutical Sciences and the Fifth Affiliated Hospital, Guangzhou Medical University, Guangzhou, China
Xinjiang Institute of Materia Medica, Urumqi, China

Bolat Makabel
Xinjiang Institute of Materia Medica, Urumqi, China

Mohamad Aljofan
Department of Biomedical Sciences, School of Medicine, Nazarbayev University, Nur-Sultan, Kazakhstan

Alireza Mosavi Jarrahi
School of Medicine, Shahid Beheshti University of Medical Sciences, Tehran, Iran

Qiujie Wang, Luna Hong, Ming Chen, Jiangting Shi, Xiaoling Lin, Linjie Huang, Tiantian Tang, Yimin Guo and Shanping Jiang
Division of Pulmonary and Critical Care Medicine, Sun Yat-sen Memorial Hospital, Sun Yat-sen University, Guangzhou, China
Guangdong Provincial Key Laboratory of Malignant Tumor Epigenetics and Gene Regulation, Medical Research Center, Sun Yat-Sen Memorial Hospital, Sun Yat-sen University, Guangzhou, China
Institute of Pulmonary Diseases, Sun Yat-sen University, Guangzhou, China

Xiaoqing Yuan
Guangdong Provincial Key Laboratory of Malignant Tumor Epigenetics and Gene Regulation, Medical Research Center, Sun Yat-Sen Memorial Hospital, Sun Yat-sen University, Guangzhou, China
Breast Tumor Center, Sun Yat-Sen Memorial Hospital, Sun Yat-Sen University, Guangzhou, China

Yishu Xue, Yan Zhou, Wuping Bao, Qiang Fu, Huijuan Hao, Lei Han, Xue Zhang, Xue Tian and Min Zhang
Department of Respiratory and Critical Care Medicine, Shanghai General Hospital, Shanghai Jiao Tong University School of Medicine, Shanghai, China

Fen Lan, Qin Li and Yang Xia
Key Laboratory of Respiratory Disease of Zhejiang Province, Department of Respiratory and Critical Care Medicine, Second Affiliated Hospital of Zhejiang University School of Medicine, Hangzhou, China

Yaling Yue
Department of Medical Oncology, Handan Central Hospital, Handan, China

Hong Shen
Department of Respiratory and Critical Care Medicine, Second Affiliated Hospital of Nanjing Medical University, Nanjing, China

Hui Shen
Department of Respiratory and Critical Care Medicine, Huzhou Central Hospital, Huzhou, China

Qiyuan Wang
Department of Radiology, Second Affiliated Hospital of Zhejiang University School of Medicine, Hangzhou, China

Xiujing Yu and Laijuan Chen
Department of Endoscopic Center, Second Affiliated Hospital of Zhejiang University School of Medicine, Hangzhou, China

Kopen Wang
Division of Pulmonary and Critical Care Medicine, Johns Hopkins University School of Medicine, Baltimore, MD, United States

Qinghua Liu
Department of Respiratory and Critical Care Medicine, Shanghai East Hospital, Tongji University, Shanghai, China

Yutong Sui, Jing Zhang, Zena Zheng and Ziwei Wang
Shenzhen Hospital, Southern Medical University, Shenzhen, China

Jiayin Liu
Department of Radiation Oncology, Harbin Medical University Cancer Hospital, Harbin, China

Zhenghu Jia
The First Affiliated Hospital, Biomedical Translational Research Institute and Guangdong Province Key Laboratory of Molecular Immunology and Antibody Engineering, Jinan University, Guangzhou, China

Ziyu Meng
NHC Key Laboratory of Hormones and Development, Tianjin Key Laboratory of Metabolic Diseases, Chu Hsien-I Memorial Hospital and Tianjin Institute of Endocrinology, Tianjin Medical University, Tianjin, China

Yicheng He, Fei Li, Chao Zhang, Xufei Du, Zhehua Shao, Wen Hua, Wen Li and Zhihua Chen
Key Laboratory of Respiratory Disease of Zhejiang Province, Department of Respiratory and Critical Care Medicine, Second Affiliated Hospital of Zhejiang University School of Medicine, Hangzhou, China

Xinwei Geng and Madiha Zahra Syeda
Department of Pharmacology, Zhejiang University School of Medicine, Hangzhou, China

Songmin Ying
Key Laboratory of Respiratory Disease of Zhejiang Province, Department of Respiratory and Critical Care Medicine, Second Affiliated Hospital of Zhejiang University School of Medicine, Hangzhou, China
Department of Pharmacology, Zhejiang University School of Medicine, Hangzhou, China

Huahao Shen
Key Laboratory of Respiratory Disease of Zhejiang Province, Department of Respiratory and Critical Care Medicine, Second Affiliated Hospital of Zhejiang University School of Medicine, Hangzhou, China
State Key Lab of Respiratory Disease, Guangzhou, China

Alicia K. Gerke
Pulmonary and Critical Care Medicine, Department of Internal Medicine, University of Iowa, Iowa City, IA, United States

Qian Han, Xiaobo Chen, Weiping Qian, Gui Zhao, Mengmeng Mao, Bingpeng Guo, Shu Xia, Shiyue Li and Qun Luo
Department of Respiratory Medicine, The First Affiliated Hospital of Guangzhou Medical University, Guangzhou, China
National Clinical Research Center for Respiratory Disease, Guangzhou Institute of Respiratory Health, Guangzhou, China

Xin Xu, Guilin Peng and Jianxing He
National Clinical Research Center for Respiratory Disease, Guangzhou Institute of Respiratory Health, Guangzhou, China
Department of Cardio-thoracic Surgery, The First Affiliated Hospital of Guangzhou Medical University, Guangzhou, China

Yingying Gu
National Clinical Research Center for Respiratory Disease, Guangzhou Institute of Respiratory Health, Guangzhou, China
Department of Pathology, Guangzhou Institute of Respiratory Health, Guangzhou, China

Xiaoqing Wang, Nanjie Xiao and Jian Guan
Department of Radiation Oncology, Nanfang Hospital, Southern Medical University, Guangzhou, China
Department of Radiation Oncology, Peking University Shenzhen Hospital, Shenzhen, China

Min Chen
Department of Radiation Oncology, Nanfang Hospital, Southern Medical University, Guangzhou, China
Department of Radiation Oncology, Peking University Shenzhen Hospital, Shenzhen, China

Wenqi Huang and Laiyu Liu
Chronic Airways Diseases Laboratory, Department of Respiratory and Critical Care Medicine, Nanfang Hospital, Southern Medical University, Guangzhou, China

Dongyong Yang and Jincheng Huang
Department of Respiratory and Critical Care Medicine, Second Affiliated Hospital of Fujian Medical University, Quanzhou, China

Gong Li
Guangdong Provincial Hospital of Traditional Chinese Medicine, Guangzhou, China

Weijian Zhang
Department of Radiation Oncology, The First Affiliation Hospital of Fujian Medical University, Fuzhou, China

Shuang Wang
Department of Pathology, Nanfang Hospital, Southern Medical University, Guangzhou, China
Department of Pathology, School of Basic Medical Sciences, Southern Medical University, Guangzhou, China

Wei Wang
Department of Thoracic Surgery, Renmin Hospital of Wuhan University, Wuhan, China

Ning-yuan Chen and Kemly Philip
Department of Biochemistry and Molecular Biology, McGovern Medical School, The University of Texas Health Science Center at Houston, Houston, TX, United States

Dewei Ren
Houston Methodist J.C. Walter Jr. Transplant Center, Houston Methodist Hospital, Houston, TX, United States

Jonathan Davies
Division of Neonatal-Perinatal Medicine, Department of Pediatrics, Baylor College of Medicine, Houston, TX, United States

Holger K. Eltzschig
Department of Anesthesiology, McGovern Medical School, The University of Texas Health Science Center at Houston, Houston, TX, United States

Michael R. Blackburn
Department of Biochemistry and Molecular Biology, McGovern Medical School, The University of Texas Health Science Center at Houston, Houston, TX, United States
UTHealth Pulmonary Center of Excellence, Houston, TX, United States

Bindu Akkanti
Divisions of Critical Care, Pulmonary and Sleep Medicine, Department of Internal Medicine, McGovern Medical School, The University of Texas Health Science Center at Houston, Houston, TX, United States

Harry Karmouty-Quintana
Divisions of Critical Care, Pulmonary and Sleep Medicine, Department of Internal Medicine, McGovern Medical School, The University of Texas Health Science Center at Houston, Houston, TX, United States
UTHealth Pulmonary Center of Excellence, Houston, TX, United States
Department of Biochemistry and Molecular Biology, McGovern Medical School, The University of Texas Health Science Center at Houston, Houston, TX, United States

Tingting Weng
Divisions of Critical Care, Pulmonary and Sleep Medicine, Department of Internal Medicine, McGovern Medical School, The University of Texas Health Science Center at Houston, Houston, TX, United States
UTHealth Pulmonary Center of Excellence, Houston, TX, United States

Shuang Bai, Rui Ye, Cuihong Wang, Pengbo Sun, Di Wang and Li Zhao
Department of Pulmonary and Critical Care Medicine, Shengjing Hospital of China Medical University, Shenyang, China

Yong Yue and Huiying Wang
Department of Radiology, Shengjing Hospital of China Medical University, Shenyang, China

Si Wu and Miao Yu
Department of Biobank, Shengjing Hospital of China Medical University, Shenyang, China

Shuhua Xi
Department of Environmental and Occupational Health, School of Public Health, China Medical University, Shenyang, China

Xianbo Wu and Xinwei Yang
1School of Sports Medicine and Health, Chegdu Sport University, Chengdu, China

Jianli Huang and Jie Wang
Guizhou University of Traditional Chinese Medicine, Guiyang, China

Yihua Xu
Chengdu University of Traditional Chinese Medicine, Chengdu, China

Minghan Sun
Central of Reproductive Medicine, Department of Obstetrics and Gynecology, School of Medicine, Sichuan Academy of Medical Sciences and Sichuan Provincial People's Hospital, University of Electronic Science and Technology of China, Chengdu, China

Jianyou Shi
Personalized Drug Therapy Key Laboratory of Sichuan Province, Sichuan Academy of Medical Science and Sichuan Provincial People's Hospital, School of Medicine of University of Electronic Science and Technology of China, Chengdu, China

Jun Duan
Department of Respiratory and Critical Care Medicine, First Affiliated Hospital of Chongqing Medical University, Chongqing, China

Jia Zeng
Department of Aviation Disease, Naval Medical Center of PLA, Second Military Medical University, Shanghai, China
Hubei Maternal and Child Health Hospital, Wuhan, China

Puyu Deng
Department of Emergency and Critical Care Medicine, Shanghai General Hospital, Shanghai Jiao Tong University School of Medicine, Shanghai, China

Zhong Ni
Department of Respiratory and Critical Care Medicine, West China Hospital, Sichuan University, Chengdu, China

Rongli Lu
Department of Pulmonary and Critical Care Medicine, Xiangya Hospital, Central South University, Changsha, China

Wenxi Xia
Department of Critical Care Medicine, West China Hospital, Sichuan University, Chengdu, China

Guoqiang Jing
Department of Pulmonary and Critical Care Medicine, Binzhou Medical University Hospital, Binzhou Medical University, Binzhou, China

Xiaoping Su
School of Basic Medicine, Wenzhou Medical University, Wenzhou Tea Mountain Higher Education Park, Wenzhou, China

Stephan Ehrmann
CHRU Tours, Médecine Intensive Réanimation, CIC INSERM 1415, CRICSTriggerSep Network, Tours France, and INSERM, Centre D'étude des Pathologies Respiratoires, Université de Tours, Tours, France

Wei Zhang
Hubei Maternal and Child Health Hospital, Wuhan, China
Department of Respiratory and Critical Care Medicine, First Affiliated Hospital, Second Military Medical University, Shanghai, China

Jie Li
Department of Cardiopulmonary Sciences, Division of Respiratory Care, Rush University Medical Center, Chicago, IL, United States

Xin Li and Shaoyu Yang
Department of Thoracic Oncology, Key Laboratory of Clinical Cancer Pharmacology and Toxicology Research of Zhejiang Province, Affiliated Hangzhou First People's Hospital, Zhejiang University School of Medicine, Hangzhou, China

Jie Huang, Kan Wu and Bing Xia
Department of Thoracic Oncology, Hangzhou Cancer Hospital, Zhejiang University School of Medicine, Hangzhou, China

Yao Qiu and Qianyun Zhang
Department of Thoracic Oncology, Nanjing Medical University Affiliated Hangzhou Hospital, Hangzhou, China

Jiaoli Wang, Limin Wang and Jian Ye
Department of Respiratory Disease, Affiliated Hangzhou First People's Hospital, Zhejiang University School of Medicine, Hangzhou, China

Shenglin Ma
Department of Thoracic Oncology, Hangzhou Cancer Hospital, Zhejiang University School of Medicine, Hangzhou, China
Cancer Center, Zhejiang University, Hangzhou, China

Xueqin Chen
Department of Thoracic Oncology, Nanjing Medical University Affiliated Hangzhou Hospital, Hangzhou, China
Department of Thoracic Oncology, Key Laboratory of Clinical Cancer Pharmacology and Toxicology Research of Zhejiang Province, Affiliated Hangzhou First People's Hospital, Zhejiang University School of Medicine, Hangzhou, China

Hongming Pan, Yong Fang and Xiaoyun Zhou
Department of Medical Oncology, School of Medicine, Sir Run Run Shaw Hospital, Zhejiang University, Hangzhou, China

Jin Sheng, Huadi Wang, Jiawei Shou, Hong Pan, Hongsen Li and Weidong Han
Department of Medical Oncology, School of Medicine, Sir Run Run Shaw Hospital, Zhejiang University, Hangzhou, China
Laboratory of Cancer Biology, Institute of Clinical Science, School of Medicine, Sir Run Run Shaw Hospital, Zhejiang University, Hangzhou, China

Xiao Liu
Department of Human Genetics, University of Chicago, Chicago, IL, United States

Yunyun Deng, Yingying Yu and Pengfei Xu
Hangzhou ImmuQuad Biotechnologies, LLC, Hangzhou, China

Tao Sun
Hangzhou ImmuQuad Biotechnologies, LLC, Hangzhou, China
Zhejiang-California International Nano-Systems Institute, Zhejiang University, Hangzhou, China

Jiajia Dong
Department of Pulmonary and Critical Care Medicine, West China Hospital, Sichuan University, Chengdu, China

Wei Li, Qi Wang, Jiahao Chen, Yue Zu, Xuedong Zhou and Qiang Guo
State Key Laboratory of Oral Diseases, National Clinical Research Center for Oral Diseases, West China Hospital of Stomatology, Sichuan University, Chengdu, China

Lingwei Wang, Danting Zhan, Kai Yang, Heng Zhang, Min Yu , Yimin Zha, Weibin Huang Rongchang Chen and Chen Qiu
The Department of Respiratory Diseases and Critic Care Unit, Shenzhen Institute of Respiratory Diseases, Shenzhen People's Hospital (The Second Clinical Medical College, Jinan University; The First Affiliated Hospital, Southern University of Science and Technology), Shenzhen, China
Shenzhen Key Laboratory of Respiratory Diseases, Shenzhen Major Respiratory Diseases's Prevention and Treatment Center, Shenzhen, China

Xiaodi Liu and Shipin Wu
Department of Infectious Diseases, Shenzhen People's Hospital (The Second Clinical Medical College, Jinan University; The First Affiliated Hospital, Southern University of Science and Technology), Shenzhen, China

Lei Li
Guangdong Provincial Key Laboratory of Brain Connectome and Behavior, CAS Key Laboratory of Brain Connectome and Manipulation, The Brain Cognition and Brain Disease Institute (BCBDI), Shenzhen Institutes of Advanced Technology, Chinese Academy of Sciences, Shenzhen-Hong Kong Institute of Brain Science-Shenzhen Fundamental Research Institutions, Shenzhen, China

Yanjiao Lu, Kun Tang, Shanshan Wang, Zhen Tian, Meijia Wang, Jianping Zhao and Jungang Xie
Department of Respiratory and Critical Care Medicine, National Clinical Research Center of Respiratory Disease, Tongji Hospital, Tongji Medical College, Huazhong University of Science and Technology, Wuhan, China

Jinkun Chen
Department of science, Western University, London, ON, Canada

Index

www.ingramcontent.com/pod-product-compliance
Lightning Source LLC
LaVergne TN
LVHW082129200926
848484LV00008B/2028
9798887405667